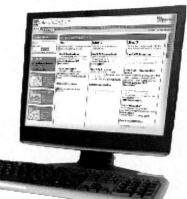

Rapid Review Series

Series Editor
Edward F. Goljan, MD

BEHAVIORAL SCIENCE, SECOND EDITION
Vivian M. Stevens, PhD; Susan K. Redwood, PhD; Jackie L. Neel, DO; Richard H. Bost, PhD; Nancy W. Van Winkle, PhD; Michael H. Pollak, PhD

BIOCHEMISTRY, THIRD EDITION
John W. Pelley, PhD; Edward F. Goljan, MD

GROSS AND DEVELOPMENTAL ANATOMY, THIRD EDITION
N. Anthony Moore, PhD; William A. Roy, PhD, PT

HISTOLOGY AND CELL BIOLOGY, SECOND EDITION
E. Robert Burns, PhD; M. Donald Cave, PhD

MICROBIOLOGY AND IMMUNOLOGY, THIRD EDITION
Ken S. Rosenthal, PhD; Michael J. Tan, MD

NEUROSCIENCE
James A. Weyhenmeyer, PhD; Eve A. Gallman, PhD

PATHOLOGY, THIRD EDITION
Edward F. Goljan, MD

PHARMACOLOGY, THIRD EDITION
Thomas L. Pazdernik, PhD; Laszlo Kerecsen, MD

PHYSIOLOGY, SECOND EDITION
Thomas A. Brown, MD

USMLE STEP 2
Michael W. Lawlor, MD, PhD

USMLE STEP 3
David Rolston, MD; Craig Nielsen, MD

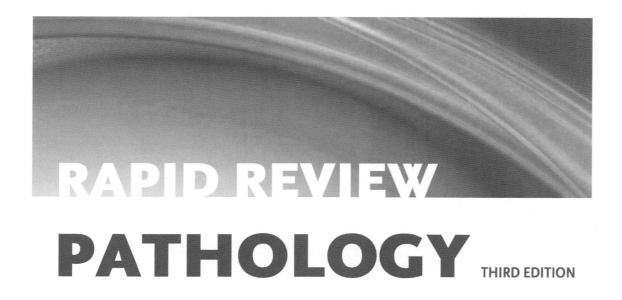

RAPID REVIEW

PATHOLOGY THIRD EDITION

Edward F. Goljan, MD

Professor
Department of Pathology
Oklahoma State University Center for Health Sciences
College of Osteopathic Medicine
Tulsa, Oklahoma

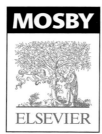

MOSBY

ELSEVIER

1600 John F. Kennedy Blvd.
Ste 1800
Philadelphia, PA 19103-2899

RAPID REVIEW: PATHOLOGY, THIRD EDITION   ISBN: 978-0-323-06862-8

Notice

Knowledge and best practice in this field are constantly changing. As new research and experience broaden our knowledge, changes in practice, treatment, and drug therapy may become necessary or appropriate. Readers are advised to check the most current information provided (i) on procedures featured or (ii) by the manufacturer of each product to be administered, to verify the recommended dose or formula, the method and duration of administration, and contraindications. It is the responsibility of the practitioner, relying on his or her own experience and knowledge of the patient, to make diagnoses, to determine dosages and the best treatment for each individual patient, and to take all appropriate safety precautions. To the fullest extent of the law, neither the Publisher nor the Editor assumes any liability for any injury and/or damage to persons or property arising out or related to any use of the material contained in this book.

Library of Congress Cataloging-in-Publication Data
Goljan, Edward F.
  Rapid review pathology / Edward F. Goljan.—3rd ed.
      p. ; cm.—(Rapid review series)
  Rev. ed. of: Pathology / Edward F. Goljan. 2nd ed. c2007.
  Includes index.
  ISBN 978-0-323-06862-8
  1. Pathology—Outlines, syllabi, etc. 2. Pathology—Examinations, questions, etc.
I. Goljan, Edward F. Pathology. II. Title. III. Title: Pathology. IV. Series: Rapid
review series.
  [DNLM: 1. Pathology—Examination Questions. 2. Pathology—Outlines. QZ 18.2
G626r 2010]
  RB120.G654 2010
  616.07—dc22

                                                                    2009022836

Acquisitions Editor: Jim Merritt
Developmental Editor: Christine Abshire
Editorial Assistant: Nicole DiCicco
Project Manager: David Saltzberg
Design Direction: Steve Stave

To all our grandchildren—Austin, Bailey, Colby, Dylan, Gabriel, PK, and those yet to come—thank you for keeping us "young at heart."

—Nannie and Poppie

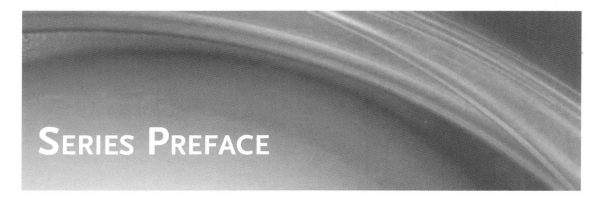

SERIES PREFACE

The First and Second Editions of the *Rapid Review Series* have received high critical acclaim from students studying for the United States Medical Licensing Examination (USMLE) Step 1 and consistently high ratings in *First Aid for the USMLE Step 1*. The new editions will continue to be invaluable resources for time-pressed students. As a result of reader feedback, we have improved upon an already successful formula. We have created a learning system, including a print and electronic package, that is easier to use and more concise than other review products on the market.

SPECIAL FEATURES

Book

- **Outline format:** Concise, high-yield subject matter is presented in a study-friendly format.
- **High-yield margin notes:** Key content that is most likely to appear on the exam is reinforced in the margin notes.
- **Visual elements:** Full-color photographs are utilized to enhance your study and recognition of key pathology images. Abundant two-color schematics and summary tables enhance your study experience.
- **Two-color design:** Colored text and headings make studying more efficient and pleasing.

New! Online Study and Testing Tool

- A minimum of **350 USMLE Step 1–type MCQs:** Clinically oriented, multiple-choice questions that mimic the current USMLE format, including high-yield images and complete rationales for all answer options.
- **Online benefits:** New review and testing tool delivered via the USMLE Consult platform, the most realistic USMLE review product on the market. Online feedback includes results analyzed to the subtopic level (discipline and organ system).
- **Test mode:** Create a test from a random mix of questions or by subject or keyword using the timed **test mode**. USMLE Consult simulates the actual test-taking experience using NBME's FRED interface, including style and level of difficulty of the questions and timing information. Detailed feedback and analysis shows your strengths and weaknesses and allows for more focused study.
- **Practice mode:** Create a test from randomized question sets or by subject or keyword for a dynamic study session. The **practice mode** features unlimited attempts at each question, instant feedback, complete rationales for all answer options, and a detailed progress report.
- **Online access:** Online access allows you to study from an internet-enabled computer wherever and whenever it is convenient. This access is activated through registration on www.studentconsult.com with the pin code printed inside the front cover.

Student Consult

- **Full online access:** You can access the complete text and illustrations of this book on www.studentconsult.com.
- **Save content to your PDA:** Through our unique Pocket Consult platform, you can clip selected text and illustrations and save them to your PDA for study on the fly!
- **Free content:** An interactive community center with a wealth of additional valuable resources is available.

ACKNOWLEDGMENT OF REVIEWERS

The publisher expresses sincere thanks to the medical students and faculty who provided many useful comments and suggestions for improving both the text and the questions. Our publishing program will continue to benefit from the combined insight and experience provided by your reviews. For always encouraging us to focus on our target, the USMLE Step 1, we thank the following:

Richard M. Awdeh, Yale University School of Medicine

Joy A. Baldwin, University of Vermont College of Medicine

John Cowden, Yale University School of Medicine

Andrew Deak, Northeastern Ohio Universities College of Medicine

Tracey DeLucia, Loyola University Chicago Stritch School of Medicine

Steven Engman, Loyola University Chicago Stritch School of Medicine

Michael Hoffman, University of Medicine and Dentistry New Jersey, Robert Wood Johnson School of Medicine

James Massullo, Northeastern Ohio Universities College of Medicine

Sarah Schlegel, University of Connecticut School of Medicine

Tina Tran, Virginia Commonwealth University School of Medicine

ACKNOWLEDGMENTS

The third edition of *Rapid Review Pathology* has been extensively revised to provide students with even more high-yield information and photographs than in previous editions. For example, there are more than double the number of high-quality, high-yield color photographs and radiographs; more than double the number of margin notes; significant additions to each of the summary tables; expanded discussions on epidemiology, clinical, and laboratory findings; and concise discussions of diagnosis and treatment for most of the diseases. Many of the photographs are grouped together in collages to provide students with an opportunity to quickly review infectious disease, dermatology, hematology, endocrinology, and many other key areas. In addition, the emphasis on margin notes and increased content in the summary tables provides the student with a "rapid review" of high-yield material for pathology examinations and USMLE and COMLEX Step 1 examinations. Furthermore, I believe that the book will be extremely useful in performing well during clinical rotations and the Step 2 examination, especially with the addition of diagnosis and treatment to the book.

As in previous editions, I especially want to thank Ivan Damjanov, MD, PhD, whose many excellent photographs have been utilized throughout the book. I highly recommend his recently published Elsevier book, *Pathophysiology*, as a companion text to the *Rapid Review Pathology* text for providing students with an even greater understanding of pathophysiologic processes in disease. I also thank Edward Klatt, MD, who graciously allowed the use of so many of his excellent images from *Robbins and Cotran Atlas of Pathology*, a resource that I also highly recommend as a source of high-quality images and supplementary learning.

Special thanks to Katie DeFrancesco, Nicole DiCicco, and Christine Abshire from Elsevier, who kept track of all the major changes in the third edition and helped facilitate the early publication of the book. In addition, I would like to thank Clay Cansler for his excellent editing of the book. Special thanks also to Karlis Sloka, DO, valued friend and teacher, whose understanding of disease processes helped me throughout the entire writing of the new edition. I want to thank Jim Merritt, Senior Acquisitions Editor of medical education, who is the inspiration and primary energy behind the entire Rapid Review Series. Thanks Jim for a job well done! Finally, I would like to thank the myriad of medical students who have sent me e-mails with encouraging words on how the book has helped them not only perform well on boards, but also become better doctors. What more could a medical educator ask for?

Edward F. Goljan, MD
"Poppie"

CONTENTS

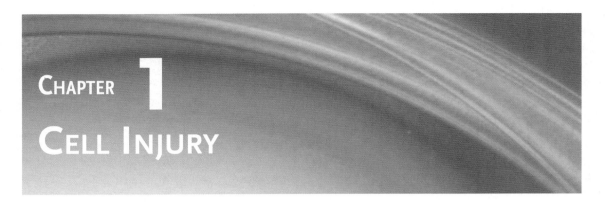

CHAPTER 1

CELL INJURY

I. Tissue Hypoxia

A. Hypoxia

1. Hypoxia refers to inadequate oxygenation of tissue.
2. Inadequate oxygen (O_2) decreases synthesis of adenosine triphosphate (ATP).
   a. ATP synthesis occurs in the inner mitochondrial membrane by the process of oxidative phosphorylation (see later).
   b. O_2 is an electron acceptor located at the end of the electron transport chain (ETC) in the oxidative pathway.
   c. A lack of O_2 or a defect in oxidative phosphorylation culminates in a decrease in ATP synthesis.
3. Several types of hypoxia produce O_2-related changes reported with arterial blood gas measurements (Table 1-1).
   - O_2 diffuses down a gradient from the alveoli, to plasma ($\uparrow Pao_2$), and to red blood cells (RBCs), where it attaches to heme groups ($\uparrow Sao_2$)

> **Pulse oximetry** is a noninvasive test for measuring Sao_2. It utilizes a probe that is usually clipped over a patient's finger. Oximetry emits light at specified wavelengths that identify oxyhemoglobin and deoxyhemoglobin, respectively. The wavelengths emitted by a pulse oximeter *cannot* identify dyshemoglobins such as methemoglobin (metHb) and carboxyhemoglobin (i.e., carbon monoxide bound to Hb, COHb), which normally decrease the Sao_2 (see later). In the presence of these dyshemoglobins, the oximeter calculates a falsely high Sao_2. Unlike the standard oximeter, a co-oximeter emits multiple wavelengths and calculates an accurate Sao_2 because it identifies metHb and COHb.

4. Clinical findings of hypoxia include cyanosis (see Fig. 10-11), confusion, cognitive impairment, and lethargy.

B. Causes of tissue hypoxia

1. Ischemia
   a. Decreased arterial blood flow or venous outflow of blood
   b. Examples—coronary artery atherosclerosis, decreased cardiac output, thrombosis of splenic vein
   c. Consequences of ischemia
      (1) Atrophy (reduction in cell/tissue mass)
      (2) Infarction of tissue (localized area of tissue necrosis)
      (3) Organ dysfunction (e.g., heart failure)
2. Hypoxemia
   - Normal ventilation and perfusion are depicted in Figure 1-1A.
   a. Decrease in Pao_2 (<40 mm Hg)
   b. Causes
      (1) Decreased inspired Po_2 (Pio_2)
         - Examples—high altitude, breathing reduced $\%O_2$ mist
      (2) Respiratory acidosis (hypoventilation)
         (a) Carbon dioxide (CO_2) retention in the lungs *always* produces a corresponding decrease in Pao_2.
         (b) Examples—depression of the medullary respiratory center (e.g., barbiturates), paralysis of the diaphragm, chronic bronchitis

---

Margin notes:

Hypoxia: inadequate oxygenation of tissue

O_2 content = (Hb g/dL × 1.34) × Sao_2 + Pao_2 × 0.003

Pulse oximeter: falsely $\uparrow Sao_2$ with metHb and COHb

Ischemia: $\downarrow$ arterial blood inflow or venous outflow

Hypoxemia: $\downarrow Pao_2$

$\uparrow$ Alveolar Pco_2 = $\downarrow$ alveolar Po_2 = $\downarrow Pao_2$ = $\downarrow Sao_2$

TABLE 1-1. **TERMINOLOGY ASSOCIATED WITH OXYGEN TRANSPORT AND HYPOXIA**

TERM	DEFINITION	CONTRIBUTING FACTORS	SIGNIFICANCE
Pao_2	Pressure keeping O_2 dissolved in the plasma of arterial blood ($0.003 \times Pao_2$)	Percentage of O_2 in inspired air, atmospheric pressure, normal O_2 exchange in lungs Driving force for movement of O_2 from capillaries into tissue by diffusion	Reduced in hypoxemia
Sao_2	Average percentage of O_2 bound to Hb	Pao_2 and valence of heme iron in each of the four heme groups Fe^{2+} binds to O_2; Fe^{3+} does not	$Sao_2 < 80\%$ produces cyanosis of skin and mucous membranes
O_2 content	Total amount of O_2 carried in blood	Hb concentration in RBCs (most important factor), Pao_2, Sao_2 Hb concentration determines total amount of O_2 delivered to tissue	Hb is the most important carrier of O_2

Fe^{2+}, ferrous iron; Fe^{3+}, ferric iron; Hb, hemoglobin; O_2, oxygen; Pao_2, partial pressure of arterial oxygen; Sao_2, arterial oxygen saturation.

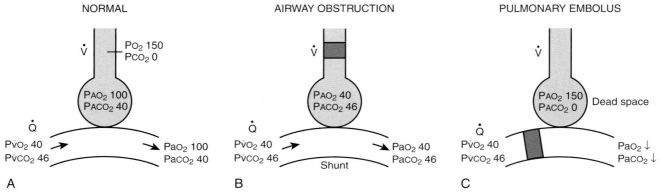

1-1: Ventilation (V)-perfusion (Q) defects. **A,** Schematic showing normal ventilation and perfusion; **B,** schematic showing ventilation defect; **C,** schematic of perfusion defect. See text for discussion. $P\overline{v}CO_2$, partial pressure of carbon dioxide in mixed venous blood; $P\overline{v}O_2$, partial pressure of oxygen in mixed venous blood. *(From Goljan EF, Sloka KI: Rapid Review Laboratory Testing in Clinical Medicine. Philadelphia, Mosby Elsevier, 2008, p 76, Fig. 3-5.)*

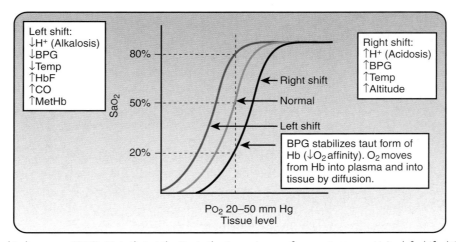

1-2: Oxygen-binding curve (OBC). Note that at the Po_2 in the tissue (ranges from 20 to 50 mm Hg) a left-shifted OBC still has an O_2 saturation (Sao_2) of 80% (only released 20% of its O_2 to tissue), a normal-shifted OBC has an Sao_2 of 50% (only released 50% of its O_2 to tissue), and a right-shifted curve has an Sao_2 of 20% (released 80% of its O_2 to tissue). 2,3-Bisphosphoglycerate (BPG) improves O_2 delivery to tissue by stabilizing the hemoglobin (Hb) in the taut form, which decreases O_2 affinity, hence facilitating the movement of O_2 from Hb into tissue by diffusion.

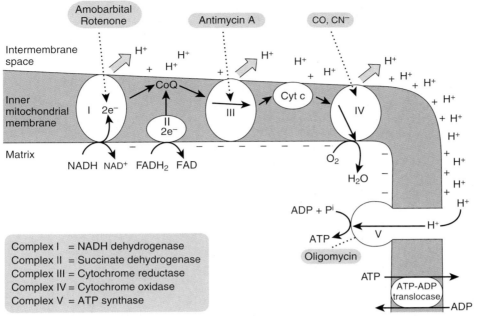

1-3: Oxidative phosphorylation. See text for discussion. *(From Pelley J, Goljan E: Rapid Review Biochemistry, 2nd ed. St. Louis, Mosby, 2007, p 81, Fig. 5-8.)*

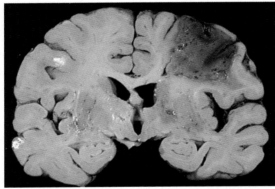

1-4: Watershed infarction showing a wedge-shaped hemorrhagic infarction at the junction of the anterior and middle cerebral arteries. *(From Damjanov I, Linder J: Anderson's Pathology, 10th ed. St. Louis, Mosby, 1996, p 375, Fig. 17-16.)*

(3) Ventilation defect (Fig. 1-1B)
  (a) Impaired O_2 delivery to alveoli
    • Example—respiratory distress syndrome (RDS) with collapse of the distal airways due to lack of surfactant
  (b) No O_2 exchange in lungs that are perfused but *not* ventilated
  (c) Diffuse disease (RDS) produces intrapulmonary shunting of blood
    • Pulmonary capillary blood has the same Po_2 and Pco_2 as venous blood returning from tissue (i.e., a large fraction of pulmonary blood flow has *not* been arterialized).
  (d) Inspired %O_2 from 0.24% to 0.28% or greater does *not* significantly increase the Pao_2.
    • This only applies to a diffuse ventilation defect involving both lungs; smaller defects are compensated for in normally ventilated lung.
(4) Perfusion defect (Fig. 1-1C)
  (a) Absence of blood flow to alveoli (e.g., pulmonary embolus)
  (b) No O_2 exchange in lungs that are ventilated but *not* perfused
  (c) Produces an increase in dead space
    • Exchange of O_2 and CO_2 does *not* occur.
  (d) Inspired %O_2 from 0.24% to 0.28% or greater increases the Pao_2.
    • Other parts of ventilated and perfused lung have normal gas exchange.

Ventilation defect: perfused but *not* ventilated; intrapulmonary shunt

Perfusion defect: ventilated but *not* perfused; ↑ dead space

Diffusion defect: interstitial fibrosis, pulmonary edema

(5) Diffusion defect
    (a) Decreased O_2 diffusion through the alveolar-capillary interface
    (b) Examples—interstitial fibrosis, pulmonary edema
(6) Ventilation, perfusion, and diffusion defects increase the difference in O_2 concentration between alveolar Po_2 (Pao_2) and arterial Po_2 (Pao_2).
    • This difference is called the alveolar-arterial (A-a) gradient (refer to Chapter 16).

3. Hemoglobin (Hb)-related abnormalities
  a. Anemia
    (1) Decreased Hb concentration (<7 g/dL)
    (2) Causes
      (a) Decreased production of Hb (e.g., iron deficiency)
      (b) Increased destruction of RBCs (e.g., hereditary spherocytosis)
      (c) Decreased production of RBCs (e.g., aplastic anemia)
      (d) Increased sequestration of RBCs (e.g., splenomegaly)

Anemia: normal Pao_2 and Sao_2

    (3) Normal Pao_2 and Sao_2
  b. Methemoglobinemia
    (1) Methemoglobin (metHb) is Hb with oxidized heme groups (Fe^{3+}).

> **Methemoglobin** is converted to the ferrous state (Fe^{2+}) by the reduced nicotinamide adenine dinucleotide (NADH) reductase system located off the glycolytic pathway in RBCs. Electrons from NADH are transferred to cytochrome b_5 and then to metHb by cytochrome b_5 reductase to produce ferrous Hb. Newborns are particularly at risk for developing methemoglobinemia after oxidant stresses (see later) owing to decreased levels of cytochrome b_5 reductase until at least 4 months of age.

    (2) Causes
      (a) Oxidant stresses
        • Examples—nitrite- and sulfur-containing drugs, sepsis, local anesthetics (e.g., benzocaine)
      (b) Congenital deficiency of cytochrome b_5 reductase

MetHb: heme Fe^{3+}; ↓ Sao_2

    (3) Pathogenesis of hypoxia
      (a) Fe^{3+} cannot bind O_2
        • Normal Pao_2, decreased Sao_2
      (b) Ferric heme groups impair unloading of O_2 by oxygenated ferrous heme.

MetHb: Rx with IV methylene blue

        • This causes a left-shifted O_2-binding curve (see later).

> Patients with **methemoglobinemia** have chocolate-colored blood (increased concentration of deoxyhemoglobin) and cyanosis. Clinically evident cyanosis occurs at metHb levels greater than 1.5 g/dL. Skin color does *not* return to normal after administration of O_2. Treatment is intravenous methylene blue, which acts as an artificial electron carrier in the reduced nicotinamide adenine dinucleotide phosphate (NADPH) metHb reductase system located in the pentose phosphate shunt.

  c. Carbon monoxide (CO) poisoning (also refer to Chapter 6)
    (1) Leading cause of death due to poisoning
    (2) Produced by incomplete combustion of carbon-containing compounds
    (3) Causes include automobile exhaust, smoke inhalation, wood stoves, methylene chloride (paint thinner).
    (4) Pathogenesis of hypoxia

CO poisoning: normal Pao_2, ↓Sao_2

      (a) CO competes with O_2 for binding sites on Hb.
        • Decreases Sao_2 *without* affecting Pao_2
      (b) CO inhibits cytochrome oxidase in the electron transport chain (ETC).
      (c) CO causes a left-shifted O_2-binding curve (OBC).
    (5) Clinical findings
      (a) Cherry-red discoloration of skin and blood
      (b) Headache (first symptom at levels of 10–20%)
      (c) Dyspnea, dizziness (levels of 20–30%)
      (d) Seizures, coma (levels of 50–60%)
      (e) Lactic acidosis due to hypoxia

Rx CO poisoning: O_2 via nonbreather mask

    (6) Treatment is O_2 via nonbreather mask or endotracheal tube (100% O_2)

d. Factors causing a left-shifted OBC
  (1) Decreased 2,3-bisphosphoglycerate (BPG)
    • Intermediate of glycolysis via conversion of 1,3-BPG to 2,3-BPG
  (2) CO, alkalosis, metHb, fetal Hb, hypothermia
  (3) These factors increase affinity of Hb for O_2 with less release of O_2 to tissue.
    • Example—at the capillary Po_2 concentration in tissue a right-shifted OBC ($\uparrow$2,3-BPG, acidosis, fever) has released most of its O_2 to tissue, but a left-shifted OBC still has most of its O_2 attached to heme groups (Fig. 1-2).

High altitude: $\uparrow$2,3-BPG synthesis; respiratory alkalosis

At **high altitudes,** the atmospheric pressure is decreased; however, the percentage of O_2 in the atmosphere remains the same (i.e., 21%). Hypoxemia stimulates peripheral chemoreceptors (e.g., carotid body) causing respiratory alkalosis, which shifts the OBC to the left. However, alkalosis activates phosphofructokinase, the rate-limiting enzyme in glycolysis, causing increased production of 1,3-BPG, which is converted to 2,3-BPG. This eventually shifts the OBC to the right, leading to increased release of O_2 to tissue.

C. Mitochondrial causes of ATP depletion
  1. Enzyme inhibition of oxidative phosphorylation (Fig. 1-3)

The **oxidative part of the pathway** in the inner mitochondrial membrane transfers donated electrons from NADH and reduced flavin adenine dinucleotide ($FADH_2$) derived from the energy cycles down the ETC to O_2. Oxygen is a strong electron acceptor located at the end of the chain on complex IV. The transfer of electrons is coupled with the transport of protons (H^+) supplied by NADH and $FADH_2$ across the inner mitochondrial membrane into the intermembranous space, which establishes both a proton and a pH gradient. The **phosphorylation part of the pathway** is the synthesis of ATP. A certain amount of heat is required to synthesize ATP. ATP synthesis occurs when the protons on the cytosolic side of the inner membrane enter small channels (proton pores) within the ATP synthase molecule (complex V) and reenter the mitochondrial matrix, where ATP is synthesized. The inner mitochondrial membrane is normally impermeable to protons except through the channel in the ATP synthase molecule. This relationship is critical to the maintenance of the proton gradient. If enzymatic reactions in electron transport are inhibited (e.g., cytochrome oxidase), the formation of protons and the proton gradient are disrupted as well, leading to a decrease in ATP synthesis.

  a. Enzyme inhibition of oxidative phosphorylation
    (1) Synthesis of ATP is decreased.
    (2) CO and cyanide (CN) inhibit cytochrome oxidase in the ETC.
    (3) CN poisoning (also refer to Chapter 6)
      (a) It may result from drugs (e.g., nitroprusside) and combustion of polyurethane products in house fires.
      (b) It produces an initial central nervous system and cardiovascular stimulation followed by CNS depression and death.
      (c) It produces lactic acidosis due to hypoxia.
      (d) It produces increased venous Po_2 and saturation.
        • Tissue *cannot* extract O_2.
      (e) Treatment involves two stages.
        • Amyl nitrite (produces metHb which combines with CN to form cyanmetHb) followed by thiosulfate (CN converted to thiocyanate)
  b. Uncoupling of oxidative phosphorylation
    (1) Uncoupling proteins carry protons in the intermembranous space through the inner mitochondrial membrane into the mitochondrial matrix without damaging the membrane.
      (a) Bypass of ATP synthase causes decreased synthesis of ATP.
      (b) Examples—thermogenin (natural uncoupler in brown fat in newborns), dinitrophenol used in synthesizing nitroglycerin
    (2) Heat normally used to synthesize ATP raises the core body temperature.
      (a) There is a danger of developing hyperthermia with dinitrophenol.
      (b) Thermogenin is useful in stabilizing body temperature in newborns.

CO and CN: inhibit cytochrome oxidase

CO and CN poisoning: house fires

Rx CN poisoning: amyl nitrite, thiosulfate

Uncouplers: thermogenin, dinitrophenol

Mitochondrial toxins: alcohol, salicylates

Agents such as **alcohol** and **salicylates** act as mitochondrial toxins. They damage the inner mitochondrial membrane, causing protons to move into the mitochondrial matrix. As with dinitrophenol, hyperthermia is a common complication in alcohol and salicylate poisoning.

D. Tissues susceptible to hypoxia
1. Watershed areas between terminal branches of major arterial blood supplies
   a. The blood supply from the two vessels does *not* overlap.
   b. Examples
      (1) Area between the distribution of the anterior and middle cerebral arteries (Fig. 1-4)
      (2) Area between the distribution of the superior and inferior mesenteric arteries (i.e., splenic flexure)
2. Subendocardial tissue
   a. Coronary vessels penetrate the epicardial surface.
   b. Subendocardial tissue receives the *least* amount of O_2.

Factors decreasing coronary artery blood flow (e.g., coronary artery atherosclerosis) produce subendocardial ischemia, which is manifested by chest pain (i.e., angina) and ST-segment depression in an electrocardiogram (ECG). Increased thickness of the left ventricle (i.e., hypertrophy) in the presence of increased myocardial demand for O_2 (e.g., exercise) can also produce subendocardial ischemia.

3. Renal cortex and medulla
   a. In the cortex, the straight portion of the proximal tubule is most susceptible to hypoxia.
      • Primary site for reclaiming bicarbonate and reabsorbing sodium
   b. In the medulla, the Na^+-K^+-2 Cl^- cotransport channel in the thick ascending limb is most susceptible to hypoxia.
      • Primary site for regenerating free water, which is necessary for normal dilution and concentration of urine.

4. Neurons in the central nervous system
   a. Examples—Purkinje cells in cerebellum, neurons in layers 3, 5, and 6 of the cerebral cortex
   b. Irreversible damage occurs ~5 minutes after global hypoxia.

5. Hepatocytes located around the central vein

In the **portal triads,** hepatic artery tributaries carrying oxygenated blood and portal vein tributaries carrying unoxygenated blood empty their blood into the liver sinusoids (mixed oxygenated and unoxygenated blood), which drain blood into the central veins (terminal hepatic venules). The central veins become the hepatic vein, which empties into the inferior vena cava. Hepatocytes closest to the portal triads (zone I) receive the most oxygen and nutrients, and those farthest from the portal triads (zone III around the central vein) receive the least amount of oxygen and nutrients. Production of free radicals from drugs (e.g., acetaminophen, see later), tissue hypoxia (e.g., shock, CO poisoning), and alcohol-related fatty change of the liver initially damage zone III hepatocytes.

E. Consequences of hypoxic cell injury
1. Decreased synthesis of ATP
2. Anaerobic glycolysis is used for ATP synthesis and is accompanied by several changes—
   a. Activation of phosphofructokinase
      • Caused by low citrate levels and increased adenosine monophosphate
   b. Net gain of 2 ATP
   c. Decrease in intracellular pH caused by an excess of lactate

      (1) Also accumulates in blood producing lactic acidosis
      (2) Denatures structural and enzymic proteins
   d. Impaired Na^+/K^+-ATPase pump
      (1) Diffusion of Na^+ and H_2O into cells causes cellular swelling.
      (2) Potentially reversible with restoration of O_2
3. Decreased protein synthesis
   • Due to detachment of ribosomes (potentially reversible)

4. Irreversible cell changes
   a. Impaired calcium (Ca^{2+})-ATPase pump
      • Normal function of the pump is to keep Ca^{2+} out of the cytosol.
   b. Increased cytosolic Ca^{2+} has two lethal effects.
      (1) Enzyme activation
         (a) Phospholipase increases cell and organelle membrane permeability.

(b) Proteases damage the cytoskeleton.
(c) Endonucleases cause fading of nuclear chromatin (karyolysis).
(2) Reentry of Ca^{2+} into mitochondria
(a) Increases mitochondrial membrane permeability
(b) Release of cytochrome *c* into the cytosol activates apoptosis (see later)

II. Free Radical Cell Injury
A. Definition of free radicals
- Unstable chemical compounds with a single unpaired electron in their outer orbital
B. Formation, function, types of free radicals (FRs)
1. Produced by—
   a. Ionizing radiation
      - Produces hydroxyl FRs
   b. Damaged mitochondria
      - Produce superoxide FRs
   c. High concentration of O_2
      (1) Produces superoxide and hydroxyl FRs
      (2) Produces hydrogen peroxide (H_2O_2)
         - A reactive oxygen species that produces hydroxyl and peroxide FRs.
   d. Oxidase reactions
      (1) NADPH oxidase in the neutrophil and monocyte cell membrane
         (a) Myeloperoxidase in a phagolysosome combines hydrogen peroxide with chloride to form bleach (hypochlorous acid).
         (b) Hypochlorous acid is a reactive oxygen species that can generate FRs.
      (2) Xanthine oxidase acting upon xanthine (degradation product of ATP)
         - Produces superoxide FRs
   e. Drugs (e.g., acetaminophen)
      - Converted to acetaminophen FRs in the liver
   f. Carbon tetrachloride
      - Converted to CCl_3 FRs in the liver
   g. Cigarette smoke
      (1) Produces quinone/hydroquinone FRs produced from tar
      (2) Produces nitric oxide (NO), an FR gas
         - NO reacts with other reactive species (e.g., isoprene) to produce additional FRs.
   h. Pollution
      - Nitrogen dioxide in car exhaust and ozone produce nitrate FRs.
   i. Metals (e.g., iron, copper)
      - Produce hydroxyl FRs (called the Fenton reaction)
   j. Nitric oxide
      - FR gas that is produced by macrophages and endothelial cells.
   k. Intima of elastic and muscular arteries
      (1) Small dense subtypes of low density lipoprotein (LDL) enter the intima and are oxidized by FRs produced by macrophages, smooth muscle cells, and endothelial cells.
      (2) Oxidized LDL contributes to formation of fatty streaks, which are progenitors of fibrous caps, the pathognomonic lesion of atherosclerosis.
2. FRs attack a molecule and "steal" its electron.
   a. The attacked molecule becomes an FR that begins a chain reaction leading to cell death.
   b. FRs primarily target nucleic acids and membrane molecules.
      (1) FRs produce DNA fragmentation and dissolution.
      (2) FRs initiate lipid peroxidation of polyunsaturated lipids in cell and mitochondrial membranes.
         (a) Lipid FRs combine with molecular O_2.
         (b) Increases membrane permeability leading to increased cytosol Ca^{2+} concentration (see section ID).
   c. FR damage accumulates with age; important in the aging process
C. Neutralization of FRs
1. Superoxide dismutase (SOD)
   - Converts superoxide free radicals to peroxide and O_2
2. Glutathione peroxidase (enhances glutathione, GSH)
   a. Located in the pentose phosphate pathway
   b. Neutralizes H_2O_2, hydroxyl, and acetaminophen FRs
3. Catalase (present in peroxisomes)
   - Degrades peroxide into O_2 and water

Margin notes:

Cytochrome *c* in cytosol: activates apoptosis (cell death)

Hydroxyl FRs: most destructive FRs

Oxidase reactions: produce superoxide FRs

Acetaminophen: drug FRs formed in liver

Iron, copper: generate hydroxyl FRs

Free radicals: damage membranes and DNA

Neutralization of FRs: SOD, GSH, vitamins C and E

4. Vitamins as antioxidants
   a. Antioxidants neutralize FRs by donating one of their own electrons.
      (1) Stops the "electron stealing" of FRs
      (2) Antioxidants remain stable and do *not* become an FR.
   b. Vitamin E (fat-soluble vitamin)
      (1) Prevents lipid peroxidation in cell membranes
      (2) Neutralizes oxidized LDL
   c. Vitamin C (water-soluble vitamin)
      (1) Neutralizes FRs produced by pollutants and cigarette smoke
         • Smokers have decreased levels of vitamin C because they are used up in neutralizing FRs derived from cigarette smoke.
      (2) Best neutralizer of hydroxyl FRs
5. Selenium
   • Neutralizes FRs in the cytosol

D. Examples of FR injury
   1. Acetaminophen FRs
      a. May cause diffuse chemical hepatitis
         (1) Liver cell necrosis initially occurs around the central veins (zone III).
            (a) Can occur at nontoxic levels in alcoholics
            (b) Produces transient decrease in functional factor VII
               • Prolongs the prothrombin time (PT)
         (2) Treatment with *N*-acetylcysteine
            • Increases synthesis of glutathione for neutralization of drug FRs.
      b. May cause renal papillary necrosis (see Chapter 19)
         • Necrosis occurs in association with the use of nonsteroidal anti-inflammatory agents.
   2. Carbon tetrachloride free radicals
      • Produce liver cell necrosis with fatty change
   3. Ischemia/reperfusion injury in acute myocardial infarction (see Chapter 10)
      a. Occurs with restoration of blood flow to ischemic myocardium
      b. Superoxide FRs and cytosolic Ca²⁺ irreversibly damage previously injured cells.
   4. Retinopathy of prematurity
      • Blindness may occur in the treatment of RDS with an O₂ concentration > 50%.
   5. Iron overload disorders
      a. Examples include hemochromatosis and hemosiderosis (see Chapter 19).
      b. Intracellular iron produces hydroxyl FRs, which damage parenchymal cells.
         • Examples of injury—cirrhosis, exocrine/endocrine pancreatic dysfunction
   6. Copper overload (Wilson's disease)
      a. Inability to excrete copper into bile
      b. Copper excess in hepatocytes increases production of hydroxyl FRs
         • Damage to hepatocytes produces cirrhosis

III. Injury to Cellular Organelles
   A. Mitochondria
      1. Release of cytochrome *c* from injured mitochondria
         • Initiates apoptosis by activating caspases in the cytosol (see later).
      2. Injurious agents include alcohol, salicylates, and increased cytosolic Ca²⁺.
         • Salicylates and alcohol produce megamitochondria (Fig. 1-5) with destruction of the cristae.
   B. Smooth endoplasmic reticulum (SER)
      1. Induction of enzymes of the liver cytochrome P-450 system
         a. May be caused by:
            • Alcohol, barbiturates, phenytoin
         b. Causes SER hyperplasia (see Fig. 1-5)
            • Increased drug detoxification with lower-than-expected therapeutic drug levels
      2. Inhibition of enzymes of the cytochrome P-450 system
         a. May be caused by:
            (1) Proton receptor blockers (e.g., omeprazole)
            (2) Macrolides (e.g., erythromycin)
            (3) Histamine blockers (e.g., cimetidine)
         b. Results in decreased drug detoxification
            • Decreased drug detoxification with higher-than-expected therapeutic drug levels

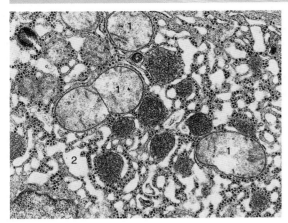

1-5: Hyperplasia of smooth endoplasmic reticulum (2) and damaged mitochondria (megamitochondria, 1) in alcoholic liver disease. (*From MacSween R, Burt A, Portmann B, et al: Pathology of the Liver, 4th ed. London, Churchill Livingstone, 2002, p 288, Fig. 6-20.*)

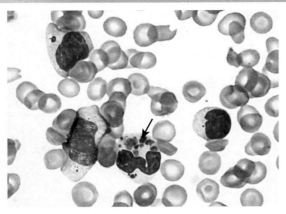

1-6: Chédiak-Higashi neutrophil (*arrow*) and lymphocytes with giant granules. See text for discussion. (*From McPherson R, Pincus M: Henry's Clinical Diagnosis and Management by Laboratory Methods, 21st ed. Philadelphia, WB Saunders, 2007, p 551, Fig. 32-7.*)

C. Lysosomes

1. Lysosome formation and function
   a. Hydrolytic enzymes synthesized by the rough endoplasmic reticulum (RER) are transported to the Golgi apparatus for post-translational modification.
   b. Modification involves attaching phosphate (via phosphotransferase) to mannose residues on hydrolytic enzymes to produce mannose 6-phosphate.
   c. The marked lysosomal enzymes attach to specific mannose 6-phosphate receptors on the Golgi membrane.
   d. Vesicles containing the receptor-bound lysosomal enzymes pinch off the Golgi membrane to form primary lysosomes in the cytosol.
   e. Fusion of additional vesicles to the primary lysosome further increases their content of hydrolytic enzymes.
   f. Small vesicles containing only the receptors pinch off the primary lysosomes and return to the Golgi apparatus to bind more marked lysosomal enzymes so the cycle can repeat itself.
   g. Lysosomal functions
      (1) Fusion with phagocytic vacuoles containing bacteria
         • These lysosomes are designated secondary or phagolysosomes.
      (2) Destruction of cell organelles (autophagy; see later)
      (3) Degradation of complex substrates (e.g., sphingolipids, glycosaminoglycans)
2. Selected lysosomal disorders
   a. Inclusion (I)-cell disease

> **Inclusion (I)-cell disease** is a rare inherited condition in which there is a defect in post-translational modification of lysosomal enzymes in the Golgi membrane. Mannose residues on newly synthesized lysosomal enzymes coming from the RER are *not* phosphorylated because of a deficiency of phosphotransferase. Without mannose 6-phosphate to direct the enzymes to lysosomes, vesicles that pinch off the Golgi membrane empty the unmarked enzymes into the extracellular space where they are degraded in the blood stream. Undigested substrates (e.g., carbohydrates, lipids, and proteins) accumulate as large inclusions in the cytosol. Symptoms include psychomotor retardation and early death.

   b. Deficiency of lysosomal enzymes involved in degradation of complex substrates characterizes the lysosomal storage diseases.
      (1) Incompletely degraded complex substrates (e.g., sphingolipids, glycosaminoglycans, glycogen) accumulate in lysosomes.
      (2) Example—Gaucher's disease with deficiency of glucocerebrosidase causes accumulation of glucocerebrosides in the lysosome.

Primary lysosomes: derive from Golgi apparatus

Phagolysosome: contain lysosomal enzymes

I-cell disease: defect in post-translational modification of lysosomal enzymes

Lysosomal storage disease: ↓ lysosomal enzymes

(3) Example—Pompe's disease with deficiency of α-1,4-glucosidase causes an accumulation of glycogen in the lysosome.
c. Chédiak-Higashi syndrome (CHS)

CHS: giant lysosomal granules; defect in formation of phagolysosomes

> **CHS** is an autosomal recessive disease with a defect in a lysosomal transport protein that affects the synthesis and maintenance and storage of secretory granules in various cells (e.g., lysosomes in leukocytes, azurophilic granules in neutrophils, dense bodies in platelets). Granules in these cells tend to fuse together to become megagranules (Fig. 1-6). In addition, there is a defect in microtubule function in neutrophils and monocytes that prevents the fusion of lysosomes with phagosomes to produce phagolysosomes. This produces a bactericidal defect. In particular, there is increased susceptibility to developing *Staphylococcus aureus* infections. Microtubular dysfunction also produces defects in chemotaxis (directed migration), which further exacerbates the susceptibility to infection.

D. Cytoskeleton
1. Normal functions of the cytoskeleton
   a. Network of protein filaments in the cytosol
      • Maintains shape of the cell and, in some cases, motility of the cell
   b. Composed of microtubules, actin filaments, intermediate filaments
   c. Microtubules are polymers composed of the protein tubulin.
   d. Actin thick and thin filaments are involved in the contractile process.
   e. Intermediate filaments are important in the integration of cell organelles.

Defect tubulin synthesis G$_2$ phase: etoposide, bleomycin B

2. Defect in synthesis of tubulin in the G$_2$ phase of the cell cycle
   • Etoposide and bleomycin

Mitotic spindle defects: vinca alkaloids, colchicine, paclitaxel

3. Mitotic spindle defects in the M phase of the cell cycle
   a. Vinca alkaloids and colchicine bind to tubulin in microtubules.
      • Interferes with the assembly of the mitotic spindle
   b. Paclitaxel enhances tubulin polymerization.
      • Interferes with disassembly of the mitotic spindle
4. Intermediate filament defects
   a. Ubiquitin, a stress protein, binds to damaged intermediate filaments.
      • Marks them for degradation in proteasomes and lysosomes in the cytosol

Ubiquitin: marker for intermediate filament degradation

   b. Mallory bodies
      • Damaged ("ubiquinated") cytokeratin intermediate filaments in hepatocytes in alcoholic liver disease (Fig. 1-7)
   c. Lewy bodies
      (1) Damaged neurofilaments in idiopathic Parkinson's disease
      (2) Eosinophilic cytoplasmic inclusions in degenerating substantia nigra neurons
5. Rigor mortis
   • Myosin heads become locked to actin filaments as a result of a lack of ATP.

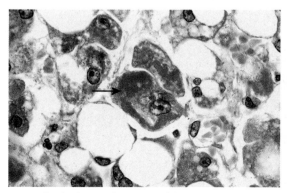

1-7: Mallory bodies. Hyaline (eosinophilic) inclusions (*arrow*) are present in the cytosol of hepatocytes. Many of the hepatocytes have vacuoles containing triglyceride. (*From Kumar V, Fausto N, Abbas A: Robbins and Cotran's Pathologic Basis of Disease, 7th ed. Philadelphia, WB Saunders, 2004, p 34, Fig. 1-34A.*)

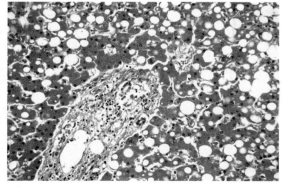

1-8: Fatty change of the liver. Vacuoles containing triglyceride are noted in most of the hepatocytes. The nucleus is displaced to the periphery. (*From Kumar V, Fausto N, Abbas A: Robbins and Cotran's Pathologic Basis of Disease, 7th ed. Philadelphia, WB Saunders, 2004, p 36, Fig. 1-36B.*)

TABLE 1-2. **SELECTED INTRACELLULAR ACCUMULATIONS**

SUBSTANCE	CLINICAL SIGNIFICANCE
Endogenous Accumulations	
Bilirubin	Kernicterus (see Fig. 15-5): fat-soluble unconjugated bilirubin derived from Rh hemolytic disease of newborn; bilirubin enters basal ganglia nuclei of brain, causing permanent damage.
Cholesterol	Xanthelasma (see Fig. 9-2B): yellow plaque on eyelid; cholesterol in macrophages Atherosclerosis (see Fig. 9-4): cholesterol-laden smooth muscle cells and macrophages (i.e., foam cells); components of fibrofatty plaques
Glycogen	Diabetes mellitus: increased glycogen in proximal renal tubule cells (cells are insensitive to insulin and become overloaded with glycogen) Von Gierke's glycogenosis: deficiency of glucose-6-phosphatase; glycogen excess in hepatocytes and renal tubular cells
Hematin	Melena: when blood is exposed to gastric acid, Hb is converted to a black pigment called hematin, which is responsible for black, tarry stools called melena, a sign of an upper GI bleed.
Hemosiderin and ferritin	Iron overload disorders (e.g., hemochromatosis; see Fig. 18-11): excess hemosiderin (breakdown product of ferritin) deposition in parenchymal cells, leading to FR damage and organ dysfunction (e.g., cirrhosis); increase in serum ferritin Pulmonary congestion: in left-sided heart failure there is pulmonary hemorrhage with phagocytosis of RBCs by alveolar macrophages. Hemosiderin is the breakdown product of RBC degradation in the macrophage (called "heart failure" cells). Responsible for rusty-colored sputum. Iron deficiency (see Fig. 11-11): decrease in ferritin and hemosiderin Anemia of chronic disease: increase in ferritin and hemosiderin
Melanin	Addison's disease (see Fig. 22-21): destruction of the adrenal cortex; hypocortisolism leads to an increase in ACTH (melanocyte-stimulating properties) causing excess synthesis of melanin and diffuse pigmentation of the skin and mucosal membranes.
Protein	Amyloid (see Figs. 3-6, 3-7): derives from different proteins (e.g., light chains, amyloid precursor protein). Stains red with Congo red and when polarized has apple green birefringence.
Triglyceride	Fatty liver (see Fig. 1-8): triglyceride in hepatocytes pushes the nucleus to the periphery.
Exogenous Accumulations	
Anthracotic pigment (see Fig. 16-18)	Coal worker's pneumoconiosis: phagocytosis of black anthracotic pigment (coal dust) by alveolar macrophages ("dust cells")
Lead	Lead poisoning: lead deposits in nuclei of proximal renal tubular cells (acid-fast inclusion) contribute to nephrotoxic changes in the proximal tubule.

ACTH, adrenocorticotropic hormone; FR, free radical; GI, gastrointestinal.

IV. Intracellular Accumulations
A. Types of accumulations (Table 1-2)
B. Fatty change in the liver
1. Cytosolic accumulation of triglyceride
   - Packaged in the very low density lipoprotein (VLDL) fraction
2. Mechanisms of fatty change
   a. Increased synthesis of triglyceride (TG)
      (1) Occurs with increased conversion of dihydroxyacetone phosphate (DHAP), an intermediate of glycolysis, to glycerol 3-phosphate (G3-P)
      - Addition of three fatty acids (FAs) to G3-P produces TG in the liver.

Most common cause of fatty change: alcohol

Fatty liver: ↑synthesis TG; ↓secretion TG

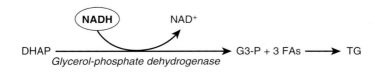

(a) Increased production of NADH from alcohol metabolism accelerates conversion of DHAP to G3-P.

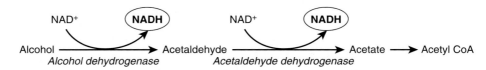

(2) Occurs with increased production of DHAP, which increases G3-P, which increases TG.
- Increased intake of carbohydrates (e.g. kwashiorkor)

G3-P: substrate for TG synthesis

(3) Increased availability of FAs increases synthesis of TG from G3-P; occurs with:
  (a) Increased synthesis of FAs from acetyl coenzyme A (acetyl CoA)
  - Acetyl CoA is the end-product of alcohol metabolism (see earlier).
  (b) Increased mobilization of FAs from TG stores in adipose tissue by activation of hormone sensitive lipase
  - Causes include alcohol and starvation.
  (c) Decreased β-oxidation of FAs in the mitochondrial matrix
  - Causes include alcohol and diphtheria toxin, which produce mitochondrial dysfunction.

b. Decreased packaging of TG into VLDL and secretion of VLDL into plasma by apolipoprotein B-100
- Example—decreased protein intake leading to decreased synthesis of apolipoprotein B-100 (e.g., kwashiorkor)

3. Morphology
  a. Normal or enlarged liver with a yellowish discoloration
  b. Clear space pushing the nucleus to the periphery (Fig. 1-8)

Fatty change in cardiac muscle: anemia, diphtheria

4. Fatty change may also occur in cardiac muscle.
  a. Causes
    (1) Severe anemia
    (2) Diphtheria
    - Exotoxin inhibits β-oxidation of FAs.
  b. Heart has a mottled appearance
    - "Tabby cat" heart, "thrush" heart

C. Iron (see Table 1-2)
  1. Ferritin
    a. Major soluble iron storage protein
    b. Synthesized and stored in bone marrow macrophages and hepatocytes
    c. Small amounts circulate in serum
    - Directly correlates with ferritin stores in the bone marrow

Serum ferritin: ↓ in iron deficiency anemia

Hemosiderin: ferritin degradation product

  2. Hemosiderin
    a. Insoluble product of ferritin degradation in lysosomes
    b. Does *not* circulate in serum
    c. Appears as golden brown granules in tissue
    d. Appears as blue granules when stained with Prussian blue (see Fig. 18-11)

D. Pathologic calcification
  1. Dystrophic calcification

Dystrophic calcification: calcification of necrotic tissue

    a. Deposition of calcium phosphate in necrotic tissue
    b. Normal serum calcium and phosphate
    c. Examples
      (1) Calcification in chronic pancreatitis (Fig. 1-9)
      (2) Calcified atherosclerotic plaque (see Fig. 9-4)
      (3) Periventricular calcification in congenital cytomegalovirus infection (see Fig. 25-24A)

  2. Metastatic calcification

Metastatic calcification: calcification of normal tissue

    a. Deposition of calcium phosphate in normal tissue
    b. Due to increased serum calcium and/or phosphate
      (1) Causes of hypercalcemia—primary hyperparathyroidism, malignancy-induced hypercalcemia
      (2) Causes of hyperphosphatemia—renal failure, primary hypoparathyroidism
      - Excess phosphate drives calcium into normal tissue.

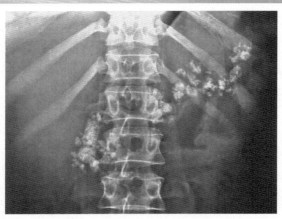

1-9: Radiograph showing multiple dystrophic calcifications in the pancreas in a patient with chronic pancreatitis. *(From Katz D, Math K, Groskin S: Radiology Secrets. Philadelphia, Hanley & Belfus, 1998, p 155, Fig. 4.)*

      c. Examples of metastatic calcification
        (1) Calcification of renal tubular basement membranes in the collecting ducts (nephrocalcinosis)
          • This can produce nephrogenic diabetes insipidus and renal failure.
        (2) Basal ganglia calcification in hypoparathyroidism

V. Adaptation to Cell Injury: Growth Alterations
  A. Atrophy
    1. Decrease in size and weight of a tissue or organ
    2. Causes of atrophy
      a. Decreased hormone stimulation
        • Example—hypopituitarism causing atrophy of target organs, such as the thyroid and adrenal cortex
      b. Decreased innervation
        • Example—skeletal muscle atrophy following loss of lower motor neurons in amyotrophic lateral sclerosis
      c. Decreased blood flow
        • Example—cerebral atrophy due to atherosclerosis of the carotid artery (Fig. 1-10A)
      d. Decreased nutrients
        • Example—total calorie deprivation in marasmus (see Fig. 7-1)
      e. Increased pressure
        (1) Example—atrophy of the renal cortex and medulla in hydronephrosis (see Fig. 19-14)
        (2) Example—thick pancreatic duct secretions in cystic fibrosis occlude the lumens causing increased luminal back-pressure and compression atrophy of the exocrine glands and tubular epithelium (Fig. 1-10B).
    3. Mechanisms of atrophy
      a. Shrinkage of cells due to increased catabolism of cell organelles (e.g., mitochondria) and reduction in cytosol
        (1) Organelles and cytosol form autophagic vacuoles.
        (2) Autophagic vacuoles fuse with primary lysosomes for enzymatic degradation.
        (3) Undigested lipids are stored as residual bodies (lipofuscin).
      b. Loss of cells by apoptosis

> **Brown atrophy** is a tissue discoloration that results from lysosomal accumulation of lipofuscin ("wear and tear" pigment). Lipofuscin is an indigestible lipid derived from lipid peroxidation of cell membranes, which may occur in atrophy and free radical damage of tissue.

  B. Hypertrophy
    1. Increase in cell size
    2. Causes of hypertrophy
      a. Increased workload
        (1) Left ventricular hypertrophy in response to an increase in afterload (resistance) or preload (volume) (Fig. 1-10C)
        (2) Skeletal muscle hypertrophy in weight training

Atrophy: ↓ size/weight of tissue or organ

Atrophy: autophagic vacuoles

Atrophy: ↑ lipofuscin in cells

Hypertrophy: ↑ cell size; ↑ workload

1-10: A, Atrophy of the brain. Note the narrow gyri and widened sulci. The meninges have been stripped from the right half of the brain. **B,** Pancreas in a patient with cystic fibrosis showing dilated ducts filled with thickened eosinophilic material. The ducts are surrounded with fibrous tissue. **C,** Left ventricular hypertrophy, showing the thickened free left ventricular wall (right side) and the thickened interventricular septum. The right ventricle wall (left side) is of normal thickness. **D,** Benign prostatic hyperplasia. The prostatic glands show infolding into the glandular spaces. **E,** Barrett's esophagus showing an extensive area of glandular metaplasia with numerous goblet cells. A small section of squamous epithelium remains on the right. **F,** Section of bronchus from a smoker showing focal squamous metaplasia (*long arrow*). Normal ciliated, pseudostratified columnar epithelium is present on the right (*short arrow*). **G,** Squamous dysplasia of the cervix, a precursor of squamous cell carcinoma. There is a lack of orientation of the squamous cells throughout the upper two thirds of the epithelium. Many of the nuclei are enlarged (*arrows*), are hyperchromatic, and have irregular nuclear margins. (*A from Kumar V, Abbas A, Fausto N, Mitchell, R: Robbins Basic Pathology, 8th ed. Philadelphia, WB Saunders, 2007, p 5, Fig. 1-4; B, D, and E from Damjanov I, Linder J: Pathology: A Color Atlas. St. Louis, Mosby, 2000, pp 169, 249, 111, Figs. 9-6, 12-32, 6-26, respectively; C and G from Kumar V, Fausto N, Abbas A: Robbins and Cotran's Pathologic Basis of Disease, 7th ed. Philadelphia, WB Saunders, 2004, pp 561, 1075, Figs. 12-3A; 22-19C, respectively; F from Corrin B: Pathology of the Lungs. London, Churchill Livingstone, 2000, p 460, Fig. 13.1.1.*)

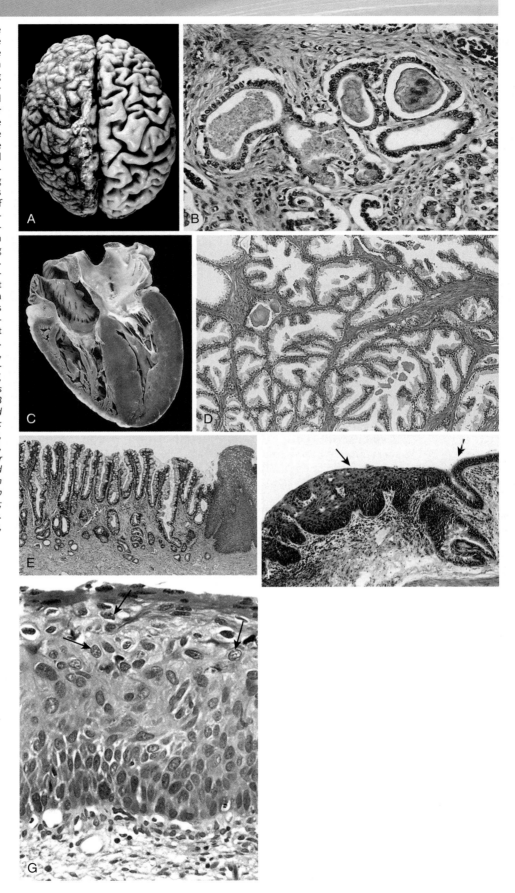

(3) Smooth muscle hypertrophy in the urinary bladder in response to urethral obstruction (e.g., prostate hyperplasia)

(4) Surgical removal of one kidney with compensatory hypertrophy (and hyperplasia) of the other kidney

  b. Cell enlargement in cytomegalovirus infections (see Fig. 16-10B)

3. Mechanisms of cardiac muscle hypertrophy

  a. Induction of genes for synthesis of growth factors, nuclear transcription, and contractile proteins

  b. Increase in cytosol, number of cytoplasmic organelles, and DNA content

C. Hyperplasia

1. Increase in the number of normal cells

2. Causes of hyperplasia

  a. Hormone stimulation

  (1) Acromegaly due to an increase in growth hormone and insulin growth factor-1 (see Fig. 22-3)

  (2) Endometrial gland hyperplasia due to hyperestrinism (see Fig. 21-20)
    • Increased risk for developing dysplasia (see later)

  (3) Benign prostatic hyperplasia due to an increase in dihydrotestosterone (Fig. 1-10D)

  (4) Gynecomastia (male breast tissue) due to increased estrogen (see Fig. 18-9)

  (5) Polycythemia due to an increase in erythropoietin

  b. Chronic irritation

  (1) Thickened epidermis from constant scratching

  (2) Bronchial mucous gland hyperplasia in smokers and asthmatics

  (3) Cirrhosis of the liver due to alcohol excess (see Fig. 18-18)

  c. Chemical imbalance

  (1) Hypocalcemia stimulates parathyroid gland hyperplasia

  (2) Iodine deficiency produces thyroid enlargement (goiter; see Fig. 22-12)
    • Combination of hypertrophy and hyperplasia

  d. Stimulating antibodies
    • Example—Graves' disease due to thyroid-stimulating antibodies (IgG) directed against thyroid-stimulating hormone receptors (see Fig. 22-9)

  e. Viral infections
    • Example—epidermal hyperplasia (wart) due to human papillomavirus

3. Mechanisms of hyperplasia

  a. Dependent on the regenerative capacity of different types of cells

  b. Labile cells (stem cells)

  (1) Divide continuously

  (2) Examples—stem cells in the bone marrow, stem cells in the crypts of Lieberkühn, and basal cells in the epidermis

  (3) May undergo hyperplasia as an adaptation to cell injury

  c. Stable cells (resting cells)

  (1) Divide infrequently, because they are normally in the G_0 (resting) phase

  (2) Must be stimulated (e.g., growth factors, hormones) to enter the cell cycle

  (3) Examples—hepatocytes, astrocytes, smooth muscle cells

  (4) May undergo hyperplasia or hypertrophy as an adaptation to cell injury

  d. Permanent cells (nonreplicating cells)

  (1) Highly specialized cells that cannot replicate

  (2) Examples—neurons and skeletal and cardiac muscle cells

  (3) May undergo hypertrophy (only muscle)

4. Increased risk for progressing into dysplasia and cancer, in some cases (see later)
    • Example–endometrial hyperplasia

D. Metaplasia

1. Replacement of one fully differentiated cell type by another
    • Substituted cells are less sensitive to a particular stress.

2. Types of metaplasia

  a. Metaplasia from squamous to glandular epithelium

  (1) Example—distal esophagus epithelium shows an increase in goblet cells and mucus-secreting cells in response to acid reflux (Fig. 1-10E)

  (2) This is called Barrett's esophagus.
    • Increased risk for developing dysplasia (see later)

  b. Metaplasia from glandular to other types of glandular epithelium

  (1) Example—pylorus and antrum epithelium shows an increase in goblet cells and Paneth cells in response to *Helicobacter pylori*–induced chronic atrophic gastritis

Hyperplasia: ↑ number of cells

Labile/stable cells: can divide

Permanent cells: cannot divide

Metaplasia: one cell type replaces another

Barrett's esophagus: glandular metaplasia, gastric reflux

(2) This is called intestinal metaplasia (see Fig. 17-14).
  • Increased risk for developing dysplasia (see later)

c. Metaplasia from glandular to squamous epithelium
  (1) Mainstem bronchus epithelium develops squamous metaplasia in response to irritants in cigarette smoke (Fig. 1-10F).
  (2) Endocervical epithelium develops squamous metaplasia in response to the acid pH in the vagina.
  (3) Both of the above alterations have an increased risk for developing dysplasia (see later).
d. Metaplasia from transitional to squamous epithelium
  (1) *Schistosoma hematobium* infection in the urinary bladder causes transitional epithelium to undergo squamous metaplasia.
  (2) Increased risk for developing dysplasia (see later)
3. Mechanism of metaplasia
  a. Stem cells have an array of progeny cells that have different patterns of gene expression.
    • Under normal physiologic conditions differentiation of these progeny cells is restricted.
  b. Metaplasia may result from reprogramming stem cells to utilize progeny cells with a different pattern of gene expression; the following signals may initiate this change:
    (1) Hormones (e.g., estrogen)
    (2) Vitamins (e.g., retinoic acid)
    (3) Chemical irritants (e.g., cigarette smoke)
  c. Metaplasia is sometimes reversible if the irritant is removed.

E. Dysplasia
  1. Disordered cell growth
    • Precursor to cancer

  2. Risk factors for dysplasia
    a. Some types of hyperplasia (see section V)
    b. Some types of metaplasia (see section V)
    c. Infection
      • Example—human papillomavirus type 16, causing squamous dysplasia of the cervix
    d. Chemicals
      • Example—irritants in cigarette smoke, causing squamous metaplasia to progress to squamous dysplasia in the mainstem bronchus
    e. Ultraviolet light
      • Example—solar damage of the skin, causing squamous dysplasia
    f. Chronic irritation of skin
      • Example—draining sinus tracts in osteomyelitis

  3. Microscopic features of dysplasia (Fig. 1-10G)
    a. Nuclear features
      (1) Increased mitotic activity, with normal mitotic spindles
      (2) Increased nuclear size and chromatin
    b. Disorderly proliferation of cells with loss of cell maturation as cells progress to the surface
  4. Dysplasia is sometimes reversible if the irritant is removed.

VI. Cell Death
  • Cell death occurs when cells or tissues are unable to adapt to injury.
  A. Necrosis
    1. Death of groups of cells, often accompanied by an inflammatory infiltrate
    2. Coagulation necrosis

      a. Preservation of the structural outline of dead cells
      b. Mechanism of coagulation necrosis
        (1) Denaturation of enzymes and structural proteins
          (a) Intracellular accumulation of lactate or heavy metals (e.g., lead, mercury)
          (b) Exposure of cells to ionizing radiation
        (2) Inactivation of intracellular enzymes prevents dissolution (autolysis) of the cell.
      c. Microscopic features (Fig. 1-11A)
        (1) Indistinct outlines of cells within dead tissue
        (2) Absent nuclei or karyolysis (fading of nuclear chromatin)
      d. Infarction

        (1) Gross manifestation of coagulation necrosis secondary to the sudden occlusion of a vessel

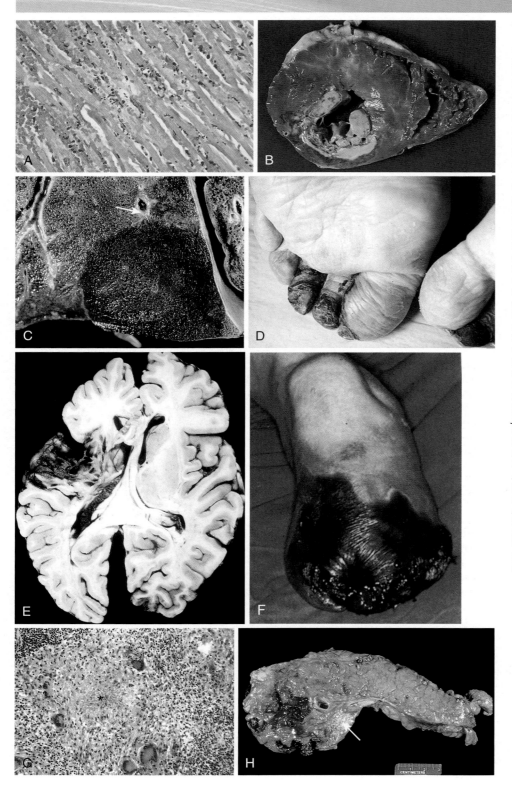

1-11: A, Acute myocardial infarction (MI) showing coagulation necrosis. This section of myocardial tissue is from a 3-day-old acute MI. The outlines of the myocardial fibers are intact; however, they lack nuclei and cross-striations. A neutrophilic infiltrate is present between some of the dead fibers. **B,** Acute MI showing a pale infarction of the posterior wall of the left ventricle (bottom left). **C,** Hemorrhagic infarction of lung. There is a roughly wedge-shaped area of hemorrhage extending to the pleural surface. The arrow shows an embolus in one of the pulmonary artery tributaries. **D,** Dry gangrene involves the first four toes. The dark black areas of gangrene are bordered by light-colored, parchment-like skin. **E,** Cerebral infarction showing liquefactive necrosis of the cerebral cortex leaving a large cystic cavity. **F,** Wet gangrene of the leg. Note the pus at the closing edges of the below-the-knee amputation site. **G,** Caseous granuloma showing a central area of acellular, necrotic material (*asterisk*) surrounded by activated macrophages (epithelioid cells), lymphocytes, and multiple multinucleated Langhans-type giant cells. **H,** Enzymatic fat necrosis in acute pancreatitis. Dark areas of hemorrhage are present in the head of the pancreas (left side), and focal areas of pale fat necrosis (*arrow*) are present in the peripancreatic fat. (*A from Damjanov I, Linder J: Pathology: A Color Atlas. St. Louis, Mosby, 2000, p 375, Fig. 17-15; B from Damjanov I, Linder J: Anderson's Pathology, 10th ed. St. Louis, Mosby, 1996, p 374, Fig. 17-13; C, E, G, and H from Kumar V, Fausto N, Abbas A: Robbins and Cotran's Pathologic Basis of Disease, 7th ed. Philadelphia, WB Saunders, 2004, pp 138, 1365, 83, 943, Figs. 4-19A, 28-16, 2-33, 19-5, respectively; D from Damjanov I: Pathology for the Health-Related Professions, 2nd ed. Philadelphia, WB Saunders, 2000, p 18, Fig. 1-24; F from Grieg JD: Color Atlas of Surgical Diagnosis. London, Mosby-Wolfe, 1996, p 6, Fig. 2-2.*)

(2) Usually wedge-shaped if dichotomously branching vessels (e.g., pulmonary artery) are occluded
(3) Pale (ischemic) type
  • Increased density of tissue (e.g., heart, kidney, spleen) prevents RBCs from diffusing through necrotic tissue (Fig. 1-11B).

(4) Hemorrhagic (red) type
  - Loose-textured tissue (e.g., lungs, small bowel) allows RBCs to diffuse through necrotic tissue (Fig. 1-11C).

Dry gangrene:
predominantly
coagulation necrosis

> **Dry gangrene** of the toes in individuals with diabetes mellitus is a form of infarction that results from ischemia. Coagulation necrosis is the primary type of necrosis that is present in the dead tissue (Fig. 1-11D).

  e. Factors influencing whether an infarction will occur in tissue
    (1) Size of the vessel that is occluded
      (a) Infarction is unlikely with obstruction of a major branch of a pulmonary artery.
      (b) Infarction is likely if a thrombus overlies an atherosclerotic plaque in a coronary artery.
    (2) State of development of a collateral circulation
      - Infarction is *less* likely if a well-developed collateral circulation is present (e.g., arcade system of the superior and inferior mesenteric arteries).
    (3) Presence of a dual blood supply
      (a) Infarction is *less* likely if a dual blood supply is present (e.g., pulmonary and bronchial arteries in the lungs).
      (b) Renal and splenic arteries have end-arteries with an inadequate network of anastomosing vessels beyond potential points of obstruction; hence, infarction is likely to occur.

Infarction less likely: dual
blood supply, collateral
circulation

    (4) Sudden onset of ischemia in an organ with preexisting disease will more likely produce an infarction.
      - Example—a pulmonary embolus will more likely produce an infarction in a patient with preexisting chronic lung or heart disease.
    (5) Tissues with a high O_2 requirement (e.g., brain, heart) are more likely to infarct than other less sensitive tissues (e.g., muscle, cartilage).
    (6) Rapidity with which a vessel is occluded often determines whether an infarction will occur.
      (a) Slow occlusion often allows time for development of a collateral circulation.
      (b) Abrupt occlusion often results in infarction.
3. Liquefactive necrosis
  a. Necrotic degradation of tissue that softens and becomes liquefied
  b. Mechanisms
    - Lysosomal enzymes released by necrotic cells or neutrophils cause liquefaction of tissue.
  c. Examples

Cerebral infarction:
liquefactive *not*
coagulative necrosis

    (1) Central nervous system infarction
      Autocatalytic effect of hydrolytic enzymes generated by neuroglial cells produces a cystic space (Fig. 1-11E).
    (2) Abscess in a bacterial infection
      - Hydrolytic enzymes generated by neutrophils liquefy dead tissue.

Wet gangrene:
predominantly
liquefactive necrosis

> Dry gangrene of the toes with a superimposed anaerobic infection (e.g., *Clostridium perfringens*) leads to acute inflammation, where liquefactive necrosis is the primary type of necrosis. This condition is called wet gangrene (Fig. 1-11F).

4. Caseous necrosis
  a. Variant of coagulation necrosis
    - Associated with acellular, cheese-like (caseous) material
  b. Mechanism
    (1) Caseous material is formed by the release of lipid from the cell walls of *Mycobacterium tuberculosis* and systemic fungi (e.g., *Histoplasma*) after immune destruction by macrophages.
    (2) Other diseases associated with granuloma formation do *not* exhibit caseation.
      - Examples—Crohn disease, sarcoidosis, foreign body giant cell reaction
  c. Microscopic features of a granuloma

Tuberculosis: most
common cause of caseous
necrosis

    - Acellular material in the center surrounded by activated macrophages, CD4 helper T cells, and multinucleated giant cells (Fig. 1-11G)

5. Enzymatic fat necrosis
   a. Peculiar to adipose tissue located around an acutely inflamed pancreas
   b. Mechanisms
      (1) Activation of pancreatic lipase (e.g., alcohol excess) causing hydrolysis of triglyceride in fat cells with release of fatty acids
      (2) Conversion of fatty acids into soap (saponification)
         • Combination of fatty acids and calcium
   c. Gross appearance
      • Chalky yellow-white deposits are primarily located in peripancreatic and omental adipose tissue (Fig. 1-11H).
   d. Microscopic appearance
      • Pale outlines of fat cells filled with basophilic-staining calcified areas
6. Traumatic fat necrosis
   a. Occurs in fatty tissue (e.g., female breast tissue) as a result of trauma
   b. *Not* enzyme-mediated
7. Fibrinoid necrosis
   a. Limited to small muscular arteries, arterioles, venules, and glomerular capillaries
   b. Mechanism
      • Deposition of pink-staining proteinaceous material in damaged vessel walls due to damaged basement membranes
   c. Associated conditions
      • Immune vasculitis (e.g., Henoch-Schönlein purpura), malignant hypertension

B. Apoptosis
1. Programmed, enzyme-mediated cell death
2. Normal and pathologic processes associated with apoptosis
   a. Destruction of cells during embryogenesis
      • Example—loss of müllerian structures in a male fetus due to Sertoli cell synthesis of müllerian inhibitory factor
   b. Hormone-dependent atrophy of tissue
      • Example—endometrial cell breakdown after withdrawal of estrogen and progesterone in the menstrual cycle
   c. Death of tumor cells and virus infected cells by cytotoxic CD8 T cells
   d. Corticosteroid destruction of lymphocytes (B and T cells)
   e. Removal of acute inflammatory cells (e.g., neutrophils) from healing sites
   f. Damage to DNA by radiation, FRs, toxins
   g. Removal of misfolded proteins
      • Examples—amyloid, β-amyloid protein, proteins in prion-related disease (Creutzfeldt-Jakob disease)
3. Mechanisms of apoptosis
   a. Extrinsic pathway
      (1) Binding of tumor necrosis factor (TNF) to its receptor
      (2) Eventual activation of caspases (see later)
   b. Intrinsic pathway
      (1) Mitochondrial leakage of cytochrome *c* into the cytosol
      (2) Eventual activation of caspases (see later)
   c. Genes regulating apoptosis via the intrinsic pathway
      (1) *BCL2* gene family
         • Located on chromosome 18
            (a) Manufactures gene products that inhibit apoptosis (i.e., antiapoptosis gene)
            (b) Gene products prevent mitochondrial leakage of cytochrome *c* into the cytosol.
      (2) *TP53* suppressor gene
            (a) Temporarily arrests the cell cycle in the G_1 phase to repair DNA damage (aborts apoptosis)
            (b) Promotes apoptosis if DNA damage is too great by activating the *BAX* apoptosis gene
               • *BAX* gene products inactivate the *BCL2* antiapoptosis gene.
   d. Caspases
      (1) Group of inactive proenzymes (proteases, endonucleases)
         • Must be activated by the extrinsic or intrinsic system to produce apoptosis
      (2) Changes in the cell

Enzymatic fat necrosis: acute pancreatitis

Traumatic fat necrosis: not enzyme-mediated

Fibrinoid necrosis: necrosis of immune-mediated disease

Apoptosis: programmed cell death

Extrinsic pathway of apoptosis: requires TNF

BCL2 gene: antiapoptosis gene

TP53 suppressor gene: "guardian" of the cell

BAX gene: apoptosis gene

Caspases: group of cysteine proteases; activation induces apoptosis

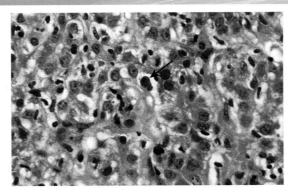

1-12: Apoptosis in viral hepatitis. The arrow shows a shrunken eosinophilic staining cell with pyknotic nucleus within a clear space. *(From Damjanov I: Pathophysiology. Philadelphia, Saunders Elsevier, 2009, p 301, Fig. 8.22.)*

(3) Activation of endonuclease leads to nuclear pyknosis ("ink dot" appearance) and fragmentation.
(4) Activation of protease leads to breakdown of the cytoskeleton.
(5) Formation of cytoplasmic buds on the cell membrane
  • Buds contain nuclear fragments, mitochondria, and condensed protein fragments.
(6) Formation of apoptotic bodies by the breaking off of cytoplasmic buds
(7) Phagocytosis of apoptotic bodies by neighboring cells or macrophages
4. Microscopic appearance of apoptosis
  a. Cell detachment from neighboring cells
  b. Deeply eosinophilic-staining cytoplasm (Fig. 1-12)
  c. Pyknotic, fragmented, or absent nucleus
  d. Minimal or no inflammatory infiltrate surrounding the cell
C. **Enzyme markers of cell death** (Box 1-1)

> Apoptosis: deeply eosinophilic cytoplasm; pyknotic nucleus

BOX 1-1   CLINICAL ENZYMOLOGY

Enzymes are protein catalysts of biologic origin that increase the rate of chemical reactions without themselves being consumed or structurally altered. **Isoenzymes** (isozymes) are multiple forms of the same enzyme that differ in stereotypical, biochemical, and immunologic properties (e.g., lactate dehydrogenase isoenzymes L_1–L_5; creatine kinase isoenzymes MM, MB, and BB). Measurement of individual isoenzymes is frequently more specific in identifying a disease than is total enzyme activity (e.g., CK-MB isoenzyme in identifying an acute myocardial infarction). **Isoforms** are subtypes of the individual isoenzymes (e.g., CK-MM isoforms).

Enzymes distribute in cell membranes (e.g., alkaline phosphatase), endoplasmic reticulum (e.g., γ-glutamyltransferase), lysosomes (e.g., muramidase), zymogen (e.g., amylase), cytoplasm (e.g., alanine aminotransferase, a transaminase), and mitochondria (e.g., aspartate aminotransferase, a transaminase).

Factors influencing the release of enzymes into body fluids include disruption or damage to the cell membrane (e.g., alanine aminotransferase, CK), increased synthesis owing to regeneration of injured cells (e.g., alkaline phosphatase), and enzyme induction in the smooth endoplasmic reticulum by drugs (e.g., alcohol and its effect on increasing γ-glutamyltransferase synthesis).

The amount of enzyme released into body fluids depends on the amount of tissue injury, the rate of diffusion out of the damaged cell, and the overall rate of catabolism or clearance of the enzyme. The following table lists important enzymes that are increased in tissue injury.

Enzyme	Diagnostic Use
Aspartate aminotransferase (AST)	Marker of diffuse liver cell necrosis (e.g., viral hepatitis)
	Mitochondrial enzyme preferentially increased in alcohol-induced liver disease
Alanine aminotransferase	Marker of diffuse liver cell necrosis (e.g., viral hepatitis)
	More specific for liver cell necrosis than AST
Creatine kinase MB	Isoenzyme increased in acute myocardial infarction or myocarditis
Amylase and lipase	Marker enzymes for acute pancreatitis
	Lipase more specific than amylase for pancreatitis
	Amylase also increased in salivary gland inflammation (e.g., mumps)

I. **Acute Inflammation (AI)**
   A. **Definition**
      1. Transient and early response to injury
      2. Involves release of chemical mediators
      3. Leads to stereotypic vessel and leukocyte responses
      4. *Not* a synonym for infection
   B. **Cardinal signs of inflammation** (Fig. 2-1)
      1. Rubor (redness) and calor (heat)
         • Histamine-mediated vasodilation of arterioles
      2. Tumor (swelling)
         a. Histamine-mediated increase in permeability of venules
         b. Synonymous with edema
            • Increased fluid in the interstitial space
      3. Dolor (pain)
         • Prostaglandin (PG) E_2 sensitizes specialized nerve endings to the effects of bradykinin and other pain mediators.
      4. Functio laesa (loss of function)
   C. **Stimuli for acute inflammation**
      1. Infections (e.g., bacterial or viral infection)
      2. Immune reactions (e.g., reaction to a bee sting)
      3. Other stimuli
         • Tissue necrosis (e.g., acute myocardial infarction), trauma, radiation, burns, foreign body (e.g., glass, splinter)
   D. **Sequential vascular events**
      1. Vasoconstriction of arterioles
         • Neurogenic reflex that lasts only seconds
      2. Vasodilation of arterioles
         a. Histamine and other vasodilators (e.g., nitric oxide) relax vascular smooth muscle, causing increased blood flow.
         b. Increased blood flow increases hydrostatic pressure.
      3. Increased permeability of venules
         a. Histamine and other mediators contract endothelial cells producing endothelial gaps.
            • Tight junctions are simpler in venules than arterioles.
         b. A transudate (protein and cell-poor fluid) moves into the interstitial tissue.
      4. Swelling of tissue (tumor, edema)
         • Net outflow of fluid surpasses lymphatic ability to remove fluid.
      5. Reduced blood flow
         • Decrease in hydrostatic pressure caused by outflow of fluid into the interstitial tissue
   E. **Sequential cellular events** (Fig. 2-2)
      • The events described will emphasize neutrophil events in acute inflammation due to a bacterial infection (e.g., *Staphylococcus aureus*).
      1. Neutrophils are the primary leukocytes in acute inflammation (Fig. 2-3).
      2. Margination
         a. RBCs aggregate into rouleaux ("stacks of coins") in venules.
         b. Neutrophils are pushed from the central axial column to the periphery (margination).

AI: chemical, vascular, cellular responses

AI: not synonymous with infection

Rubor, calor, tumor: histamine-mediated

Mast cells: release preformed histamine

Neutrophils: primary leukocytes in acute inflammation

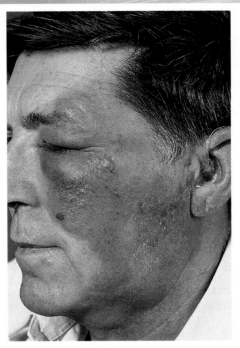

2-1: Signs of acute inflammation. The patient has erysipelas of the face due to group A streptococcus. Signs of acute inflammation that are present in the photograph include redness (rubor) and swelling (tumor). The infection is associated with warm skin (calor) and pain (dolor). *(From Forbes C, Jackson W: Color Atlas and Text of Clinical Medicine, 2nd ed. St. Louis, Mosby, 2003, p 37, Fig. 1-106.)*

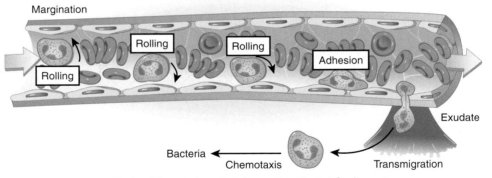

2-2: Neutrophil events in acute inflammation. See text for discussion.

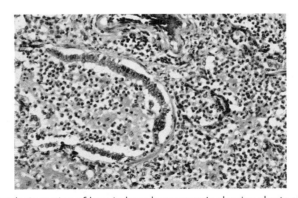

2-3: Acute inflammation. Histologic section of lung in bronchopneumonia showing sheets of neutrophils with multilobed nuclei. *(From Damjanov I: Pathology for the Health-Related Professions, 2nd ed. Philadelphia, WB Saunders, 2000, p 182, Fig. 8-8.)*

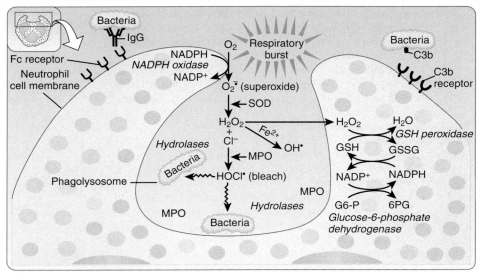

2-4: Oxygen-dependent myeloperoxidase system. A series of biochemical reactions occurs in the phagolysosome, resulting in the production of hypochlorous free radicals (bleach; HOCl·) that destroy bacteria. Fe^{2+}, reduced iron; GSH, reduced glutathione; G6-P, glucose 6-phosphate; GSSG, oxidized glutathione; H_2O_2, peroxide; MPO, myeloperoxidase; NADP, oxidized form of nicotinamide adenine dinucleotide phosphate; NADPH, reduced nicotinamide adenine dinucleotide phosphate; OH·, hydroxyl free radical; 6PG, 6-phosphogluconate; SOD, superoxide dismutase.

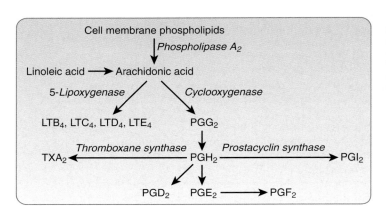

2-5: Arachidonic acid metabolism. Arachidonic acid is released from membrane phospholipids. It is converted into prostaglandins (PGs), thromboxane A_2 (TXA_2), and leukotrienes (LTs). See text for further discussion.

3. Rolling
   a. Due to activation of selectin adhesion molecules on the surface of neutrophils and endothelial cells
   b. Neutrophils loosely bind to selectins and "roll" along the endothelium.
4. Adhesion
   a. Adhesion molecules firmly bind neutrophils to endothelial cells.
      (1) Neutrophils in the peripheral blood are subdivided into a circulating pool and a marginating pool (already attached to endothelial cells).
      (2) Normally, ~50% of peripheral blood neutrophils are in the circulating pool and ~50% in the marginating pool.
      (3) This distribution can be altered by activating or inactivating neutrophil adhesion molecules (see later).
   b. Neutrophil adhesion molecules
      (1) β_2-Integrins (CD11a:CD18)
      (2) Adhesion molecule activation is mediated by C5a and leukotriene B_4 (LTB_4).
      (3) Catecholamines, corticosteroids, and lithium inhibit activation of adhesion molecules.
         (a) Peripheral blood neutrophil count (neutrophilic leukocytosis) is increased.
         (b) Normal marginating pool is now part of the circulating pool.

Selectins: responsible for "rolling" of neutrophils

β_2-Integrins: neutrophil adhesion molecules

Neutrophil leukocytosis: catecholamines, corticosteroids, lithium

(4) Endotoxins enhance activation of adhesion molecules.

    (a) Peripheral blood neutrophil count (neutropenia) is decreased.

    (b) Normal circulating pool is now part of the marginating pool.

  c. Endothelial cell adhesion molecules

    (1) Intercellular adhesion molecule (ICAM) and vascular cell adhesion molecule (VCAM) bind to integrins on the surface of neutrophils.

    (2) ICAM and VCAM activation is mediated by interleukin 1 (IL-1) and tumor necrosis factor (TNF).

  d. Leukocyte adhesion deficiency (LAD)

    (1) Autosomal recessive disorders

    (2) LAD type 1 is a deficiency of CD11a:CD18.

    (3) LAD type 2 is a deficiency of a selectin that binds neutrophils.

    (4) Clinical findings

      (a) Delayed separation of the umbilical cord (~1 month)

        • Neutrophil enzymes are important in cord separation.

      (b) Severe gingivitis, poor wound healing, peripheral blood neutrophilic leukocytosis (loss of marginating pool)

5. Transmigration (diapedesis)

  a. Neutrophils dissolve the basement membrane and enter interstitial tissue.

  b. Fluid rich in proteins and cells (i.e., exudate) accumulates in interstitial tissue.

  c. Functions of exudate

    (1) Dilutes bacterial toxins

    (2) Provides opsonins (IgG, C3b) to assist in phagocytosis

6. Chemotaxis

  a. Neutrophils follow chemical gradients that lead to the infection site.

  b. Chemotactic mediators bind to neutrophil receptors.

    • Mediators include C5a, LTB_4, bacterial products, and interleukin (IL) 8.

  c. Binding causes the release of calcium, which increases neutrophil motility.

7. Phagocytosis

  a. Multistep process, consisting of three steps

    (1) Opsonization

    (2) Ingestion

    (3) Killing

  b. Opsonization

    (1) Opsonins attach to bacteria (or foreign bodies).

      (a) Opsonins include IgG, C3b fragment of complement, and other proteins (e.g., C-reactive protein).

      (b) Neutrophils have membrane receptors for IgG and C3b.

    (2) Opsonization enhances neutrophil recognition and attachment to bacteria.

    (3) Bruton's agammaglobulinemia is an opsonization defect.

  c. Ingestion

    (1) Neutrophils engulf (phagocytose) and then trap bacteria in phagocytic vacuoles.

    (2) Primary lysosomes empty hydrolytic enzymes into phagocytic vacuoles producing phagolysosomes.

    • In Chédiak-Higashi syndrome (refer to Chapter 1), a defect in microtubule function prevents phagolysosome formation.

  d. Bacterial killing

    (1) O_2-dependent myeloperoxidase (MPO) system (Fig. 2-4)

      (a) Only present in neutrophils and monocytes (*not* macrophages)

      (b) Production of superoxide free radicals ($O_2^{\bullet}$)

        • Reduced nicotinamide adenine dinucleotide phosphate (NADPH) oxidase converts molecular O_2 to $O_2^{\bullet}$, which releases energy called the respiratory, or oxidative, burst.

      (c) Production of peroxide (H_2O_2)

        • Superoxide dismutase converts $O_2^{\bullet}$ to H_2O_2, which is neutralized by glutathione peroxidase.

      (d) Some peroxide is converted to hydroxyl free radicals by iron.

      (e) Production of bleach ($HOCl^{\bullet}$)

        • MPO combines H_2O_2 with chloride (Cl^-) to form hypochlorous free radicals ($HOCl^{\bullet}$), which kill bacteria.

      (f) Chronic granulomatous disease and MPO deficiency are examples of diseases that have a defect in the O_2-dependent MPO system.

Chronic granulomatous disease (CGD) is an X-linked recessive (XR) disorder (65% of cases) or autosomal recessive disorder (35% of cases). The X-linked type is characterized by deficient NADPH oxidase in the cell membranes of neutrophils and monocytes. The reduced production of $O_2^{\cdot}$ results in an absent respiratory burst. Catalase-positive organisms that produce H_2O_2 (e.g., *Staphylococcus aureus*) are ingested but *not* killed, because the catalase degrades H_2O_2. Myeloperoxidase is present, but HOCl· is *not* synthesized because of the absence of H_2O_2. Catalase-negative organisms (e.g., *Streptococcus* species) are ingested and killed when myeloperoxidase combines H_2O_2 with Cl to form HOCl·. Granulomatous inflammation occurs in tissue, because the neutrophils, which can phagocytose bacteria but not kill most of them, are eventually replaced by cells associated with chronic inflammation, mainly lymphocytes and macrophages. Macrophages fuse together to form multinucleated giant cells. Patients have severe infections involving lungs, skin, visceral organs, and bones. The classic screening test for CGD is the nitroblue tetrazolium (NBT) test. In this test, leukocytes are incubated with a colorless NBT dye, which is converted to a blue color if the respiratory burst is intact. This test has been replaced by a more sensitive test involving oxidation of dihydrorhodamine to fluorescent rhodamine. Bone marrow transplantation is the treatment of choice for the XR type of CGD.

Myeloperoxidase (MPO) deficiency, an autosomal recessive disorder, differs from CGD in that both $O_2^{\cdot}$ and H_2O_2 are produced (normal respiratory burst). However, the absence of MPO prevents synthesis of HOCl·.

(g) Deficiency of NADPH (e.g., glucose-6-phosphate dehydrogenase deficiency) produces a microbicidal defect.

> MPO deficiency: normal respiratory burst

(2) O_2-independent system
  (a) Refers to bacterial killing from substances located in leukocyte granules
  (b) Examples—lactoferrin (binds iron necessary for bacterial reproduction) and major basic protein (eosinophil product that is cytotoxic to helminths)

F. Chemical mediators (Table 2-1)
  1. They derive from plasma, leukocytes, local tissue, bacterial products.
   • Example—arachidonic acid mediators are released from membrane phospholipids in macrophages, endothelial cells, and platelets (Fig. 2-5).
  2. They have short half-lives (e.g., seconds to minutes).
  3. They may have local and systemic effects.
   • Example—histamine may produce local signs of itching or systemic signs of anaphylaxis.
  4. They have diverse functions.
   a. Vasodilation
    • Examples—histamine, nitric oxide, PGI_2
   b. Vasoconstriction
    • Example—thromboxane A_2 (TXA_2)
   c. Increase vessel permeability
    • Examples—histamine, bradykinin, LTC_4-D_4-E_4, C3a and C5a (anaphylatoxins)
   d. Produce pain
    • Examples—PGE_2, bradykinin
   e. Produce fever
    • Examples—PGE_2, IL-1, TNF
   f. Chemotactic
    • Examples—C5a, LTB_4, IL-8

> Histamine: most important chemical mediator of acute inflammation

> Chemical mediators: short half-lives

G. Types of acute inflammation
  • Location, cause, and duration of inflammation determine the morphology of an inflammatory reaction.
  1. Purulent (suppurative) inflammation
   a. Localized proliferation of pus-forming organisms, such as *Staphylococcus aureus* (e.g., skin abscess; Fig. 2-6)
   b. *S. aureus* contains coagulase, which cleaves fibrinogen into fibrin and traps bacteria and neutrophils.
  2. Fibrinous inflammation
   a. Due to increased vessel permeability, with deposition of a fibrin-rich exudate
   b. Often occurs on the serosal lining of the pericardium, peritoneum, or pleura
    • Danger of adhesions
   c. Example—fibrinous pericarditis (Fig. 2-7)

> *S. aureus*: most common cause of a skin abscess

TABLE 2-1. **SOURCES AND FUNCTIONS OF CHEMICAL MEDIATORS**

MEDIATOR	SOURCE(S)	FUNCTION(S)
Arachidonic acid metabolites		
Prostaglandins	Macrophages, endothelial cells, platelets PGH_2: major precursor of PGs and thromboxanes	PGE_2: vasodilation, pain, fever PGI_2: vasodilation; inhibition of platelet aggregation
Thromboxane A_2	Platelets Converted from PGH_2 by thromboxane synthase	Vasoconstriction, platelet aggregation
Leukotrienes (LTs)	Leukocytes Converted from arachidonic acid by lipoxygenase-mediated hydroxylation	LTB_4: chemotaxis and activation of neutrophil adhesion molecules LTC_4, LTD_4, LTE_4: vasoconstriction, increased venular permeability, bronchoconstriction Zileuton inhibits 5-lipoxygenase: $\downarrow$ synthesis LTB_4, LTC_4, LTD_4, LTE_4 Montelukast leukotriene receptor antagonist: $\downarrow$ synthesis LTC_4, LTD_4, LTE_4
Bradykinin	Product of kinin system activation by activated factor XII	Vasodilation, increased venular permeability, pain
Chemokines	Leukocytes, endothelial cells	Activate neutrophil chemotaxis
Complement	Synthesized in liver (acute phase reactant)	C3a, C5a (anaphylatoxins): stimulate mast cell release of histamine C3b: opsonization C5a: activation of neutrophil adhesion molecules, chemotaxis C5–C9 (membrane attack complex): cell lysis
Cytokines		
IL-1, TNF	Macrophages (main source), monocytes, dendritic cells, endothelial cells	Initiate PGE_2 synthesis in anterior hypothalamus, leading to production of fever Activate endothelial cell adhesion molecules Increase liver synthesis of acute-phase reactants, such as ferritin, coagulation factors (e.g., fibrinogen), and C-reactive protein Increase release of neutrophils from bone marrow (neutrophil leukocytosis) TNF is a promoter of apoptosis (refer to Chapter 1)
IL-6		Increase liver synthesis of acute phase reactants
IL-8		Chemotaxis
Histamine	Mast cells (primary cell), platelets, enterochromaffin cells	Vasodilation, increased venular permeability
Nitric oxide (NO)	Macrophages, endothelial cells Free radical gas released during conversion of arginine to citrulline by NO synthase	Vasodilation, bactericidal
Serotonin	Platelets	Vasodilation, increased venular permeability, increases collagen synthesis

IL, interleukin; PG, prostaglandin; TNF, tumor necrosis factor.

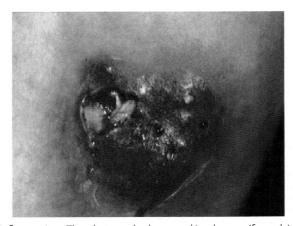

2-6: Purulent (suppurative) inflammation. The photograph shows a skin abscess (furuncle) due to *Staphylococcus aureus.* Abscesses are pus-filled nodules located in the dermis. Note the multiple draining sinus tracts filled with pus. *(From Bouloux P: Self-Assessment Picture Tests: Medicine, Vol. 1. London, Mosby-Wolfe, 1997, p 33, Fig. 66.)*

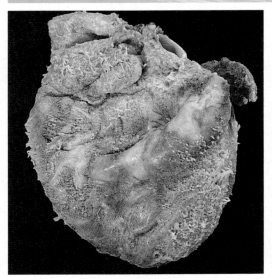

2-7: Fibrinous inflammation. The surface of the heart is covered by a shaggy, fibrinous exudate. *(From Damjanov I, Linder J: Pathology: A Color Atlas. St. Louis, Mosby, 2000, p 25, Fig. 1-59.)*

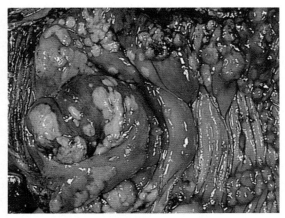

2-8: Pseudomembranous inflammation. There is necrosis and a yellow exudate covering the mucosal surface of the colon due to a toxin produced by *Clostridium difficile*. *(From Grieg JD: Color Atlas of Surgical Diagnosis. London, Mosby-Wolfe, 1996, p 202, Fig. 26-10.)*

3. Serous inflammation
   a. Thin, watery exudate
      • Insufficient amount of fibrinogen to produce fibrin
   b. Examples–blister in second-degree burns, viral pleuritis
4. Pseudomembranous inflammation
   a. Bacterial toxin-induced damage of the mucosal lining, producing a shaggy membrane composed of necrotic tissue
   b. Example—pseudomembranes associated with *Clostridium difficile* in pseudomembranous colitis (Fig. 2-8)
      • *Corynebacterium diphtheriae* produces a toxin causing pseudomembrane formation in the pharynx and trachea.

> Pseudomembranous inflammation: diphtheria, *Clostridium difficile*; noninvasive bacteria

H. **Role of fever in inflammation**
   1. Right-shifts oxygen-binding curve
      • More O_2 is available for the O_2-dependent MPO system.
   2. Provides a hostile environment for bacterial and viral reproduction

> Fever is good!

I. **Factors involved in the termination of acute inflammation**
   1. Short half-life of inflammatory mediators
   2. Lipoxins
      a. Anti-inflammatory mediators
      b. Derive from arachidonic acid metabolites (e.g., LXA_4, LXB_4)
      c. Inhibit transmigration and chemotaxis
      d. Signal macrophages to phagocytose apoptotic bodies
   3. Resolvins
      a. Synthesized from omega-3 fatty acids
      b. Inhibit production and recruitment of inflammatory cells to the site of inflammation
   4. Clearance of neutrophils by apoptosis

> Clearance of neutrophils in AI: apoptosis

J. **Consequences of acute inflammation**
   1. Complete resolution
      a. Occurs with mild injury to cells that have the capacity to enter the cell cycle (e.g., labile and stable cells)
      b. Examples—first-degree burn, bee sting
   2. Tissue destruction and scar formation
      a. Occurs with extensive injury or damage to permanent cells
      b. Example—third-degree burns
   3. Formation of abscesses
      • Example—lung abscess in bronchopneumonia
   4. Progression to chronic inflammation

II. Chronic Inflammation

A. Definition
- Inflammation of prolonged duration (weeks to years) that most often results from persistence of an injury-causing agent

B. Causes of chronic inflammation
1. Infection
   - Examples—tuberculosis, leprosy, hepatitis C
2. Autoimmune disease
   - Examples—rheumatoid arthritis, systemic lupus erythematosus
3. Sterile agents
   - Examples—silica, uric acid, silicone in breast implants

C. Morphology
1. Cell types
   - Monocytes and macrophages (key cells), lymphocytes and plasma cells, eosinophils (Fig. 2-9)
2. Necrosis
   - *Not* as prominent a feature as in acute inflammation
3. Destruction of parenchyma
   - Loss of functional tissue, with repair by fibrosis
4. Formation of granulation tissue
   a. Highly vascular tissue composed of blood vessels and activated fibroblasts
      (1) Blood vessels derive from preexisting blood vessels (i.e., angiogenesis)
      (2) Essential for normal wound healing
      (3) Precursor for scar tissue
   b. Fibronectin is required for granulation tissue formation.
      (1) Cell adhesion glycoprotein located in the extracellular matrix (ECM)
         - Binds to collagen, fibrin, and cell surface receptors (e.g., integrins)
      (2) Chemotactic factor that attracts fibroblasts (synthesize collagen) and endothelial cells (form new blood vessels, angiogenesis)
         - Vascular endothelial growth factor (VEGF) and basic fibroblast growth factor (FGF) are important in angiogenesis.
5. Comparison of acute and chronic inflammation (Table 2-2)
6. Granulomatous inflammation
   a. Specialized type of chronic inflammation
   b. Causes
      (1) Infections
         (a) Examples—tuberculosis and systemic fungal infection (e.g., histoplasmosis)
         (b) Usually associated with caseous necrosis (i.e., soft granulomas)
            - Caseation is due to lipid released from the cell wall of dead pathogens.

Marginal notes:

Infection: most common cause of chronic inflammation

Monocytes and macrophages: primary leukocytes in chronic inflammation

Granulation tissue: converted to scar tissue

Fibronectin: key adhesion glycoprotein in ECM

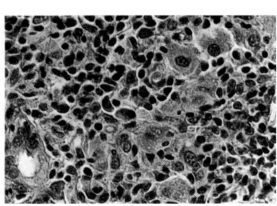

2-9: Chronic inflammation. This tissue shows an infiltrate of predominantly lymphocytes and plasma cells (cells with eccentric nucleus and perinuclear clearing). *(From Gitlin M, Strauss R: Atlas of Clinical Hepatology. Philadelphia, WB Saunders, 1995, p 59, Fig. 5-11.)*

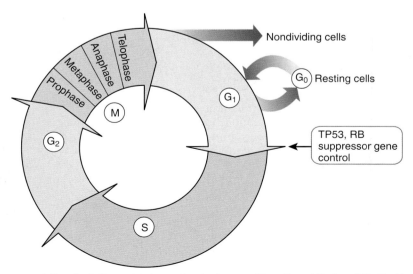

2-10: Cell cycle. Refer to the description in the text. *(From Burns ER, Cave MD: Rapid Review: Histology and Cell Biology. St. Louis, Mosby, 2004, p 36, Fig. 3-5.)*

TABLE 2-2. **COMPARISON OF ACUTE AND CHRONIC INFLAMMATION**

FEATURE	ACUTE INFLAMMATION	CHRONIC INFLAMMATION
Pathogenesis	Microbial pathogens, trauma, burns	Persistent acute inflammation, foreign bodies (e.g., silicone, glass), autoimmune disease, certain types of infection (e.g., tuberculosis, leprosy)
Primary cells involved	Neutrophils	Monocytes/macrophages (key cells), B and T lymphocytes, plasma cells, fibroblasts
Primary mediators	Histamine (key mediator), prostaglandins, leukotrienes	Cytokines (e.g., IL-1), growth factors
Necrosis	Present	Less prominent
Scar tissue	Absent	Present
Onset	Immediate	Delayed
Duration	Few days	Weeks, months, years
Outcome	Complete resolution, progression to chronic inflammation, abscess formation	Scar tissue formation, disability, amyloidosis (refer to Chapter 3)
Main immunoglobulin	IgM	IgG
Serum protein electrophoresis effect	Mild hypoalbuminemia	Polyclonal gammopathy; greater degree of hypoalbuminemia
Peripheral blood leukocyte response	Neutrophilic leukocytosis	Monocytosis

  (2) Noninfectious causes
   (a) Examples—sarcoidosis and Crohn's disease
   (b) Noncaseating (i.e., hard granulomas)
 c. Morphology
  (1) Pale, white nodule with or without central caseation
  (2) Usually well-circumscribed (see Fig. 1-11G)
  (3) Cell types
   (a) Epithelioid cells (activated macrophages), mononuclear (round cell) infiltrate (CD4 helper T cells, or T_H cells of the T_H1 type)
   (b) Multinucleated giant cells formed by fusion of epithelioid cells
    • Nuclei usually located at the periphery
  (4) TNF-α is important in the formation and maintenance of tuberculous and systemic fungal granulomas.
   (a) TNF-α and γ-interferon recruit cells for granuloma formation (see later).
   (b) TNF-α inhibitors cause the breakdown of granulomas leading to dissemination of disease.
  (5) Pathogenesis of a tuberculous granuloma (Box 2-1)
III. **Tissue Repair**
 A. **Factors involved in tissue repair**
  1. Parenchymal cell regeneration
  2. Repair by connective tissue (fibrosis)
 B. **Parenchymal cell regeneration**
  1. Depends on the ability of cells to replicate
   a. Labile cells (e.g., stem cells in epidermis) and stable cells (e.g., fibroblasts) can replicate (refer to Chapter 1).

Cell types in tuberculous granuloma: macrophages and CD4 helper T cells

Epithelioid cells: macrophages activated by γ-interferon from CD4 T_H cells

TNF-α: important in formation and maintenance of granulomas

BOX 2-1 SEQUENCE OF FORMATION OF A TUBERCULOUS GRANULOMA

• The tubercle bacillus *Mycobacterium tuberculosis* undergoes phagocytosis by alveolar macrophages (processing of bacterial antigen).
• Macrophages present antigen to CD4 T cells in association with class II antigen sites.
• Macrophages release interleukin (IL) 12 (stimulates naïve T_H cells to produce T_H1 class memory cells) and IL-1 (causes fever; activates T_H1 cells).
• T_H1 cells release IL-2 (stimulates T_H1 proliferation), γ-interferon (activates macrophages to kill tubercle bacillus; epithelioid cells), and migration inhibitory factor (causes macrophages to accumulate).
• Lipids from killed tubercle bacillus lead to caseous necrosis.
• Activated macrophages fuse and become multinucleated giant cells.

b. Permanent cells *cannot* replicate.
- Cardiac and striated muscle are replaced by scar tissue (fibrosis).

2. Depends on factors that stimulate parenchymal cell division and migration
- Stimulatory factors include loss of tissue and production of growth factors (Table 2-3).

3. Cell cycle (Fig. 2-10)
a. Phases of the cell cycle
(1) G_0 phase
- Resting phase of stable parenchymal cells

(2) G_1 phase
- Synthesis of RNA, protein, organelles, and cyclin D

(3) S (synthesis) phase
- Synthesis of DNA, RNA, protein

(4) G_2 phase
- Synthesis of tubulin, which is necessary for formation of the mitotic spindle

(5) M (mitotic) phase
- Two daughter cells are produced.

b. Regulation of the G_1 checkpoint (G_1 to S phase)
(1) Most critical phase of the cell cycle
(2) Control proteins include cyclin-dependent kinase 4 (Cdk4) and cyclin D
(a) Growth factors activate nuclear transcribing proto-oncogenes to produce cyclin D and Cdk4.
(b) Cyclin D binds to Cdk4, forming a complex causing the cell to enter the S phase.

(3) *RB* (retinoblastoma) suppressor gene
(a) RB protein product arrests the cell in the G_1 phase.
(b) Cdk4 phosphorylates the RB protein causing the cell to enter the S phase.

(4) *TP53* suppressor gene
(a) TP53 protein product arrests the cell in the G_1 phase by inhibiting Cdk4.
- Prevents RB protein phosphorylation and, if necessary, provides time for repair of DNA in the cell

(b) In the event that there is excessive DNA damage, the *BAX* gene is activated.
- *BAX* gene inhibits the *BCL2* antiapoptosis gene (refer to Chapter 1) causing release of cytochrome *c* from the mitochondria and apoptosis of the cell.

4. Restoration to normal
a. Requires preservation of the basement membrane
b. Requires a relatively intact ECM (i.e., collagen, adhesive proteins)
- Laminin, the key adhesion protein in the basement membrane, interacts with type IV collagen, cell surface receptors, and components in the ECM.

Margin notes:

G_1 phase: most variable phase in cell cycle

G_1 to S phase: most critical phase in cell cycle

Genes controlling G_1 to S phase: *RB* and *TP53* suppressor genes

BAX gene: activation by *TP53* initiates apoptosis

Laminin: key adhesion glycoprotein in basement membrane

TABLE 2-3. FACTORS INVOLVED IN TISSUE REPAIR

FACTOR	FUNCTION(S)
Growth Factors	
Vascular endothelial cell growth factor (VEGF)	Stimulates angiogenesis
Basic fibroblast growth factor (BFGF)	Stimulates angiogenesis
Epidermal growth factor (EGF)	Stimulates keratinocyte migration Stimulates granulation tissue formation
Platelet-derived growth factor (PDGF)	Stimulates proliferation of smooth muscle, fibroblasts, endothelial cells
Transforming growth factor-β (TGF-β)	Chemotactic for macrophages, lymphocytes, fibroblasts
Hormones	
Insulin growth factor-1 (IGF-1)	Stimulates synthesis of collagen Promotes keratinocyte migration
Interleukins (IL)	
IL-1	Chemotactic for neutrophils Stimulates synthesis of metalloproteinases (i.e., trace metal containing enzymes) Stimulates synthesis and release of acute phase reactants from the liver

C. Repair by connective tissue (fibrosis)

1. Occurs when injury is severe or persistent
   - Tissue in a third-degree burn *cannot* be restored to normal owing to loss of skin, basement membrane, and connective tissue infrastructure.
2. Steps in repair
   a. Requires neutrophil transmigration to liquefy injured tissue and then macrophage transmigration to remove the debris
   b. Requires formation of granulation tissue
      - Accumulates in the ECM and eventually produces dense fibrotic tissue (scar)
   c. Requires the initial production of type III collagen
      (1) Collagen is the major fibrous component of connective tissue.
      (2) Tropocollagen, the structural unit of collagen, is a triple helix of α-chains.
         (a) Tropocollagen undergoes extensive posttranslational modification.
         (b) Hydroxylation reactions in the rough endoplasmic reticulum convert proline to hydroxyproline and lysine to hydroxylysine.
            - Ascorbic acid is required in these hydroxylation reactions.
         (c) Hydroxyproline residues produce bonds that stabilize the triple helix in the tropocollagen molecule.
         (d) Hydroxylysine residues are oxidized to form an aldehyde residue that produces covalent cross-links at staggered intervals between adjacent tropocollagen molecules.
            - Lysyl oxidase is a metalloproteinase enzyme containing copper.
         (e) Cross-linking increases the overall tensile strength of collagen (also elastic tissue).
            - Type I collagen in skin, bone, and tendons has the greatest tensile strength.
         (f) Cross-linking increases with age.
            - This leads to decreased elasticity of skin, joints, and blood vessels.
         (g) Decreased cross-linking (e.g., vitamin C deficiency) reduces the tensile strength of collagen.
            - In vitamin C deficiency, the structurally weakened collagen is responsible for a bleeding diathesis (e.g., bleeding into skin and joints) and poor wound healing (refer to Chapter 7).

Margin notes:

Granulation tissue: essential for normal connective tissue repair.

Lysyl oxidase: cross-links ↑ tensile strength

Ascorbic acid: hydroxylates proline and lysine

Copper: cofactor in lysyl oxidase

EDS: defects in type I and III collagen

Ehlers-Danlos syndrome (EDS) consists of a group of mendelian disorders characterized by defects of type I and type III collagen synthesis and structure. Clinical findings include hypermobile joints, aortic dissection (most common cause of death), bleeding into the skin (ecchymoses), rupture of the bowel, and poor wound healing (Fig. 2-11).

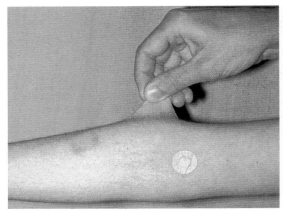

2-11: Ehlers-Danlos syndrome. The patient shows extreme hyperelasticity of the skin. *(From Forbes C, Jackson W: Color Atlas and Text of Clinical Medicine, 2nd ed. St. Louis, Mosby, 2003, p 150, Fig. 3-112.)*

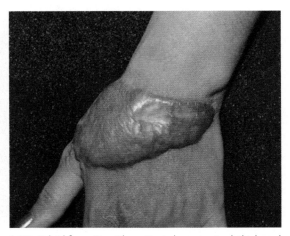

2-12: Keloid formation. The patient shows a raised, thickened scar over the dorsum of the hand. *(From Lookingbill D, Marks J: Principles of Dermatology, 3rd ed. Philadelphia, WB Saunders, 2000, p 115, Fig. 8-5A.)*

BOX 2-2	WOUND HEALING BY PRIMARY AND SECONDARY INTENTION

Primary Intention

Day 1: Fibrin clot (hematoma) develops. Neutrophils infiltrate the wound margins. There is increased mitotic activity of basal cells of squamous epithelium in the apposing wound margins.

Day 2: Squamous cells from apposing basal cell layers migrate under the fibrin clot and seal off the wound after 48 hours. Macrophages emigrate into the wound.

Day 3: Granulation tissue begins to form. Initial deposition of type III collagen begins but does *not* bridge the incision site. Macrophages replace neutrophils.

Days 4–6: Granulation tissue formation peaks, and collagen bridges the incision site.

Week 2: Collagen compresses blood vessels in fibrous tissue, resulting in reduced blood flow. Tensile strength is ~10%.

Month 1: Collagenase remodeling of the wound occurs (breaks peptide bonds), with replacement of type III collagen by type I collagen. Tensile strength increases, reaching ~80% within 3 months. Scar tissue is devoid of adnexal structures (e.g., hair, sweat glands) and inflammatory cells.

Secondary Intention

Typically, these wounds heal differently from primary intention:

More intense inflammatory reaction than primary healing

Increased amount of granulation tissue formation than in primary healing

Wound contraction caused by increased numbers of myofibroblasts

---

Zinc: cofactor in collagenase

> d. Dense scar tissue produced from granulation tissue must be remodeled.
> > (1) Remodeling increases the tensile strength of scar tissue.
> > (2) Metalloproteinases (collagenases) replace type III collagen with type I collagen, increasing tensile strength to approximately 80% of the original.
>
> 3. Primary and secondary intention wound healing (Box 2-2)
> > a. Healing by primary intention
> > > (1) Approximation of wound edges by sutures
> > > (2) Used for clean surgical wounds
> > b. Healing by secondary intention
> > > (1) Wound remains open
> > > (2) Used for gaping or infected wounds

D. Factors that impair healing

Infections: most common cause of impaired wound healing

> 1. Persistent infection
> > a. Most common cause of impaired wound healing
> > b. *Staphylococcus aureus* is the most common pathogen.
> > c. Nosocomial and community-acquired methicillin-resistant *Staphylococcus aureus* wound infections are increasing.
> > > (1) Vancomycin is used for treating nosocomial infections.
> > > (2) Trimethoprim-sulfamethoxazole is used for treating community acquired infections.
> 2. Metabolic disorders
> > • Example—diabetes mellitus increases susceptibility to infection by decreasing blood flow to tissue and increasing tissue levels of glucose.
> 3. Nutritional deficiencies
> > a. Decreased protein (e.g., malnutrition)

Vitamin C deficiency: ↓ cross-linking of tropocollagen→ ↓ tensile strength

> > b. Vitamin C deficiency
> > c. Trace metal deficiency
> > > (1) Copper deficiency leads to decreased cross-linking in collagen (also in elastic tissue).
> > > (2) Zinc deficiency leads to defects in removal of type III collagen in wound remodeling.
> > > > • Type III collagen has decreased tensile strength, which impairs wound healing.

Glucocorticoids: prevent scar formation

> 4. Glucocorticoids
> > a. Interfere with collagen formation and decrease tensile strength
> > b. Useful clinically in preventing excessive scar formation
> > > • Example–dexamethasone is used along with antibiotics to prevent scar formation in bacterial meningitis.

Keloids: excess type III collagen

Keloids, the raised scars caused by excessive synthesis of type III collagen, are common in blacks and may occur as the result of third-degree burns. Microscopically, keloids appear as irregular, thick collagen bundles that extend beyond the confines of the original injury (Fig. 2-12).

E. Repair in other tissues
  1. Liver
      a. Mild injury (e.g., hepatitis A)
          (1) Regeneration of hepatocytes
          (2) Restoration to normal is possible if cytoarchitecture is intact.
      b. Severe or persistent injury (e.g., hepatitis C)
          (1) Regenerative nodules develop that lack sinusoids and portal triads.
          (2) Increased fibrosis occurs around regenerative nodules (see Fig. 18-8)
              • Potential for cirrhosis
  2. Lung
      a. Type II pneumocytes are the key repair cells of the lung.
      b. They replace damaged type I and type II pneumocytes.
      c. They synthesize surfactant.
  3. Brain
      a. Astrocytes proliferate in response to an injury (e.g., brain infarction).
          • This is called gliosis.
      b. Microglial cells (macrophages) are scavenger cells that remove debris (e.g., myelin).
  4. Peripheral nerve transection
      a. Distal degeneration of the axon (called wallerian degeneration) and myelin sheath
      b. Proximal axonal degeneration up to the next node of Ranvier
      c. Macrophages and Schwann cells phagocytose axonal/myelin debris.
      d. Muscle undergoes atrophy in ~15 days.
      e. Nerve cell body undergoes central chromatolysis.
          (1) Nerve cell body swells.
          (2) Nissl bodies (composed of rough endoplasmic reticulum and free ribosomes) disappear centrally.
          (3) Nucleus is peripheralized.
      f. Schwann cells proliferate in the distal stump.
      g. Axonal sprouts develop in the proximal stump and extend distally using Schwann cells for guidance.
      h. Regenerated axon grows 2 to 3 mm/day.
      i. Axon becomes remyelinated.
      j. Muscle is eventually reinnervated.
  5. Heart
      a. Cardiac muscle is permanent tissue.
      b. Damaged muscle is replaced by noncontractile scar tissue.

IV. Laboratory Findings Associated with Inflammation
  A. Leukocytes
      1. Acute inflammation (e.g., bacterial infection)
          a. Absolute neutrophilic leukocytosis (Fig. 2-13)

Severe injury liver: regenerative nodules and fibrosis

Lung injury: type II pneumocyte is repair cell

Brain injury: proliferation of astrocytes and microglial cells

Peripheral nerve transection: Schwann cell key cell in reinnervation

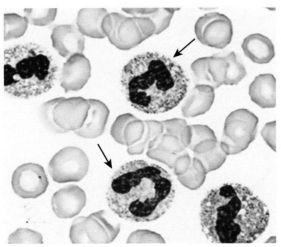

2-13: Absolute leukocytosis with left shift. Arrows point to band (stab) neutrophils, which exhibit prominence of the azurophilic granules (toxic granulation). Vacuoles in the cytoplasm represent phagolysosomes. *(From Hoffbrand AV: Color Atlas: Clinical Hematology, 3rd ed. St. Louis, Mosby, 2000, p 115, Fig. 7-11A.)*

(1) Accelerated release of neutrophils from the bone marrow
(2) Mediated by IL-1 and TNF
b. Left shift
   • Defined as greater than 10% band (stab) neutrophils or the presence of earlier precursors (e.g., metamyelocytes)
c. Toxic granulation
   • Prominence of azurophilic granules (primary lysosomes) in neutrophils
d. Increase in serum IgM
   (1) Peaks in 7 to 10 days
   (2) Isotype switching (μ heavy chain replaced by γ heavy chain) in plasma cells to produce IgG peaks in 12 to 14 days.
2. Chronic inflammation (e.g., tuberculosis, rheumatoid arthritis)
   a. Absolute monocytosis
   b. Increase in serum IgG
3. Table 2-4 summarizes cells involved in inflammation (Fig. 2-14A to D).

IgM: predominant immunoglobulin in acute inflammation

IgG: predominant immunoglobulin in chronic inflammation

TABLE 2-4. **SUMMARY OF LEUKOCYTES**

CELL	CHARACTERISTICS
Neutrophil (see Fig. 2-13)	Key cell in acute inflammation. Receptors for IgG and C3b: important in phagocytosis of opsonized bacteria. Bone marrow neutrophil pools Mitotic pool: myeloblasts, promyelocytes, myelocytes Post-mitotic pool: metamyelocytes, band neutrophils (stabs), segmented neutrophils Peripheral blood neutrophil pools Marginating pool: adherent to the endothelium; account for ~50% of peripheral blood pool Circulating pool: measured in complete blood cell count (CBC); account for ~50% of peripheral blood pool Causes neutrophilic leukocytosis Infections (e.g., acute appendicitis) Sterile inflammation with necrosis (e.g., acute myocardial infarction) Drugs inhibiting neutrophil adhesion molecules: corticosteroids, catecholamines, lithium
Monocytes and macrophages (see Figs. 2-14A; 12-2D):	Key cells in chronic inflammation Receptors for IgG and C3b Monocytes become macrophages: fixed (e.g., macrophages in red pulp), wandering (e.g., alveolar macrophages) Functions: phagocytosis, process antigen, enhance host immunologic response (secrete cytokines like IL-1, TNF) Causes of monocytosis: chronic inflammation, autoimmune disease, malignancy
B cells and T cells (see Figs. 2-14B; 12-2C)	Peripheral blood lymphocyte count: T cells 60–70%, B cells 10–20% of the total B cell function: become plasma cells when antigenically stimulated T cell functions: cellular immunity (type IV HSR), cytokines regulate B cells, defense against intracellular pathogens (e.g., tuberculosis) Causes of B/T lymphocytosis: viral infections
Plasma cells (see Fig. 2-14C)	Antibody producing cells derived from B cells Morphology: well-developed rough endoplasmic reticulum (site of protein synthesis). Bright blue cytoplasmic staining with Wright-Giemsa. Nucleus eccentrically located and has perinuclear clearing.
Mast cells and basophils (see Fig. 12-2B)	Release mediators in acute inflammation and allergic reactions (type I HSR) Receptors for IgE Early release reaction: release of preformed mediators (i.e., histamine, chemotactic factors, proteases) Late phase reaction: new synthesis and release of PGs and LTs, which enhance and prolong the acute inflammatory process.
Eosinophils (see Figs. 2-14D, 12-2A)	Receptors for IgE Red granules contain crystalline material; become Charcot-Leyden crystals in the sputum of asthmatics. Preformed chemical mediators in granules Major basic protein (MBP) kills invasive helminths. Histaminase neutralizes histamine. Arylsulfatase neutralizes leukotrienes. Functions Modulate type I HSR by neutralizing histamine and leukotrienes Destruction of invasive helminths: IgE receptors interact with IgE coating the surface of invasive helminths→ antibody dependent cytotoxicity reaction (type II HSR) causes the release of MBP→ kills helminth Causes of eosinophilia Type I HSR reactions: allergic rhinitis, bronchial asthma. Invasive helminthic infections *excluding* pinworms and adult worms in ascariasis, which are not invasive

HSR, hypersensitivity reaction; IL, interleukin; LT, leukotriene; PG, prostaglandin; TNF, tumor necrosis factor.

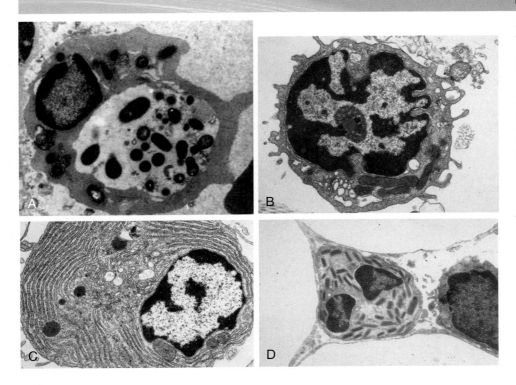

2-14: **A,** Macrophage. Note the phagocytic debris in the cytosol. **B,** Lymphocyte. Note the large nucleus and scant cytoplasm. **C,** Plasma cell. Note the extensive rough endoplasmic reticulum and globules of immunoglobulin in the cytosol. **D,** Eosinophil. Note the crystalline material in the cytosol that becomes Charcot-Leyden crystals in sputum of asthmatics. *(A, B, C, D courtesy of William Meek, Ph.D., Professor and Vice Chairman of Anatomy and Cell Biology, Oklahoma State University, Center for Health Sciences, Tulsa, Oklahoma.)*

4. Peripheral blood effects of corticosteroid therapy
   a. Absolute neutrophilic leukocytosis
     • Inhibits activation of neutrophil adhesion molecules
   b. Lymphopenia
     (1) Sequesters B and T lymphocytes in lymph nodes
     (2) Signal for apoptosis of lymphocytes
   c. Eosinopenia
     • Sequesters eosinophils in lymph nodes

B. Erythrocyte sedimentation rate (ESR)
   • ESR is the rate (mm/hour) of settling of RBCs in a vertical tube.
   1. ESR is increased in acute and chronic inflammation (e.g., rheumatoid arthritis).
   2. Plasma factor or RBC factors that promote rouleaux formation increase the ESR (Fig. 2-15).
     a. Increase in fibrinogen (acute-phase reactant) in plasma decreases negative charge in RBCs, promoting rouleaux formation.
     b. Anemia promotes rouleaux formation.
       • Abnormally shaped RBCs (e.g., sickle cells) do *not* produce rouleaux.

Corticosteroid effect in blood: ↑ neutrophils; ↓ lymphocytes and eosinophils

↑ ESR: ↑ fibrinogen, anemia

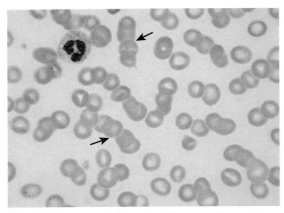

2-15: Rouleaux formation. The arrows show red blood cells stacked like coins. *(From Goldman L, Ausiello D: Cecil's Textbook of Medicine, 23rd ed. Philadelphia, Saunders/ Elsevier, 2008, p 1175, Fig. 161-19.)*

C. C-reactive protein (CRP)

CRP: marker of necrosis and disease activity

1. Acute-phase reactant
2. Clinical usefulness
   a. Sensitive indicator of necrosis associated with acute inflammation
      • CRP is increased in inflammatory (disrupted) atherosclerotic plaques and bacterial infections.
   b. Excellent monitor of disease activity (e.g., rheumatoid arthritis)

D. Serum protein electrophoresis (SPE) in inflammation (Fig. 2-16)

Proteins in serum are separated into individual fractions by SPE. Charged proteins placed in a buffered electrolyte solution will migrate toward one or the other electrode when a current is run through the solution. Proteins with the most negative charges (e.g., albumin) migrate to the positive pole, or anode, and those with the most positive charges (e.g., γ-globulins) remain at the negatively charged pole, or cathode. Beginning at the anode, proteins separate into five major peaks on cellulose acetate—albumin, followed by α_1-, α_2-, β-, and γ-globulins. The γ-globulins in decreasing order of concentration are IgG, IgA, and IgM (IgD and IgE are in very low concentration).

SPE acute inflammation: ↓ albumin; no alteration in γ-globulin peak

1. Acute inflammation (see Fig. 2-16A)
   a. Slight decrease in serum albumin
      (1) Catabolic effect of inflammation
      (2) Amino acids are used by the liver to synthesize acute phase reactants.
   b. Normal γ-globulin peak
      • Serum IgM is increased in acute inflammation; however, it does *not* alter the configuration of the γ-globulin peak.
2. Chronic inflammation (see Fig. 2-16B)
   a. Greater decrease in serum albumin than in acute inflammation
   b. Increase in γ-globulins due to increase in IgG

Polyclonal gammopathy: sign of chronic inflammation

   • Diffuse increase in the γ-globulin peak is due to many clones of benign plasma cells producing IgG (i.e., polyclonal gammopathy).

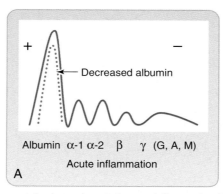

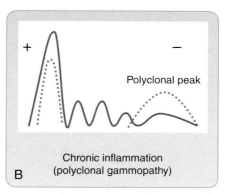

2-16: Serum protein electrophoresis in acute inflammation (**A**) and chronic inflammation (**B**). Refer to the text for discussion.

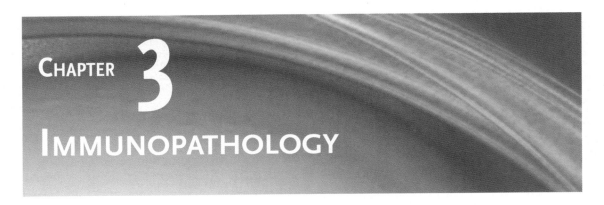

CHAPTER 3

IMMUNOPATHOLOGY

I. **Cells of the Immune System** (Table 3-1)
   A. **Innate (natural, nonspecific) immunity**
      1. Nonspecific defense system against microbial pathogens
      2. Does *not* confer long-lasting immunity against pathogens
      3. Types of effector cells
         a. Phagocytic cells (e.g., neutrophils, macrophages)
         b. Natural killer (NK) cells
         c. Dendritic cells
         d. Microglial cells (macrophage of the central nervous system)
         e. Eosinophils, mast cells
         f. Mucosal epithelial cells, endothelial cells
      4. Toll-like receptors (TLRs) in innate immunity
         a. TLRs are membrane proteins located on the above effector cells.
         b. TLRs recognize non-self antigens (molecules) commonly shared by pathogens.
            (1) Called pathogen-associated molecular patterns (PAMPs)
            (2) Examples of PAMPs
               (a) Endotoxin in gram-negative bacteria
               (b) Peptidoglycan in gram-positive bacteria
         c. PAMPs are *not* present on normal host effector cells.
         d. Interaction of TLRs on effector cells with PAMPs
            (1) Initiates intracellular transmission of activating signals to nuclear factor (NF)κβ
               • NFκβ is the "master switch" to the nucleus.
            (2) Genes are encoded for mediator production.
            (3) Mediators are released into the serum or spinal fluid.
            (4) Innate immunity mediators
               (a) Nitric oxide
               (b) Cytokines (tumor necrosis factor, interleukin 1)
               (c) Adhesion molecules for neutrophils (e.g., selectins)
               (d) Reactive oxygen species (e.g., peroxide)
               (e) Antimicrobial peptides
               (f) Chemokines
   B. **Acquired (specific) immunity**
      1. Antigen-dependent activation and expansion of lymphocytes
      2. B lymphocytes produce antibodies (i.e., humoral immune response).
         a. IgM synthesis begins at birth.
            • Presence of IgM at birth may indicate congenital infection (e.g., cytomegalovirus).
         b. IgG synthesis begins at ~2 months.
            • Presence of IgG at birth is maternally derived IgG.
      3. T cells are involved in cell-mediated immune responses.
II. **Major Histocompatibility Complex (MHC)**
   A. **Overview**
      1. Known collectively as the human leukocyte antigen (HLA) system
      2. Located on short arm of chromosome 6
      3. Gene products are coded for on different loci (see later).
      4. Gene products are membrane-associated glycoproteins.
         • Located on all nucleated cells with the *exception* of mature RBCs
      5. HLA genes and their subtypes are transmitted to children from their parents.

Innate immunity:
first defense against
pathogens

Natural killer cells: large
granular lymphocytes in
peripheral blood

TLRs: recognize non-self
antigens on pathogens

NFκβ: "master switch" to
the nucleus

IgM and IgG synthesis:
begin after birth

TABLE 3-1. **TYPES OF IMMUNE CELLS**

CELL TYPE	DERIVATION	LOCATION	FUNCTION
T cells CD4 (helper) CD8 (cytotoxic/suppressor)	Bone marrow lymphocyte stem cells mature in thymus	Peripheral blood and bone marrow, thymus, paracortex of lymph nodes, Peyer's patches	CD4 cells: secrete cytokines (IL-2 → proliferation of CD4/CD8 T cells; IFN-γ → activation of macrophages); help B cells become antibody-producing plasma cells CD8 cells: kill virus-infected, neoplastic, and donor graft cells
B cells	Bone marrow stem cells	Peripheral blood and bone marrow, germinal follicles in lymph nodes, Peyer's patches	Differentiate into plasma cells that produce immunoglobulins to kill encapsulated bacteria (e.g., *Streptococcus pneumoniae*) Act as APCs that interact with CD4 cells
Natural killer cells	Bone marrow stem cells	Peripheral blood (large granular lymphocytes)	Kill virus-infected and neoplastic cells Release IFN-γ
Macrophages	Conversion of monocytes into macrophages in connective tissue	Connective tissue; organs (e.g., alveolar macrophages, lymph node sinuses)	Involved in phagocytosis and cytokine production Act as APCs to T cells
Dendritic cells	Bone marrow stem cells	Skin (Langerhans' cells), germinal follicles	Act as APCs to T cells

APC, antigen-presenting cell; IFN, interferon; IL, interleukin.

B. Class I antigens
1. Coded by HLA-A, -B, and -C genes
2. Recognized by CD8 T cells and natural killer cells
   • Altered class I antigens (e.g., virus-infected cell) lead to destruction of the cell.

C. Class II antigens

APCs: B cells, macrophages, dendritic cells

1. Coded by HLA-DP, -DQ, and -DR genes
2. Present on antigen-presenting cells (APCs)
   • B cells, macrophages, dendritic cells
3. Recognized by CD4 T cells

D. HLA association with disease

HLA-B27: ankylosing spondylitis

1. HLA-B27 with ankylosing spondylitis
2. HLA-DR2 with multiple sclerosis
3. HLA-DR3 and -DR4 with type 1 diabetes mellitus

E. Applications of HLA testing
1. Transplantation workup
   • Close matches of HLA-A, -B, and -D loci in both the donor and graft recipient increase the chance of graft survival.
2. Determining disease risk
   • Example—HLA-B27–positive individuals have an increased risk of ankylosing spondylitis.

III. Hypersensitivity Reactions (HSRs)

A. Type I (immediate) hypersensitivity

Type I hypersensitivity: IgE activation of mast cells

   • IgE antibody–mediated activation of mast cells (effector cells) produces an inflammatory reaction.
1. IgE antibody production (sensitization)
   a. Allergens (e.g., pollen, drugs) are first processed by APCs (macrophages or dendritic cells).
   b. APCs interact with CD4 T$_H$2 cells, causing interleukins (ILs) to stimulate B-cell maturation.
   c. IL-4 causes plasma cells to switch from IgM to IgE synthesis.
   d. IL-5 stimulates the production and activation of eosinophils.

Mast cell activation: allergens cross-link allergen-specific antibodies

2. Mast cell activation (re-exposure)
   a. Allergen-specific IgE antibodies are bound to mast cells.
   b. Allergens cross-link IgE antibodies specific for the allergen on mast cell membranes.
   c. IgE triggering causes mast cell release of preformed mediators.
      (1) Early phase reaction with release of histamine, chemotactic factors for eosinophils, proteases
      (2) Produces tissue swelling and bronchoconstriction

   d. Late phase reaction
      (1) Mast cells synthesize and release prostaglandins and leukotrienes.
      (2) Enhances and prolongs acute inflammatory reaction

Mast cells: early and late phase reactions

> Desensitization therapy involves repeated injections of increasingly greater amounts of allergen, resulting in production of IgG antibodies that attach to allergens and prevent them from binding to mast cells.

   3. Tests used to evaluate type I hypersensitivity
      a. Scratch test (best overall sensitivity)
         • Positive response is a histamine-mediated wheal-and-flare reaction after introduction of an allergen into the skin.
      b. Radioimmunosorbent test
         • Detects specific IgE antibodies in serum that are against specific allergens
   4. Clinical examples of type I hypersensitivity (Table 3-2)

B. Type II (cytotoxic) hypersensitivity
   • Antibody-dependent cytotoxic reactions
   1. Complement-dependent reactions
      a. Lysis (IgM-mediated)
         (1) Antibody (IgM) directed against antigen on the cell membrane activates the complement system, leading to lysis of the cell by the membrane attack complex.
         (2) Example—IgM types of cold immune hemolytic anemias (refer to Chapter 13)
         (3) Example—transfusion of group A blood (contains anti-B-IgM antibodies) into a group B individual (refer to Chapter 15)
      b. Lysis (IgG-mediated)
         (1) IgG attaches to basement membrane/matrix → activates complement system → C5a is produced (chemotactic factor) → recruitment of neutrophils/monocytes to the activation site → release of enzymes, reactive oxygen species → damage to tissue
         (2) Example—Goodpasture's syndrome with IgG antibodies directed against pulmonary and glomerular capillary basement membranes (refer to Chapter 19)
         (3) Example—acute rheumatic fever with IgG antibodies directed against antigens in heart, skin, brain, subcutaneous tissue, joints (refer to Chapter 10)
      c. Phagocytosis
         (1) Fixed macrophages (e.g., in spleen) phagocytose hematopoietic cells (e.g., RBCs) coated by IgG antibodies or complement (C3b).

Anaphylactic shock: potentially fatal type I hypersensitivity reaction

Type II hypersensitivity: antibody-dependent cytotoxic reactions

TABLE 3-2. HYPERSENSITIVITY REACTIONS

REACTION	PATHOGENESIS	EXAMPLES
Type I	IgE-dependent activation of mast cells	Atopic disorders: hay fever, eczema, hives, asthma, reaction to bee sting Drug hypersensitivity: penicillin rash or anaphylaxis
Type II	Antibody-dependent reaction	Complement-dependent reactions Lysis (IgM mediated): ABO mismatch, cold immune hemolytic anemia Lysis (IgG mediated): Goodpasture's syndrome, PA Phagocytosis: warm (IgG) autoimmune hemolytic anemia, ABO and Rh hemolytic disease of newborn, ITP Complement-independent reactions Antibody (IgG)-dependent cell-mediated cytotoxicity: natural killer cell destruction of neoplastic and virus-infected cells Antibody (IgE)-dependent cell-mediated cytotoxicity: eosinophil destruction of helminths Antibodies directed against cell surface receptors: myasthenia gravis, Graves' disease
Type III	Deposition of antigen-antibody complexes	Systemic lupus erythematosus (DNA–anti-DNA) Serum sickness (horse antithymocyte globulin-antibody) Poststreptococcal glomerulonephritis
Type IV	Antibody-independent T cell–mediated reactions	Delayed type: tuberculous granuloma; PPD reaction, MS Cell-mediated cytotoxicity: killing of tumor cells and virus-infected cells; contact dermatitis (e.g., poison ivy, nickel)

ITP, idiopathic thrombocytopenic purpura; MS, multiple sclerosis; PA, pernicious anemia; PPD, purified protein derivative

(2) Example—warm (IgG) immune hemolytic anemia (refer to Chapter 13)

(3) Example—ABO hemolytic disease of the newborn (refer to Chapter 15)

- Group O mother has anti-A,B-IgG antibodies that cross the placenta and attach to fetal blood group A or B red blood cells.

2. Complement-independent reactions

a. Antibody (IgG)-dependent cell-mediated cytotoxicity

(1) Cells are coated by IgG → leukocytes (neutrophils, monocyte, NK cells) bind to IgG → activated cells release inflammatory mediators causing lysis of the cells

(2) Example—killing virus-infected cells or tumor cells

b. Antibody (IgE)-dependent cell-mediated cytotoxicity

- Helminth in tissue is coated by IgE antibodies → eosinophil IgE receptors attach to the IgE → eosinophils release major basic protein, which kills the helminth

Myasthenia gravis, Graves' disease: antibodies against receptors; type II HSR

c. IgG autoantibodies directed against cell surface receptors → impair function of the receptor (e.g., anti-acetylcholine receptor antibodies in myasthenia gravis) or stimulate function (e.g., anti-thyroid-stimulating hormone receptor antibodies in Graves' disease)

3. Tests used to evaluate type II hypersensitivity

a. Direct Coombs' test detects IgG and C3b attached to RBCs.

b. Indirect Coombs' test detects antibodies (e.g., anti-D) in serum.

4. Clinical examples of type II hypersensitivity (see Table 3-2)

C. Type III (immunocomplex) hypersensitivity

Type III hypersensitivity: complement activation by circulating antigen-antibody complexes

- Activation of the complement system by circulating antigen-antibody complexes (e.g., DNA–anti-DNA complexes)

1. First exposure to antigen

- Synthesis of antibodies

2. Second exposure to antigen

a. Deposition of antigen-antibody complexes

b. Complement activation, producing C5a, which attracts neutrophils that damage tissue

3. Arthus reaction

a. Localized immunocomplex reaction

b. Example—farmer's lung from exposure to thermophilic actinomycetes, or antigens, in air

Antibody-mediated hypersensitivity reactions: types I, II, and III

4. Test used to evaluate type III hypersensitivity

a. Immunofluorescent staining of tissue biopsies

b. Example—glomeruli in glomerulonephritis

5. Clinical examples of type III hypersensitivity (see Table 3-2)

D. Type IV hypersensitivity

Type IV hypersensitivity: cellular immunity

- Antibody-independent T cell–mediated reactions (cellular-mediated immunity, CMI)

1. Functions of CMI

a. Control of infections caused by viruses, fungi, helminths, mycobacteria, intracellular bacterial pathogens

b. Graft rejection

c. Tumor surveillance

2. Types of reactions

DRH: CD4 cells interact with macrophages; TB granuloma

a. Delayed reaction hypersensitivity (DRH)

- CD4 cells interact with macrophages (APCs with MHC class II antigens), resulting in cytokine injury to tissue (refer to Chapter 2).

CD8 T cell mediated: altered class I antigens; contact dermatitis

b. Cell-mediated cytotoxicity

(1) CD8 T cells interact with altered MHC class I antigens on neoplastic, virus-infected, or donor graft cells, causing cell lysis.

(2) Contact dermatitis

- CD8 T cells attack antigens in skin (e.g., poison ivy, nickel).

3. Test used to evaluate type IV hypersensitivity

a. Patch test to confirm contact dermatitis

- Example—suspected allergen (e.g., nickel) placed on an adhesive patch is applied to the skin to see if a skin reaction occurs.

b. Skin reaction to *Candida*

c. Quantitative count of T cells

d. Various mitogenic assays

4. Clinical examples of type IV hypersensitivity (see Table 3-2)

IV. **Transplantation Immunology**
   A. **Factors enhancing graft viability**
      1. ABO blood group compatibility between recipients and donors
      2. Absence of preformed anti-HLA cytotoxic antibodies in recipients
         • People must have previous exposure to blood products to develop anti-HLA cytotoxic antibodies.
      3. Close matches of HLA-A, -B, and -D loci between recipients and donors
      4. Chance of a sibling in a family having another sibling with a 0, 1, or 2 haplotype match is illustrated in Figure 3-1.
   B. **Types of grafts**
      1. Autograft (i.e., self to self)
         • Associated with the best survival rate
      2. Syngeneic graft (isograft)
         • Between identical twins
      3. Allograft
         • Between genetically different individuals of the same species

   The fetus is an allograft that is *not* rejected by the mother. Trophoblastic tissue may prevent maternal T cells from entering fetus.

      4. Xenograft
         a. Between two species
         b. Example—transplant of heart valve from pig to human
   C. **Types of rejection**
      • Transplantation rejection involves a humoral or cell-mediated host response against MHC antigens in the donor graft.
      1. Hyperacute rejection
         a. Irreversible reaction occurs within minutes.
         b. Pathogenesis
            (1) ABO incompatibility or action of preformed anti-HLA antibodies in the recipient directed against donor antigens in vascular endothelium
            (2) Type II hypersensitivity reaction

ABO blood group compatibility: most important requirement for successful transplantation

Autograft: best survival rate

Fetus: allograft not rejected by mother

Hyperacute rejection: irreversible; type II hypersensitivity reaction

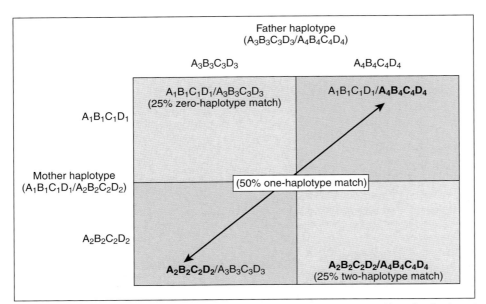

3-1: Chance of a sibling with haplotype $A_2B_2C_2D_2/A_4B_4C_4D_4$ having a 0-, 1-, or 2-haplotype match in a family where the father is haplotype $A_3B_3C_3D_3/A_4B_4C_4D_4$ and the mother is haplotype $A_1B_1C_1D_1/A_3B_3C_3D_3$. Note that there is a 25% chance for a 2-haplotype match ($A_2B_2C_2D_2/A_4B_4C_4D_4$), a 25% chance for a 0-haplotype match ($A_1B_1C_1D_1/A_3B_3C_3D_3$), and a 50% chance of a 1-haplotype match ($A_2B_2C_2D_2/A_3B_3C_3D_3$) or ($A_1B_1C_1D_1/A_4B_4C_4D_4$). Using a parent as a transplant donor is considered a 1-haplotype match. An identical 2-haplotype is rarely achieved owing to crossing over between the individual loci during meiosis when homologous chromosomes line up close to each other. *(From Goljan EF: Star Series: Pathology. Philadelphia, WB Saunders, 1998, p 63, Fig. 4-2.)*

c. Pathologic finding
  • Vessel thrombosis
d. Example—blood group A person receives a blood group B heart.
2. Acute rejection
  a. Most common transplant rejection
  b. Reversible reaction that occurs within days to weeks
     (1) Type IV cell-mediated hypersensitivity
        (a) Host CD4 T cells release cytokines, resulting in activation of host macrophages, proliferation of CD8 T cells, and destruction of donor graft cells.
        (b) Extensive interstitial round cell lymphocytic infiltrate in the graft, edema, and endothelial cell injury
     (2) Antibody-mediated type II hypersensitivity reaction
        (a) Cytokines from CD4 T cells promote B-cell differentiation into plasma cells, producing anti-HLA antibodies that attack vessels in the donor graft.
        (b) Vasculitis with intravascular thrombosis in recent grafts
        (c) Intimal thickening with obliteration of vessel lumens in older grafts

Acute rejection: most common type; type IV and type II hypersensitivity

> **Acute rejection** is potentially reversible with immunosuppressive agents, such as cyclosporine (blocks CD4 T-cell release of IL-2), OKT3 (monoclonal antibody against T-cell antigen recognition site), and corticosteroids (lymphotoxic). Immunosuppressive therapy is associated with an increased risk of cervical squamous cell cancer, malignant lymphoma, and squamous cell carcinoma of the skin (most common cancer).

3. Chronic rejection
  a. Irreversible reaction that occurs over months to years
  b. Pathogenesis
     (1) Not well characterized
     (2) Involves continued vascular injury with ischemia to tissue
  c. Blood vessel damage with intimal thickening and fibrosis

Chronic rejection: irreversible

Immunosuppressive therapy: danger of squamous cell carcinoma

D. Graft-versus-host (GVH) reaction
  1. Causes
     a. Potential complication in bone marrow (85% of cases) and liver transplants
     b. Potential complication in blood transfusions given to patients with a T-cell immunodeficiency and newborns
  2. Pathogenesis
     a. Donor cytotoxic T cells recognize host tissue as foreign
     b. Proliferate in host tissue and produce severe organ damage
  3. Clinical findings
     a. Bile duct necrosis (jaundice)
     b. Gastrointestinal mucosa ulceration (bloody diarrhea)
     c. Dermatitis
  4. Treatment
     a. Treat with anti-thymocyte globulin or monoclonal antibodies *before* grafting
     b. Cyclosporine reduces the severity of the reaction.

GVH reaction: jaundice, diarrhea, dermatitis

E. Types of transplants (Table 3-3)

Corneal transplants: best allograft survival rate

V.   **Autoimmune Diseases**
  • Autoimmune dysfunction is associated with a loss of self-tolerance, resulting in immune reactions directed against host tissue.
  A. Mechanisms of autoimmunity
     1. Release of normally sequestered antigens (e.g., sperm)
     2. Imbalance favoring CD4 T helper cells over CD8 T suppressor cells

TABLE 3-3. SOME TYPES OF TRANSPLANTS

TYPE OF TRANSPLANT	COMMENTS
Cornea	Best allograft survival rate Danger of transmission of Creutzfeldt-Jakob disease
Kidney	Better survival with kidney from living donor than from cadaver
Bone marrow	Graft contains pluripotential cells that repopulate host stem cells Host assumes donor ABO group Danger of graft-versus-host reaction and cytomegalovirus infection

3. Sharing of antigens between host and pathogen (mimicry)
  - Example—group A streptococcus antigens are similar to antigens in the human heart and other tissues in rheumatic fever.
4. Alteration of self-antigens by drugs or by a pathogen
  a. Drug example—methyldopa alters Rh antigens on the surface of RBCs
  b. Pathogen example—coxsackievirus alters β-islet cells
5. Abnormal immune response genes on chromosome 6 (Ir genes)
6. Polyclonal activation of B lymphocytes
  - Polyclonal activators include Epstein-Barr virus, cytomegalovirus, endotoxins

B. Classification of autoimmunity
1. Organ-specific disorders
  a. Addison's disease
    - Immune destruction of the adrenal cortex (refer to Chapter 22)
  b. Pernicious anemia
    - Immune destruction of parietal cells in the stomach (refer to Chapter 11)
  c. Hashimoto's thyroiditis
    - Immune destruction of the thyroid (refer to Chapter 22)
2. Systemic examples
  a. Systemic lupus erythematosus (SLE; see later)
  b. Rheumatoid arthritis (refer to Chapter 23)
  c. Systemic sclerosis (see later)

C. Laboratory evaluation of autoimmune disease
1. Serum antinuclear antibody (ANA) test
  a. Most useful screening test for autoimmune diseases
  b. Antinuclear antibodies are directed against various nuclear antigens.
    (1) DNA
      - Anti-double-stranded (ds) antibodies present in SLE patients who have renal disease
    (2) Histones
      - Antihistone antibodies present in drug-induced lupus
    (3) Acidic proteins
      (a) Anti-Smith (Sm) present in SLE
      (b) Anti-ribonucleoprotein antibodies present in systemic sclerosis
    (4) Nucleolar antigens
      - Anti-nucleolar antibodies present in systemic sclerosis
  c. Serum ANA is a fluorescent antibody test.
    (1) Provides a pattern of immunofluorescence
      (a) Patterns include speckled, homogeneous, nucleolar, and rim
      (b) Rim pattern correlates with anti-dsDNA antibodies and the presence of renal disease in SLE
    (2) Provides a titer of the antibody
2. Specific antibody tests
  a. Utilized in documenting organ-specific autoimmune diseases
  b. Example—antibodies directed against the proton pump in parietal cells in pernicious anemia
3. Summary of autoantibodies in Table 3-4

D. Systemic lupus erythematosus
  - Connective tissue disease that mainly affects the blood, joints, skin, and kidneys
1. Occurs predominantly in women of childbearing age
2. Pathogenesis
  a. Genetic
    (1) There is an increased risk for developing SLE in family members.
    (2) Genetic links appear to be located on chromosome 6.
  b. Environmental factors are important in exacerbating SLE or triggering its initial onset.
    (1) Examples
      (a) Infectious agents (viruses, bacteria)
      (b) Ultraviolet light
      (c) Estrogen
      (d) Medications
      (e) Extreme stress
    (2) These factors cause destruction of cells leading to antibodies directed against various nuclear antigens (see earlier).

Organ-specific disorders: Addison's disease, pernicious anemia

Systemic autoimmune disorders: SLE, rheumatoid arthritis

Serum ANA: antibodies against DNA, histones, acidic proteins, nucleoli

Anti-dsDNA: SLE with glomerulonephritis

Rim pattern: associated with anti-dsDNA antibodies

SLE: genetic + environmental factors

TABLE 3-4. **AUTOANTIBODIES IN AUTOIMMUNE DISEASE**

AUTOANTIBODIES	DISEASE	TEST SENSITIVITY (%)
Anti-acetylcholine receptor	Myasthenia gravis	>85
Anti–basement membrane	Goodpasture's syndrome	>90
Anticentromere	CREST syndrome	50–90
Antiendomysial IgA	Celiac disease	95
Antigliadin IgA	Celiac disease	80
Antihistone	Drug-induced lupus	90–95
Anti-insulin	Type 1 diabetes	50
Anti–islet cell		75–80
Anti–intrinsic factor	Pernicious anemia	60
Anti–parietal cell		90
Antimicrosomal	Hashimoto's thyroiditis	97
Anti-Smith (Sm)	Systemic lupus erythematosus	30
Anti-SS-A (Ro)	Sjögren's syndrome	70–95
	Systemic lupus erythematosus	25–50
Anti-SS-B (La)	Sjögren's syndrome	60–90
Antithyroglobulin	Hashimoto's thyroiditis	85
Anti–tissue transglutaminase IgA	Celiac disease	98
Anti-topoisomerase	Systemic sclerosis	30
Antimitochondrial	Primary biliary cirrhosis	90–100
Antimyeloperoxidase	Microscopic polyangiitis	80 (p-ANCA)
Antinuclear	Systemic lupus erythematosus Systemic sclerosis Dermatomyositis	99 70–90 <30
Antiproteinase 3	Wegener's granulomatosis	>90 (c-ANCA)
Anti-ribonucleoprotein	MCTD	85
Anti-TSH receptor	Graves' disease	85

c-ANCA, cytoplasmic antineutrophil cytoplasmic antibody; CREST, calcinosis, Raynaud's phenomenon, esophageal dysfunction, sclerodactyly, telangiectasia; MCTD, mixed connective tissue disease; p-ANCA, perinuclear antineutrophilic cytoplasmic antibody.

(3) Autoantibodies are present many years before the diagnosis of SLE, indicating that cell damage occurs prior to onset of symptoms.
  c. An allele of STAT4 is associated with increased risk for developing SLE (also rheumatoid arthritis).
    (1) STAT4 is part of a family of transcription factors.
    (2) Protein products of STAT4 are essential for mediating responses to IL-12 in lymphocytes and in regulating the differentiation of T helper cells.
  3. Clinical findings
    a. Hematologic
      • Autoimmune hemolytic anemia, thrombocytopenia, leukopenia
    b. Lymphatic
      (1) Generalized painful lymphadenopathy
      (2) Splenomegaly
    c. Musculoskeletal
      • Small-joint inflammation (e.g., hands) with absence of joint deformity
    d. Skin
      (1) Immunocomplex deposition along basement membrane
        • Produces liquefactive degeneration
      (2) Malar butterfly rash (Fig. 3-2A)
    e. Renal
      • Diffuse proliferative glomerulonephritis (most common glomerulonephritis)

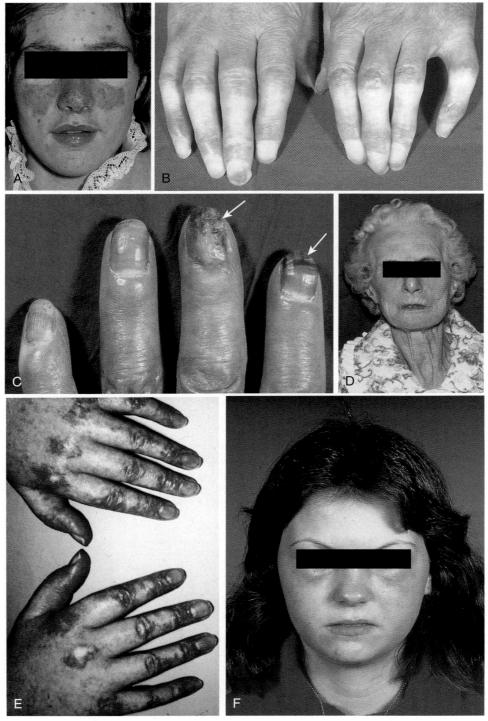

3-2: A, Malar rash in systemic lupus erythematosus showing the butterfly-wing distribution. **B,** Raynaud's phenomenon: Raynaud's phenomenon in systemic sclerosis is due to a digital vasculitis. The usual color changes are white (this patient) to blue to red. It is one of the first signs of systemic sclerosis. **C,** Systemic sclerosis. The skin is erythematous and tightly bound. The fingertips are tapered (called sclerodactyly) and have digital infarcts (*arrows*) due to fibrosis of the digital vessels. **D,** Systemic sclerosis. Note the thinned lips and characteristic radial furrowing around the mouth giving a pursed-lip appearance. This is due to increased deposition of collagen in the subcutaneous tissue. There are also dilatations of small vessels (telangiectasia) on the face. **E,** Dermatomyositis. Note the characteristic purple papules overlying the knuckles and proximal and distal interphalangeal joints. **F,** Dermatomyositis. Note the characteristic swelling and red-mauve discoloration below the eyes. (*A from Forbes C, Jackson W: Color Atlas and Text of Clinical Medicine, 2nd ed. St. Louis, Mosby, 2003, Fig. 3-77; B from Savin JA, Hunter JAA, Hepburn NC: Diagnosis in Color: Skin Signs in Clinical Medicine. London, Mosby-Wolfe, 1997, p 205, Fig. 8.43; C, D, and F courtesy of R.A. Marsden, MD, St. George's Hospital, London; E from Firestein G, Budd RC, Harris ED, Jr: Kelley's Textbook of Rheumatology, 8th ed. Philadelphia, WB Saunders, 2008, Fig. 47-9.*)

Most common cardiac
finding in SLE: fibrinous
pericarditis with effusion

f. Cardiovascular
   (1) Fibrinous pericarditis with or without effusion
   (2) Libman-Sacks endocarditis (sterile vegetations on mitral valve; 18% of cases)
g. Respiratory
   (1) Interstitial fibrosis of lungs
   (2) Pleural effusion with friction rub
h. Pregnancy-related
   (1) Complete heart block in newborns
      • Caused by IgG anti-SS-A (Ro) antibodies crossing the placenta
   (2) Recurrent spontaneous abortions
      • Caused by antiphospholipid antibodies (refer to Chapter 14)
4. Drug-induced lupus erythematosus
   a. Associated drugs
      • Procainamide, hydralazine

Procainamide: most
common drug associated
with drug-induced lupus

Drug-induced lupus:
antihistone antibodies

   b. Features that distinguish drug-induced lupus from SLE
      (1) Antihistone antibodies
      (2) Low incidence of renal and CNS involvement
      (3) Disappearance of symptoms when the drug is discontinued
5. Laboratory testing for SLE

Screen for SLE: serum
ANA

   a. Serum antinuclear antibody (ANA)
      (1) Serum ANA is the best screening test for SLE (sensitivity 99%).
         • False negative test results (have SLE but test is negative) are uncommon.
      (2) Specificity of serum ANA is only 80%.
         • False positive results due to other autoimmune diseases (e.g., systemic sclerosis)
   b. Anti-dsDNA antibodies and anti-Sm antibodies
      (1) Tests used to confirm the diagnosis of SLE
         • They have high specificity for diagnosing SLE (i.e., few false positive results)
      (2) Specificity for anti-dsDNA is 99% and 100% for anti-Sm.

Confirm SLE: anti-dsDNA
and anti-Sm antibodies

   c. Anti-Ro antibodies are positive in 25% to 50% of cases.
   d. Antiphospholipid antibodies (refer to Chapter 14)
      (1) Lupus anticoagulant and anticardiolipin antibodies
      (2) Damage vessel endothelium, producing vessel thrombosis
      (3) Increased incidence of strokes and recurrent spontaneous abortions

Anticardiolipin antibodies may produce a false positive syphilis serologic test by cross-reacting with cardiolipin in the rapid plasma reagin (RPR) and venereal disease research laboratory (VDRL) tests.

LE cell: neutrophil with
phagocytosed, altered
DNA

   e. Lupus erythematosus (LE) cell
      (1) Neutrophil containing phagocytosed altered DNA
      (2) Sensitivity 76% and specificity 97%
   f. Serum complement
      • Usually decreased because of activation of complement system by immunocomplexes
   g. Immunofluorescence testing
      (1) Immunocomplexes at the dermal-epidermal junction in skin biopsies
         • Immunofluorescent studies identify complexes in a band-like distribution along the dermal-epidermal junction (called *band test*).
      (2) Immunofluorescence studies of kidney biopsies to identify glomerulonephritis.
6. Prognosis
   a. Improved survival due to advances in diagnosis and treatment (see later)
      • Over 90% now survive for 10 years or more
   b. Most common cause of death is infection due to immunosuppression.

Treatment for SLE depends on the organ systems that are involved. Joint pain and serositis are generally controlled with NSAIDs. Treatment modalities used for cutaneous disease include topical corticosteroids, antimalarial agents, sunscreen, and immunosuppressive drugs (e.g., methotrexate or azathioprine). Renal disease is treated with cyclophosphamide. Autoimmune hemolytic anemia and thrombocytopenia are initially treated with corticosteroids; other drugs or splenectomy may be required if corticosteroids are ineffective. Tumor necrosis factor-α inhibitors are also being used in treating SLE; however, there is a danger for disseminated infections (refer to Chapter 2).

E. Systemic sclerosis (scleroderma)
- Excessive production of collagen that primarily targets the skin (scleroderma), gastrointestinal tract, lungs, and kidneys

Systemic sclerosis: excess collagen deposition, digital vasculitis

1. Occurs predominantly in women of childbearing age
2. Pathogenesis
   a. Small-vessel endothelial cell damage produces blood vessel fibrosis and ischemic injury.
   b. T-cell release of cytokines results in excessive collagen synthesis.
   c. Stimulatory autoantibodies against platelet-derived growth factor
3. Clinical findings
   a. Raynaud's phenomenon (Fig. 3-2B; refer to Chapter 9)

Raynaud's phenomenon: most common initial sign of systemic sclerosis

   (1) Sequential color changes (white to blue to red) caused by digital vessel vasculitis and fibrosis
      - Most common initial complaint (70% of cases)
   (2) Tapered fingers often with digital infarcts (Fig. 3-2C)
   b. Skin
   (1) Skin atrophy and tissue swelling beginning in the fingers and extending proximally
   (2) Parchment-like appearance
   (3) Extensive dystrophic calcification in subcutaneous tissue
   (4) Tightened facial features (e.g., radial furrowing around the lips) (Fig. 3-2D)
   c. Gastrointestinal
   (1) Dysphagia for solids and liquids
      (a) No peristalsis in the lower two thirds of the esophagus (smooth muscle replaced by collagen)
      (b) Lower esophageal sphincter relaxation with reflux
   (2) Small bowel
      (a) Loss of villi (malabsorption)
      (b) Wide-mouthed diverticula (bacterial overgrowth)
      (c) Dysmotility (cramps and diarrhea)
   d. Respiratory

Systemic sclerosis: respiratory failure most common cause of death

   (1) Interstitial fibrosis
   (2) Respiratory failure (most common cause of death)
   e. Renal
   (1) Vasculitis involving arterioles (i.e., hyperplastic arteriolosclerosis) and glomeruli
   (2) Infarctions, malignant hypertension
4. Laboratory findings in systemic sclerosis
   a. Serum ANA is positive in 70% to 90% of cases.
   b. Anti-topoisomerase antibody is positive in 30% of cases.
      - Extractable nuclear antibody to Scl 70.

Systemic sclerosis: anti-topoisomerase antibodies

5. CREST syndrome
   - Limited sclerosis
   a. Clinical findings
   (1) C—calcification, centromere antibody
   (2) R—Raynaud's phenomenon (see Fig. 3-2B)
   (3) E—Esophageal dysmotility
   (4) S—sclerodactyly (i.e., tapered, claw-like fingers; see Fig. 3-2C)
   (5) T—telangiectasias (i.e., multiple punctate blood vessel dilations)
   b. Laboratory findings
      - Anticentromere antibodies in 50% to 90% of cases

CREST syndrome = calcinosis, Raynaud's phenomenon, esophageal dysfunction, sclerodactyly, telangiectasia

6. Treatment
   - D-Penicillamine; recombinant human relaxin

F. Dermatomyositis (DM; with skin involvement) and polymyositis (PM; no skin involvement)
1. Occurs predominantly in women 40 to 60 years of age
2. Associated with risk of malignant neoplasms (15–20% of cases), particularly lung cancer
3. Pathogenesis
   a. DM is associated with antibody-mediated damage.
   b. PM is associated with T cell–mediated damage.
4. Clinical findings
   a. Muscle pain and atrophy
      - Shoulders are commonly involved.
   b. Heliotrope eyelids or "raccoon eyes" (purple-red eyelid discoloration; Fig. 3-2E)

DM/PM: heliotrope eyes; Gottron's patches

DM/PM: ↑ serum creatine kinase

MCTD: anti-ribonucleoprotein antibodies

c. Purple papules over the knuckles and proximal interphalangeal joints (see Fig 3-2F)
   • Called Gottron's patches
5. Laboratory findings
   a. Serum ANA is positive in <30% of cases.
   b. Increased serum creatine kinase
   c. Muscle biopsy shows a lymphocytic infiltrate.
G. **Mixed connective tissue disease (MCTD)**
   1. Signs and symptoms similar to SLE, systemic sclerosis, and PM
   2. Renal disease is uncommon.
   3. Anti-ribonucleoprotein antibodies are positive in almost 100% of cases.

VI. **Immunodeficiency Disorders**
   • Defects in B cells, T cells, complement, or phagocytic cells
   A. **Risk factors for immune disorders**
      1. Prematurity
      2. Autoimmune diseases (e.g., systemic lupus erythematosus)
      3. Lymphoproliferative disorders (e.g., malignant lymphoma)
      4. Infections (e.g., human immunodeficiency virus, HIV)
      5. Immunosuppressive drugs (e.g., corticosteroids)
   B. **Congenital immunodeficiency disorders** (Table 3-5)
      1. B-cell disorders
         • Recurrent encapsulated bacterial infections (e.g., *Streptococcus pneumoniae*)

IgA deficiency: most common congenital immunodeficiency

TABLE 3-5. **CONGENITAL IMMUNODEFICIENCY DISORDERS**

DISEASE	DEFECT(S)	CLINICAL FEATURES
B-Cell Disorders		
Bruton's agammaglobulinemia	Failure of pre-B cells to become mature B cells; Mutated tyrosine kinase; X-linked recessive disorder	SP infections; Maternal antibodies protective from birth to age 6 months; ↓ Immunoglobulins
IgA deficiency	Failure of IgA B cells to mature into plasma cells	SP infections; giardiasis; Anaphylaxis if exposed to blood products that contain IgA; ↓ IgA and secretory IgA
Common variable immunodeficiency	Defect in B-cell maturation to plasma cells; Adult immunodeficiency disorder	Sinopulmonary infections (90–100%), GI infections (e.g., *Giardia*), pneumonia, autoimmune disease (ITP, AIHA), malignancy (25%); Common pathogens: *Actinomyces israeli, Streptococcus pneumoniae, Haemophilus influenzae*; chronic infections—*Staphylococcus aureus, Pseudomonas aeruginosa*; ↓ Immunoglobulins
T-Cell Disorder		
DiGeorge syndrome	Failure of third and fourth pharyngeal pouches to develop; Thymus and parathyroid glands fail to develop	Hypoparathyroidism (tetany); absent thymic shadow on radiograph; PCP; Danger of GVH reaction
Combined B- and T-Cell Disorders		
Severe combined immunodeficiency (SCID)	Adenosine deaminase deficiency (15%); autosomal recessive disorder; adenine toxic to B and T cells; ↓ deoxynucleoide triphosphate precursors for DNA synthesis; Other disorders: stem cell defect	Defective CMI; ↓ Immunoglobulins; Treatment: gene therapy, bone marrow transplant (patients with SCID do *not* reject allografts)
Wiskott-Aldrich syndrome	Progressive deletion of B and T cells; X-linked recessive disorder	Symptom triad: eczema, thrombocytopenia, SP infections; Associated risk of malignant lymphoma; Defective CMI; ↓ IgM, normal IgG, ↑ IgA and IgE
Ataxia-telangiectasia	Mutation in DNA repair enzymes; Thymic hypoplasia; Autosomal recessive disorder	Cerebellar ataxia, telangiectasias of eyes and skin; ↑ Risk of lymphoma and/or leukemia; adenocarcinoma; ↑ Serum α-fetoprotein; ↓ IgA 50-80%, ↓ IgE, IgM low molecular weight variety, ↓ IgG2 or total IgG; ↓ T cell function

AIHA, autoimmune hemolytic anemia; CMI, cell-mediated immunity; GI, gastrointestinal; GVH, graft-versus-host; ITP, idiopathic thrombocytopenic purpura; PCP, *Pneumocystis jiroveci* pneumonia; SP, sinopulmonary.

2. T-cell disorders
  • Recurrent infections caused by intracellular pathogens (fungi, viruses, protozoa)
3. Combined B- and T-cell disorders
C. Acquired immunodeficiency syndrome
  1. Modes of transmission
    a. Sexual transmission (~75% of cases)
      (1) Man-to-man transmission by anal intercourse is the most common cause in the United States.
      (2) Heterosexual transmission is the most common cause in developing countries.
      (3) Virus enters blood vessels or dendritic cells in areas of mucosal injury.
    b. Intravenous drug abuse
      • Rate of HIV infection is markedly increasing in female sex partners of male intravenous drug abusers.
    c. Other modes of transmission
      (1) Vertical transmission
        (a) Transplacental route, blood contamination during delivery, breast-feeding
        (b) Most pediatric cases of AIDS are due to transmission of virus from mother to child.
      (2) Accidental needlestick
        (a) Risk per accident is 0.3%.
        (b) Most common mode of infection in health care workers
      (3) Blood products
    d. Body fluids containing HIV
      (1) Blood, semen, breast milk
      (2) Virus *cannot* enter intact skin or mucosa.
  2. Etiology
    a. RNA retrovirus
    b. HIV-1 is the most common cause in the United States.
    c. HIV-2 is the most common cause in developing countries.
  3. Pathogenesis
    a. HIV envelope protein (gp120) attaches to the CD4 molecule of T cells.
    b. HIV infects CD4 T cells, causing direct cytotoxicity.
    c. Infection of non–T cells
      (1) Can infect monocytes and macrophages in tissue (e.g., lung, brain)
      (2) Can infect dendritic cells in mucosal tissue
        • Dendritic cells transfer virus to B-cell germinal follicles.
      (3) Macrophages and dendritic cells are reservoirs for virus.
        • Loss of cell-mediated immunity
    d. Reverse transcriptase
      (1) Converts viral RNA into proviral double-stranded DNA
      (2) DNA is integrated into the host DNA.
  4. HIV and AIDS testing (Table 3-6)
  5. Clinical findings
    a. Acute phase
      • Mononucleosis-like syndrome 3 to 6 weeks after infection

Margin notes:

AIDS: most common acquired immunodeficiency disease worldwide

AIDS: most common cause of death due to infection worldwide

Pediatric AIDS: most due to vertical transmission

Risk per unit of blood is 1 per 2 million units of blood transfused.

HIV: cytotoxic to CD4 T cells; loss of cell-mediated immunity

Anti-gp120: detected in ELISA test screen
Western blot: confirms HIV

TABLE 3-6. LABORATORY TESTS USED IN HIV AND AIDS

TEST	USE	COMMENTS
ELISA	Screening test	Detects anti-gp120 antibodies Sensitivity ~100% Positive within 3–5 weeks; all in 3 months
Western blot	Confirmatory test	Used if ELISA is positive or indeterminate Positive test: presence of p24 antigen and gp41 antibodies and either gp120 or gp160 antibodies Specificity ~100%
p24 antigen	Indicator of active viral replication Present before anti-gp120 antibodies	Positive prior to seroconversion and when AIDS is diagnosed (two distinct peaks)
CD4 T-cell count	Monitoring immune status	Useful in determining when to initiate HIV treatment and when to administer prophylaxis against opportunistic infections
HIV viral load	Detection of actively dividing virus Marker of disease progression	Most sensitive test for diagnosis of acute HIV before seroconversion

AIDS, acquired immunodeficiency syndrome; ELISA, enzyme-linked immunosorbent assay; HIV, human immunodeficiency virus.

b. Latent (chronic) phase
   (1) Asymptomatic period 2 to 10 years after infection
   (2) CD4 T-cell count greater than 500 cells/mm³
   (3) Viral replication occurs in dendritic cells (reservoir cells) in germinal follicles of lymph nodes.
     • Cytotoxic T cells control but do *not* clear HIV reservoirs.
c. Early symptomatic phase
   (1) CD4 T-cell count 200 to 500 cells/mm³
   (2) Generalized lymphadenopathy
   (3) Non–AIDS-defining infections, including hairy leukoplakia, or Epstein-Barr virus (EBV)–caused glossitis, oral candidiasis
   (4) Fever, weight loss, diarrhea
     • Most common CNS fungal infection in AIDS: cryptococcosis
d. AIDS (Table 3-7)
   (1) Criteria
     • HIV-positive with CD4 T-cell count of 200 cells/mm³ or less or an AIDS-defining condition
   (2) Most common AIDS-defining infections
     • *Pneumocystis jiroveci* pneumonia (Fig. 3-3), systemic candidiasis
   (3) AIDS-defining malignancies
     • Kaposi's sarcoma (Fig. 3-4), Burkitt's lymphoma (EBV), primary CNS lymphoma (EBV)

Margin notes:

Reservoir cell for HIV: follicular dendritic cells in lymph nodes

Most common malignancy in AIDS: Kaposi's sarcoma

CMV: most common cause of blindness in AIDS

TABLE 3-7. ORGAN SYSTEMS AFFECTED BY AIDS

ORGAN SYSTEM	CONDITION	COMMENTS
Central nervous system (CNS)	AIDS dementia complex (see Fig. 25-24C)	Caused by HIV Multinucleated microglial cells reservoir of virus
	Primary CNS lymphoma	Caused by EBV Most common extranodal site for lymphoma
	Cryptococcosis (see Fig. 25-26A)	Cause of CNS fungal infection
	Toxoplasmosis (see Fig. 25-26E)	Cause of space-occupying lesions
	CMV retinitis (see Fig. 25-40M)	Cause of blindness
Gastrointestinal	Esophagitis	Caused by *Candida*, herpesvirus, CMV
	Colitis	Caused by *Cryptosporidium*, CMV
Hepatobiliary	Biliary tract infection	Caused by CMV
Renal	Focal segmental glomerulosclerosis	Causes hypertension and nephrotic syndrome
Respiratory	Pneumonia	Caused by *Pneumocystis jiroveci* and *Streptococcus pneumoniae*
Skin	Kaposi's sarcoma	Caused by HHV-8
	Bacillary angiomatosis	Caused by *Bartonella henselae*

CMV, cytomegalovirus; EBV, Epstein-Barr virus; HHV-8, human herpesvirus type 8.

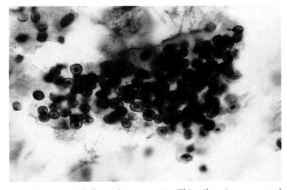

3-3: *Pneumocystis jiroveci* pneumonia. This silver-impregnated cytologic smear prepared from bronchial washings in an HIV-positive patient contains numerous *P. jiroveci* cysts. Some cysts look like crushed ping-pong balls. *(From Damjanov I, Linder J: Pathology: A Color Atlas. St. Louis, Mosby, 2000, p 56, Fig. 4-22B.)*

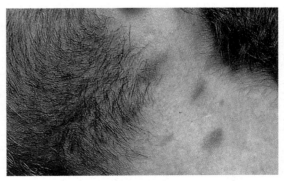

3-4: Kaposi's sarcoma in HIV. Skin lesions are raised, red, and nonpruritic. *(From Forbes C, Jackson W: Color Atlas and Text of Clinical Medicine, 2nd ed. St. Louis, Mosby, 2003, Fig. 1-48.)*

       (4) Causes of death
         • Disseminated infections (cytomegalovirus, *Mycobacterium avium* complex)

Death in AIDS: disseminated infection

     e. Immunologic abnormalities
       (1) Lymphopenia (low CD4 T-cell count)
       (2) Cutaneous anergy (defect in cell-mediated immunity)
       (3) Hypergammaglobulinemia (due to polyclonal B-cell stimulation by EBV)
       (4) CD4:CD8 ratio < 1
     f. CD4 count and risk for certain diseases
       (1) 700 to 1500: normal
       (2) 200 to 500: oral thrush, herpes zoster (shingles), hairy leukoplakia
       (3) 100 to 200: *Pneumocystis jiroveci* pneumonia, dementia
       (4) Below 100: toxoplasmosis, cryptococcosis, cryptosporidiosis
       (5) Below 50: CMV retinitis, *Mycobacterium avium* complex, progressive multifocal leukoencephalopathy, primary central nervous system lymphoma
  6. Pregnant women with AIDS
     • Treatment with a reverse transcriptase inhibitor reduces transmission to newborns to less than 8%.

D. Complement system disorders
  1. Overview
     a. Synthesized in the liver
     b. Augment natural host immune defense
       • Acute phase reactant (refer to Chapter 2)
     c. Circulate as inactive proteins
       (1) Activated by IgM, IgG-antigen complexes, endotoxin
         • Complement: only cleavage products are functional
       (2) Only complement cleavage products are functional.
     d. Functions complement cleavage products
       (1) C3a, C5a (anaphylatoxins)

C3a, C5a: anaphylatoxins

         • Stimulate mast cell release of histamine
       (2) C3b

C3b: opsonization

         • Opsonization
       (3) C5a

C5a: activate neutrophil adhesion molecules; chemotaxis

         (a) Activation of neutrophil adhesion molecules
         (b) Neutrophil chemotaxis
       (4) C5-C9 (membrane attack complex, MAC)

C5-C9: cell lysis

         • Cell lysis
  2. Complement pathways (Fig. 3-5)
     a. Classic pathway
       (1) Contains complement components C1, C4, C2
       (2) C1 esterase inhibitor
         (a) Inactivates the protease activity of C1
           • Protease normally cleaves C2 and C4 to produce C4b2b complex (C3 convertase)
         (b) Inhibitor is deficient in hereditary angioedema

Hereditary angioedema: deficiency C1 esterase inhibitor

     b. Alternative pathway
       • Contains complement components factor B, properdin, factor D
     c. Membrane attack complex (C5-C9)
       • Final common pathway for both the classic and alternative pathways.
     d. Decay accelerating factor (DAF)
       (1) Present on cell membranes
       (2) Enhances degradation of C3 convertase and C5 convertase
       (3) Protects the cell against MAC destruction
       (4) Deficient in paroxysmal nocturnal hemoglobinuria (PNH) (refer to Chapter 11)

DAF: deficient in PNH

  3. Testing of the complement system
     a. Total hemolytic complement assay (CH_{50})
       • Tests functional ability of both complement systems
     b. Tests indicating activation of classic system
       (1) Decreased C4, C3
       (2) Normal factor B

Classical pathway activation: decreased C4, C3; normal factor B

     c. Tests indicating activation of alternative system
       (1) Decreased factor B, C3
       (2) Normal C4

Alternative pathway activation: decreased factor B, C3; normal C4

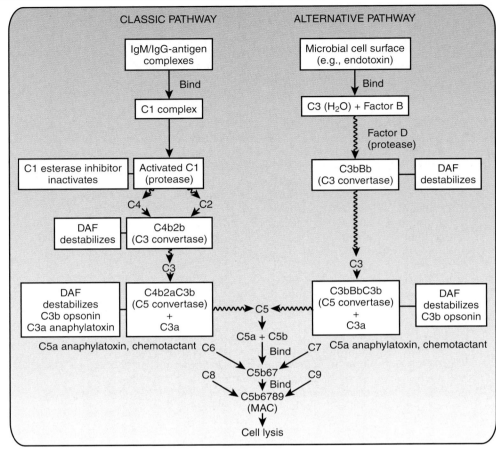

3-5: Complement cascade. Refer to the text for discussion. DAF, decay accelerating factor; MAC, membrane attack complex.

      d. Tests indicating activation of both systems
        • Decreased C4, factor B, C3
    4. Summary of complement disorders (Table 3-8)

VII. Amyloidosis
A. Amyloid
    1. Fibrillar protein that forms deposits in interstitial tissue, resulting in organ dysfunction
    2. Characteristics
      a. Linear, nonbranching filaments in a β-pleated sheet
      b. Apple green–colored birefringence in polarized light with Congo red stain of tissue (Fig. 3-6)
      c. Eosinophilic staining with H&E (hematoxylin and eosin) stain (Fig. 3-7)

Amyloid: apple green birefringence in polarized light

TABLE 3-8. COMPLEMENT DISORDERS

DISORDER	COMMENTS
Hereditary angioedema	Autosomal dominant disorder with deficiency of C1 esterase inhibitor Continued C1 activation decreases C2 and C4 and increases their cleavage products, which have anaphylatoxic activity Normal C3 Swelling of face and oropharynx
C2 deficiency	Most common complement deficiency Association with septicemia (usually *Streptococcus pneumoniae*) and lupus-like syndrome in children
C6-C9 deficiency	Increased susceptibility to disseminated *Neisseria gonorrhoeae* or *N. meningitidis* infections
Paroxysmal nocturnal hemoglobinuria	Acquired stem cell disease Defect in molecule anchoring decay accelerating factor (DAF), which normally degrades C3 and C5 convertase on hematopoietic cell membranes Complement-mediated intravascular lysis of red blood cells (hemoglobinuria), platelets, and neutrophils

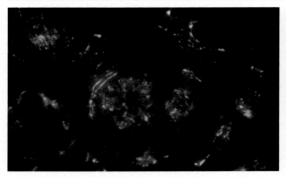

3-6: Amyloidosis: This Congo red–stained section of glomerulus and tubules reveals apple-green birefringence under polarized light in areas with amyloid deposition. *(From Kern WF, Silva FG, Laszik ZG, et al: Atlas of Renal Pathology. Philadelphia, Saunders, 1999, p 225, Fig. 19-17.)*

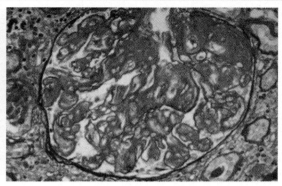

3-7: Amyloidosis: This hematoxylin and eosin–stained slide of a glomerulus shows eosinophilic acellular amyloid material in the glomerular tuft and capillary walls. *(From Kern WF, Silva FG, Laszik ZG, et al: Atlas of Renal Pathology. Philadelphia, Saunders, 1999, p 225, Fig. 19-20.)*

TABLE 3-9. COMMON TYPES OF AMYLOIDOSIS AND ASSOCIATED CLINICAL FINDINGS

TYPE OF AMYLOIDOSIS	CLINICAL FINDINGS
Primary and secondary	Nephrotic syndrome, renal failure (common cause of death) Arrhythmia, heart failure Macroglossia, malabsorption Hepatosplenomegaly Carpal tunnel syndrome
Senile cerebral	Dementia (Alzheimer's type) caused by toxic Aβ deposits in neurons Amyloid precursor protein coded by chromosome 21 Associated with Down syndrome

    d. Derived from various proteins
   3. Major types of amyloid proteins
    a. Amyloid light (AL) chain
     • Derived from light chains (e.g., Bence Jones protein)
    b. Amyloid-associated (AA)
     • Derived from serum-associated amyloid, an acute phase reactant (refer to Chapter 2)
    c. β-Amyloid (Aβ)
     • Derived from amyloid precursor protein (protein product of chromosome 21)

> β-Amyloid is associated with Alzheimer's disease in Down syndrome.

B. Types of amyloidosis (Table 3-9)
   1. Systemic
    a. Similar tissue involvement in both primary and secondary types
    b. Primary amyloidosis
     (1) AL amyloid disposition
     (2) Associated with multiple myeloma (30% of cases)
    c. Secondary (reactive)
     (1) AA amyloid
     (2) Associated with chronic inflammation (e.g., rheumatoid arthritis, tuberculosis)
   2. Localized
    a. Confined to a single organ (e.g., brain)
    b. Alzheimer's disease
     (1) Aβ
     (2) Most common cause of dementia
   3. Hereditary
    • Autosomal recessive disorder involving AA amyloid (e.g., familial Mediterranean fever)

C. Pathogenesis
    • Abnormal folding of normal or mutant proteins

> Amyloid: abnormal folding of protein

D. Techniques used to diagnose amyloidosis
   1. Immunoelectrophoresis (to detect light chains) in primary amyloidosis
   2. Tissue biopsy (e.g., adipose, rectum)

CHAPTER 4

WATER, ELECTROLYTE, ACID-BASE, AND HEMODYNAMIC DISORDERS

I. **Water and Electrolyte Disorders**
  A. **Body fluid compartments**
    1. Total body water (TBW) is ~60% of the body weight in kg (Fig. 4-1).
      a. TBW distribution
        (1) Intracellular fluid (ICF) compartment
          • Equals ~40% of body weight in kg
        (2) Extracellular fluid (ECF) compartment
          • Equals ~20% of body weight in kg
        (3) ECF is subdivided into the interstitial and vascular compartments.
      b. Sodium (Na^+) is the major ECF cation.
        • Chloride (Cl^-) major anion
      c. Potassium (K^+) is the major ICF cation.
        • Phosphate (PO_4^{2-}) major cation.
    2. Plasma osmolality (POsm)
      a. Osmolality is the number of solutes in plasma (i.e., tonicity of ECF).
        (1) Isotonic state = normal POsm
        (2) Hypotonic state = decreased POsm
        (3) Hypertonic state = increased POsm
      b. POsm = 2 (serum Na^+) + serum glucose/18 + serum blood urea nitrogen (BUN)/2.8 = 275–295 mOsm/kg
        • POsm roughly correlates with the serum Na^+ concentration.
      c. Urea diffuses freely between ECF and ICF.
        (1) Nephrologists frequently use the term effective osmolality (EOsm).
          • Excludes urea from the calculation, because it does *not* affect the osmotic gradient
        (2) EOsm = 2 (serum Na^+) + serum glucose/18
    3. Na^+ and glucose are limited to the ECF (impermeant solutes).
      a. Changes in their concentration produce an osmotic gradient.
        (1) Water shifts between the ECF and ICF compartments by osmosis.
        (2) Water moves from a low to a high solute concentration.
        (3) Water shifts do *not* occur with alterations in urea concentration.
          • Urea is a permeant solute and diffuses between the ECF and ICF.
      b. Hyponatremia (decreased POsm) causes water to shift from ECF to ICF (Fig. 4-2A).
      c. Hypernatremia and hyperglycemia (increased POsm) cause water to shift from ICF to ECF (Fig. 4-2B).
  B. **Isotonic, hypotonic, and hypertonic disorders**
    1. Serum Na^+ concentration (mEq/L) reflects the ratio of total body Na^+ (TBNa^+) to total body water (TBW).
      a. Serum Na^+ ~ TBNa^+/TBW
        • TBNa^+ is the sum total of all the ECF Na^+ (vascular space and interstitial space); unlike serum Na^+, which is the amount of Na^+ in a liter of serum/plasma in the vascular compartment.

Compartment sizes: ICF > ECF; interstitial > vascular

Na^+, K^+: major ECF and ICF cations, respectively

EOsm = 2 (serum Na^+) + serum glucose/18

Osmosis: H_2O moves between ECF and ICF; controlled by serum Na^+

Serum Na^+ ~ TBNa^+/TBW

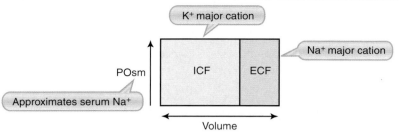

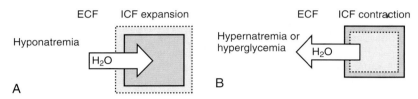

4-1: Body fluid compartments. See text for discussion.

4-2: Osmotic shifts in hyponatremia (**A**) and hypernatremia or hyperglycemia (**B**). See text for discussion.

b. Evaluation of TBNa⁺ status
  (1) Decreased TBNa⁺ produces signs of volume depletion.
    (a) Dry mucous membranes (Fig. 4-3)
    (b) Decreased skin turgor (i.e., skin tenting when the skin is pinched)
    (c) Drop in blood pressure and increase in pulse when sitting up from a supine position (i.e., positive tilt test)
  (2) Increased TBNa⁺ may produce body cavity effusions (e.g., ascites) and dependent pitting edema (Fig. 4-4).
    (a) Dependent pitting edema is due to an excess of Na⁺-containing fluid in the interstitial space (>2–3 liters).

↓ TBNa⁺: signs of volume depletion

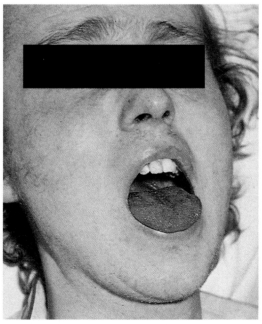

4-3: Patient with signs of volume depletion. The mucosal surface of the tongue is dry. Additional findings on examination were hypotension, tachycardia, and decreased skin turgor. *(From Forbes C, Jackson W: Color Atlas and Text of Clinical Medicine, 2nd ed. St. Louis, Mosby, 2003, Fig. 7-90.)*

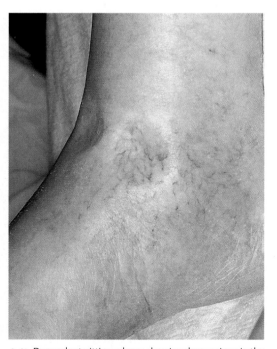

4-4: Dependent pitting edema showing depressions in the skin around the ankle. Pitting edema is due to an increase in vascular hydrostatic pressure or a decrease in vascular oncotic pressure (hypoalbuminemia). *(From Forbes C, Jackson W: Color Atlas and Text of Clinical Medicine, 2nd ed. St. Louis, Mosby, 2003, Fig. 5-8.)*

- Due to the low protein content in edema fluid, fluid obeys the law of gravity and moves to the most dependent portion of the body (e.g., ankles, if the person is standing).
    (b) An alteration in Starling pressures must be present to produce pitting edema and body effusions.

Fluid movement across a capillary/venule wall into the interstitial space is driven by Starling pressures (*not* osmosis). The net direction of fluid movement depends on which Starling pressure is dominant. An increase in plasma hydrostatic pressure or a decrease in plasma oncotic pressure (i.e., serum albumin) causes fluid to diffuse out of capillaries and venules and into the interstitial space, resulting in dependent pitting edema and body cavity effusions.

(3) An increase in TBNa$^+$ increases plasma hydrostatic pressure.
- Due to an increase in plasma volume
(4) An increase in TBNa$^+$ increases the weight of the patient.
- The most common cause of an increase in weight in a hospitalized patient is an increase in TBNa$^+$.
(5) Normal TBNa$^+$ is associated with normal skin turgor and hydration.
2. Isotonic fluid disorders (Table 4-1)
    a. Isotonic loss of fluid
        (1) Isotonic net loss of Na$^+$ and H$_2$O ($\downarrow$TBNa$^+$/$\downarrow$TBW)
        (2) POsm and serum Na$^+$ are normal.
        - The arrows represent the magnitude of change in TBNa$^+$ and TBW.
        (3) There is *no* osmotic gradient or fluid shift between ECF and ICF.
        - ECF volume contracts; however, the ICF volume remains normal.
        (4) Signs of volume depletion are present.
        (5) Examples include adult diarrhea, loss of whole blood.

Normal (isotonic) saline (0.9%) approximates plasma tonicity (POsm). It is infused in patients to maintain the blood pressure when there is a significant loss of sodium-containing fluid (e.g., blood loss, diarrhea, sweat). As expected, some of the normal saline enters the interstitial compartment and some remains in the vascular compartment, the latter being responsible for the increase in blood pressure. Other solutions that are used that are more expensive include Ringer's lactate and 5% albumin (remains in the vascular compartment).

    b. Isotonic gain of fluid
        (1) Isotonic net gain of Na$^+$ and H$_2$O ($\uparrow$TBNa$^+$/$\uparrow$TBW)
        (2) POsm and serum Na$^+$ are normal.
        (3) There is *no* osmotic gradient or fluid shift between ECF and ICF.
        - ECF volume expands; however, the ICF volume remains normal.
        (4) Pitting edema and body cavity effusions may be present.
        (5) Example is excessive infusion of isotonic saline.
3. Hypotonic fluid disorders (see Table 4-1)
    a. Hyponatremia (decreased POsm) is always present.
        (1) Osmotic gradient is present.
        (2) Water shifts to the ICF compartment (expands).
    b. Hypertonic loss of Na$^+$
        (1) Net loss of Na$^+$ in excess of water ($\downarrow\downarrow$TBNa$^+$/$\downarrow$TBW)
        (2) POsm and serum Na$^+$ are decreased
        (3) ECF volume contracts and ICF volume expands.
        (4) Signs of volume depletion are present.
        (5) Examples—causes of increased renal loss of Na$^+$ include loop diuretic, Addison's disease, 21-hydroxylase deficiency

In an alcoholic, rapid intravenous fluid correction of hyponatremia with saline may result in central pontine myelinolysis (see Fig. 25-28), an irreversible demyelinating disorder. However, as a general rule, all intravenous replacement of sodium-containing fluids should be given slowly over the first 24 hours regardless of the cause of the underlying serum sodium imbalance.

    c. Gain of pure water
        (1) Net gain in only water (TBNa$^+$/$\uparrow\uparrow$TBW)

Margin notes (left column):

$\uparrow\uparrow$ TBNa$^+$: pitting edema, body cavity effusions

Starling pressure alterations: control water movement in ECF compartment

$\uparrow$ Weight of patient in hospital: $\uparrow$TBNa$^+$

Isotonic loss: $\downarrow$TBNa$^+$/$\downarrow$TBW; loss whole blood, secretory diarrhea (e.g., cholera)

Isotonic gain: $\uparrow$TBNa$^+$/$\uparrow$TBW; excessive infusion isotonic saline

Isotonic loss or gain: serum Na$^+$ normal

Hypotonic disorders: hyponatremia always present; ICF expansion

Gain in fluid: ECF always expands

Loss in fluid: ECF always contracts

Hypertonic loss: $\downarrow\downarrow$TBNa$^+$/$\downarrow$TBW; loop diuretic, Addison's disease, 21-hydroxylase deficiency

Central pontine myelinolysis: rapid correction of hyponatremia with saline

TABLE 4-1. ISOTONIC AND HYPOTONIC DISORDERS

COMPARTMENT ALTERATION	POsm/Na+	ECF VOLUME	ICF VOLUME	CONDITIONS
Normal ECF and ICF volume	Normal	Normal	Normal	Normal hydration
Normal ECF and ICF				
Isotonic net loss Na+ + H₂O Isotonic loss 	Normal ↓TBNa+/↓TBW	Contracted	Normal	Adult diarrhea Loss whole blood
Isotonic net gain Na+ + H₂O Isotonic gain 	Normal ↑TBNa+/↑TBW	Expanded	Normal	Excessive isotonic saline
Net loss Na+ in excess of H₂O Hypertonic loss of Na+ 	Decreased ↓↓TBNa+/↓TBW	Contracted	Expanded	Loop diuretics Addison's disease 21-Hydroxylase deficiency
Net gain in only water Gain of water 	Decreased TBNa+/↑↑TBW	Expanded	Expanded	SIADH Compulsive water drinker
Net gain in H₂O in excess of Na+ Hypotonic gain of Na+ 	Decreased ↑TBNa+/↑↑TBW	Expanded Starling pressure alteration	Expanded	Right-sided heart failure Cirrhosis Nephrotic syndrome

ECF, extracellular fluid; ICF, intracellular fluid; POsm, plasma osmolality; SIADH, syndrome of inappropriate antidiuretic hormone; TB total body; TBW total body water.

(2) Decreased POsm and serum Na+
(3) Expansion of ECF and ICF volumes
(4) Normal skin turgor
(5) Examples—syndrome of inappropriate secretion of antidiuretic hormone (syndrome of inappropriate antidiuretic hormone [SIADH], e.g., small cell carcinoma of the lung), compulsive water drinking

d. Hypotonic gain of Na+
  (1) Net gain in H₂O in excess of Na+ (↑TBNa+/↑↑TBW)
  (2) Decreased POsm and serum Na+
  (3) Expansion of the ECF and ICF volumes
  (4) Caused by pitting edema states with Starling pressure alterations
    (a) Right-sided heart failure with increase in venous hydrostatic pressure
    (b) Cirrhosis and nephrotic syndrome with decrease in plasma oncotic pressure

Hypotonic gain of water:
TBNa+/↑↑TBW; SIADH

Hypotonic gain water +
Na+: ↑TBNa+/↑↑TBW

Pitting edema states: right-side heart failure, cirrhosis, nephrotic syndrome; cardiac output decreased

In these pitting edema states, the cardiac output is decreased, which causes the release of catecholamines, activation of the renin-angiotensin-aldosterone system, stimulation of ADH release, and increased renal retention of Na+. The kidney reabsorbs a slightly hypotonic, Na+-containing fluid ($\uparrow$TBNa+/$\uparrow\uparrow$TBW). Because these pitting edema states have alterations in Starling pressures, the Na+-containing fluid is redirected into the interstitial space, causing pitting edema and body cavity effusions. Unfortunately, the cardiac output remains decreased, until the cause of the decreased cardiac output is corrected.

Hypertonic disorder: hypernatremia or hyperglycemia; ICF contraction

4. Hypertonic fluid disorders (Table 4-2)
    a. Increased POsm is most often due to hypernatremia or hyperglycemia.
        (1) Osmotic gradient is present.
        (2) Water shifts from the ICF (contracts) to the ECF.
    b. Hypotonic loss of Na+
        (1) Net loss of H$_2$O in excess of Na+ ($\downarrow$TBNa+/$\downarrow\downarrow$TBW)
        (2) POsm and serum Na+ increased
        (3) Contraction of the ECF and ICF volumes
        (4) Signs of volume depletion
        (5) Examples—sweating, osmotic diuresis (e.g., glucosuria)

Hypotonic loss Na+ + water: $\downarrow$TBNa+/$\downarrow\downarrow$TBW; osmotic diuresis, sweating

    c. Loss of pure water
        (1) Net loss of only H$_2$O (TBNa+/$\downarrow\downarrow$TBW)
        (2) POsm and serum Na+ increased

TABLE 4-2. HYPERTONIC DISORDERS

COMPARTMENT ALTERATION	POsm/Na+	ECF VOLUME	ICF VOLUME	CONDITIONS
Net loss of H$_2$O in excess of Na+ Hypotonic loss of Na+ 	Increased $\downarrow$TBNa+/$\downarrow\downarrow$TBW	Contracted	Contracted	Osmotic diuresis: glucose Sweating
Net loss of only water Loss of water 	Increased TBNa+/$\downarrow\downarrow$TBW	Contracted (mild)	Contracted	Insensible water loss: fever Diabetes insipidus
Net gain in Na+ in excess of H$_2$O Hypertonic gain of Na+ 	Increased $\uparrow\uparrow$TBNa+/$\uparrow$TBW	Expanded	Contracted	Infusion of a Na+-containing antibiotic Infusion of NaHCO$_3$
Hyperglycemia Hyperglycemia 	Increased $\uparrow$Glucose $\downarrow$Na+ (dilutional effect)	Contracted	Contracted	Diabetic ketoacidosis Hyperosmolar nonketotic coma (type 2 diabetes)

ECF, extracellular fluid; ICF, intracellular fluid; POsm, plasma osmolality; TB, total body; TBW total body water.

(3) Contraction of the ECF and ICF volumes
   • ECF contraction is mild, because there has been no loss of Na^+.
(4) Normal skin turgor
(5) Examples
   (a) Diabetes insipidus, due to loss of antidiuretic hormone (ADH) or refractoriness to ADH
   (b) Insensible water loss (e.g., fever)
      • Water evaporates from the warm skin surface.
d. Hypertonic gain of Na^+
   (1) Net gain in Na^+ in excess of H_2O ($\uparrow\uparrow$TBNa$^+$/$\uparrow$TBW)
   (2) POsm and serum Na^+ increase.
   (3) ECF volume expands and ICF volume contracts.
   (4) Pitting edema and body cavity effusions may be present.
   (5) Examples include infusion of $NaHCO_3$ or Na^+-containing antibiotics.
e. Hypertonic state due to hyperglycemia
   • Examples—diabetic ketoacidosis (DKA), hyperosmolar nonketotic coma
   (1) Water shifts from the ICF to the ECF compartment.
      (a) Dilutional effect on serum Na^+ causes hyponatremia.
      (b) Increased POsm (due to hyperglycemia) and hyponatremia (dilutional)
      (c) Water does *not* remain in the ECF, because glucose in urine acts as an osmotic diuretic causing loss of water and Na^+.
   (2) Signs of volume depletion
      • Glucosuria produces a hypotonic loss of water and Na^+ (osmotic diuresis), causing signs of volume depletion.
C. Volume control (Box 4-1)

Hypotonic loss of water: TBNa$^+$/$\downarrow\downarrow$TBW; diabetes insipidus; insensible water loss

Hypertonic gain: $\uparrow\uparrow$TBNa$^+$/$\uparrow$TBW; excess $NaHCO_3$, infusion Na^+-containing antibiotic

Diabetic ketoacidosis: hypertonic state with dilutional hyponatremia; osmotic diuresis

---

BOX 4-1   VOLUME CONTROL

Protection of the intravascular volume is paramount to normal survival. Maintenance of the extracellular fluid (ECF) volume involves the integration of factors that (1) control thirst (e.g., increased POsm and angiotensin II [ATII]), (2) activate the renin-angiotensin-aldosterone (RAA) system (e.g., reduced renal blood flow, sympathetic nervous system stimulation), (3) stimulate the baroreceptors in the arterial circulation (e.g., decreased effective arterial blood volume), (4) increase free water reabsorption to concentrate the urine (e.g., antidiuretic hormone), and (5) increase renal reabsorption of Na^+ and water.

Effective Arterial Blood Volume
Effective arterial blood volume (EABV) is a conceptual term that refers to that portion of the ECF that is in the vascular space. In most instances, it correlates directly with the ECF volume and TBNa$^+$ status of the individual (i.e., $\downarrow$ EABV // $\downarrow$ ECF/$\downarrow$ TBNa$^+$ or $\uparrow$ EABV // $\uparrow$ ECF/$\uparrow$TBNa$^+$). However, in edema states, where there is an alteration in Starling pressures (e.g., right-sided heart failure), the redistribution of fluid (a transudate) from the intravascular compartment into the interstitial fluid compartment increases the total ECF volume at the expense of reducing the venous return of blood to the right side of the heart, reducing cardiac output, and reducing EABV ($\downarrow$ EABV // $\uparrow$ ECF/$\uparrow$ TBNa$^+$). Hence, an increase in total ECF volume does *not* always correlate with an increase in the EABV.

Baroreceptors and the Renin-Angiotensin-Aldosterone System
Control of the EABV is monitored by the pressure impacting upon the high pressure arterial baroreceptors located in the aortic arch and carotid sinus, and the flow of blood to the renal arteries. When the baroreceptors are activated by a decreased EABV, signals are sent to the medulla to increase sympathetic tone leading to release of catecholamines resulting in vasoconstriction of peripheral resistance arterioles (increases diastolic blood pressure), venoconstriction (increases venous return to the heart), increases heart rate (chronotropic effect), and increases cardiac contractility (inotropic effect). Signals are also sent to the supraoptic and paraventricular nuclei in the hypothalamus to synthesize and release antidiuretic hormone (ADH, vasopressin), the latter from nerve endings located in the posterior pituitary. ADH enhances the reabsorption of free water (fH_2O; water without electrolytes) from the collecting tubules in the kidneys and is a potent vasoconstrictor of the peripheral resistance vessels. Finally, the RAA system is activated owing to reduced blood flow to the juxtaglomerular (JG) apparatus located in the afferent arterioles and by direct sympathetic stimulation of the JG apparatus with subsequent release of the enzyme renin. Renin initiates the following reaction sequence: it cleaves renin substrate (angiotensinogen) into **angiotensin I** (ATI), which is converted by pulmonary **angiotensin converting enzyme** (ACE) into **angiotensin II** (ATII). ATII has a threefold function:

Continued

BOX 4-1   VOLUME CONTROL —cont'd

1. Vasoconstriction of peripheral resistance arterioles
2. Stimulation of aldosterone synthesis and release from the zona glomerulosa (increases Na^+ reabsorption in exchange for potassium ions [K^+] and hydrogen ions [H^+])
3. Direct stimulation of the thirst center in the brain

All of these events are an attempt to increase the EABV before medical intervention.

In contradistinction, when there is an increase in EABV, there are many counterregulatory mechanisms that come into play to eliminate the excess fluid prior to medical intervention. An increase in EABV is associated with a corresponding increase in cardiac output. This stretches the arterial baroreceptors, which triggers cessation of sympathetic outflow from the medulla. This, in turn, leads to inhibition of ADH synthesis and release, vasodilation of peripheral resistance arterioles, decreased cardiac contraction, inhibition of the RAA system, and decreased renal retention of Na^+ and water. Other counterregulatory factors also come into play including **atrial natriuretic peptide** (ANP), **prostaglandin E$_2$**, and **brain natriuretic peptide (BNP)**. ANP is released from the left and right atria in response to atrial distention (e.g., left- and/or right-sided heart failure). ANP has multiple functions including (1) suppression of ADH release, (2) inhibition of the effect of ATII on stimulating thirst and aldosterone secretion, (3) vasodilation of the peripheral resistance vessels, (4) direct inhibition of Na^+ reabsorption in the kidneys (diuretic effect), and (5) suppression of ren n release. Prostaglandin E$_2$ (1) inhibits ADH, (2) blocks Na^+ reabsorption in the kidneys, and (3) is a potent intrarenal vasodilator that offsets the vasoconstrictive effects of ATII and the catecholamines. BNP increases in the blood when the right and/or left ventricles are volume overloaded (e.g., left- and/or right-sided heart failure).

Renal Mechanisms in Volume Regulation

The response of the kidney to volume alterations is closely integrated with many of the events previously described. The reabsorption of solutes from the proximal tubules is dependent on the **filtration fraction** (FF) in the glomerulus in concert with Starling pressures that are operative in the peritubular capillaries. The FF is the fraction of the **renal plasma flow** (RPF) that is filtered across the glomerular capillaries into the tubular lumen. It is calculated by dividing the **glomerular filtration rate** (GFR) by the RPF (FF = GFR ÷ RPF). Normally, the FF is ~20%, with the remaining 80% of the RPF entering the efferent arterioles, which divide to form the intricate peritubular capillary microcirculation. Because prostaglandin E$_2$, a vasodilator, controls the afferent arteriolar blood flow into the glomerulus and ATII, a vasoconstrictor, monitors the efferent arteriolar blood flow leaving the glomerulus, the FF is significantly affected by alterations in their concentrations. Starling pressures in the peritubular capillaries determine how much of the fluid from the proximal tubule is reabsorbed back into the ECF compartment. A low peritubular capillary hydrostatic pressure (P_H) coupled with a high oncotic pressure (P_O) is responsible for enhancing the reabsorption of solutes from the tubular lumen into the tubular cell out into the lateral intercellular space, and into the peritubular capillary (A). This occurs when the EABV is decreased (e.g., ECF volume depletion, or hypovolemia). A high P_H coupled with a low P_O results in the loss of solutes in the urine in conditions when the EABV is increased (B; e.g., ECF volume overload, or hypervolemia). When hypovolemia is present in the ECF, the EABV is reduced and the FF s increased ($\uparrow$FF = $\downarrow$GFR ÷ $\downarrow\downarrow$RPF), hence increasing the filtered load of Na^+ and other solutes. The P_H is decreased and the P_O is increased, resulting in the reabsorption of the filtered Na^+ plus other solutes into the ECF compartment (e.g., urea) in isosmotic proportions. The above mechanism is so effective that a **random urine Na^+** (UNa$^+$) measurement is usually < 20 mEq/L and is often 0 when hypovolemia is extreme. In the presence of an increased EABV, or hypervolemia, the FF is decreased ($\downarrow$FF = $\uparrow$GFR ÷ $\uparrow\uparrow$RPF), the filtered load of Na^+ and other solutes is decreased, the P_H is increased and the P_O is decreased, hence favoring loss of the filtered Na^+ plus other solutes (e.g., urea, uric acid) in the urine (random UNa$^+$ > 20 mEq/L).

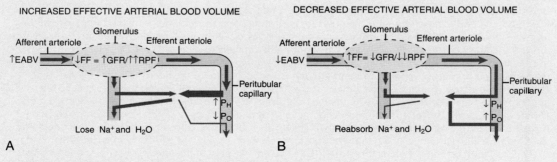

INCREASED EFFECTIVE ARTERIAL BLOOD VOLUME

DECREASED EFFECTIVE ARTERIAL BLOOD VOLUME

From Goljan EF: Star Series: Pathology. Philadelphia, WB Saunders, 1998, p 77, Fig. 5-2.

D. Correlation of nephron cotransporters and pumps with electrolyte disorders

1. Proximal renal tubule
   a. Primary site for Na^+ reabsorption
      (1) Na^+ reabsorption is increased when cardiac output is decreased.
         (a) $\downarrow$ EABV $\rightarrow$ $\uparrow$ FF $\rightarrow$ $P_O > P_H$
         (b) Examples—congestive heart failure, cirrhosis, hypovolemia
      (2) Na^+ reabsorption is decreased when cardiac output is increased.
         (a) $\uparrow$ EABV $\rightarrow$ $\downarrow$ FF $\rightarrow$ $P_H > P_O$
         (b) Examples—mineralocorticoid excess, isotonic gain in fluid
   b. Primary site for reclamation of bicarbonate (HCO_3^-; Fig. 4-5)
      • Mechanism for reabsorbing some of the filtered HCO_3^- back into the blood
      (1) Hydrogen ions (H^+) in tubular cells are exchanged for Na^+ in the urine.
      (2) H^+ combines with filtered HCO_3^- to form H_2CO_3 in the brush border of the proximal tubules.
      (3) Carbonic anhydrase (c.a.) dissociates H_2CO_3 to H_2O and CO_2
         • CO_2 and H_2O are reabsorbed into proximal renal tubular cells.
      (4) H_2CO_3 is re-formed in the proximal renal tubular cells.
         • H_2CO_3 dissociates into H^+ and HCO_3^-.

> Proximal tubule: reabsorb Na^+, reclaim HCO_3^-
>
> $\downarrow$ EABV $\rightarrow$ $\downarrow$ FF $\rightarrow$ $P_O > P_H$
>
> $\uparrow$ EABV $\rightarrow$ $\downarrow$ FF $\rightarrow$ $P_H > P_O$

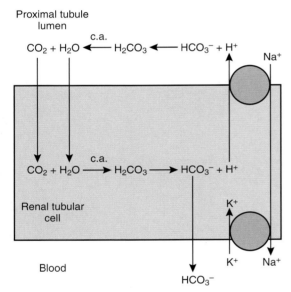

4-5: Reclamation of bicarbonate in the proximal tubule. See text for description. c.a., carbonic anhydrase. *(From Goljan EF, Sloka KI: Rapid Review Laboratory Testing in Clinical Medicine. St. Louis, Mosby Elsevier, 2008, p 32, Fig. 2-5.)*

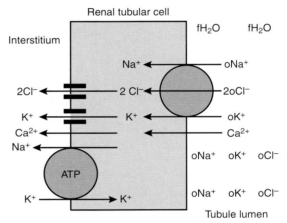

4-6: Sodium, potassium, chloride cotransporter in the medullary segment of the thick ascending limb. See text for description. ATP, adenosine triphosphate; f, free; o, obligated. *(From Goljan EF, Sloka KI: Rapid Review Laboratory Testing in Clinical Medicine. St. Louis, Mosby Elsevier, 2008, p 34, Fig. 2-6.)*

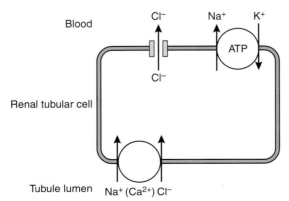

4-7 Sodium-chloride cotransporter in the early distal tubule. See text for description. ATP, adenosine triphosphate. *(From Goljan EF, Sloka KI: Rapid Review Laboratory Testing in Clinical Medicine. St. Louis, Mosby Elsevier, 2008, p 35, Fig. 2-7.)*

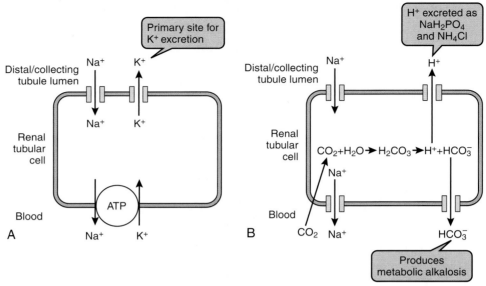

4-8 Sodium-potassium channels (**A**) and sodium-hydrogen ion channels (**B**) in the late distal and collecting duct. See text for description. ATP, adenosine triphosphate. *(From Goljan EF, Sloka KI: Rapid Review Laboratory Testing in Clinical Medicine. St. Louis, Mosby Elsevier, 2008, p 36, Fig. 2-8.)*

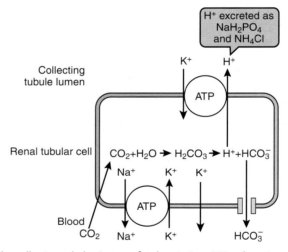

4-9: H+/K+-ATPase pump in the collecting tubule. See text for description. ATP, adenosine triphosphate. *(From Goljan EF, Sloka KI: Rapid Review Laboratory Testing in Clinical Medicine. St. Louis, Mosby Elsevier, 2008, p 37, Fig. 2-9.)*

     (5) HCO_3^- is reabsorbed into the blood.
     (6) An Na^+/K^+-ATPase pump moves Na^+ into the blood.
  c. Clinical effect of lowering renal threshold for reclaiming HCO_3^-
     (1) Example—normal threshold is lowered from the normal of 24 mEq/L to 15 mEq/L.
     (2) This results in loss of more of the filtered HCO_3^- than normal.
       (a) Urine pH > 5.5 (alkalinizing effect of increased HCO_3^-)
       (b) Urine loss of HCO_3^- occurs until serum HCO_3^- matches the renal threshold.

Carbonic anhydrase
inhibitor: causes proximal
renal tubular acidosis

Carbonic anhydrase inhibitors (e.g., acetazolamide) lower the renal threshold for reclaiming HCO_3^-. HCO_3^- combines with Na^+ to form $NaHCO_3$, which is excreted, hence acting as a proximal tubule diuretic. Loss of HCO_3^- produces metabolic acidosis (see later).

  d. Clinical effect of raising renal threshold for reclaiming HCO_3^-
     (1) Example—volume depletion associated with vomiting
     (2) Increased threshold means that proportionately more of the filtered HCO_3^- is reclaimed.

- Increased reclamation of HCO_3^- is the most important factor contributing to the increase in serum HCO_3^- that defines metabolic alkalosis (see later).

In **heavy metal poisoning** with lead or mercury, the proximal tubule cells undergo coagulation necrosis, which produces a nephrotoxic acute tubular necrosis (refer to Chapter 19). All of the normal proximal renal tubule functions are destroyed resulting in a loss of sodium (hyponatremia), glucose (hypoglycemia), uric acid (hypouricemia), phosphorus (hypophosphatemia), amino acids, bicarbonate (type II proximal renal tubular acidosis), and urea in the urine. This is called the Fanconi syndrome.

Heavy metal poisoning: produces Fanconi syndrome

2. Thick ascending limb (TAL; medullary segment)
   a. Primary function is to generate free water (fH_2O)
      - Secondary function is to reabsorb calcium (Ca^{2+})
   b. Generation of fH_2O primarily occurs in the active Na^+-K^+-$2Cl^-$ cotransporter (Fig. 4-6).
   c. Water proximal to the cotransporter is obligated (o).
      (1) Water is normally bound to Na^+ (oNa^+), K^+ (oK^+), and Cl^- (oCl^-).
      (2) Obligated water must accompany every Na^+, K^+, or Cl^- excreted in urine.
      (3) Obligated water *cannot* be reabsorbed by ADH, only fH_2O.
   d. Cotransporter separates oH_2O from Na^+, K^+, and Cl^-.
      (1) Water left behind in the urine is fH_2O.
         (a) fH_2O is entirely free of electrolytes.
         (b) Reabsorption of fH_2O concentrates the urine.
         (c) Loss of fH_2O in the urine dilutes urine.
      (2) Urine Osm (UOsm) is ~150 mOsm/kg distal to the TAL medullary segment.
   e. A Na^+/K^+-ATPase pump moves reabsorbed Na^+ into the interstitium.
   f. Reabsorbed Cl^- and K^+ diffuse through channels into the interstitium.
   g. Ca^{2+} is also reabsorbed by the cotransporter.
   h. Cl^- binding site in Na^+-K^+-$2Cl^-$ cotransporter is inhibited by loop diuretics.

Na^+-K^+-$2Cl^-$ cotransporter: generates free water

Cl^- binding site in Na^+-K^+-$2Cl^-$ cotransporter: inhibited by loop diuretics
Loop diuretic: hyponatremia, hypokalemia, metabolic alkalosis

Loop diuretics (e.g., furosemide) are the mainstay for the treatment of congestive heart failure and hypercalcemia. They decrease TBNa$^+$ and TBW (see above) and also decrease reabsorption of Ca^{2+} by the Na^+-K^+-$2Cl^-$ cotransporter. The drug attaches to the Cl^- binding site of the cotransporter, which not only inhibits reabsorption of Na^+, K^+, and Cl^- but also impairs the generation of fH_2O. The electrolytes are lost in the urine as obligated water. Because the normal dilution process is impaired, patients must be warned against consuming excess amounts of water. Loop diuretics also result in a hypertonic loss of Na^+ in the urine (see above) which, along with impaired dilution, may produce hyponatremia. Additional electrolyte abnormalities include hypokalemia and metabolic alkalosis (see later).

3. Na^+-Cl^- cotransporter in the early distal tubule
   a. Function is to reabsorb Na^+ and Ca^{2+}.
   b. Na^+ and Ca^{2+} share the same site for reabsorption (Fig. 4-7).
      - Parathyroid hormone (PTH)-enhanced Ca^{2+} reabsorption
   c. Na^+/K^+-ATPase pump moves Na^+ into the blood.
      - Cl^- diffuses through a channel into the blood.
   d. Thiazides inhibit the Cl^- site in the Na^+-Cl^- cotransporter.

Thiazides: inhibit Cl^- site in Na^+-Cl^- cotransporter

Thiazide diuretic: hyponatremia, hypokalemia, metabolic alkalosis, hypercalcemia

Thiazides in addition to being a diuretic are the mainstay for the treatment of hypertension in blacks and the elderly. Both patient populations have renal retention of Na^+ as the primary cause of the hypertension (refer to Chapter 8). Thiazides are also used in the treatment of hypercalciuria in Ca^{2+} renal stone formers (refer to Chapter 19). The drug attaches to the Cl^- site and inhibits Na^+ and Cl^- reabsorption. This leaves the Na^+ channel open for Ca^{2+} reabsorption.

Hyponatremia may occur due to a hypertonic loss of sodium (see earlier) in the urine. Additional electrolyte abnormalities include hypokalemia and metabolic alkalosis (see later). Hypercalcemia may also be a complication; however, this is uncommon and is more likely to occur if the patient has primary hyperparathyroidism with an increase in PTH.

4. Na^+ and K^+ channels in the late distal tubule and collecting ducts
   a. Aldosterone-enhanced pump functions to reabsorb Na^+ and excrete K^+.
   b. Na^+ diffuses into the cell (Fig. 4-8A).

c. K$^+$ diffuses out of the cell to maintain electroneutrality.
  • Primary site for K$^+$ excretion
d. Na$^+$/K$^+$-ATPase pump moves Na$^+$ into the blood.
e. Effect of K$^+$ depletion (hypokalemia, Fig. 4-8B)
  (1) Hydrogen (H$^+$) ions are excreted into the lumen in exchange for Na$^+$.
  (2) HCO$_3^-$ is reabsorbed into the ECF causing metabolic alkalosis.

Hypokalemia: increased risk for metabolic alkalosis

Amiloride and triamterene: diuretics with K$^+$-sparing effect

Amiloride and **triamterene** are diuretics with K$^+$-sparing effect. They bind to the luminal membrane Na$^+$ channels, hence inhibiting Na$^+$ reabsorption and K$^+$ excretion.

f. Effect of increased distal delivery of Na$^+$ from loop/thiazide diuretics acting proximal to this channel
  (1) Augmented Na$^+$ reabsorption and K$^+$ excretion
  (2) May produce hypokalemia, if K$^+$ supplements are *not* taken
  (3) May produce metabolic alkalosis if H$^+$ exchanges with Na$^+$ (see earlier)
5. H$^+$/K$^+$-ATPase pump (Fig. 4-9)
  a. Located in the collecting tubule; primary site for excretion of H$^+$ ions
  b. H$^+$ ions are secreted into the lumen and K$^+$ is reabsorbed.
  c. H$^+$ combines with HPO$_4^{2-}$ to produce NaH$_2$PO$_4$ (titratable acidity).
  d. H$^+$ also combines with NH$_3$ and Cl$^-$ to produce NH$_4$Cl.
    • Most effective way of removing excess H$^+$ ions
  e. Both titratable acid and NH$_4$Cl acidify the urine.
  f. HCO$_3^-$ is synthesized and reabsorbed into the ECF.
    • Primary site for regenerating (synthesizing) HCO$_3^-$

Spironolactone: aldosterone inhibitor; K$^+$ sparer

Spironolactone is a diuretic with a K$^+$-sparing effect. It inhibits aldosterone, which results in a loss of Na$^+$ in the urine (see Fig. 4-8A) and retention of K$^+$ in the blood (K$^+$-sparer). Hyperkalemia may occur in some cases. H$^+$ is retained, which produces metabolic acidosis in some cases (see Fig. 4-9).

An **angiotensin converting enzyme (ACE) inhibitor** is important in the treatment of congestive heart failure. Inhibition of the enzyme causes a decrease in angiotensin II (ATII) and aldosterone. ATII is normally a vasoconstrictor of peripheral resistance arterioles, which increases afterload (resistance the heart must contract against). Aldosterone normally reabsorbs sodium and increases preload (volume in the left ventricle). Therefore, an ACE inhibitor decreases both afterload and preload. The inhibition of aldosterone is short-lived and is frequently counterbalanced by the use of spironolactone.

6. Electrolyte changes in Addison's disease (also refer to Chapter 22)
  a. Most often due to autoimmune destruction of the adrenal cortex
  b. Pathogenesis of electrolyte abnormalities
    • Deficiency of aldosterone and other mineralocorticoids
  c. Clinical findings
    (1) Hyponatremia and hyperkalemia
      (a) Due to inhibition of Na$^+$ reabsorption and K$^+$ excretion (see Fig. 4-8A)
      (b) Hypertonic loss of Na$^+$ in the urine
        • Signs of volume depletion
    (2) Retention of H$^+$ ions, which produces metabolic acidosis
      • Due to dysfunction of the H$^+$/K$^+$-ATPase pump (see Fig. 4-9)

Addison's disease: hyponatremia, hyperkalemia, metabolic acidosis

7. Primary aldosteronism (Conn's syndrome; also refer to Chapter 22)
  a. Epidemiology
    • Benign adenoma arising in the zona glomerulosa
  b. Pathogenesis of electrolyte abnormalities
    (1) Enhanced activity of aldosterone channels and pumps (see Fig. 4-8A)
      • Increased Na$^+$ reabsorption and H$^+$ and K$^+$ excretion
    (2) Increased reabsorption of Na$^+$ causes hypernatremia.
    (3) Increased excretion of K$^+$ causes hypokalemia.
      • Hypokalemia produces severe muscle weakness (see later).
    (4) Increased excretion of H$^+$ (see Fig. 4-8B)
      • Causes increased synthesis and reabsorption of HCO$_3^-$ (metabolic alkalosis)

Primary aldosteronism: hypernatremia, hypokalemia, metabolic alkalosis

c. Effect of excess Na^+ in the ECF
    (1) Increases plasma volume
        (a) Increases stroke volume, which increases systolic blood pressure
        (b) Increases peritubular capillary hydrostatic pressure (P_H)
           • Prevents the proximal tubule from reabsorbing Na^+
    (2) Increases renal blood flow
        • Inhibits the renin-angiotensin-aldosterone system causing a decrease in plasma renin activity (PRA)
    (3) Excess Na^+ enters smooth muscle cells of peripheral resistance arterioles.
        (a) Na^+ opens up Ca^{2+} channels causing vasoconstriction of smooth muscle cells.
        (b) Increased total peripheral resistance increases the diastolic blood pressure.

Primary aldosteronism: low plasma renin type of hypertension

d. Summary of clinical findings
    (1) Hypertension
        • Due to retention of Na^+ (refer to Chapter 9)
    (2) Polyuria and muscle weakness
        • Complication of hypokalemia (see later)
    (3) Hypernatremia, hypokalemia, metabolic alkalosis
    (4) Decreased PRA
    (5) Absence of pitting edema and effusions
        (a) Due to excessive loss of Na^+ in the urine from inhibition of proximal reabsorption of Na^+ (called the escape mechanism)
        (b) Although $TBNa^+$ is increased, the amount of Na^+-containing fluid in the interstitial space is *not* enough to produce pitting edema.

Primary aldosteronism: absence of pitting edema

e. Treatment is surgery.

8. Bartter's syndrome
  a. Epidemiology
    • Majority of cases occur in children
  b. Pathogenesis
    (1) Renal defect in Cl^- reabsorption in the Na^+-K^+-$2Cl^-$ cotransporter
        • Similar to the mechanism of a loop diuretic
    (2) Loss of Na^+, K^+, and Cl^- ions in the urine
        • Hypertonic loss of Na^+ causes hyponatremia.
    (3) Augmented exchange of Na^+ and excretion of K^+ in distal/collecting tubules
        • Causes hypokalemia and metabolic alkalosis (see earlier)
    (4) Hypokalemia stimulates increased prostaglandin synthesis in the kidneys
        (a) Stimulates hyperplasia of the juxtaglomerular apparatus
        (b) Increased renin causes hyperaldosteronism.

Bartter's syndrome: normotensive

c. Clinical findings
    (1) Patients are normotensive (*not* hypertensive).
        • Due to vasodilation of peripheral resistance arterioles by prostaglandin
    (2) Muscle weakness due to hypokalemia
    (3) Increased PRA
        • Decreased PRA in primary aldosteronism.

Bartter's syndrome: hypokalemia, metabolic alkalosis; ↑ aldosterone and PRA

d. Treatment
    (1) K^+-sparing diuretic
        • Corrects K^+ loss
    (2) Nonsteroidal anti-inflammatory drug
        • Decreases prostaglandin synthesis

E. Dilution and concentration of urine

1. Normal dilution
  a. UOsm in the late distal tubule/collecting ducts is ~150 mOsm/kg.
    (1) Most of the water is fH_2O.
    (2) Small amount of water is obligated water (oH_2O) accompanying solute
  b. Decreased POsm inhibits ADH release from the posterior pituitary.
    • Absence of ADH results in a loss of fH_2O in the urine.
  c. Positive free water clearance (CH_2O)
    (1) $CH_2O = V - COsm$
        • V is the volume of urine in mL/min and COsm is obligated water.
    (2) $COsm = UOsm \times V/POsm$
    (3) Positive CH_2O indicates dilution.
        • Loss of fH_2O is greater than obligated water.

+CH_2O: indicates dilution; absence of ADH

(4) Example—urine volume 10 mL, POsm 250 mOsm/kg, UOsm 150 mOsm/kg
  - COsm = 150 × 10/250 = 6 mL, CH_2O = 10 − 6 = 4 mL

d. Syndrome of inappropriate ADH (SIADH; also refer to Chapter 22)

(1) Epidemiology

(a) Ectopic production of ADH
  - Small cell carcinoma of lung is the most common cause of SIADH.

(b) Drugs that enhance ADH effect
  - Chlorpropamide, cyclophosphamide, phenothiazines, narcotics

(c) CNS injury, lung infections (e.g., TB)

(d) Accounts for nearly 50% of hyponatremia in hospitalized patients

(2) Pathophysiology of electrolyte abnormalities

(a) Urine is always concentrated, because ADH is always present.
  - Negative CH_2O; UOsm is greater than POsm

(b) Hypotonic gain of water produces a dilutional hyponatremia (see section IB).

(c) Increased plasma volume increases peritubular capillary hydrostatic pressure (P_H).
  - Decreased proximal tubular cell reabsorption of Na^+ with random urine Na^+ > 40 mEq/L

(3) Clinical findings

(a) Mental status abnormalities from cerebral edema

(b) Mild SIADH treated by restricting water.

(c) Acute SIADH treated by combination of slow intravenous drip of hypertonic saline and intravenous furosemide.

> **Demeclocycline** is often used when a patient has a small cell carcinoma of the lung. The drug inhibits the effect of ADH on the collecting tubules (acquired nephrogenic diabetes insipidus), causing loss of fH_2O in the urine. It is unnecessary to restrict water while the patient is taking the drug.

2. Normal concentration

a. Increased POsm stimulates ADH synthesis and release.

b. ADH reabsorbs fH_2O and concentrates the urine.

c. Negative CH_2O clearance

(1) fH_2O is reabsorbed back into the blood.
  - Loss of obligated water is greater than fH_2O.

(2) Example—urine volume 10 mL, POsm 300 mOsm/kg, UOsm 900 mOsm/kg
  - COsm = 900 × 10/300 = 30 mL, CH_2O = 10 − 30 = −20 mL

d. Electrolyte abnormalities in diabetes insipidus (also refer to Chapter 22)

(1) Epidemiology

(a) Central diabetes insipidus (CDI) is absence of ADH.
  - Causes—CNS trauma and tumors

(b) Nephrogenic diabetes insipidus (NDI) is refractoriness to ADH.
  - Causes—drugs (e.g., demeclocycline, lithium) and hypokalemia (see later)

(2) Pathogenesis of electrolyte abnormalities

(a) Urine is always diluted and never concentrated.
  - Continual loss of fH_2O

(b) Positive CH_2O

(3) Clinical and laboratory findings

(a) Increased thirst and polyuria

(b) Hypernatremia due to a loss of water (TBNa$^+$/↓↓TBW).

(c) POsm > 295 mOsm/kg and UOsm < 500 mOsm/kg

(4) Treatment

(a) CDI is treated with desmopressin acetate.

(b) NDI is treated with thiazides.
  - Volume depletion decreases polyuria.

C. Potassium (K^+) disorders

1. Functions of potassium

a. Regulation of neuromuscular excitability and muscle contraction

b. Regulation of insulin secretion

(1) Hypokalemia inhibits insulin secretion.

(2) Hyperkalemia stimulates insulin secretion.

SIADH: small cell carcinoma of lung most common cause

SIADH: serum Na^+ < 120 mEq/L; dilution disorder

Serum Na^+ is usually < 120 mEq/L (136–145 mEq/L).

Treatment of SIADH: restrict water

−CH_2O: concentration; presence of ADH

oCH_2O: chronic renal failure; no concentration or dilution

CDI and NDI: hypernatremia, polyuria; concentration disorder

CDI: desmopressin ↑ UOsm (concentration); NDI: desmopressin no significant ↑ in UOsm

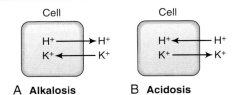

4-10: Potassium (K^+) shifts related to alkalosis (**A**) and acidosis (**B**). See text for discussion.

2. Control of potassium
   a. Aldosterone
      (1) Increases the excretion of K^+ and H^+ in the late distal and collecting tubules (see Fig. 4-8A)
      (2) Increases reabsorption of K^+ by the H^+/K^+-ATPase pump in the collecting tubules (see Fig. 4-9)
   b. Arterial pH
      (1) In general, alkalosis causes H^+ to move out of cells and K^+ into cells (Fig. 4-10A).
         • Potential for hypokalemia
      (2) In general, acidosis causes H^+ to move into cells (for buffering) and K^+ out of cells (Fig. 4-10B).
         • Potential for hyperkalemia
      (3) Exception—in diarrhea, there is a loss of K^+ and HCO_3^- in the stool, the former producing hypokalemia and the latter metabolic acidosis.
3. Hypokalemia (serum $K^+ < 3.5$ mEq/L)
   a. Causes of hypokalemia (Table 4-3)
   b. Clinical findings
      (1) Muscle weakness
         • Due to changes in the intracellular/extracellular K^+ membrane potential
      (2) U waves on an electrocardiogram (ECG; Fig. 4-11)
      (3) Polyuria
         (a) Collecting tubules are refractory to ADH (i.e., nephrogenic diabetes insipidus).
         (b) Tubule cells become distended with fluid (called vacuolar nephropathy).
      (4) Rhabdomyolysis
         • Hypokalemia inhibits insulin, which decreases muscle glycogenesis, leading to rhabdomyolysis.
4. Hyperkalemia (serum $K^+ > 5$ mEq/L)
   a. Causes (Table 4-4)
   b. Clinical findings
      (1) Ventricular arrhythmias
         • Severe hyperkalemia (e.g., 7–8 mEq/L) causes the heart to stop in diastole.
      (2) Peaked T waves on an ECG (Fig. 4-12)
         • Due to accelerated repolarization of cardiac muscle

pH changes: may cause shift of K^+ into or out of ICF

Insulin, β_2-agonist (e.g., albuterol): may shift K^+ into cell; hypokalemia
Digitalis, β-blocker, succinylcholine: may shift K^+ out of the cell; hyperkalemia
Loop and thiazide diuretics: most common cause of hypokalemia
Hypokalemia: ECG shows U wave

Renal failure: most common cause of hyperkalemia

Pseudohyperkalemia: RBC hemolysis from difficult venipuncture

Hyperkalemia: ECG shows peaked T waves

TABLE 4-3. CAUSES OF HYPOKALEMIA

PATHOGENESIS	CAUSES
Decreased intake	Occurs in elderly patients, those with eating disorders
Transcellular shift (intracellular)	Alkalosis (intracellular shift of K^+) Drugs enhancing Na^+/K^+-ATPase pump: insulin, β_2-agonists (e.g., albuterol)
Gastrointestinal loss	Diarrhea (~30 mEq/L in stool) Laxatives Vomiting (~5 mEq/L in gastric juice)
Renal loss	Loop and thiazide diuretics (most common cause): excessive exchange of Na^+ for K^+ in late distal and collecting tubules Osmotic diuresis: glucosuria Mineralocorticoid excess: primary aldosteronism, 11-hydroxylase deficiency, Cushing syndrome (excessive exchange of Na^+ for K^+ in late distal and collecting tubules), glycyrrhizic acid (licorice, chewing tobacco), secondary aldosteronism (cirrhosis, congestive heart failure, nephrotic syndrome; decreased cardiac output decreases blood flow and activates renin-angiotensin-aldosterone system)

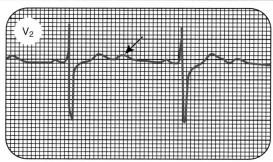

4-11: Electrocardiogram showing hypokalemia. A positive wave after the T wave is called a U wave (*arrow*). U waves are a sign of hypokalemia. *(From Goldman L, Bennet JC: Cecil Textbook of Medicine, 21st ed. Philadelphia, Saunders, 1999, Fig 102-7.)*

LEAD V$_3$

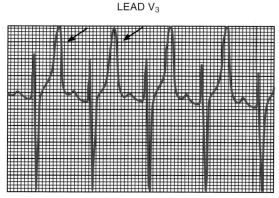

4-12: Electrocardiogram showing hyperkalemia. Arrows show peaked T waves, which are a sign of hyperkalemia. *(From Goldman L, Bennet JC: Cecil Textbook of Medicine, 21st ed. Philadelphia, Saunders, 1999, Fig 102-8A.)*

Chronic bronchitis due to smoking: common cause of respiratory acidosis

Respiratory acidosis: Paco$_2$ > 45 mm Hg

Full compensation: rarely occurs

(3) Muscle weakness
- Hyperkalemia partially depolarizes the cell membrane which interferes with membrane excitability.

II. **Acid-Base Disorders**
    A. **Primary alterations in arterial Pco$_2$ (Paco$_2$ = 33–45 mm Hg)**
        1. Respiratory acidosis
            a. Causes of respiratory acidosis (Table 4-5)
            b. Pathogenesis
                (1) Alveolar hypoventilation with retention of CO$_2$
                (2) Paco$_2$ > 45 mm Hg
                - $\downarrow$ pH ~ $\uparrow$ HCO$_3^-$/$\uparrow\uparrow$Pco$_2$
            c. Metabolic alkalosis is compensation
                (1) Serum HCO$_3^-$ $\leq$ 30 mEq/L in acute respiratory acidosis
                (2) Serum HCO$_3^-$ > 30 mEq/L (indicates renal compensation) in chronic respiratory acidosis

Compensation refers to respiratory and renal mechanisms that bring the arterial pH close to but *not* into the normal pH range (7.35–7.45). In primary respiratory acidosis and alkalosis, compensation is metabolic alkalosis and metabolic acidosis, respectively. In primary metabolic acidosis and alkalosis, compensation is respiratory alkalosis and respiratory acidosis, respectively. When the expected compensation remains in the normal range, an uncompensated disorder is present. If compensation moves outside the normal range but does *not* bring pH into the normal range, a partially compensated disorder is present. When compensation brings the pH into the normal range, full compensation is present, which rarely occurs.

TABLE 4-4. **CAUSES OF HYPERKALEMIA**

PATHOGENESIS	CAUSES
Tissue breakdown	Iatrogenic (e.g., venipuncture); pseudohyperkalemia Rhabdomyolysis (rupture of muscle)
Increased intake	Increased intake of salt substitute Infusion of old blood K$^+$-containing antibiotics
Transcellular shift (extracellular)	Acidosis Drugs inhibiting Na$^+$/K$^+$-ATPase pump: β-blocker (e.g., propranolol), digitalis toxicity, succinylcholine
Decreased renal excretion	Renal disease: renal failure (most common cause), interstitial nephritis (legionnaires' disease; lead poisoning) Mineralocorticoid deficiency: Addison's disease, 21-hydroxylase deficiency, hyporeninemic hypoaldosteronism (destruction of juxtaglomerular apparatus) Drugs: spironolactone (inhibits aldosterone); triamterene, amiloride (inhibit Na$^+$ channels)

TABLE 4-5. CAUSES OF RESPIRATORY ACIDOSIS AND ALKALOSIS

ANATOMIC SITE	RESPIRATORY ACIDOSIS	RESPIRATORY ALKALOSIS
CNS respiratory center	Depression of center: trauma, barbiturates	Overstimulation: anxiety, high altitude, normal pregnancy (estrogen/progesterone effect), salicylate poisoning, endotoxic (septic) shock, cirrhosis
Upper airway	Obstruction: acute epiglottitis (*Haemophilus influenzae*), croup (parainfluenza virus)	
Muscles respiration	Paralysis: ALS, phrenic nerve injury, Guillain-Barré syndrome, poliomyelitis, hypokalemia, hypophosphatemia ($\downarrow$ ATP)	Rib fracture: hyperventilation from pain
Lungs	Obstructive disease: chronic bronchitis, cystic fibrosis Other: pulmonary edema, ARDS, RDS, severe bronchial asthma	Restrictive disease: sarcoidosis, asbestosis Others: pulmonary embolus, mild bronchial asthma

ALS, amyotrophic lateral sclerosis; ARDS, acute respiratory distress syndrome; ATP, adenosine triphosphate; RDS, respiratory distress syndrome.

    d. Calculation of expected compensation in acute respiratory acidosis
      (1) Sometimes calculations help in identifying whether there is more than one primary acid-base disorder in a patient (called a mixed disorder; see later).
      (2) If the calculated expected compensation closely approximates the measured compensation, a single primary disorder is present.
      (3) If there is an obvious disparity between calculated expected compensation and measured compensation, another primary disorder is also present.
      (4) In acute respiratory acidosis, expected HCO_3^- compensation $= 0.1 \times \Delta P_{CO_2}$ (difference from normal of 40 mm Hg)
      (5) Example—pH 7.2, P_{CO_2} 74 mm Hg, HCO_3^- 27 mEq/L
        (a) Expected HCO_3^- compensation $= 0.1 \times (74 - 40) = 3.4$ mEq/L increase above normal
        (b) Expected HCO_3^- compensation $= 24$ mEq/L (mean HCO_3^-) $+ 3.4 = 27.4$ mEq/L
          • Note that measured and expected calculated HCO_3^- values are similar; therefore, a single disorder is present.
    e. Calculation of expected compensation in chronic respiratory acidosis
      (1) Expected HCO_3^- compensation $= 0.4 \times \Delta P_{CO_2}$
      (2) Example—pH 7.34, P_{CO_2} 60 mm Hg, HCO_3^- 32 mEq/L
        (a) Expected HCO_3^- compensation $= 0.4 \times (60 - 40) = 8$ mEq/L increase above normal
        (b) Expected HCO_3^- compensation $= 24 + 8 = 32$ mEq/L
          • Note that measured and expected calculated HCO_3^- values are similar; therefore, a single disorder is present.
    f. Clinical findings
      (1) Somnolence
      (2) Cerebral edema (vasodilation of cerebral vessels)
  2. Respiratory alkalosis
    a. Causes of respiratory alkalosis (see Table 4-5)
    b. Pathogenesis
      (1) Alveolar hyperventilation with elimination of CO_2
      (2) $Paco_2 < 33$ mm Hg
        • $\uparrow$ pH ~ $\downarrow HCO_3^-/\downarrow\downarrow P_{CO_2}$
    c. Metabolic acidosis is compensation.
      (1) Serum $HCO_3^- \geq 18$ mEq/L in acute respiratory alkalosis
      (2) Serum $HCO_3^- < 18$ mEq/L but > 12 mEq/L (indicates renal compensation) in chronic respiratory alkalosis
    d. Calculation of expected compensation in acute respiratory alkalosis
      (1) Expected HCO_3^- compensation $= 0.2 \times \Delta Paco_2$ (difference from normal of 40 mm Hg)
      (2) Example: pH 7.56, $Paco_2$ 24 mm Hg, HCO_3^- 21 mEq/L
        (a) Expected HCO_3^- compensation $= 0.2 \times (40 - 24) = 3.2$ mEq/L less than the normal

Formulas: help recognize single versus multiple acid-base disorders

Anxiety: most common cause of respiratory alkalosis

Respiratory alkalosis: $Paco_2 < 33$ mm Hg

(b) Expected HCO_3^- compensation = 24 mEq/L (mean HCO_3^-) – 3.2 = 20.8 mEq/L
  • Note that measured and expected calculated HCO_3^- values are similar; therefore, a single disorder is present.

  e. Calculation of expected compensation in chronic respiratory alkalosis
  (1) Expected HCO_3^- = 0.5 × $\Delta Paco_2$
  (2) Example: pH 7.47, $Paco_2$ 18 mm Hg, HCO_3^- 13 mEq/L
    (a) Expected HCO_3^- compensation = 0.5 × (40 – 18) = 11 mEq/L less than the normal
    (b) Expected HCO_3^- compensation = 24 – 11 = 13 mEq/L
      • Note that measured and expected calculated HCO_3^- values are similar; therefore, a single disorder is present.

  f. Clinical findings
  (1) Light-headedness and confusion
  (2) Signs of tetany
    (a) Thumb adduction into the palm (carpopedal spasm)
    (b) Perioral twitching when the facial nerve is tapped (Chvostek sign)
    (c) Perioral numbness and tingling

Tetany: commonly occurs in acute respiratory alkalosis

Alkalosis increases the number of negative charges on albumin (more COO^- groups on acidic amino acids). Therefore, calcium is displaced from the ionized calcium fraction and is bound to albumin, causing a decrease in ionized calcium levels and signs of tetany (refer to Chapter 22).

B. Primary alterations in HCO_3^- (22–28 mEq/L)
  • Applies to venous and arterial bicarbonate
  1. Metabolic acidosis
    a. Pathogenesis
    (1) Serum HCO_3^- < 22 mEq/L
      • ↓ pH ~ ↓↓ HCO_3^-/↓ Pco_2
    (2) Addition of an acid (increased AG type)
    (3) Loss of HCO_3^- or inability to synthesize HCO_3^- (normal AG type)
    b. Respiratory alkalosis is compensation.
    c. Calculation of the expected compensation in metabolic acidosis (either type)
    (1) Expected $Paco_2$ = 1.2 × ΔHCO_3^- +/– 2
      • ΔHCO_3^- is measured HCO_3^- subtracted from the mean HCO_3^- of 24 mEq/L.
    (2) Example: pH 7.27, $Paco_2$ 27 mm Hg, HCO_3^- 12 mEq/L
      (a) Expected $Paco_2$ compensation = 1.2 × (24 – 12) = 14.4 mm Hg less than the normal
      (b) Expected $Paco_2$ = 40 (mean $Paco_2$) – 14.4 = 25.6 mm Hg (23.6–27.6)
        • Note that measured $Paco_2$ is within the calculated range; therefore, only a single disorder is present.
    d. Increased anion gap (AG) type
    (1) Formula for calculating anion gap:
      (a) AG = serum Na^+ – (serum Cl^- + serum HCO_3^-) = 12 mEq ± 2, where the 12 mEq/L represent the anions that are *not* accounted for in the formula (e.g., phosphate, albumin, sulfate).
      (b) Therefore, if the AG is greater than 12 mEq/L ± 2, there must be additional anions present that should *not* be there (e.g., lactate, salicylate, acetoacetate, β-hydroxybutyrate anions).
    (2) In increased AG metabolic acidosis, excess H^+ ions of an acid (e.g., lactic acid) are buffered by HCO_3^-, which decreases the serum HCO_3^-.
    (3) HCO_3^- loss due to buffering is counterbalanced by the anions of the acid (e.g., lactate anions), which maintains electroneutrality.
      • Example—for every HCO_3^- ion that is lost, there is a lactate anion to replace it.
    (4) Example—serum Na^+ 130 mEq/L (135–147), serum Cl^- 88 mEq/L (95–105), serum HCO_3^- 10 mEq/L (22–28)
      • AG = 130 – (88 + 10) = 32 mEq/L (12 mEq/L ± 2).
    (5) Causes of increased AG metabolic acidosis (Table 4-6)

Metabolic acidosis: HCO_3^- < 22 mEq/L

↑ AG metabolic acidosis: anions of acid replace buffered HCO_3^-

Lactic acidosis: most common ↑ AG metabolic acidosis; e.g., anaerobic glycolysis in shock

TABLE 4-6. CAUSES OF INCREASED ANION GAP METABOLIC ACIDOSIS

CAUSES	PATHOGENESIS
Lactic acidosis	Most common type Any cause of tissue hypoxia with concomitant anaerobic glycolysis: e.g., shock, CN poisoning, CO poisoning, severe hypoxemia ($Pao_2 < 35\,mm\,Hg$), CHF, severe anemia (Hb < 6 g/dL) Alcoholism: pyruvate is converted to lactate from the excess of NADH in alcohol metabolism. Liver disease: liver normally converts lactate to pyruvate. Liver disease (e.g., hepatitis, cirrhosis) causes lactate to accumulate in the blood. Drugs: e.g., phenformin
Ketoacidosis	Diabetic ketoacidosis (type 1 diabetes mellitus): accumulation of AcAc and β-OHB Alcoholism: acetyl CoA in alcohol metabolism is converted to ketoacids. Increase in NADH causes AcAc to convert to β-OHB, which is *not* detected with standard tests for ketone bodies. Starvation
Renal failure	Retention of organic acids: e.g., sulfuric and phosphoric acids
Salicylate poisoning	Salicylic acid is an acid. It is also a mitochondrial toxin that uncouples oxidative phosphorylation leading to tissue hypoxia and lactic acidosis. In some cases, excess salicylate overstimulates the CNS respiratory center producing a primary respiratory alkalosis.
Ethylene glycol poisoning	Ethylene glycol is in antifreeze. It is converted to glycolic and oxalic acid by alcohol dehydrogenase. Oxalate anions combine with calcium to produce calcium oxalate crystals that obstruct the renal tubules causing renal failure. IV infusion of ethanol decreases the metabolism of ethylene glycol, because alcohol dehydrogenase is preferentially metabolizing alcohol. Unmetabolized ethylene glycol is removed by hemodialysis. Another treatment is the use of 4-methylpyrazole, which inhibits alcohol dehydrogenase. Osmolal gap > 10 mOsm/kg.
Methyl alcohol poisoning	Methyl alcohol is present in windshield washer fluid, Sterno, and solvents for paints. It is converted into formic acid by alcohol dehydrogenase. Formic acid damages the optic nerve causing optic neuritis and the potential for permanent blindness. IV infusion of ethanol decreases the metabolism of methyl alcohol, because alcohol dehydrogenase is preferentially metabolizing alcohol. Another treatment is the use of 4-methylpyrazole, which inhibits alcohol dehydrogenase. Osmolal gap > 10 mOsm/kg.

AcAc, acetoacetate; β-OHB, β-hydroxybutyrate; CHF, congestive heart failure; CN, cyanide; CO, carbon monoxide; Hb, hemoglobin; IV, intravenous; NADH, reduced form of nicotinamide adenine dinucleotide.

Calculation of the osmolal gap is useful in evaluating causes of an increased AG metabolic acidosis. The plasma osmolality (POsm) is calculated as follows: POsm = 2 (serum Na^+) + serum glucose/18 + serum blood urea nitrogen/2.8 + serum ethanol (mg/dL)/4.6 (if the patient is drinking ethanol) and is then subtracted from the measured POsm. A difference of <10 mOsm/kg is normal. A difference of >10 mOsm/kg is highly suspicious for methanol or ethylene glycol poisoning.

e. Normal AG metabolic acidosis
  (1) Due to a loss of HCO_3^- or an inability to synthesize (regenerate) or reclaim HCO_3^- in the kidneys
  (2) Cl^- anions increase to counterbalance the loss of HCO_3^- anions in order to maintain electroneutrality.
    • Produces a hyperchloremic normal AG metabolic acidosis
  (3) Example—serum Na^+ 136 mEq/L, serum Cl^- 110 mEq/L, serum HCO_3^- 14 mEq/L
    (a) AG = 136 − (110 + 14) = 12 mEq/L.
    (b) Drop of 10 mEq/L of HCO_3^- from normal (24 − 14 = 10) is counterbalanced by a gain of 10 mEq/L of Cl^- ions (100 + 10 = 110), hence the term hyperchloremic normal AG metabolic acidosis.
  (4) Causes of normal AG metabolic acidosis (Table 4-7)
f. Clinical findings
  (1) Hyperventilation (Kussmaul breathing)
  (2) Warm shock
    • Acidosis vasodilates peripheral resistance arterioles.
  (3) Osteoporosis
    • Bone buffers excess H^+ ions.

Normal AG metabolic acidosis: Cl^- anions replace HCO_3^-

TABLE 4-7. **CAUSES OF NORMAL ANION GAP METABOLIC ACIDOSIS**

CAUSE	PATHOGENESIS
Diarrhea	Most common cause in children Loss of HCO_3^- in stool: HCO_3^- is secreted from the pancreas to alkalinize the gastric meal
Cholestyramine	Binds HCO_3^- as well as bile salts, vitamins, and some drugs
Drainage of bile or pancreatic secretions	Bile and pancreatic secretions contain large amounts of HCO_3^-
Type I distal renal tubular acidosis	Inability to regenerate HCO_3^- in the H^+/K^+-ATPase pump in the collecting tubules. Excess H^+ ions in the blood combine with Cl^- anions. Hypokalemia is severe. Inability to secrete H^+ ions decreases titratable acidity and NH_4Cl causing the urine pH to be > 5.5. Causes: amphotericin, light chains in multiple myeloma Rx: oral administration of HCO_3^-
Type II proximal renal tubular acidosis	Renal threshold for reclaiming HCO_3^- is lowered from a normal of ~24 mEq/L to ~15 mEq/L Urine pH is initially > 5.5 due to loss of filtered HCO_3^- in the urine. When the serum HCO_3^- is equal to the renal threshold, the proximal tubules reclaim HCO_3^- causing the urine pH to drop to < 5.5. Hypokalemia may occur due to K^+ binding to HCO_3^-. Causes: carbonic anhydrase inhibitors (most common cause), primary hyperparathyroidism ($\uparrow$ PTH, $\downarrow$ proximal tubule HCO_3^- reclamation), proximal tubule nephrotoxic drugs/chemicals (e.g., aminoglycosides, heavy metals). Rx: thiazides to produce volume depletion, which increases the renal threshold for reclaiming HCO_3^-
Type IV renal tubular acidosis	Due to destruction of the JG apparatus: e.g., hyaline arteriolosclerosis of afferent arterioles in DM, acute or chronic tubulointerstitial inflammation (e.g., legionnaires' disease) Produces hyporeninemic hypoaldosteronism Only RTA with hyperkalemia: due to hypoaldosteronism

DM, diabetes mellitus; JG, juxtaglomerular; PTH, parathyroid hormone; RTA, renal tubular acidosis; Rx, treatment.

Loop and thiazide diuretics: most common cause of metabolic alkalosis
Metabolic alkalosis: $HCO_3^- > 28$ mEq/L

2. Metabolic alkalosis
   a. Causes of metabolic alkalosis (Table 4-8)
   b. Pathogenesis
      (1) Due to a loss of H^+ ions or a gain in HCO_3^-
      (2) Serum $HCO_3^- > 28$ mEq/L
        • pH ~ $\uparrow\uparrow HCO_3^- / \uparrow PCO_2$
   c. Respiratory acidosis is compensation.
   d. Calculation of expected compensation in metabolic alkalosis
      (1) Expected $PaCO_2 = 0.7 \times \Delta HCO_3^- \pm 2$
      (2) Example: pH 7.58, $PaCO_2$ 49 mm Hg, HCO_3^- 39 mEq/L
        (a) Expected $PaCO_2$ compensation = $0.7 \times (39 - 24)$ = 10.5 greater than the normal
        (b) Expected $PaCO_2$ compensation = 40 + 10.5 = 50.5 mm Hg (48.5–52.5)
          • Note that measured $PaCO_2$ is within the calculated range; therefore, only a single disorder is present.

TABLE 4-8. **CAUSES OF METABOLIC ALKALOSIS**

CAUSE	PATHOGENESIS
Vomiting	Loss of hydrochloric acid. For every H^+ ion lost in the vomitus there is a corresponding HCO_3^- in the blood. This causes metabolic alkalosis; however, it is filtered by the kidney and must be reclaimed in order to maintain the increase in serum HCO_3^-. Volume depletion from excessive vomiting increases proximal tubule reclamation of HCO_3^- (renal threshold for reclaiming HCO_3^- is increased). Correction of volume depletion with 0.9% normal saline corrects the alkalosis (chloride-responsive), because the renal threshold returns to normal and the excess filtered HCO_3^- is lost in the urine.
Mineralocorticoid excess	Gain in HCO_3^- Enhanced function of aldosterone-mediated Na^+-H^+ channels in the late distal and collecting ducts increases the synthesis of HCO_3^- leading to metabolic alkalosis (see Fig. 4-8); infusion of 0.9% normal saline does *not* correct the metabolic alkalosis (chloride-resistant). Causes: primary aldosteronism, 11-hydroxylase deficiency, Cushing syndrome
Thiazide and loop diuretics	Gain in HCO_3^- Block in Na^+ reabsorption leads to augmented late distal and collecting tubule reabsorption of Na^+ and excretion of H^+, the latter increasing synthesis of HCO_3^-, leading to metabolic alkalosis (see Fig. 4-8); volume depletion also increases the proximal tubule reclamation of HCO_3^-, which maintains the metabolic alkalosis.

e. Clinical findings
(1) Increased risk for ventricular arrhythmias
(2) Metabolic alkalosis left-shifts the oxygen-binding curve and its compensation, respiratory acidosis, decreases arterial Po_2 causing hypoxia in cardiac muscle, which precipitates ventricular arrhythmias.

C. Mixed acid-base disorders
1. Blend of two or more primary acid-base disorders occurring at the same time
2. Clues that suggest a mixed disorder
   a. Presence of a normal pH due to a combination of a primary acidosis and a primary alkalosis
      (1) Salicylate intoxication, particularly in adults
         (a) Salicylic acid produces a primary metabolic acidosis.
         (b) Salicylates overstimulate the respiratory center causing primary respiratory alkalosis.
      (2) Patient with chronic bronchitis who is taking a loop diuretic
         (a) Chronic bronchitis produces a primary respiratory acidosis.
         (b) Loop diuretics produce a primary metabolic alkalosis.
   b. Extreme acidemia due to a primary metabolic acidosis plus a primary respiratory acidosis
      • Example—cardiorespiratory arrest with primary respiratory acidosis (no ventilation) and primary metabolic acidosis (lactic acidosis from hypoxia)
3. Examples of how formulas help to identify a mixed disorder
   a. pH 7.26, $Paco_2$ 38 mm Hg, HCO_3^- 17 mEq/L
      (1) Presumptive diagnosis: metabolic acidosis ($HCO_3^- < 22$ mEq/L) without compensation ($Paco_2$ in normal range)
      (2) Formula for calculating expected compensation in metabolic acidosis
         (a) Expected $Paco_2 = 1.2 \times \Delta HCO_3^- \pm 2$
         (b) Expected $Paco_2 = 1.2 \times (24 - 17) = 8.4$ mm Hg less than the normal value
         (c) Expected $Paco_2 = 40$ (mean $Paco_2$) $- 8.4 = 31.6$ (29.6–33.6)
         (d) The measured $Paco_2$ is 38 mm Hg, which is higher than it should be, indicating that a respiratory acidosis (retention of CO_2) must also be present as a primary disorder.
   b. pH 7.38, $Paco_2$ 70 mm Hg, HCO_3^- 41 mEq/L
      (1) Presumptive diagnosis: mixed disorder (because the pH is normal) with chronic respiratory acidosis ($Paco_2 > 45$ mm Hg, $HCO_3^- > 30$ mEq/L) and primary metabolic alkalosis ($HCO_3^- > 28$ mEq/L)
      (2) Using either the formula for metabolic alkalosis or chronic respiratory acidosis will prove the presence of a mixed disorder.
      (3) Using the chronic respiratory acidosis formula (expected $HCO_3^- = 0.4 \times \Delta Paco_2$)
         (a) Expected HCO_3^- compensation $= 0.4 \times (70 - 40) = 12$ mEq/L increase above normal
         (b) Expected HCO_3^- compensation $= 24 + 12 = 36$ mEq/L
         (c) Measured HCO_3^- is 41 mEq/L, which is higher than the expected compensation indicating the presence of an additional primary metabolic alkalosis (more HCO_3^- than there should be for compensation).
      (4) Using the metabolic alkalosis formula (expected $Paco_2 = 0.7 \times \Delta HCO_3^- \pm 2$)
         (a) Expected $Paco_2 = 0.7 \times (41 - 24) = 11.9$ mm Hg increase from the normal
         (b) Expected $Paco_2 = 40 + 11.9 = 51.9$ mm Hg (49.9–53.9)
         (c) The measured $Paco_2$ is 70 mm Hg, which is much higher than it should be indicating the presence of an additional primary respiratory acidosis.

D. Selected electrolyte profiles (Table 4-9)
E. Selected arterial blood gas profiles (Table 4-10)

III. Edema
• Presence of increased fluid in the interstitial space of the ECF compartment
A. Types of edema fluid
1. Transudate
   a. Protein-poor (<3 g/dL) and cell-poor fluid
   b. Produces dependent pitting edema and body cavity effusions
   c. Associated with an alteration in Starling pressures (see section IB1)
2. Exudate
   a. Protein-rich (>3 g/dL) and cell-rich (e.g., neutrophils) fluid
   b. Produces swelling of tissue but *no* pitting edema

Clues for mixed disorder: normal pH; extreme change in pH

Salicylate intoxication: often mixture of primary metabolic acidosis and primary respiratory alkalosis; normal pH

pH defines what is the primary disorder versus what is the compensation.

Edema: excess fluid in interstitial space

Transudate: protein-poor and cell-poor fluid

Pitting edema: transudate; ↑ hydrostatic pressure and/or ↓ oncotic pressure

Exudate: protein-rich and cell-rich fluid

TABLE 4-9. **SELECTED ELECTROLYTE PROFILES**

SERUM NA⁺ (mEq/L)	SERUM K⁺ (mEq/L)	SERUM Cl⁻ (mEq/L)	SERUM HCO₃⁻ (mEq/L)	DISCUSSION
136–145	3.5–5.0	95–105	22–28	Normal ranges
118	3.0	84	22	SIADH: dilutional effect of excess water on all electrolytes
128	5.9	96	20	Addison's disease: lack of aldosterone causes loss of Na⁺ (hyponatremia), retention of K⁺ (hyperkalemia), and decreased synthesis of HCO₃⁻ (metabolic acidosis; see Fig. 4-8)
130	2.9	80	36	Vomiting: loss of Na⁺ and K⁺ in vomitus (hyponatremia, hypokalemia); volume depletion causes increased reclamation of HCO₃⁻ in proximal tubule (metabolic alkalosis; see Fig. 4-5)
				Loop and thiazide diuretics: hypertonic loss Na⁺ in urine (hypernatremia); augmented exchange of Na⁺ for K⁺ (hypokalemia) and increased regeneration of HCO₃⁻ (metabolic alkalosis, see Fig. 4-8)
152	2.8	110	33	Mineralocorticoid excess: primary aldosteronism; augmented exchange of Na⁺ for K⁺ (hypernatremia, hypokalemia), and increased synthesis of HCO₃⁻ (metabolic alkalosis, see Fig. 4-8)

SIADH, syndrome of inappropriate antidiuretic hormone.

TABLE 4-10. **SELECTED ARTERIAL BLOOD GAS PROFILES**

pH	Paco₂ (mm HG)	HCO₃⁻ (mEq/L)	DISCUSSION
7.35–7.45	33–45	22–28	Normal ranges
7.00	52	13	Mixed disorder (extreme acidemia): primary metabolic acidosis (HCO₃⁻ < 22 mEq/L), primary respiratory acidosis (Paco₂ > 45 mm Hg) *Example:* cardiorespiratory arrest
7.20	74	28	Acute respiratory acidosis, uncompensated (Paco₂ > 45 mm Hg, HCO₃⁻ < 30 mEq/L) *Example:* CNS respiratory center depression (e.g., barbiturate poisoning)
7.33	60	31	Chronic respiratory acidosis with partially compensated metabolic alkalosis (Paco₂ > 45 mm Hg, HCO₃⁻ > 30 mEq/L) *Examples:* chronic bronchitis, cystic fibrosis
7.28	28	12	Metabolic acidosis with partially compensated respiratory alkalosis (HCO₃⁻ < 22 mEq/L, Paco₂ < 33 mm Hg) *Examples:* disorders associated with increased and normal anion gap metabolic acidosis
7.42	22	14	Mixed disorder (normal pH): primary metabolic acidosis (HCO₃⁻ < 22 mEq/L), primary respiratory alkalosis (Paco₂ < 33 mm Hg) *Examples:* salicylate poisoning, septic shock
7.50	47	35	Metabolic alkalosis with partially compensated respiratory acidosis (HCO₃⁻ > 28 mEq/L, Paco₂ > 45 mm Hg) *Causes:* loop/thiazide diuretics, vomiting, mineralocorticoid excess
7.56	24	21	Acute respiratory alkalosis with partially compensated metabolic acidosis (Paco₂ < 33 mm Hg, HCO₃⁻ < 22 mEq/L) *Causes:* anxiety, pulmonary embolus, normal pregnancy

3. Lymphedema
   a. Protein-rich fluid
   b. Nonpitting edema
4. Glycosaminoglycans
   a. Increase in hyaluronic acid and chondroitin sulfate
   b. Nonpitting edema called myxedema

B. Pathophysiology of edema
1. Alteration in Starling pressure
   a. Produces a transudate
   b. Clinical examples of increased vascular hydrostatic pressure
      (1) Pulmonary edema in left-sided heart failure
      (2) Peripheral pitting edema in right-sided heart failure (see Fig. 4-4)
      (3) Portal hypertension in cirrhosis producing ascites (see Fig. 18-9)
   c. Clinical examples of decreased vascular plasma oncotic pressure (hypoalbuminemia)
      (1) Malnutrition with decreased protein intake (see Fig. 7-1, left)
      (2) Cirrhosis with decreased synthesis of albumin
      (3) Nephrotic syndrome with increased loss of protein in urine (>3.5 g/24 hours)
      (4) Malabsorption with decreased reabsorption of protein
   d. Renal retention of sodium and water
      (1) Increases hydrostatic pressure (increased plasma volume)
      (2) Decreases oncotic pressure (dilutional effect on albumin)
      (3) Examples—acute renal failure, glomerulonephritis
2. Increased vascular permeability
   a. Produces an exudate
   b. Example—acute inflammation (e.g., tissue swelling following a bee sting)
3. Lymphatic obstruction
   a. Produces lymphedema
   b. Examples
      (1) Lymphedema following modified radical mastectomy and radiation (see Fig. 9-8)
      (2) Filariasis due to *Wuchereria bancrofti*
      (3) Scrotal and vulvar lymphedema due to lymphogranuloma venereum
      (4) Breast lymphedema (inflammatory carcinoma) due to blockage of subcutaneous lymphatics by malignant cells (see Fig. 21-39F)
4. Increased synthesis of extracellular matrix components (e.g., glycosaminoglycans)
   a. T-cell cytokines stimulate fibroblasts to synthesize glycosaminoglycans.
   b. Example—pretibial myxedema and exophthalmos in Graves' disease (see Fig. 22-11)

IV. Thrombosis
- A thrombus is an intravascular mass attached to the vessel wall and is composed of varying proportions of coagulation factors, RBCs, and platelets.

A. Pathogenesis of thrombi
1. Endothelial cell injury
   - Due to turbulent blood flow at arterial bifurcations or overlying atherosclerotic plaques; cigarette smoke
2. Stasis of blood flow
   - Sluggish blood flow due to prolonged bed rest or sitting (e.g., long airplane flight)
3. Hypercoagulability
   a. Activation of coagulation system
   b. Causes of hypercoagulability
      (1) Hereditary or acquired factor deficiencies (refer to Chapter 14)
         - Example—hereditary antithrombin III deficiency or acquired deficiency due to oral contraceptives
      (2) Antiphospholipid syndrome (refer to Chapter 14)
         - Due to lupus anticoagulant and/or anticardiolipin antibodies

B. Types of thrombi
1. Venous thrombi
   a. Pathogenesis
      (1) Stasis
         (a) Procoagulants (e.g., tissue thromboplastin) released from damaged endothelium cause localized activation of the coagulation system.
         (b) Fibrin is produced, which forms a mesh around RBCs, platelets, and white blood cells in the stagnant blood within the vessel to produce a thrombus.
      (2) Hypercoagulable state

Pitting edema: right-sided heart failure due to ↑ hydrostatic pressure; cirrhosis due to ↓ oncotic pressure

Lymphedema: lymphatic obstruction after modified radical mastectomy and radiation

Endothelial cell injury: arterial thrombi

Stasis of blood flow: venous thrombi

b. Sites
  (1) Deep vein in the lower extremity below the knee
  (2) Other sites
    • Superficial saphenous, hepatic, and renal veins; dural sinuses
c. Composition
  (1) Adherent, occlusive, dark red fibrin clot (see previous)
    • Contains entrapped RBCs (primary component), white blood cells, and platelets
  (2) In the lower extremities, they propagate (extend) toward the heart.
    • Danger of pulmonary artery embolization once they reach the femoral vein
d. Anticoagulants heparin and warfarin prevent formation of venous thrombi (refer to Chapter 14).
  (1) Anticoagulants do *not* dissolve the thrombus; they only prevent further formation of a thrombus.
  (2) The fibrinolytic system (plasmin) is responsible for dissolution of the thrombus.
2. Arterial thrombi
  a. Pathogenesis
    (1) Endothelial cell injury due to turbulent blood flow
      • Platelets adhere to areas of injury.
    (2) Hypercoagulable state
  b. Sites
    (1) Elastic and muscular arteries
    (2) Majority of thrombi overlie disrupted atherosclerotic plaques
      • Example—coronary artery thrombosis (Fig. 4-13)
  c. Composition of thrombi in muscular arteries and aortic branches
    (1) Adherent, usually occlusive, gray-white fibrin clot composed of platelets
    (2) Aspirin and other inhibitors of platelet aggregation prevent formation of these thrombi (refer to Chapter 14).
  d. Composition of thrombi in the heart chambers and aorta
    (1) Laminated thrombi with alternating pale and red areas (lines of Zahn)
      (a) Pale areas are composed of platelets held together by fibrin.
      (b) Red areas are composed predominantly of RBCs held together by fibrin.
      (c) Mixed type of thrombus
    (2) Examples of thrombi in the heart chambers
      (a) Thrombus in left ventricle due to a transmural myocardial infarction (mural thrombus)
      (b) Thrombus in left atrium in patients with mitral stenosis complicated by atrial fibrillation
    (3) Thrombi in the aorta usually develop in aneurysms.
      • Example—abdominal aortic aneurysm (see Fig. 9-4)

Most common site for venous thrombosis: deep vein in lower extremity below the knee

Composition venous thrombus: entrapped RBCs, platelets, white blood cells

Heparin and warfarin: anticoagulants that prevent venous thrombosis

Composition of arterial thrombus: fibrin clot composed of platelets

Aspirin: prevents formation of arterial thrombi

Mixed thrombus: prevented by aspirin along with anticoagulant therapy

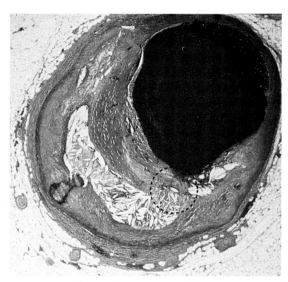

4-13: Coronary artery thrombosis. In this specially stained cross-section of a coronary artery, collagen is blue and the thrombus is red. The red thrombus in the vessel lumen is composed of platelets held together by fibrin. Directly beneath the thrombus is a fibrous plaque, which stains blue. Beneath the plaque is necrotic atheromatous debris. The circle shows disruption of the fibrous plaque with cholesterol crystals extending through the wall to the lumen. *(From Damjanov I, Linder J: Pathology: A Color Atlas. St. Louis, Mosby, 2000, p 21, Fig. 1-44.)*

(4) Aspirin along with anticoagulant therapy helps to prevent these types of mixed thrombi.
  e. Clinical findings in arterial thrombosis
    (1) Infarction (e.g., acute myocardial infarction, stroke)
    (2) Embolization
  3. Postmortem clot
    a. Fibrin clot of plasma (resembles chicken fat) *without* entrapped cells
    b. It is *not* attached to the vessel wall.
V. **Embolism**
  • Detached mass (e.g., clot, fat, gas) that is carried through the blood to a distant site
  A. **Pulmonary thromboembolism** (refer to Chapter 16)
    1. Site of origin
      a. Majority originate from the femoral vein (extension of deep vein thrombus).
      b. Others originate from the pelvic veins or vena cava.
    2. Clinical findings
      a. Sudden death
        • Due to a saddle embolus occluding the major pulmonary artery branches (see Fig. 16-15)
      b. Pulmonary infarction
        (1) Small thromboemboli occlude medium-sized or small pulmonary arteries (see Fig. 1-11C).
        (2) Less than 10% of thromboemboli produce infarction.
          • Due to dual blood supply of the lungs: pulmonary artery, bronchial artery (refer to Chapter 16)
      c. Paradoxic embolism
        • Venous thromboembolus passes through an atrial septal defect into the systemic circulation.
  B. **Systemic embolism**
    • Emboli traveling in the arterial system
    1. Causes of systemic embolism
      a. Thrombi from the left side of the heart (80% of cases)
        (1) Mural thrombus in left ventricle following acute myocardial infarction
        (2) Thrombus in the left atrium in mitral stenosis
          • Atrial fibrillation predisposes to atrial clot formation and embolization.
      b. Atrial myxoma, vegetations from aortic or mitral valve
    2. Sites of embolism
      a. Lower extremities (most common)
      b. Brain (via the middle cerebral artery)
      c. Small bowel (via the superior mesenteric artery)
      d. Spleen and kidneys
    3. Clinical findings
      a. Pale infarctions in the digits, spleen, and kidneys
      b. Hemorrhagic infarctions in the brain and small bowel (see Chapter 1)
  C. **Fat embolism**
    1. Causes
      a. Most often due to traumatic fracture of the long bones (e.g., femur) or pelvis
      b. Other causes include trauma to fat-laden tissues (liposuction), fatty liver.
    2. Pathogenesis
      a. Microglobules of fat from the bone marrow gain access to the microvasculature.
      b. Microglobules eventually obstruct the microvasculature in the brain, lungs, kidneys, and other sites.
        • Produces ischemia and hemorrhage
      c. Fatty acids derived from breakdown of the microglobules damage vessel endothelium.
        • Platelet thrombi develop in areas of endothelial injury.
    3. Clinical findings
      a. Symptoms begin 24 to 72 hours after trauma.
      b. Restlessness, delirium, coma
      c. Dyspnea, tachypnea
        (1) Fat microglobules in pulmonary capillaries cause hypoxemia.
        (2) Massive perfusion defect

Pulmonary thromboembolism: majority originate in femoral veins

Pulmonary infarction uncommon: due to dual blood supply—pulmonary arteries, bronchial arteries

Systemic embolism: majority originate in left side of heart

Fat embolism: fracture of long bones

Fat embolism: dyspnea, petechia over chest/upper extremities

　　　　d. Petechiae commonly develop over the chest and upper extremities.
　　　　　　• Due to thrombocytopenia from platelet adhesion to microglobules of fat
　　　　e. Death results in less than 10% of cases.
　　4. Diagnosis
　　　　a. Usually a clinical diagnosis based on above findings
　　　　b. Search for fat globules in urine, pulmonary alveolar lavage, spinal fluid
　　5. Treatment is supportive
　　　　• Maintain good arterial oxygenation

D. Amniotic fluid (AF) embolism
　　1. Occurs during labor or immediately post-partum
　　2. Pathogenesis
　　　　a. Tears in placental membranes or uterine veins
　　　　b. Infusion of amniotic fluid into the maternal circulation
　　　　　　• Leads to cardiorespiratory collapse (? anaphylactic reaction to fetal antigens) and disseminated intravascular coagulation (procoagulants in AF)
　　3. Clinical findings

Amniotic fluid embolism: abrupt onset dyspnea, hypotension, bleeding (DIC)

　　　　a. Abrupt onset of dyspnea, cyanosis, hypotension, and bleeding
　　　　　　(1) Dyspnea is due to pulmonary edema or acute respiratory distress syndrome.
　　　　　　(2) Bleeding is due to disseminated intravascular coagulation (DIC).
　　　　b. Diagnosis is most often confirmed at autopsy.
　　　　　　• Fetal squamous cells are present in the pulmonary vessels.
　　　　c. Maternal mortality rate varies from 60% to 80%.
　　　　　　• Most women who survive have permanent neurologic impairment.
　　4. Treatment is supportive.

E. Decompression sickness
　　1. Form of gas embolism
　　2. Scuba and deep sea diving is the most common cause.
　　3. Pathogenesis
　　　　a. Atmospheric pressure increases by 1 for every 33 feet of descent into water.
　　　　b. Nitrogen gas is forced out of the alveoli and dissolves in blood and tissues.
　　　　c. Rapid ascent causes nitrogen to expand and form gas bubbles in tissue and vessel lumens.

Decompression sickness: nitrogen gas bubbles occlude vessel lumens

　　4. Clinical findings
　　　　a. Pain develops in joints, muscles, and bones.
　　　　　　• Called "the bends"
　　　　b. Pneumothorax (refer to Chapter 16)
　　　　　　(1) Complication of a sudden rise to the surface
　　　　　　(2) Due to rupture of a preexisting subpleural or intrapleural bleb
　　　　　　(3) Causes dyspnea and pleuritic chest pain
　　　　c. Pulmonary embolus
　　　　　　(1) Pressure on the veins in the lower extremities produces stasis and thrombus formation.
　　　　　　(2) Pulmonary thromboembolism occurs
　　　　　　(3) Causes dyspnea and pleuritic chest pain

Pneumothorax, pulmonary embolism, aseptic necrosis: complications of scuba diving

　　　　d. Chronic changes
　　　　　　• Aseptic necrosis in bones (femur, tibia, humerus) from bone infarctions
　　5. Treatment
　　　　• Recompression (nitrogen forced back into tissue) followed by slow decompression

VI. Shock
　　• Shock is reduced perfusion of tissue, which results in impaired oxygenation of tissue.

A. Types of shock
　　1. Hypovolemic shock

Hypovolemic shock: most often caused by blood loss

　　　　a. Due to excessive fluid loss (e.g., blood, sweat)
　　　　b. Hemorrhage
　　　　　　(1) Loss of greater than 20% of blood volume (~1000 mL) results in shock.
　　　　　　(2) *No* initial effect on hemoglobin and hematocrit concentration
　　　　　　　　(a) Absolute neutrophilic leukocytosis is the first hematologic sign.
　　　　　　　　(b) Infusion of 0.9% saline immediately uncovers the RBC deficit.
　　　　　　(3) Plasma is replaced first with fluid from the interstitial space.
　　　　　　　　• Uncovers the RBC deficit within hours to days

(4) RBC response in the bone marrow begins in 5 to 7 days.
c. Pathophysiology of hypovolemic shock
   (1) Decreased cardiac output (CO)
      • Due to decreased volume of blood
   (2) Decreased left ventricular end-diastolic pressure (LVEDP)
   (3) Increased peripheral vascular resistance (PVR)
      • Due to vasoconstriction of arterioles from catecholamines, ADH, and angiotensin II, which are released in response to the decreased CO
   (4) Decreased mixed venous oxygen content (MVO_2)
      (a) Best indicator of tissue hypoxia
      (b) Measured in the right side of the heart with a Swan-Ganz catheter
      (c) Indicates the degree of extraction of O_2 from the blood delivered to tissue
      (d) In hypovolemic shock, decreased blood flow through the microcirculation leads to increased extraction of O_2 from the blood and a decreased MVO_2.
d. Clinical findings in hypovolemic shock
   (1) Cold, clammy skin due to vasoconstriction of skin vessels
   (2) Hypotension; rapid, weak pulse (compensatory response to decreased CO)
2. Cardiogenic shock
a. Most commonly caused by an acute myocardial infarction
b. Pathophysiology of cardiogenic shock
   (1) Decreased CO
      • Due to decreased force of contraction in the left ventricle
   (2) Increased LVEDP
      • Blood accumulates in the left ventricle.
   (3) Increased PVR
      • Same mechanism as in hypovolemic shock
   (4) Decreased MVO_2
      • Same mechanism as in hypovolemic shock
c. Clinical findings in cardiogenic shock
   • Chest pain followed by signs similar to hypovolemic shock
3. Septic shock
a. Septicemia is most commonly due to gram-negative pathogens (e.g., *Escherichia coli*).
b. Pathogenesis
   (1) Endotoxins damage endothelial cells.
      • Causes the release of vasodilators such as nitric oxide and prostaglandin I_2
   (2) Endotoxins activate the alternative complement pathway.
      • Anaphylatoxins (C3a and C5a) are produced, which stimulate mast cell release of histamine (vasodilator)
   (3) Interleukin 1 and tumor necrosis factor (TNF) are released from macrophages.
      (a) Activate neutrophil adhesion molecules, causing neutrophil adherence to pulmonary capillaries
      (b) Circulating neutrophil pool becomes part of the marginating neutrophil pool (refer to Chapter 2).
      (c) High levels of TNF contribute to the vascular leakage syndrome.
         • Important in the pathophysiology of acute respiratory distress syndrome
c. Pathophysiology of septic shock
   (1) Initial increase in CO
      • Due to rapid blood flow through dilated peripheral resistance arterioles, causing increased return of blood to the heart
   (2) Decreased LVEDP
      • Due to neutrophil transmigration through the pulmonary capillaries into alveoli producing noncardiogenic pulmonary edema
   (3) Decreased PVR
      • Due to vasodilation of peripheral resistance arterioles
   (4) Increased MVO_2
      • Tissues are unable to extract O_2, because of the increased blood flow.
d. Clinical findings in septic shock
   (1) Warm skin, due to vasodilation of skin vessels
   (2) Bounding pulse, due to increased CO
   (3) Acute respiratory distress syndrome
      • Due to neutrophil transmigration into alveoli

MVO_2: best indicator of tissue hypoxia

Hypovolemic shock: ↓CO, ↓LVEDP, ↑PVR, ↓MVO_2

Cardiogenic shock: most often caused by acute myocardial infarction

Cardiogenic shock: ↓CO, ↑LVEDP, ↑PVR, ↓MVO_2

Septic shock: most often caused by sepsis due to *E. coli*

Septic shock (initial phase): ↑CO, ↓LVEDP, ↓PVR, ↑MVO_2

TABLE 4-11. **SUMMARY OF PATHOPHYSIOLOGIC FINDINGS IN HYPOVOLEMIC, CARDIOGENIC, AND SEPTIC SHOCK**

TYPE OF SHOCK	CO	PVR	LVEDP	MVO$_2$
Hypovolemic	↓	↑	↓	↓
Cardiogenic	↓	↑	↑	↓
Endotoxic (septic)	↑	↓	↓	↑

CO, cardiac output; LVEDP, left ventricular end-diastolic pressure; MVO$_2$, mixed venous oxygen content; PVR, peripheral vascular resistance.

(4) Disseminated intravascular coagulation
  • Due to activation of the intrinsic and extrinsic coagulation system
4. Summary of pathophysiologic findings in shock (Table 4-11)
B. Complications associated with shock
  1. Ischemic acute tubular necrosis
    • Coagulation necrosis of proximal tubule cells and cells in the thick ascending limb

Multiorgan dysfunction: most common cause of death in shock

  2. Multiorgan dysfunction
    • Most common cause of death
  3. Lactic acidosis due to tissue hypoxia

5
GENETIC AND DEVELOPMENTAL DISORDERS

I. **Mutations**
- Mutations are a permanent change in DNA.
   A. **Point mutations**
      - Mutation involving a change in a single nucleotide base within a gene
      1. Silent mutation (Fig. 5-1A)
         - Altered DNA codes for the *same* amino acid without changing the phenotypic effect
      2. Missense mutation (Fig. 5-1B)
         - Altered DNA codes for a *different* amino acid, which changes the phenotypic effect

Missense mutation: sickle cell disease/trait

> In both **sickle cell trait** and **sickle cell disease**, a missense mutation occurs when adenine replaces thymidine, causing valine to replace glutamic acid in the sixth position of the β-globin chain. As a result, RBCs spontaneously sickle in the peripheral blood if the amount of sickle hemoglobin is greater than 60%.

      3. Nonsense mutation (Fig. 5-1C)
         - Altered DNA codes for a stop codon that causes premature termination of protein synthesis

β-Thalassemia major: nonsense mutation with stop codon

> In β-**thalassemia major**, a nonsense mutation produces a stop codon that causes premature termination of DNA transcription of the β-globin chain. Consequently, there is no synthesis of hemoglobin A ($\alpha_2\beta_2$), resulting in a microcytic anemia.

   B. **Frameshift mutation**
      1. Insertion or deletion of one or more nucleotides shifts the reading frame of the DNA strand
      2. Example—in Tay-Sachs disease, a four-base insertion results in an altered DNA code leading to formation of a stop codon leading to decreased synthesis of hexosaminidase (Fig. 5-2).

Frameshift mutation: Tay-Sachs disease

   C. **Trinucleotide repeat disorders**
      1. Errors in DNA replication
         - Cause amplification of a sequence of three nucleotides (e.g., CAG), which disrupts gene function
      2. Associated with anticipation
         a. Increasing severity of clinical disease in each successive generation
         b. Caused by the addition of more trinucleotide sequences during gametogenesis
         c. Female carriers may be symptomatic
            - Occurs if they have more paternally (than maternally) derived X chromosomes with trinucleotide repeats
         d. Examples—fragile X syndrome, Huntington's disease, Friedreich's ataxia, myotonic dystrophy

Anticipation: additional trinucleotide repeats increase disease severity in future generations

II. **Mendelian Disorders**
- Usually single-gene mutations
   A. **Autosomal recessive (AR) disorders**
      1. Inheritance pattern (Fig. 5-3)
         a. Individuals must be homozygous for the mutant recessive gene (aa) to express the disorder.

Most common type of mendelian disorder: autosomal recessive

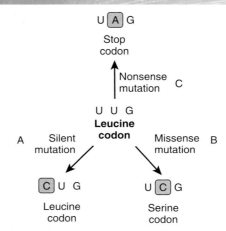

5-1: Point mutations: silent mutation (A), missense mutation (B), nonsense mutation (C). See text for discussion. (From Pelley JW, Goljan E: Rapid Review Biochemistry, 2nd ed. St. Louis, Mosby Elsevier, 2007, p 190, Fig. 10-11.)

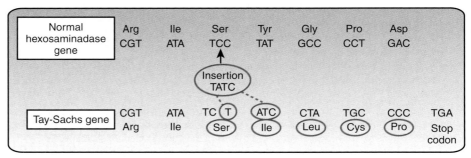

5-2: Frameshift mutation. See text for discussion.

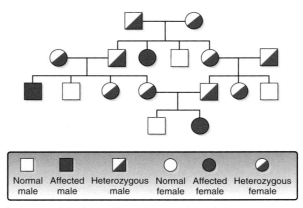

5-3: Pedigree of an autosomal recessive disorder. Both parents must have the mutant gene to transmit the disorder to their children. On average, 25% of the children of heterozygous parents are normal, 50% are asymptomatic heterozygous carriers, and 25% have the disorder.

b. Homozygotes are symptomatic early in life.
c. Heterozygous individuals (Aa) are asymptomatic carriers.
  • The dominant gene (A) overrides the mutant recessive gene (a).
d. Both parents must be heterozygous to transmit the disorder.
  • Example—Aa × Aa → AA, Aa, Aa, aa (25% without disorder; 50% asymptomatic carriers; 25% with disorder)

AR inheritance: both parents must have mutant gene.

Cystic fibrosis (CF) is an AR disorder with a carrier rate of 1/25. To calculate the prevalence of CF in the population, the number of couples at risk of having a child with CF (1/25 × 1/25, or 1/625) is multiplied by the chance of having a child with CF (1/4). Prevalence of CF = 1/625 × 1/4, or 1/2500. Note how it is possible to calculate the carrier rate if given the prevalence of the disease by dividing 1/2500 by 4 to get the number of couples at risk and then taking the square root of 1/625 to get the carrier rate of 1/25.

TABLE 5-1. PROTEIN DEFECTS ASSOCIATED WITH SELECTED MENDELIAN DISORDERS

PROTEIN TYPE	SPECIFIC PROTEIN	DISORDER	INHERITANCE PATTERN
Enzyme	C1 esterase inhibitor deficiency Glucose-6-phosphate dehydrogenase	Hereditary angioedema Glucose-6-phosphate dehydrogenase deficiency	Autosomal dominant X-linked recessive
Structural	Sickle hemoglobin Ankyrin Dystrophin	Sickle cell disease Hereditary spherocytosis Duchenne's muscular dystrophy	Autosomal recessive Autosomal dominant X-linked recessive
Transport	Cystic fibrosis transmembrane regulator	Cystic fibrosis	Autosomal recessive
Receptor	Low-density lipoprotein receptor	Familial hypercholesterolemia	Autosomal dominant
Growth regulating	Neurofibromin	Neurofibromatosis	Autosomal dominant
Hemostasis	Factor VIII	Hemophilia A	X-linked recessive

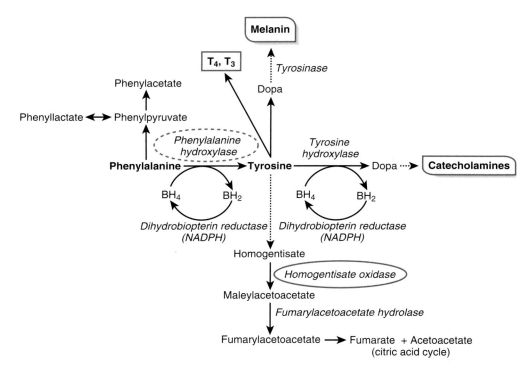

5-4: Alkaptonuria. In alkaptonuria, there is a deficiency of homogentisic oxidase with proximal accumulation of homogentisic acid, which turns black upon oxidation. *(From Pelley JW, Goljan E: Rapid Review Biochemistry, 2nd ed. St. Louis, Mosby Elsevier, 2007, p 139, Fig. 8-4.)*

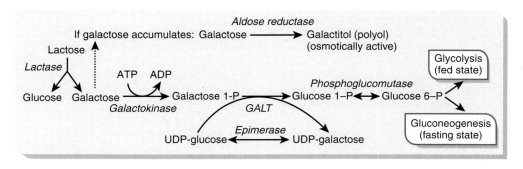

5-5: Galactosemia: See Table 5-2 for information. GALT, galactose-1-phosphate uridyltransferase; P, phosphate; UDP, uridine diphosphate. *(From Pelley JW, Goljan E: Rapid Review Biochemistry, 2nd ed. St. Louis, Mosby Elsevier, 2007, p 104, Fig. 6-10.)*

  2. AR protein defects (Table 5-1)
  3. Inborn errors of metabolism (Figs. 5-4 to 5-7 and Table 5-2)
     a. Most metabolic disorders are due to an enzyme deficiency.
     b. Substrate and intermediates proximal to the enzyme block increase.
     c. Intermediates and the end-product distal to the enzyme block decrease.

Most AR disorders involve enzyme deficiencies.

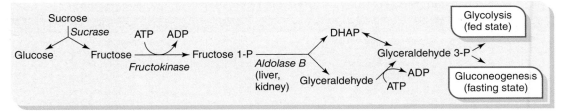

5-6: Hereditary fructose intolerance. See Table 5-2 for information. DHAP, dihydroxyacetone phosphate; P, phosphate. *(From Pelley JW, Goljan E: Rapid Review Biochemistry, 2nd ed. St. Louis, Mosby Elsevier, 2007, p 104, Fig. 6-11.)*

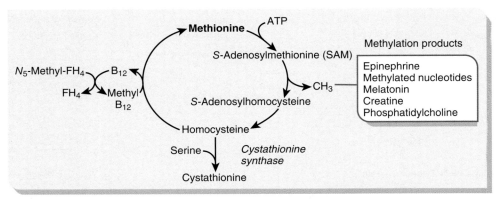

5-7: Homocystinuria. See text for discussion. CH₃, methyl group. *(From Pelley JW, Goljan E: Rapid Review Biochemistry, 2nd ed. St. Louis, Mosby Elsevier, 2007, p 143, Fig. 8-5.)*

PKU: ↑ phenylalanine, ↓ tyrosine

Phenylketonuria (PKU, see Fig. 5-4) is characterized by a deficiency of phenylalanine hydroxylase, causing an increase in the substrate phenylalanine and a decrease in the product tyrosine. In individuals with PKU, phenylalanine is further metabolized into neurotoxic phenylketones and acids that produce mental retardation and urine with a musty odor.

d. Glycogenoses
   (1) Pathogenesis
      (a) Increase in glycogen synthesis (e.g., von Gierke's disease)
      (b) Inhibition of glycogenolysis (e.g., debranching enzyme deficiency)
      (c) Increase in normal or structurally abnormal glycogen
   (2) Clinical findings
      (a) Organ dysfunction (e.g., restrictive heart disease, Pompe's disease).
      (b) Fasting hypoglycemia
         • Decrease in gluconeogenesis (e.g., glucose-6-phosphatase deficiency, von Gierke's disease) or liver glycogenolysis (e.g., liver phosphorylase deficiency)
e. Lysosomal storage diseases (Table 5-3 and Figs. 5-8 and 5-9)
   • Enzyme deficiencies lead to accumulation of undigested substrates (e.g., glycosaminoglycans, sphingolipids) in lysosomes
4. Other AR disorders
   • Hematochromatosis, 21-hydroxylase deficiency, Wilson's disease, thalassemia
B. Autosomal dominant (AD) disorders
   1. Inheritance pattern
      a. One dominant mutant gene (A) is required to express the disorder.
         (1) Heterozygotes (Aa) express the disorder.
         (2) Homozygotes (AA) are often spontaneously aborted.
         (3) Example—Aa × aa → Aa, Aa, aa, aa (50% with disorder; 50% without disorder)
      b. Some disorders arise by new mutations involving either an egg or a sperm.
   2. AD protein defects (see Table 5-1)
      • Enzyme deficiencies are relatively uncommon.

Von Gierke's disease: glucose-6-phosphatase deficiency (gluconeogenic enzyme)

Most common AR disorder: hemochromatosis

AD inheritance: heterozygotes with dominant mutant gene express disease

TABLE 5-2. SELECTED INBORN ERRORS OF METABOLISM

ERROR	DEFICIENT ENZYME	ACCUMULATED SUBSTRATE (S)	COMMENTS
Alkaptonuria (see Fig. 5-4)	Homogentisate oxidase Homogentisate →* Maleylacetoacetate	Homogentisate	Black urine (when exposed to light) and cartilage, degenerative arthritis
Galactosemia (see Fig. 5-5)	GALT Galactose 1-P →* Glucose 1-P Glucose	Galactose 1-phosphate (toxic to liver, CNS) Galactose (in urine) Galactitol (alcohol sugar, increase produces osmotic damage)	Mental retardation, cirrhosis, hypoglycemia (decrease in gluconeogenic substrate), cataracts (osmotic damage) Avoid dairy products (galactose derives from lactose)
Hereditary fructose intolerance (see Fig. 5-6)	Aldolase B Fructose 1-P →* G-3P + DHAP → Glucose	Fructose 1-phosphate (toxic substrate)	Cirrhosis, hypoglycemia (decrease in gluconeogenic substrates), hypophosphatemia (used up in phosphorylating fructose) Avoid fructose (e.g., honey) and sucrose (glucose + fructose)
Homocystinuria (see Fig. 5-7)	Cystathionine synthase Homocysteine → Cystathionine	Homocysteine and methionine	Mental retardation, vessel thrombosis; lens dislocation, arachnodactyly (similar to Marfan syndrome; genetic heterogeneity)
Maple syrup urine disease	Branched chain α-ketoacid dehydrogenase Isoleucine → AcCoA + Succinyl CoA Leucine → AcCoA + AcAc Valine → Succinyl CoA	Leucine, valine, isoleucine, and their ketoacids	Mental retardation, seizures, feeding problems, sweet-smelling urine
Phenylketonuria (see Fig. 5-4);	Phenylalanine hydroxylase Phenylalanine → Tyrosine	Phy Neurotoxic by-products	Mental retardation, microcephaly, mousy odor (Phy converted into phenylacids), decreased pigmentation (melanin derives from tyrosine) Must be exposed to Phy (milk) *before* Phy is increased) Restrict phenylalanine; avoid sweeteners containing Phy (e.g., Nutrasweet) Add tyrosine to diet Pregnant women with PKU must be on Phy-free diet or newborns will be mentally retarded at birth
"Malignant" phenylketonuria (see Fig. 5-4)	Dihydropterin reductase	Phy Neurotoxic by-products	Similar to PKU Inability to metabolize tryptophan or tyrosine, which both require BH_4. This ↓ synthesis of neurotransmitters (serotonin and dopamine, respectively). Neurologic problems occur despite adequate dietary therapy. Restrict phenylalanine in diet. Administer L-dopa and 5-hydroxytryptophan to replace neurotransmitters. Administer BH_4.
McArdle's disease	Muscle phosphorylase Glycogen → Glucose	Glycogen	Glycogenosis, muscle fatigue; no lactic acid increase with exercise
Pompe's disease	α-1,4-Glucosidase (lysosomal enzyme)	Glycogen	Glycogenosis, cardiomegaly with early death
Von Gierke's disease	Glucose-6-phosphatase (gluconeogenic enzyme) Glucose-6P → Glucose → Glycogen	Glucose 6-phosphate	Glycogenosis, enlarged liver and kidneys, hypoglycemia (no response to glucagon or other gluconeogenesis stimulators)

*Site of enzyme activity.
AcAc, acetoacetate; AcCoA, acetyl CoA; DHAP, dihydroxyacetone phosphate; GALT, galactose-1-phosphate uridyltransferase; G-3P, glyceraldehyde 3-phosphate; Phy, phenylalanine; PKU, phenylketonuria.

TABLE 5-3. **SELECTED LYSOSOMAL STORAGE DISORDERS**

DISORDER	DEFICIENT ENZYME	ACCUMULATED SUBSTRATE	CLINICAL FINDINGS
Gaucher's disease (adult type) (see Fig. 13-14)	Glucocerebrosidase	Glucocerebroside	Hepatosplenomegaly; fibrillar-appearing macrophages in liver, spleen, and bone marrow
Hurler's syndrome (see Fig. 5-9)	α-L-Iduronidase	Dermatan and heparan sulfate	Mental retardation, coarse facial features, short neck, corneal clouding, coronary artery disease X-linked recessive form (Hunter's syndrome) is milder
Niemann-Pick disease (see Fig. 13-15)	Sphingomyelinase	Sphingomyelin	Mental retardation, hepatosplenomegaly, foamy macrophages
Tay-Sachs disease	Hexosaminidase	GM₂ ganglioside	Mental retardation, muscle weakness, cherry-red macula, blindness

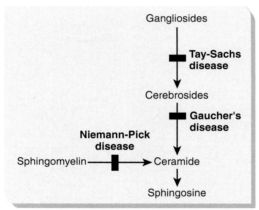

5-8: Sphingolipid degeneration. See Table 5-3 for discussion of selected sphingolipidoses. *(From Pelley JW, Goljan E: Rapid Review Biochemistry, 2nd ed. St. Louis, Mosby Elsevier, 2007, p 104, Fig. 6-11.)*

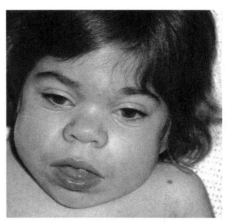

5-9: Hurler syndrome. Note the coarse facial features and short neck. *(From Seidel HM, Ball JW, Danis JE, Benedict GW: Mosby's Guide to Physical Examination, 6th ed. St. Louis, Mosby Elsevier, 2006, p 273, Fig. 10-26.)*

3. Characteristics
   a. Delayed manifestations of disease
      (1) Symptoms and signs may *not* occur early in life.
      (2) Example—in adult polycystic kidney disease, cysts are *not* present at birth.
   b. Penetrance
      (1) Complete penetrance (Fig. 5-10A)
         • All individuals with the mutant gene express the disorder (e.g., familial polyposis).
      (2) Reduced penetrance (Fig. 5-10B)
         (a) Individuals with the mutant gene are phenotypically normal.
         (b) They transmit the disorder to their offspring (e.g., Marfan syndrome; see Fig. 9-6A).
   c. Variable expressivity
      • All individuals with the mutant gene express the disorder but at different levels of severity.
4. Other AD disorders
   • Huntington's disease, osteogenesis imperfecta, achondroplasia, tuberous sclerosis
C. X-linked recessive (XR) disorders
   1. Inheritance pattern (Fig. 5-11)
      a. Males must have the mutant recessive gene on the X chromosome to express the disorder.

Reduced penetrance: individual with mutant gene does *not* express the disease; transmits to children

Most common AD disorder: von Willebrand disease

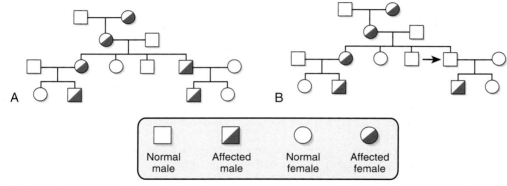

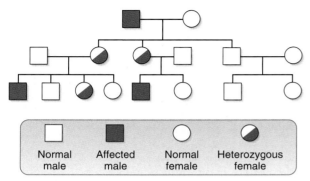

5-10: Pedigrees showing complete and reduced penetrance in an autosomal dominant disorder. Complete penetrance (**A**) means that all individuals with the mutant gene express the disorder. Reduced penetrance (**B**) means that an individual has the mutant gene but does *not* express the disorder (*arrow*). The unaffected father has transmitted the disorder to his son.

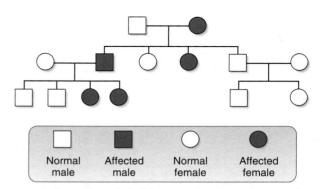

5-11: Pedigree of an X-linked recessive disorder. The affected male transmits the mutant gene on the X chromosome to both of his daughters and none of his sons. Both daughters are asymptomatic heterozygous carriers of the mutant gene. The daughter with four children has transmitted the mutant gene to 50% of her sons.

5-12: Pedigree of an X-linked dominant disorder. In these rare disorders, female carriers and males with the mutant dominant gene express the disorder. The distribution is similar to that of X-linked recessive disorders, *except* that carrier females are symptomatic.

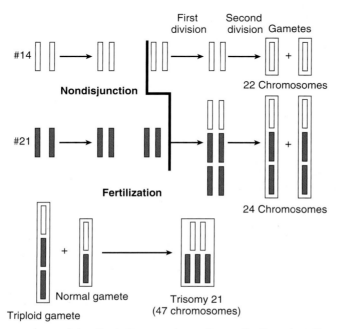

5-13: Pathogenesis of trisomy 21 by nondisjunction in Down syndrome. See text for discussion. *(From Goljan EF: Star Series: Pathology. Philadelphia, WB Saunders, 1998, p 133, Fig. 7-1.)*

b. Affected males (XY) transmit the mutant gene to all of their daughters.
  (1) Males are homozygous for the mutant gene.
  (2) Example—XY × XX → XX, XX, XY, XY
  (3) Daughters (XX) are usually asymptomatic carriers.
c. Asymptomatic female carriers (X mutant gene) transmit the disorder to 50% of their male offspring.
  • Example—XX × XY → XX, XX, XY, XY
d. In rare cases, female carriers can be symptomatic.
  (1) Maternally derived X chromosomes (without the mutant gene) are preferentially inactivated.
    • Only paternally derived X chromosomes with the mutant gene remain.
  (2) Offspring of a symptomatic male and asymptomatic female carrier
    • Example—XX × XY → XX, XX, XY, XY
e. Some XR disorders may arise as new mutations.

XR inheritance: asymptomatic female carrier transmits mutant gene to 50% of sons

2. XR protein defects (see Table 5-1)
  • Enzymes are the most common type of protein affected in XR disorders.
3. Fragile X syndrome
  a. Trinucleotide repeat disorder
  b. Clinical findings
    (1) Mental retardation
      (a) Most common mendelian disorder that causes mental retardation
      (b) 50% of female carriers may develop mental retardation.
    (2) Phenotypic changes
      • Long face, large mandible, everted ears
    (3) Macro-orchidism (enlarged testes) at puberty
    (4) Diagnosis
      (a) DNA analysis to identify trinucleotide repeats (best test)
      (b) Fragile X chromosome study

Most common X-linked disorder: fragile X syndrome

4. Lesch-Nyhan syndrome
  a. Deficiency of hypoxanthine-guanine phosphoribosyltransferase (HGPRT)
    • Normally involved in salvaging the purines hypoxanthine and guanine
  b. Clinical findings
    • Mental retardation, hyperuricemia, self-mutilation
5. Other XR disorders
  • Testicular feminization, chronic granulomatous disease, Bruton's agammaglobulinemia

D. X-linked dominant (XD) disorders
1. Inheritance pattern
  • Same as XR *except* the dominant mutant gene causes disease in males and females (Fig. 5-12)
2. Vitamin D–resistant rickets
  a. Defect in renal and gastrointestinal reabsorption of phosphate
  b. Causes defective bone mineralization (i.e., osteomalacia)
3. Alport's syndrome
  • Hereditary glomerulonephritis with nerve deafness

XD inheritance: female carriers are symptomatic

III. Chromosomal Disorders
A. General considerations
1. Most human cells are diploid (46 chromosomes).
  a. Autosomes: 22 pairs
  b. Sex chromosomes (XX in females and XY in males): 1 pair
2. Gametes, the products of meiosis, are haploid (23 chromosomes).
3. Lyon hypothesis
  a. In females, one of the two X chromosomes is randomly inactivated.
    • Inactivation occurs in the embryonic period of development.
  b. The inactivated X chromosome is called a Barr body.
    (1) The Barr body is attached to the nuclear membrane of cells.
    (2) They are visible in squamous cells obtained by scraping the buccal mucosa.
  c. Normal females have one Barr body, and normal males have none.
  d. Inactivation accounts for the parental derivation of the X chromosomes in females.
    • ~50% of X chromosomes are paternal and ~50% are maternal.

Barr body: inactivated X chromosome

Barr body: attached to nuclear membrane

Number of Barr bodies = number of X chromosomes − 1

B. Chromosomal alterations
- Numeric or structural abnormalities of autosomes or sex chromosomes
1. Nondisjunction
   a. Unequal separation of chromosomes in the first phase of meiosis
   b. Results in 22 or 24 chromosomes in the egg or sperm
2. Examples—Turner's syndrome (22 + 23 = 45 chromosomes), Down syndrome (24 + 23 = 47 chromosomes, trisomy; Fig. 5-13)
3. Mosaicism
   a. Nondisjunction of chromosomes during mitotic division in the early embryonic period
   b. Two chromosomally different cell lines are derived from a single fertilized egg.
   c. Most often involves sex chromosomes (e.g., Turner's syndrome)
4. Translocation
   a. Transfer of chromosome parts between nonhomologous chromosomes
   b. Balanced translocation
      - Translocated fragment is functional.
   c. Robertsonian translocation
      - Balanced translocation between two acrocentric chromosomes (e.g., chromosomes 14 and 21)

> In one type of **Down syndrome**, the mother of an affected child has 45 (not 46) chromosomes because of a robertsonian translocation between the long arms of chromosomes 21 and 14. This produces one long chromosome (14;21). The mother also has one chromosome 14 and one chromosome 21. The father has the normal 46 chromosomes. The affected child has 46 chromosomes with three functional 21 chromosomes including chromosome (14;21) and chromosome 21 from the mother and chromosome 14 and chromosome 21 from the father (Fig. 5-14).

5. Deletion
   a. Loss of a portion of a chromosome
   b. Cri du chat syndrome
      (1) Loss of the short arm of chromosome 5
      (2) Clinical findings
         - Mental retardation, cat-like cry, ventricular septal defect

C. Disorders involving autosomes
1. Down syndrome
   a. Causes
      (1) Nondisjunction (95% of cases, trisomy 21)

Nondisjunction: unequal separation of chromosomes in meiosis

Mosaicism: nondisjunction in mitosis

Cri du chat syndrome: deletion short arm chromosome 5

Down syndrome: most cases due to nondisjunction

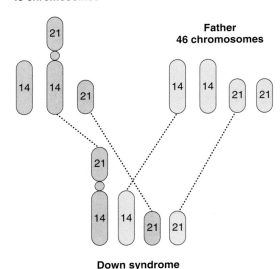

**Mother
45 chromosomes**

**Father
46 chromosomes**

**Down syndrome
46 chromosomes**

5-14: Robertsonian translocation. See text for description.

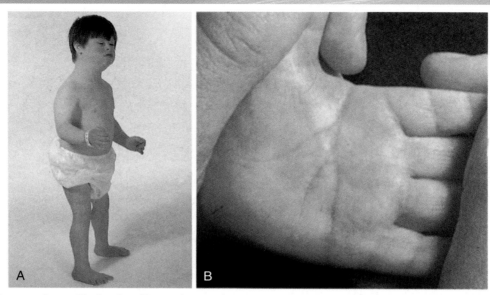

5-15: Down syndrome. The facial profile (**A**) shows a short stature and a small head with small nose and ears. The hand (**B**) shows a single palmar (simian) crease. *(From Forbes C, Jackson W: Color Atlas and Text of Clinical Medicine, 2nd ed. St. Louis, Mosby, 2003, Figs. 7-168 and 7-172.)*

Advanced maternal age: increased risk for bearing offspring with trisomy syndromes

Most common genetic cause of mental retardation: Down syndrome

Down syndrome: duodenal atresia, Hirschsprung's

Down syndrome: Alzheimer's disease at young age

Edward's syndrome: trisomy 18

Patau's syndrome: trisomy 13

Turner's syndrome: 45,X karyotype

      (2) Robertsonian translocation (4% of cases)
      (3) Mosaicism (1% of cases)
  2. Risk factors
    a. Increased maternal age is a risk factor.
    b. Occurs in 1 in 25 live births in women over 45 years of age
    c. Clinical findings
      (1) General
        (a) Most common genetic cause of mental retardation
        (b) Epicanthic folds, flat facial profile, macroglossia (Fig. 5-15A)
        (c) Simian crease (Fig. 5-15B)
      (2) Combined atrial and ventricular septal defects (cushion defects)
        • Major factor affecting survival in early childhood
      (3) Increased risk of Hirschsprung's disease and duodenal atresia
      (4) Increased risk of leukemia
        • Acute lymphoblastic leukemia most commonly
      (5) Alzheimer's disease by 35 years of age in most cases
        • Major factor affecting survival in older individuals
      (6) Sterility in all males
      (7) Females have a 50% chance of having a child with Down syndrome.
  2. Edwards' syndrome
    a. Trisomy 18
    b. Clinical findings
      (1) Mental retardation
      (2) Clenched hands with overlapping fingers
      (3) Ventricular septal defect (VSD)
      (4) Early death
  3. Patau's syndrome
    a. Trisomy 13
    b. Clinical findings
      (1) Mental retardation
      (2) Cleft lip and palate
      (3) Polydactyly, VSD, cystic kidneys
      (4) Early death
  D. Disorders involving sex chromosomes
    1. Turner's syndrome
      a. Causes
        (1) Nondisjunction
          • 45,X karyotype (~60% of cases)

(2) Mosaicism
- 45,X/46,XX karyotype (~40% of cases)

b. Clinical and laboratory findings
  (1) Short stature
    (a) Cardinal finding
    (b) Normal growth hormone and insulin-like growth factor
  (2) Lymphedema in hands and feet in infancy
    - Webbed neck is caused by dilated lymphatic channels (cystic hygroma) (Fig. 5-16).
  (3) Preductal coarctation and bicuspid aortic valve
  (4) Streak gonads
    (a) Ovaries replaced by fibrous stroma
    (b) Ovaries devoid of oocytes by 2 years of age
      - All patients with a 45,X karyotype are infertile.
    (c) Increased risk for developing ovarian dysgerminoma

Webbed neck: cystic hygroma

Turner's syndrome: "menopause before menarche"

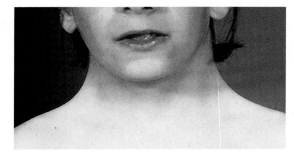

5-16: Turner's syndrome is characterized by a webbed neck. Other findings include short stature, primary amenorrhea, and delayed secondary sex characteristics (e.g., underdeveloped breasts). *(From Bouloux P-M: Self-Assessment Picture Tests: Medicine, Vol. 1. St. Louis, Mosby, 1996, p 45.)*

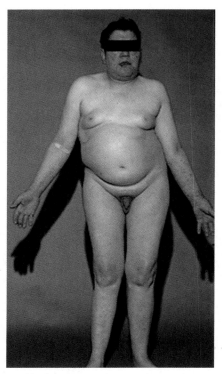

5-17: Klinefelter's syndrome is characterized by female secondary sex characteristics, including gynecomastia (breast development) and a female distribution of pubic hair. The legs are disproportionately long. *(From Bouloux P-M: Self-Assessment Picture Tests: Medicine, Vol. 1. St. Louis, Mosby, 1996, p 82.)*

Most common genetic cause of primary amenorrhea: Turner's syndrome

(5) Primary amenorrhea with delayed sexual maturation
    (a) Decreased estradiol and progesterone
    (b) Increased follicle-stimulating hormone (FSH) and luteinizing hormone (LH)
(6) Normal intelligence, horseshoe kidney, hypothyroidism
(7) No Barr bodies

2. Klinefelter's syndrome
  a. Cause
    (1) Nondisjunction
    (2) XXY karyotype
  b. Clinical and laboratory findings (Fig. 5-17)
    (1) Female secondary sex characteristics at puberty
      (a) Persistent gynecomastia
      (b) Soft skin
      (c) Female hair distribution
    (2) Delayed sexual maturation (hypogonadism)
      (a) Testicular atrophy (decreased testicular volume)
      (b) Fibrosis of seminiferous tubules
        • Absence of spermatogenesis (azoospermia); loss of Sertoli cells

Klinefelter's syndrome: ↓ testosterone and inhibin; ↑ LH and FSH, respectively

      (c) Leydig cell hyperplasia
    (3) Disproportionately long legs, learning disabilities
    (4) Decreased inhibin (loss of Sertoli cells)
      (a) Causes increased FSH (loss of negative feedback with inhibin)
      (b) Increased FSH causes increased synthesis of aromatase in Leydig cells.
    (5) Decreased testosterone
      (a) Aromatase converts testosterone to estradiol; estradiol causes feminization.
      (b) Increased LH (loss of negative feedback with testosterone)
    (6) One Barr body

XYY syndrome: paternal nondysjunction; aggressive behavior

3. XYY syndrome
  a. Caused by paternal nondisjunction
  b. Associated with aggressive (sometimes criminal) behavior
  c. Normal gonadal function

IV. Other Patterns of Inheritance
  A. Multifactorial (polygenic) inheritance
    1. Combination of multiple minor gene mutations plus environmental factors

Polygenic disorders are more common than mendelian and chromosomal disorders.

    2. Examples of multifactorial inheritance
      a. Open neural tube defects
        • Associated with decreased maternal folate levels
      b. Type 2 diabetes mellitus
        • Associated with obesity, which downregulates insulin receptor synthesis
  B. Mitochondrial DNA disorders (Fig. 5-18)
    1. Function of mitochondrial DNA
      • Codes for enzymes involved in mitochondrial oxidative phosphorylation reactions
    2. Inheritance pattern

Mitochondrial DNA disorders: associated with maternal inheritance; ova have mutant gene

      a. Affected females transmit the mutant gene to all their children.
        • Ova contain mitochondria with the mutant gene.

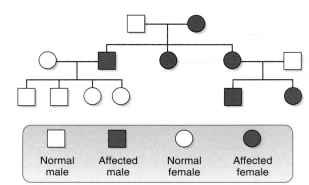

5-18: Pedigree showing transmission of mitochondrial DNA. Affected females transmit the disorder to all their children, whereas affected males do not.

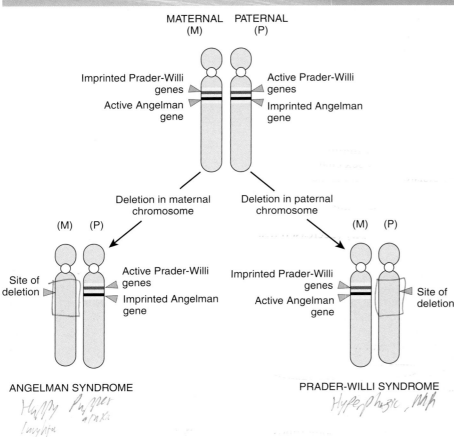

MATERNAL   PATERNAL
(M)   (P)

Imprinted Prader-Willi genes

Active Angelman gene

Active Prader-Willi genes

Imprinted Angelman gene

Deletion in maternal chromosome

Deletion in paternal chromosome

(M)   (P)

Site of deletion

Active Prader-Willi genes

Imprinted Angelman gene

(M)   (P)

Imprinted Prader-Willi genes

Active Angelman gene

Site of deletion

ANGELMAN SYNDROME

PRADER-WILLI SYNDROME

5-19: Genetics of Angelman and Prader-Willi syndromes. See text for discussion. *(From Kumar V, Abbas AK, Fausto N, Mitchell RN: Robbins Basic Pathology, 8th ed. Philadelphia, Saunders Elsevier, 2007, p 251, Fig. 7-18.)*

b. Affected males do *not* transmit the mutant gene to any of their children.
   • Sperm lose their mitochondria during fertilization.
3. Examples—Leber's hereditary optic neuropathy, myoclonic epilepsy

C. Genomic imprinting
1. Inheritance pattern
   a. Inheritance depends on whether the mutant gene is of maternal or paternal origin.
   b. Examples—Prader-Willi syndrome and Angelman syndrome
2. Pathogenesis (Fig. 5-19)
   a. Normal changes in maternal chromosome 15 during gametogenesis
      (1) Prader-Willi gene is inactivated by methylation (imprinted).
      (2) Angelman gene is demethylated (activated).
   b. Normal changes in paternal chromosome 15 during gametogenesis
      (1) Prader-Willi gene is demethylated (activated).
      (2) Angelman gene is imprinted (inactivated).
   c. Microdeletion of the entire gene site on paternal chromosome 15
      (1) Causes Prader-Willi syndrome
      (2) Complete loss of Prader-Willi gene activity
         (a) Loss of activated Prader-Willi gene on paternal chromosome 15
         (b) Inactivated Prader-Willi gene on maternal chromosome 15
   d. Microdeletion of the entire gene site on maternal chromosome 15
      (1) Causes Angelman syndrome
      (2) Complete loss of Angelman gene activity
         (a) Loss of activated Angelman gene on maternal chromosome 15
         (b) Inactivated Angelman gene on paternal chromosome 15
3. Clinical findings in Prader-Willi syndrome
   a. Mental retardation, short stature, hypotonia at birth
   b. Obesity (tendency to overeat), hypogonadism
4. Clinical findings in Angelman syndrome
   a. Mental retardation
   b. Wide-based gait (resembles a marionette)
   c. Inappropriate laughter ("happy puppet" syndrome)

Genomic imprinting: inheritance depends whether mutant gene of maternal or paternal origin

Prader-Willi syndrome: microdeletion on paternal chromosome 15

Angelman syndrome: microdeletion on maternal chromosome 15

V. **Disorders of Sex Differentiation**
   A. **Normal sex differentiation**
      1. Absence of the Y chromosome
         a. Germinal tissue differentiates into ovaries.
         b. Wolffian (mesonephric) duct structures undergo apoptosis.
      2. Presence of the Y chromosome
         a. Germinal tissue differentiates into testes.
         b. Müllerian inhibitory factor (MIF) causes müllerian tissue to undergo apoptosis.
            • MIF is synthesized in the Sertoli cells.
         c. Function of fetal testosterone
            (1) Develops the wolffian duct structures
            (2) Epididymis, seminal vesicles, vas deferens
         d. 5α-Reductase converts testosterone to dihydrotestosterone (DHT).
         e. Functions of fetal DHT
            (1) Develops the prostate gland
            (2) Develops the external male genitalia
               • Genitalia is phenotypically female *before* DHT is produced.
   B. **True hermaphrodite**
      1. Fetus has both male and female gonads.
      2. Karyotype is usually 46,XX.
   C. **Pseudohermaphrodite**
      1. Phenotype and genotype do *not* match.
      2. Male pseudohermaphrodite
         a. Genotypic male (XY with testes)
         b. Phenotypic female
         c. Example—testicular feminization
      3. Female pseudohermaphrodite
         a. Genotypic female (XX with ovaries)
         b. Phenotypic male
         c. Example—virilization in adrenogenital syndrome
   D. **Testicular feminization (androgen insensitivity syndrome)** (Fig. 5-20)
      1. XR disorder with a defective androgen receptor
         • Fetal DHT and testosterone are unable to function without a receptor.

Y chromosome: determines the genetic sex of an individual

Testicular feminization: most common cause of male pseudohermaphroditism

Testicular feminization: defective androgen receptors

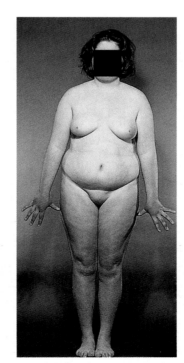

5-20: Testicular feminization. The patient is genotypically male, but phenotypically female. The vagina ended as a blind pouch. *(From Forbes C, Jackson W: Color Atlas and Text of Clinical Medicine, 2nd ed. St. Louis, Mosby, 2003, p 321, Fig. 7-55.)*

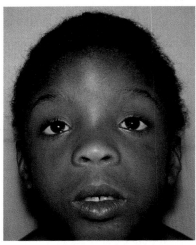

5-21: Fetal alcohol syndrome. Note the wide-spread eyes, inner epicanthal folds, short nose, hirsute forehead, and thin upper lip. *(From Zitelli: B: Atlas of Pediatric Physical Diagnosis, 3rd ed. St. Louis, Mosby, 1997.)*

    2. Clinical and laboratory findings
        a. Testicles are present in the inguinal canal or abdominal cavity.
        b. Müllerian structures are absent because MIF is present.
          • Absence of fallopian tubes, uterus, cervix, upper vagina
        c. Male accessory structures are absent.
          • *No* testosterone effect on the wolffian duct structures → *no wolffian,*
        d. External genitalia remain female.
          (1) *No* DHT effect → *External male genetalia*   *Müllerian = MIF*
          (2) Vagina ends as a blind pouch.
        e. Hormone levels
          (1) Normal male levels of testosterone and DHT
          (2) Slightly increased luteinizing hormone levels
          (3) Slightly increased serum estradiol levels
            • Estrogen activity is unopposed, because estrogen receptors are present.
    3. Majority of patients are reared female.

VI. Congenital Anomalies
    • Known to occur in 3% to 5% of all newborns.
    A. Types of errors in morphogenesis
        1. Malformations
          a. Disturbances in the morphogenesis (development) of an organ
          b. Occur between the third and ninth weeks of embryogenesis
            • Most susceptible period is fourth to fifth weeks.
          c. Causes
            • Multifactorial (e.g., drugs, infection)
          d. Examples—open neural tube defects (see Figs. 25-6 and 25-7), congenital heart disease, cleft lip/palate (see Fig. 17-1)
        2. Deformations
          a. Extrinsic disturbances in fetal development
          b. Occur between the ninth week and term after fetal organs have developed
          c. Most often due to restricted movement in uterine cavity
            • Examples—oligohydramnios, uterus with leiomyomas, twin pregnancies

Oligohydramnios (decreased amniotic fluid) from decreased production of fetal urine (e.g., renal agenesis, cystic disease of the kidneys) restricts fetal movement in the uterine cavity. As a result, newborns have flat facial features (Potter's facies), underdevelopment of the chest wall, and clubfeet.

        3. Agenesis
          a. Complete absence of an organ resulting from absence of the anlage (primordial tissue)
          b. Example—renal agenesis

Sidebar notes:

Testicular feminization: vagina ends as blind pouch

Malformation: disturbance in morphogenesis in embryonic period

Malformation: open neural tube defect, cleft lip/palate

Deformation: extrinsic disturbance in fetal development

Deformation: oligohydramnios causing Potter's facies, clubfeet

            4. Aplasia
                a. Anlage is present but *never* develops.
                b. Example—lung aplasia with tissue containing rudimentary ducts and connective tissue
            5. Hypoplasia
                a. Anlage develops incompletely, but the tissue is histologically normal.
                b. Example—microcephaly
            6. Atresia
                a. Incomplete formation of a lumen
                b. Example—duodenal atresia (see Fig. 17-22)
        B. Causes of congenital anomalies
            1. Majority are unknown
            2. Multifactorial
                • Combination of genetic and environmental factors
            3. Environmental factors
                a. Maternal disorders
                    (1) Diabetes mellitus
                        (a) Increased risk of neural tube defects and congenital heart disease
                        (b) Maternal hyperglycemia causes fetal macrosomia.
                            • Hyperinsulinemia in the fetus increases muscle mass and stores of fat in
                              the adipose tissue.
                    (2) Systemic lupus erythematosus
                        • Newborn may develop congenital heart block if the mother has anti-Ro
                          antibodies.
                    (3) Hypothyroidism
                        • Newborn may develop cretinism.
                b. Drugs and chemicals (Table 5-4; Fig. 5-21)
                c. Congenital infections (Table 5-5)
                    (1) Newborn has an increase in cord blood IgM.
                        • IgM normally is *not* synthesized in the fetus unless there is a congenital
                          infection.
                    (2) Vertical transmission; routes of transmission:
                        (a) Transplacental (most common route)
                        (b) Birth canal
                        (c) Breast-feeding
                d. Ionizing radiation
        C. Pathogenesis of congenital anomalies
            1. Timing of teratogenic insult
                a. Malformations occur during the embryonic period (between third and ninth weeks).
                b. Deformations occur during the fetal period (ninth week to term).
            2. Alterations during key steps in morphogenesis
                a. Mutations may occur in genes normally involved in morphogenesis.
                    • Example—mutations of the *HOX* gene alter development of craniofacial
                      structures.

Margin notes:

Congenital anomalies: genetic + environmental factors

Maternal diabetes: macrosomia— hyperinsulinemia ↑ muscle mass and fat

Alcohol: most common teratogen (fetal alcohol syndrome)

Most common pathogen causing a congenital infection: cytomegalovirus

TORCH syndrome = *t*oxoplasmosis, *o*ther agents, *r*ubella, *c*ytomegalovirus, *h*erpes simplex virus

Retinoic acid in pregnancy: disrupts *HOX* gene function (craniofacial, CNS, cardiovascular defects)

TABLE 5-4. TERATOGENS ASSOCIATED WITH CONGENITAL DEFECTS

TERATOGEN	DEFECT
Alcohol (see Fig. 5-21)	Mental retardation (leading cause in Western Hemisphere), microcephaly, VSD ASD, attention deficit, diagnostic facial features (thinning of upper lip, flattening of grove between nose and upper lip, small eye openings)
Cocaine	Microcephaly, low birth weight, renal agenesis, congenital heart disease
DES	Vaginal and/or cervical clear cell carcinoma, müllerian defects
Phenytoin	Nail and distal phalanx hypoplasia, cleft lip and/or palate, neuroblastoma, bleeding (vitamin K deficiency)
Isotretinoin	Hearing defects, missing ear lobes, visual impairment, facial dysmorphism, mental retardation
Thalidomide	Amelia (absent limbs), phocomelia (seal-like limbs), deafness
Tobacco	IUGR, low birth weight
Valproate	Neural tube defects (valproate is a folate antagonist), autism
Warfarin	Nasal hypoplasia, agenesis corpus callosum, fetal bleeding and death

ASD, atrial septal defect; DES, diethylstilbestrol; IUGR, intrauterine growth retardation; VSD, ventricular septal defect.

TABLE 5-5. CONGENITAL INFECTIONS ASSOCIATED WITH CONGENITAL DEFECTS

INFECTION	TRANSMISSION	CLINICAL FINDINGS
Cytomegalovirus (see Fig. 25-24A)	Transplacental	Deafness, IUGR, CNS calcification (periventricular) Culture urine (best fluid to culture), urine cytologic findings: intranuclear inclusions
Herpes simplex type 2	Birth canal	IUGR, vesicular lesions or scarring, keratoconjunctivitis, microcephaly
Rubella	Transplacental	Deafness (sensorineural), PDA, cataract, thrombocytopenia ("blueberry muffin" rash), hepatomegaly
Syphilis (see Fig. 17-2E)	Transplacental	Occurs after 20 weeks' gestation Hepatitis, saddle nose, blindness, peg teeth
Toxoplasmosis	Transplacental	Blindness (chorioretinitis), deafness (sensorineural), CNS calcification (basal ganglia), IUGR, hydrocephalus, hepatosplenomegaly Pregnant woman should avoid cat litter, raw meat
Varicella	Transplacental	Limb defects, mental retardation, blindness (chorioretinitis), cataracts, skin scars
HIV	Transplacental, birth canal, breast feeding	Oral thrush, recurrent bacterial infections, intracranial calcification, failure to thrive

IUGR, intrauterine growth retardation; PDA, patent ductus arteriosus.

b. Alterations in cell proliferation, migration, and apoptosis

Pregnant women should *not* be treated for acne with retinoic acid. Retinoic acid disrupts the function of the *HOX* gene, leading to craniofacial, central nervous system, and cardiovascular defects.

VII. Selected Perinatal and Infant Disorders
A. Stillbirth
1. Birth of a dead child
2. Most often caused by an abruptio placentae
   - Premature separation of the placenta because of a retroplacental blood clot
3. Other causes
   - Maternal diabetes, infection, Rh hemolytic disease of newborn

Stillbirth: most often caused by abruptio placentae

B. Spontaneous abortion (miscarriage)
1. Termination of a pregnancy *before* 20 weeks
2. Most common complication in early pregnancy
3. Most often caused by a fetal karyotypic abnormality
   - Usually trisomy 16 in ~50% of cases
4. Predisposing factors
   a. Advanced maternal age
   b. Infections (e.g., *Streptococcus agalactiae*, *Listeria monocytogenes*)
   c. Tobacco, alcohol use

Spontaneous abortion: frequently caused by trisomy 16

C. Sudden infant death syndrome (SIDS)
- Sudden and unexpected death of an apparently healthy infant from 1 month to 1 year of age
1. Epidemiology
   a. Most common cause of death of an infant younger than 1 year old in developed countries
   b. Most deaths occur between 2 and 4 months of age.
      - 90% occur in infants under 6 months
   c. Death usually occurs during sleep.
2. Pathogenesis
   a. No single cause
   b. Maternal risk factors
      - Examples—smoking, young age
   c. Infant risk factors
      - Examples—prematurity, sleeping prone, neural developmental delay, brainstem defect increasing risk for not being able to be aroused from slow wave sleep
3. Autopsy findings
   a. Nonspecific signs of tissue hypoxia are present.
   b. Thickened pulmonary arteries

SIDS: majority of deaths occur before age 6 months

c. Petechiae on the pleura and epicardium

d. Microscopic changes of hypoxia in the brainstem (e.g., arcuate nucleus)

D. Prematurity and intrauterine growth retardation (IUGR)

1. Newborn classification based on weight and gestational age

a. Appropriate for gestational age (AGA)

b. Small for gestational age (SGA)

- Highest mortality rate

c. Large for gestational age (LGA)

- Usually due to maternal diabetes mellitus

2. Prematurity

a. Gestational age less than 37 weeks

- Usually weigh less than 2500 g

b. Most common cause of neonatal death and morbidity

c. Risk factors

(1) Premature rupture of membranes

(2) Chorioamnionitis (e.g., *Streptococcus agalactiae*)

(3) Placental abnormalities

(4) Twin pregnancies

d. Complications

(1) Respiratory distress syndrome (RDS, decreased surfactant)

(2) Necrotizing enterocolitis (intestinal ischemia)

(3) Intraventricular hemorrhage

3. IUGR usually occurs in SGA infants.

- Defined as <10% of predicted fetal weight for gestational age

a. Maternal factors

(1) Most common cause of IUGR in SGA infants

(2) Examples—preeclampsia, poor nutrition, drug addiction, alcoholism, smoking

b. Fetal causes

(1) Chromosomal disorders, congenital malformations, congenital infections

(2) Symmetric growth retardation

- Affects all organ systems equally

c. Placental causes

(1) Abruptio placentae, placental infarction

(2) Asymmetric growth retardation

- Example—the brain is spared relative to visceral organs such as the liver.

d. Ultrasonography is a common initial step in the workup of IUGR.

e. About 85% of IUGR infants have oligohydramnios.

(1) Blood flow from peripheral organs (kidneys) is diverted to the brain.

(2) Renal perfusion and urinary flow rates are reduced in IUGR infants.

E. Neonatal period

1. First 4 weeks of life

2. Majority of deaths in childhood occur during this period.

3. Common causes of death include RDS and congenital anomalies.

VIII. Diagnosis of Genetic and Developmental Disorders

A. Amniocentesis

- Used to identify prenatal genetic defects

B. Ultrasound

- Used to rule out neural tube defects

C. Maternal triple marker screen

1. α-Fetoprotein (AFP)

a. Increased in neural tube defects

b. Causally related to folate deficiency prior to conception

2. Human chorionic gonadotropin (hCG)

- Levels vary with gestational age.

LGA: most often due to maternal diabetes

Prematurity: most common cause neonatal death/morbidity

IUGR: maternal factors most often responsible in SGA infants

IUGR: often have oligohydramnios

Open neural tube defect: folate deficiency prior to conception; ↑ AFP

3. Urine for unconjugated estriol
   - Excellent marker of fetal, placental, or maternal dysfunction
4. Triple marker findings in Down syndrome
   a. AFP decreased
   b. hCG increased
   c. Urine estriol decreased

Triple marker for Down
syndrome: ↓ AFP, ↑ hCG,
↓ urine estriol

D. **Genetic analysis**
1. Chromosome karyotyping
   - Identifies numeric and structural abnormalities
2. DNA polymerase chain reaction
   - Amplifies DNA fragments harboring abnormal gene loci
3. Restriction fragment length polymorphism (RFLP)
   - Identifies abnormal gene when the exact site is unknown

IX. **Aging**
A. **Theories**
1. Stochastic theory
   a. Cumulative injury to cell membranes and DNA due to free radical injury
   b. Increased cross-linking of proteins
      - Decreases elasticity
   c. Accumulation of errors in protein synthesis adversely affects cellular function.
2. Programmed
   - Apoptosis genes are programmed to kill cells at a set time.
B. **Age-dependent changes**
   - Refers to changes that are inevitable with age (Table 5-6)
C. **Age-related changes**
   - Refers to changes that have a greater incidence with age but are *not* inevitable (Table 5-7)

Age-dependent: inevitable
with age; e.g., ↓ GFR,
prostate hyperplasia

Age-related: common but
not inevitable with age;
e.g., Alzheimer's disease,
systolic hypertension

TABLE 5-6. AGE-DEPENDENT CHANGES

SYSTEM	DESCRIPTION
Auditory	Presbycusis: sensorineural hearing loss, particularly at high frequency Otosclerosis: fusion of ear ossicles producing conductive hearing loss
Cardiovascular	Loss of elasticity in aorta (increases systolic pressure)
Central nervous	Cerebral atrophy with mild forgetfulness Impaired sleep patterns such as insomnia, early wakening Decreased dopaminergic synthesis: parkinsonian-like gait
Female reproductive	Breast and vulvar atrophy Decreased estrogen and progesterone: ↑ FSH and LH, respectively
Gastrointestinal	Decreased gastric acidity: predisposes to *Helicobacter pylori* infection Decreased colonic motility: constipation predisposing to diverticulosis
General	Increased body fat: decreased number insulin receptors (glucose intolerance)
Immune	Decreased skin response to antigens (called anergy)
Male reproductive	Prostate hyperplasia: predisposes to urinary retention Prostate cancer
Musculoskeletal	Osteoarthritis in weight-bearing joints
Renal	Decreased GFR: increased risk of drug toxicity from slow clearance of drugs
Respiratory	Mild obstructive pattern in pulmonary function tests: e.g., increased TLC Mild hypoxemia and increased A-a gradient
Skin	Decreased skin elasticity due to increased cross-bridging of collagen Senile purpura over the dorsum of the hands and lower legs
Visual	Cataracts: visual impairment, increased risk for falls Presbyopia: inability to focus on near objects

A-a, alveolar-arterial; FSH, follicle-stimulating hormone; GFR, glomerular filtration rate; LH, luteinizing hormone; TLC, total lung capacity.

TABLE 5-7. **AGE-RELATED CHANGES**

SYSTEM	DESCRIPTION
Cardiovascular	Atherosclerosis: increased risk for coronary artery disease, peripheral vascular disease, strokes Aortic stenosis: most common valvular abnormality in the elderly Systolic hypertension: due to loss of aortic elasticity
Central nervous	Alzheimer's disease: most common cause of dementia in people older than 65 years Parkinson's disease Subdural hematomas: due to falls
Endocrine	Type 2 diabetes mellitus
Female reproductive	Increased incidence of cancers of the breast, endometrium, ovary
Gastrointestinal	Increased incidence of colorectal cancer
Immune	MGUS: most common cause of monoclonal gammopathy
Musculoskeletal	Osteoporosis: vertebral column in females and femoral head in males
Renal/lower urinary tract	Renovascular hypertension secondary to atherosclerosis Urinary incontinence
Respiratory	Pneumonia: usually *Streptococcus pneumoniae* Primary lung cancer: particularly in smokers
Skin	UVB-induced cancers: e.g., basal cell carcinoma (most common) Actinic (solar) keratosis: precursor for squamous cell carcinoma Pressure sores: pressure on capillaries is the most important risk factor
Visual	Macular degeneration: most common cause of blindness in the elderly

MGUS, monoclonal gammopathy of undetermined significance; UVB, ultraviolet light B.

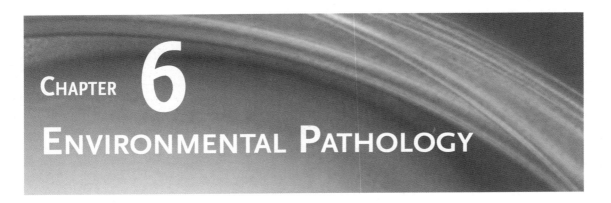

I. Chemical Injury

- The two leading causes of illness and death in the United States are tobacco and alcohol use.

A. Tobacco use

1. Tobacco is the leading cause of premature death in the United States.
2. The rate of cigarette smoking is increasing in females and decreasing in males.
3. Chemical components of tobacco
   a. Nicotine
      (1) Rapidly absorbed
      (2) Most addictive chemical in tobacco smoke
      (3) Cotinine is the most important metabolite of nicotine.
         - Screening test in blood or urine for detecting nicotine
   b. Polycyclic hydrocarbons are the primary carcinogens.
4. Smokeless tobacco (e.g., chewing tobacco)
   a. Can cause nicotine addiction and cancer
   b. Risk for squamous cell cancer of buccal mucosa and gums
5. Passive (secondhand) smoke inhalation
   a. Greatest impact on children
      (1) Increased risk of respiratory and middle ear infections
      (2) Exacerbates asthma
   b. Increased risk for lung cancer and coronary artery disease
6. Systemic effects associated with tobacco use (Table 6-1)
7. Beneficial effects of smoking cessation
   a. Live longer, regardless of age, than those who continue to smoke
      - If cessation *before* age 50, reduction in risk of dying in next 15 years is cut in half compared with those who continue to smoke.
   b. Lower risk for cardiovascular disease
      - Approaches nonsmoker after 15 years
   c. Lower risk for lung cancer
      - Approaches nonsmoker after 15 years
   d. Lower risk for stroke
      - Approaches nonsmoker after 5 to 15 years
   e. Other benefits
      (1) Reduced risk for cancers of the mouth, larynx, esophagus, pancreas, kidney, and urinary bladder
      (2) Improved pulmonary function regardless of severity of the disease
      (3) Reduced risk for pneumonia, influenza, and bronchitis

B. Alcohol abuse

1. Alcohol metabolism
   a. Absorption occurs in the stomach (25%)
   b. Metabolism occurs in the stomach and liver
      - Alcohol dehydrogenase is the rate-limiting enzyme.
   c. Important products of alcohol metabolism (Fig. 6-1)
      (1) Reduced nicotinamide adenine dinucleotide (NADH)
         (a) Causes conversion of pyruvate to lactate
         (b) Causes conversion of acetoacetate to β-hydroxybutyrate
         (c) Causes conversion of dihydroxyacetone phosphate to glycerol 3-phosphate

Smoking: most important preventable cause of disease and death in United States

Cotinine: metabolite of nicotine; used for screening

Nicotine patch: effective in treating ulcerative colitis

Alcohol metabolism: ↑ NADH is key to lab abnormalities

TABLE 6-1. SYSTEMIC EFFECTS ASSOCIATED WITH TOBACCO USE

SYSTEM	EFFECTS
Cardiovascular	AMI Sudden cardiac death Peripheral vascular disease Hypertension
Central nervous	Strokes: intracerebral bleeding, subarachnoid hemorrhage
Gastrointestinal	Increased risk for oropharyngeal cancer: squamous cell carcinoma Increased risk for upper, midesophageal cancer: squamous cell carcinoma Increased risk for stomach cancer: adenocarcinoma Gastroesophageal reflux disease: decreases tone of LES Delayed healing of peptic ulcers Increased risk for pancreatic cancer: adenocarcinoma
General	Low birth weight in newborns, IUGR Neutrophilic leukocytosis: decreased activation of neutrophil adhesion molecules Decreased concentration of ascorbic acid (used up in neutralizing hydroxyl free radicals) and β-carotenes
Genitourinary	Increased risk for cervical cancer: squamous cell carcinoma ? Decreased free testosterone in males (↑ sex-hormone binding globulin) Decreased estrogen in females (early menopause) Increased risk for kidney cancer: renal cell carcinoma Increased risk for urinary bladder cancer: transitional cell carcinoma
Hematologic	Increased risk for acute myelogenous leukemia
Integument	Increased facial wrinkling
Musculoskeletal	Osteoporosis: due to decreased estrogen in females and decreased free testosterone in males
Respiratory	Increased risk for laryngeal cancer: squamous cell carcinoma Chronic obstructive pulmonary disease: chronic bronchitis, emphysema Increased risk for lung cancer: squamous cell carcinoma, small cell carcinoma, some types of adenocarcinoma
Special senses	Decreased sense of smell and taste Blindness: macular degeneration Cataracts

AMI, acute myocardial infarction; IUGR, intrauterine growth retardation; LES, lower esophageal sphincter.

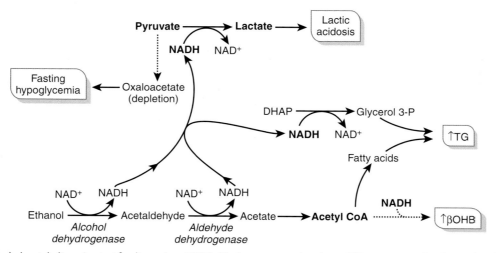

6-1: Alcohol metabolism. See text for discussion. DHAP, dihydroxyacetone phosphate; NAD⁺, nicotinamide adenine dinucleotide; NADH, reduced nicotinamide adenine dinucleotide; βOHB, β-hydroxybutyric acid; TG, triglyceride. (*From Pelley JW, Goljan EF: Rapid Review Biochemistry, 2nd ed. St. Louis, Mosby, 2007, p 172, Fig. 9-6.*)

(2) Acetyl coenzyme A (acetyl CoA)
    (a) Used to synthesize fatty acids for triglyceride synthesis
    (b) Used to synthesize ketoacids
  d. Alcohol induction of the cytochrome P-450 enzyme system
    • Increases alcohol metabolism, which increases the tolerance for alcohol
  e. Legal blood alcohol limit for driving
    • Ranges from 80 to 100 mg/dL

2. Risk factors for alcohol-related disease
   a. Amount
   b. Duration
   c. Female sex
      (1) Decreased gastric alcohol dehydrogenase levels
         • Causes higher alcohol levels in women than in men, even after drinking the same amount of alcohol
      (2) Genetic susceptibility
3. Systemic effects associated with alcohol abuse (Table 6-2)
4. Laboratory findings in alcohol abuse
   a. Fasting hypoglycemia
      • Excess NADH causes pyruvate (substrate for gluconeogenesis) to convert to lactate.
   b. Increased anion gap metabolic acidosis
      (1) Lactic acidosis
      (2) β-Hydroxybutyric ketoacidosis
         (a) Excess acetyl CoA is converted to β-hydroxybutyrate.
         (b) *Not* detected with urine dipstick or blood test for ketone bodies
   c. Other findings
      (1) Hyperuricemia (potential for developing gout)
         • Lactic acid and β-hydroxybutyric acid compete with uric acid for excretion in the proximal tubules.
      (2) Hypertriglyceridemia
         • Increased production of glycerol 3-phosphate, the key substrate for triglyceride synthesis in the liver
      (3) Serum aspartate aminotransferase (AST) greater than serum alanine aminotransferase (ALT) in liver disease (90% sensitivity, 75% specificity)
         • Alcohol is a mitochondrial toxin that causes release of AST, which is located in the mitochondria.
      (4) Increased serum γ-glutamyltransferase (GGT; 75% sensitivity, 90% specificity)
         • Alcohol induces hyperplasia of the smooth endoplasmic reticulum causing increased synthesis of GGT.

Margin notes:

Women: less gastric alcohol dehydrogenase than men

Alcohol abuse: most common cause of thiamine deficiency

↑ Anion gap metabolic acidosis in alcohol abuse: lactic acid, β-hydroxybutyric acid

Alcohol liver disease: AST > ALT; ↑ GGT

TABLE 6-2. **SYSTEMIC EFFECTS ASSOCIATED WITH ALCOHOL ABUSE**

SYSTEM	EFFECTS
Cardiovascular	Dilated cardiomyopathy: due to thiamine deficiency Hypertension: vasopressor effects due to increase in catecholamines
Central nervous system	CNS depressant: particularly cerebral cortex and limbic system Wernicke's syndrome: confusion, ataxia, nystagmus due to thiamine deficiency Korsakoff's psychosis: memory deficits due to thiamine deficiency Cerebellar atrophy: due to loss of Purkinje cells Cerebral atrophy: due to loss of neurons Central pontine myelinolysis: due to rapid intravenous fluid correction of hyponatremia in an alcoholic
Gastrointestinal	Oropharyngeal and upper to midesophageal cancer: squamous cell carcinoma Acute hemorrhagic gastritis Mallory-Weiss syndrome: tear of distal esophagus due to retching Boerhaave's syndrome: rupture of distal esophagus due to retching Esophageal varices: caused by portal vein hypertension in alcoholic cirrhosis Acute and chronic pancreatitis
General	Fetal alcohol syndrome: mental retardation, microcephaly, atrial septal and ventricular septal defects
Genitourinary	Testicular atrophy: decreased testosterone, decreased spermatogenesis Increased risk for spontaneous abortion
Hematopoietic	Folate deficiency: decreased reabsorption in jejunum; macrocytic anemia Acquired sideroblastic anemia: microcytic anemia due to defect in heme synthesis Anemia chronic disease: most common anemia in alcoholics
Hepatobiliary	Fatty liver, alcoholic hepatitis, cirrhosis Hepatocellular carcinoma: preexisting cirrhosis
Integument	Porphyria cutanea tarda: photosensitive bullous skin lesions
Musculoskeletal	Rhabdomyolysis: direct alcohol effect on muscle
Peripheral nervous system	Peripheral neuropathy: due to thiamine deficiency

TABLE 6-3. SELECTED DRUGS OF ABUSE AND THEIR EFFECTS

DRUG	DESCRIPTION	TOXIC EFFECTS
Cocaine	Stimulant	Mydriasis, tachycardia, hypertension Associated risk of AMI, CNS infarction, perforation of nasal septum (intranasal use)
Heroin	Opiate	Miotic pupils, noncardiogenic pulmonary edema (frothing from mouth), focal segmental glomerulosclerosis (nephrotic syndrome) Granulomatous reactions in skin and lungs from material used to "cut" (dilute) drug
Marijuana *(Cannabis)**	THC-containing psychoactive stimulant	Red conjunctivae, euphoria, delayed reaction time
MPTP	By-product of synthesis of meperidine	Irreversible Parkinson's disease: cytotoxic to neurons in nigrostriatal dopaminergic pathways

*Used medically to decrease nausea and vomiting associated with chemotherapy and to decrease intraocular pressure in glaucoma.
AMI, myocardial infarction; MPTP, 1-methyl-4-phenyl-1,2,3,6-tetrahydropyridine; THC, Δ9-tetrahydrocannabinol.

C. **Other drugs of abuse**
- Sedatives, stimulants, hallucinogens (Table 6-3)
1. CNS effects of long-term drug abuse
   a. Damage to neurotransmitter receptor sites
   b. Cerebral atrophy (e.g., alcohol)
2. Complications of intravenous drug use (IVDU)
   a. Hepatitis B
   b. HIV
   c. Infective endocarditis (tricuspid/aortic valves)
   - Caused by *Staphylococcus aureus*
   d. Tetanus
   - Complication of "skin popping" using a dirty needle
D. **Adverse effects of therapeutic drug use** (Table 6-4)
1. Acetaminophen
   a. Conversion to free radicals in the liver
   b. May result in damage to the liver (e.g., fulminant hepatitis)
   c. May result in damage to the kidneys (e.g., renal papillary necrosis)
2. Aspirin (acetylsalicylic acid) overdose
   a. General symptoms
   - Tinnitus, vertigo, change in mental status (confusion, seizures), tachypnea
   b. Acid-base disorders
      (1) Respiratory alkalosis may occur initially (within 12–24 hours).
         (a) Due to direct stimulation of the respiratory center
         (b) Respiratory acidosis may occur as a late finding.
      (2) Shift to metabolic acidosis with an increased anion gap
      - Occurs more often in children
      (3) Mixed primary respiratory alkalosis and metabolic acidosis
      - Occurs more often in adults
   c. Hyperthermia
      (1) Salicylates damage the inner mitochondrial membrane.
      (2) Oxidative energy is released as heat, *not* as adenosine triphosphate.
   d. Hemorrhagic gastritis, fulminant hepatitis
3. Disorders associated with exogenous estrogen *without* progestin
   a. Cancer (adenocarcinoma)
   - Endometrium, breast
   b. Venous thromboembolism
      (1) Estrogen decreases synthesis of antithrombin III (ATIII).
      - ATIII normally neutralizes activated coagulation factors.
      (2) Estrogen increases synthesis of factors I (fibrinogen), V, and VIII.
   c. Intrahepatic cholestasis with jaundice
   d. Cardiovascular effects
   - Myocardial infarction (MI), stroke
4. Disorders associated with oral contraceptives
   - Contain estrogen and progestin

Hepatitis B: most common systemic complication of IVDU

Salicylate poisoning: danger of hyperthermia

Both acetaminophen and aspirin cause fulminant hepatitis.

Unopposed estrogen: thrombogenic, carcinogenic, cholestasis

TABLE 6-4. **ADVERSE REACTIONS ASSOCIATED WITH THERAPEUTIC DRUG USE**

REACTION	DRUG(S)
Blood Dyscrasias	
Aplastic anemia	Chloramphenicol, alkylating agents
Hemolytic anemia	Penicillin, methyldopa, quinidine
Macrocytic anemia	Methotrexate (most common), phenytoin, oral contraceptives, 5-fluorouracil
Platelet dysfunction	Aspirin, other NSAIDs
Thrombocytopenia	Heparin (most common cause in hospital), quinidine
Cardiac	
Dilated cardiomyopathy	Doxorubicin, daunorubicin
Central Nervous System	
Tinnitus, vertigo	Salicylates
Cutaneous	
Angioedema	ACE inhibitors ($\uparrow$ bradykinin)
Maculopapular rash	Penicillin
Photosensitive rash	Tetracycline
Urticaria	Penicillin
Gastrointestinal	
Hemorrhagic gastritis	Iron, salicylates
Hepatic	
Cholestasis	Oral contraceptives, estrogen, anabolic steroids
Fatty change	Amiodarone, tetracycline, methotrexate
Hepatic adenoma	Oral contraceptives, anabolic steroids
Liver necrosis	Acetaminophen (most common), isoniazid, salicylates, halothane, iron
Pulmonary	
Asthma	Aspirin, other NSAIDs
Interstitial fibrosis	Bleomycin, busulfan, nitrofurantoin, methotrexate
Systemic	
Drug-induced lupus	Procainamide, hydralazine

ACE, angiotensin-converting enzyme.

a. Cancer
  (1) Breast (adenocarcinoma)
  (2) Cervix (squamous cell carcinoma)
b. Venous thromboembolism
  • Similar pathogenesis to estrogen without progestin
c. Folate deficiency
  • Decreases jejunal reabsorption of folate
d. Hypertension
  • Due to increased synthesis of angiotensinogen
e. Hepatic adenoma
  • Risk of intraperitoneal hemorrhage
f. Intrahepatic cholestasis with jaundice
g. Cholesterol gallstones
  • Estrogen increases cholesterol excretion in bile.
  E. **Injuries caused by environmental chemicals** (Table 6-5)
  F. **Injuries caused by arthropods and reptiles** (Table 6-6 and Fig. 6-2)
II. **Physical Injury**
  A. **Mechanical injury**
    1. Types of skin wounds
      a. Contusion (bruise)
        • Blunt force injury to blood vessels with subsequent escape of blood into tissue
      b. Abrasion
        • Superficial excoriation of the epidermis
      c. Laceration
        • Jagged tear with intact bridging blood vessels, nerves, and connective tissue
    2. Incision
      • Wound with sharp margins with severed bridging blood vessels

Oral contraceptives: $\downarrow$ risk for endometrial and ovarian cancer (only surface type)

Oral contraceptives: most common cause of hypertension in young women

Bee/wasp/hornet sting: most common cause of death due to a venomous bite

TABLE 6-5. ENVIRONMENTAL CHEMICALS AND ASSOCIATED TOXIC EFFECTS

CHEMICAL	SOURCE	TOXIC EFFECTS/TREATMENT
Arsenic	Pesticides, contaminated ground water	Inhibits enzymes that require lipoic acid as a cofactor (e.g., pyruvate dehydrogenase) causing increased conversion of pyruvate to lactate. Severe headaches, abdominal pain, diarrhea, delirium, convulsions, transverse bands in nails (Mees lines), death. Squamous cell carcinoma of skin, liver angiosarcoma, lung cancer *Treatment*: chelating agents: succimer (2,3-dimercaptosuccinic acid) or dimercaprol (BAL)
Asbestos (refer to Chapter 16)	Insulation, roofing material	Primary lung cancer, mesothelioma
Benzene	Solvent	Acute leukemia, aplastic anemia
Carbon monoxide (CO) (refer to Chapter 1)	Automobile exhaust, house fires, generators	Headache (first sign), cherry-red skin, coma ↓ O_2 saturation, normal Pao_2; lactic acidosis (due to hypoxia) *Treatment*: O_2 via nonbreather mask or endotracheal tube (100% O_2)
Cyanide (CN) (refer to Chapter 1)	House fires	Odor of bitter almonds; coma, seizures, heart dysfunction, metabolic acidosis (serum lactate >10 mmol/L), due to inhibition of cytochrome oxidase in ETC and subsequent shift to anaerobic glycolysis as only ATP source *Treatment*: amyl nitrite (produces metHb which combines with CN to form cyanmetHb) followed by thiosulfate (CN converted to thiocyanate)
Ethylene glycol (refer to Chapter 4)	Antifreeze End-product: oxalic acid	Increased anion gap metabolic acidosis Acute renal failure *Treatment*: IV infusion of ethanol or 4-methylpyrazole (see Table 4-6 for discussion)
Isopropyl alcohol	Rubbing alcohol End-product: acetone	Fruity odor to breath (acetone); can progress into deep coma Does *not* produce increased anion gap like ethanol, methanol, ethylene glycol but does increase osmolal gap (refer to Chapter 4) *Treatment*: hemodialysis
Lead (refer to Chapter 11)	Lead-based paint, batteries, metal casting	Microcytic anemia with coarse basophilic stippling, nephrotoxicity in proximal tubule *Treatment*: chelating agents: succimer, dimercaprol (BAL), EDTA
Mercury	Fish most important source	Diarrhea, constricted visual fields, nephrotoxicity in proximal tubule, tachycardia, hyperhidrosis (↑ sweating), peripheral neuropathy, hypertension *Treatment*: chelating agents: succimer, penicillamine, or dimercaprol (BAL)
Methanol (refer to Chapter 4)	Windshield-washer fluid End-product: formic acid	Increased anion gap metabolic acidosis Blindness due to optic atrophy *Treatment*: IV infusion of ethanol or 4-methylpyrazole (see Table 4-6 for discussion)
Organophosphates	Pesticides	Salivation, lacrimation, urinary/fecal incontinence, diaphoresis, blurred vision, hypotension, bradycardia, muscle fasiculations Decreased serum and RBC cholinesterase levels *Treatment*: atropine; pralidoxime has also been used
Polyvinyl chloride	Plastics industry	Liver angiosarcoma

ATP, adenosine triphosphate; BAL, British anti-lewisite; EDTA, ethylenediamine-tetraacetic acid; ETC, electron transport chain.

a. Gunshot wounds
   (1) Contact wounds
   (2) Stellate-shaped

Contact gunshot wound: fouling

b. Contain soot and gunpowder (fouling)
c. Intermediate-range wounds
   • Powder tattooing (stippling) of the skin around the entrance site

Intermediate range wound powder tattooing

d. Long-range wounds
   • *No* powder tattooing
e. Exit wounds
   • Typically larger and more irregular than entrance wounds

Motor vehicle collisions: most common cause of accidental death in people ages 1 to 39 years

3. Motor vehicle collisions
  a. Frequently cause mechanical injury
  b. Frequently alcohol-related
4. Shaken baby syndrome
  a. More than 50% of deaths in child abuse are due to this syndrome.

TABLE 6-6. INJURIES CAUSED BY ARTHROPODS AND REPTILES

AGENT	VENOM	TOXIC EFFECTS/TREATMENT
Coral snake (elapid)	Neurotoxin: binds to presynaptic nerve terminals and acetylcholine	Snake has "red on yellow" bands (red and yellow kill a fellow); "red on black" is a harmless scarlet king snake (red and black friend of jack) Toxic effects: paralysis (diplopia, respiratory muscles), fixed and contracted pupils; death by respiratory failure *Treatment*: elapid antivenin
Rattlesnake, copperhead, water moccasin (crotalids)	Venom cytohemoneurotoxic	Toxic effects: local edema/pain with progressive development of ecchymoses and bleeding into tissue, shock, DIC *Treatment*: avoid tourniquets and suction/incision kits; constriction bands above bite to reduce venous/lymphatic flow but maintain pulse; sheep antivenin (equine discontinued) with monospecific antibodies.
Latrodectus (black widow spider) (see Fig. 6-2A)	Latrotoxin (acts through Ca²⁺-mediated channels to cause release of acetylcholine and norepinephrine from nerve terminals)	Painful bite followed by increasing local pain; small erythematous macule develops within an hour which develops into a "target" lesion with a pale center surrounded by erythema; severe muscle cramps/spasms develop in trunk, thighs, and abdomen, the latter simulating an acute abdomen; hypertension may occur. *Treatment*: supportive; *Latrodectus* antivenom is available
Loxosceles (brown recluse spider) (see Fig. 6-2B)	Necrotoxins	Initially painless bite; painful reddish blister in several hours that develops a bluish discoloration in 24 hours; extensive skin necrosis occurs over next 3–4 days, with eschar formation by the end of the first week; may become infected; surgical débridement may be necessary. *Treatment*: supportive measures; antibiotics if necessary
Scorpion (see Fig. 6-2C)	Neurotoxin	Poisonous species in southwestern U.S. deserts (*Centruroides* sp.) Toxic effects: initially has painful sting followed by numbness, hypertension, ascending motor paralysis leading to death. May cause acute pancreatitis. *Treatment*: supportive; antivenom (goat serum) only with severe toxicity
Bees, wasps, hornets	Histamine and other components	As a group, they are the most common cause of death due to a venomous bite in the United States. Reactions range from localized erythema and swelling to an anaphylactic reaction (dyspnea, wheezing, inspiratory stridor [laryngeal swelling], shock, death) *Treatment*: epinephrine 0.3–0.5 mL of 1:1000 concentration intramuscularly in adults; 0.01 mg/kg in children; long-term management: insect sting kit with premeasured epinephrine; skin desensitization
Fire ants	Insoluble alkaloid	Swarm when provoked and attack in great numbers; painful bites with papules becoming sterile pustules in several hours; necrosis, scarring, secondary infection can occur; death may occur in some cases. *Treatment*: local wound care; desensitization is available

DIC, disseminated intravascular coagulation.

    b. Majority are <1 year old
    c. Characteristic signs
      (1) Retinal hemorrhages
      (2) Multiple fractures of long bones
      (3) Subdural hematomas
B. Thermal injury
  1. Burns
    a. First-degree
      (1) Painful partial-thickness burns (e.g., sunburn)
      (2) Heal without scarring
    b. Second-degree
      (1) Painful partial-thickness burns
      (2) Damage to entire epidermis
      (3) Blister formation
      (4) Usually heal without scarring
    c. Third-degree
      (1) Painless full-thickness burns

Shaken baby syndrome: retinal hemorrhages

First- and second-degree burns: no permanent scarring

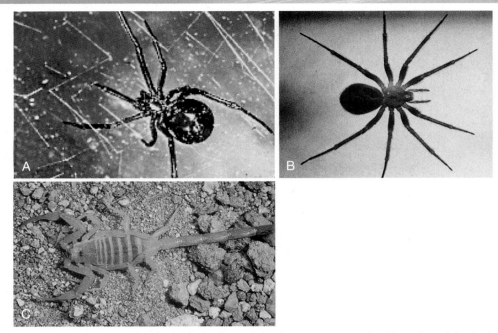

6-2: **A,** Black widow spider. Note the glossy black color and the characteristic ventral red hourglass abdominal marking. **B,** Brown recluse spider. Note the yellow-brown body and violin-shaped dark brown marking on the dorsal surface of the spider. **C,** Scorpion. *Centuroides* species are the most poisonous scorpions in the United States. (*A from Goldstein BG: Practical Dermatology, 2nd ed. St. Louis, Mosby, 1997, p 69, Fig. 6-11; **B,** courtesy of Professor H. Schenone, from Peters W: A Colour Atlas of Arthropods in Clinical Medicine. London, Wolfe, 1992; **C,** courtesy of Dr. J.C. Cockendolpher, from Peters W: A Colour Atlas of Arthropods in Clinical Medicine. London, Wolfe, 1992.)*

(2) Extensive necrosis of epidermis and adnexa
(3) Scarring is inevitable.
  (a) Keloids (exaggerated scars) commonly occur.
  (b) Potential for developing squamous cell carcinoma
(4) Healing of epithelial surface
  • Proliferation of residual epithelium located at burn margins and lining adnexal structures
d. Complications
(1) Infection
  • Sepsis due to *Pseudomonas aeruginosa* is the most common cause of death in burn patients.
(2) Curling's ulcers (stomach)
2. Minor heat syndromes
a. Heat edema
(1) Mild swelling of feet, ankles, and hands
(2) Cutaneous vasodilation with pooling of blood in gravity-dependent extremities
(3) Occurs in the elderly nonacclimatized individuals; healthy travelers coming from cold to hot environment
(4) Self-limited
b. Heat cramps (Table 6-7)
(1) Painful, involuntary spasmodic contractions of muscle
  (a) Usually starts in calves but may progress to other muscle groups
  (b) Due to deficiency of sodium, potassium, and fluids in muscle fibers

Most common cause of death in burn patients: sepsis caused by Pseudomonas aeruginosa

TABLE 6-7. **HEAT INJURIES***

TYPE OF INJURY	BODY TEMPERATURE	SKIN	MENTAL STATUS
Heat cramps	37°C (98.6°F)	Moist and cool	Normal
Heat exhaustion	≤40°C (104°F)	Sweating	Normal
Heat stroke	>40°C (>104°F)	Dry (anhidrosis)	Impaired consciousness CNS dysfunction

*Heat injury is exacerbated by high humidity.

(2) May occur in individuals sweating profusely without proper fluid replacement

(3) Treatment
- Commercially available electrolyte solution drinks

c. Heat exhaustion (see Table 6-7)

(1) Significant volume depletion (salt and water depletion) with or without increase in body temperature

(a) Orthostatic hypotension, dizziness, headache, nausea/vomiting

(b) Core temperature variable; normal to 40°C (104°F)

(c) No anhidrosis (absence of sweating); normal mental status examination

(2) Laboratory studies

(a) Hemoconcentration (e.g., ↑ hemoglobin/hematocrit)

(b) Variable serum Na$^+$ depending on previous intake
- Hypernatremia (no intake), normal, or hyponatremia (patient drank water without electrolytes)

(3) Treatment

(a) Intravenous volume and electrolyte replacement

(b) May progress to heat stroke if not treated promptly

3. Major heat syndrome: heat stroke (see Table 6-7)

a. Similar presentation as heat exhaustion, except the following

(1) Core body temperature > 40°C (104°F)

(2) Anhidrosis; mental status (e.g., do not know time, date) and CNS dysfunction (e.g., ataxia, cerebral edema, seizures)

b. Treatment

(1) High-flow O$_2$; intravenous fluids (normal saline, Ringer's lactate)

(2) Rapid cooling to < 40°C (104°F)

4. Frostbite

a. Pathogenesis

(1) Localized tissue injury caused by direct damage (e.g., ice crystallization in cells)

(2) Indirect damage (e.g., vasodilation, thrombosis)

b. Clinical findings

(1) Loss of pain sensation or burning/tingling sensation

(2) Discoloration of the skin; waxy appearance; cold to the touch

(3) Left untreated, skin gradually darkens (becomes completely black) and blisters

c. Treatment principles

(1) Pre-thaw: stabilize core body temperature; rehydration

(2) Thaw: immerse in circulating water 37°C to 40°C; ibuprofen

(3) Post-thaw: dry and elevate body part

C. Electrical injury

1. Produced by alternating current (AC) and direct current (DC)

a. AC is more dangerous than DC.

b. AC produces tetanic contractions.

c. DC produces a single shock.

d. Wet skin decreases resistance, which increases current.

e. Dry skin increases resistance, which decreases current.

f. Tissue damage increases with increased voltage and duration of exposure.

g. Current moving from the left arm to the right leg

(1) Most dangerous route, because it affects the heart

(2) Death results from cardiorespiratory arrest.

2. Lightning injury

a. 100 to 200 deaths/year

b. Hair on end; buzzing

c. Mortality rate 30% with direct strike

D. Drowning

1. Common cause of death in children from 1 to 14 years of age

2. Terminology

a. Drowning refers to death by suffocation from immersion in liquid.

b. Near drowning is defined as survival following asphyxia secondary to submersion.

c. Diving reflex occurs in water that is colder than 20°C (70°F).

(1) Bradycardia

Heat exhaustion: ≤ 40°C (<104°F); no anhidrosis/no mental status changes

Heat stroke: > 40°C (>104°F), anhidrosis (absence of sweating), impaired consciousness

AC more dangerous than DC

(2) Peripheral vasoconstriction
- Shunts blood to more vital areas.

(3) Blood shifting
- Shift to thoracic cavity to prevent lung collapse

(4) Allows both conscious and unconscious person to survive longer without O_2

d. Wet drowning

Most common drowning: wet drowning

(1) ~90% of cases

(2) Initial laryngospasm on contact with water followed by relaxation and aspiration of water

e. Dry drowning is characterized by intense laryngospasm *without* aspiration.

3. Pathophysiology

a. Lung aspiration of fresh water (90% of cases)

(1) Due to its hypotonicity, water is reabsorbed from the alveoli into the pulmonary circulation.

(2) Plasma is diluted causing hemolysis of RBCs (hemoglobinuria), hyponatremia, hyperkalemia.

(3) Electrolyte abnormalities precipitate ventricular fibrillation.
- Most common cause of death

(4) Hemoglobinuria can produce acute renal failure.

b. Lung aspiration of salt water (10% of cases)

(1) Salt water is more isotonic to blood (no RBC hemolysis).

(2) Cause of death is asphyxia from pulmonary edema.

E. High altitude injury

1. General

a. O_2 concentration 21%

b. Decreased barometric pressure

High altitude: O_2 concentration 21%, ↓ atmospheric pressure

c. Hypoxemic stimulus to chemoreceptors increases the respiratory rate producing respiratory alkalosis.
- Decrease in $Paco_2$ causes a corresponding increase in Pao_2.

d. Respiratory alkalosis activates glycolysis.

(1) Increased synthesis of 2,3-bisphosphoglycerate

High altitude: respiratory alkalosis; right-shifted OBC

(2) Right-shifts O_2-binding curve (OBC)
- Increases release of O_2 to tissue

2. Acute mountain sickness

a. Usually occurs at above 8000 feet (2440 m) elevation

b. Risk factors

(1) Increased rate of ascent

(2) Extreme altitude

c. Clinical findings

(1) Headache (most common)

(2) Fatigue, dizziness, anorexia, insomnia

(3) Acute pulmonary edema
- Noncardiogenic (exudate)

(4) Acute cerebral edema
- Ataxia, stupor, coma

d. Treatment
- Immediate descent (if severe complications)

III. Radiation Injury

A. Ionizing radiation injury
- Examples—x-rays, γ-rays

1. Pathophysiology

a. Injury correlates with type of radiation, cumulative dose, and amount of surface area exposed.

Ionizing radiation: damage to DNA

b. Direct or indirect DNA injury occurs via formation of hydroxyl free radicals.

2. Tissue susceptibility

a. Most radiosensitive tissues (highest mitotic activity)

Lymphoid tissue: most sensitive to radiation

(1) Lymphoid tissue (most sensitive)

(2) Bone marrow

(3) Mucosa of gastrointestinal tract, germinal tissue

b. Least radiosensitive tissues

Bone: least sensitive tissue to radiation

(1) Bone (least sensitive)

(2) Brain, muscle, skin

3. Radiation effects in different tissues
   a. Hematopoietic
      (1) Lymphopenia (first change)
      (2) Thrombocytopenia
      (3) Bone marrow hypoplasia
   b. Vascular
      (1) Thrombosis (early), fibrosis (late)
      (2) Ischemic damage
   c. Epidermal
      (1) Acute effects are erythema, edema, blistering.
      (2) Chronic effect is radiodermatitis.
         • Potential for squamous cell carcinoma
   d. Gastrointestinal
      (1) Acute effect is diarrhea.
      (2) Chronic effects are adhesions with potential for bowel obstruction.
4. Cancers caused by radiation
   a. Acute leukemia (most common)
   b. Papillary carcinoma of the thyroid
   c. Osteogenic sarcoma
B. Nonionizing radiation
1. Ultraviolet light B (UVB) is most damaging
   a. Pathogenesis
      (1) Pyrimidine dimers distort the DNA helix (see Fig. 8-4).
      (2) Inactivation of the *TP53* suppressor gene
      (3) Activation of the *RAS* oncogene
   b. General effects
      (1) Sunburn
      (2) Actinic (solar) keratosis (see Fig. 24-7A)
         • Precursor of squamous cell carcinoma (2–5% of cases)
      (3) Corneal burns from skiing
   c. Cancers
      (1) Basal cell carcinoma (most common) (see Fig. 24-7B)
      (2) Squamous cell carcinoma (see Fig. 24-7D), malignant melanoma (see Fig. 24-5H)
2. Effects of other types of radiation
   a. Laser radiation
      • Third-degree burns
   b. Microwave radiation
      • Skin burns, cataracts, sterility
   c. Infrared radiation
      • Skin burns, cataracts

Total body radiation: lymphopenia first hematologic sign

Acute leukemia: most frequent type of cancer caused by radiation

UVB: increase in pyrimidine dimers distorts DNA helix

Basal cell carcinoma: most common UVB light–related skin cancer

I. **Nutrient and Energy Requirements in Humans**
   A. **Recommended dietary allowance (RDA)**
      1. Optimal dietary intake of nutrients that under ordinary conditions will keep the general population in good health
      2. Varies with sex, age, body weight, diet, and physiologic status
   B. **Daily energy expenditure (DEE)**
      1. Factors influencing DEE
         a. Basal metabolic rate (BMR)
         b. Thermic effect of food
         c. Physical activity
      2. BMR
         a. Accounts for ~60% of DEE
         b. Energy consumption involved in normal body functions
            • Examples—cardiac function, maintaining ion pumps
         c. Body weight is the most important factor determining BMR.
         d. Thyroid function alters the BMR.
            • BMR is increased or decreased in hyperthyroidism and hypothyroidism, respectively.
      3. Thermic effect of foods
         • Energy used in digestion, absorption, and distribution of nutrients
      4. Degree of physical activity

II. **Dietary Fuels**
   A. **Carbohydrates**
      1. Glucose
         a. Stored primarily as glycogen in liver and muscle
         b. RBCs use only glucose for energy.
         c. Complete oxidation produces 4 kcal/g.
      2. Enzymatic digestion
         a. Begins in the mouth (amylase)
         b. Pancreatic amylase
            • In chronic pancreatitis, carbohydrates are *not* malabsorbed due to predigestion by salivary amylase.
         c. Brush border intestinal enzymes (disaccharidases)
            (1) Hydrolyze lactose (galactose + glucose), maltose (glucose + glucose), and sucrose (fructose + glucose)
            (2) Disaccharidases produce glucose, galactose, and fructose.
   B. **Proteins**
      1. Amino acids are substrates for gluconeogenesis.
         a. Transaminases remove amine groups to form corresponding α-ketoacid.
         b. Examples—alanine becomes pyruvate, aspartate becomes oxaloacetic acid
      2. Digestion
         a. Begins in the stomach (pepsin and acid)
         b. Pancreatic proteases (e.g., trypsin) and peptidases release amino acids.
      3. Complete oxidation produces 4 kcal/g.
   C. **Fats**
      1. Triglycerides
         a. Major dietary lipids
         b. Major source of energy for cells *except* RBCs and brain

---

BMR: most important factor in determining daily energy expenditure

BMR: ↓ hypothyroidism, ↑ hyperthyroidisim

Carbohydrate digestion: begins in the mouth; 4 kcal/g

Disaccharidases: produce glucose, galactose, fructose

Amino acids: substrates for gluconeogenesis

Protein digestion: begins in the stomach; pepsin and acid

2. Essential fatty acids (FAs)
   a. Linolenic acid (ω-3) is cardioprotective.
   b. Linoleic acid (ω-6) is required for synthesis of arachidonic acid.
   c. Deficiency of essential fatty acids
      (1) Scaly dermatitis, hair loss
      (2) Poor wound healing
3. Digestion of dietary triglyceride (TG)
   a. Occurs primarily in the small intestine
      (1) Hydrolyzed by pancreatic lipase
         • Produces monoglycerides (MGs) and FAs
      (2) Bile salts/acid produce micelles to enhance reabsorption by villi.
         • Contain MGs, FAs, fat-soluble vitamins, and cholesterol esters
      (3) Intestinal cells resynthesize TG and package it into chylomicrons, which enter the blood.
         • Formation and secretion of chylomicrons requires apolipoprotein B48.
   b. Complete oxidation produces 9 kcal/g.

III. Protein-Energy Malnutrition (PEM)
A. Kwashiorkor
1. Pathogenesis
   a. Inadequate protein intake
   b. Adequate caloric intake consisting mainly of carbohydrates
   c. Protein in liver and other organs (i.e., visceral protein) is decreased.
   d. Muscle protein (i.e., somatic protein) is relatively unchanged.
2. Clinical findings (Fig. 7-1, left)
   a. Pitting edema and ascites
      • Caused by hypoalbuminemia and loss of plasma oncotic pressure

Margin notes:

Essential FAs: linolenic, linoleic acids

Fat digestion: begins in the small intestine

Fat digestion: pancreas → bile salts/acids → intestinal cells

Kwashiorkor: inadequate protein intake

Pitting edema is characteristic of kwashiorkor

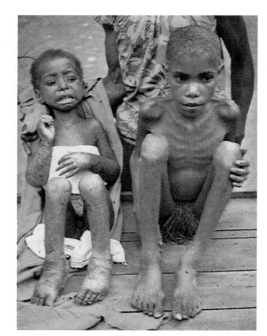

7-1: Kwashiorkor and marasmus. *Left,* Child with kwashiorkor, showing dependent pitting edema involving the lower legs. *Right,* Child with marasmus, showing "broomstick" extremities with loss of muscle mass and subcutaneous tissue. *(From Forbes C, Jackson W: Color Atlas and Text of Clinical Medicine, 2nd ed. St. Louis, Mosby, 2003, p 343, Fig. 7-138.)*

7-2: Anorexia nervosa. Note the loss of muscle and subcutaneous tissue consistent with total calorie deprivation. *(From Forbes C, Jackson W: Color Atlas and Text of Clinical Medicine, 2nd ed. St. Louis, Mosby, 2003, p 344, Fig. 7-141.)*

Kwashiorkor: fatty liver; ↓ apoB synthesis

b. Fatty liver
(1) Caused by decreased synthesis of apolipoproteins
(2) Apolipoprotein B-100 is required for assembly and secretion of very low density lipoproteins (VLDLs) in the liver.
c. Diarrhea
• Caused by loss of the brush border enzymes and parasitic infections
d. Anemia and defects in cell-mediated immunity (CMI)

B. Marasmus

Marasmus: total calorie deprivation

1. Pathogenesis
a. Dietary deficiency of both protein and calories
b. Decrease in somatic protein (muscle protein)

2. Clinical findings (see Fig. 7-1, right)

Extreme muscle wasting is common in marasmus.

a. Extreme muscle wasting ("broomstick extremities")
(1) Breakdown of muscle protein for energy
(2) Loss of subcutaneous fat
b. Growth retardation; anemia; defects in CMI

IV. Eating Disorders and Obesity

A. Anorexia nervosa

1. Pathogenesis
a. Self-induced starvation leading to PEM (Fig. 7-2)

Anorexia nervosa: distorted body image

b. Distorted body image
2. Clinical findings
a. Secondary amenorrhea
(1) Decreased gonadotropin-releasing hormone
• Caused by excessive loss of body fat and weight

Anorexia nervosa: secondary amenorrhea; osteoporosis

(2) Decreased serum gonadotropins produces hypoestrinism.
b. Osteoporosis
(1) Caused by hypoestrinism
• Estrogen normally enhances osteoblastic activity and inhibits osteoclastic activity.
(2) Lack of estrogen leads to decreased osteoblastic activity and increased osteoclastic activity.
c. Increased lanugo (fine, downy hair)
d. Increased hormones associated with stress (e.g., cortisol, growth hormone)

Most common cause of death in anorexia nervosa: ventricular arrhythmia

e. Most common cause of death is ventricular arrhythmia

B. Bulimia nervosa

1. Pathogenesis
• Bingeing with self-induced vomiting
2. Clinical findings
a. Complications of vomiting
(1) Acid injury to tooth enamel
(2) Hypokalemia and metabolic alkalosis

Vomiting in bulimia nervosa: produces hypokalemic metabolic alkalosis

b. Ventricular arrhythmia is the most common cause of death.

C. Obesity

BMI: weight (kg)/height (m²)

1. Body mass index (BMI) ≥ 30 kg/m² (normal, 18.5–24.9 kg/m²)
a. BMI = weight (kg)/height (m²)
b. Other factors than body weight
(1) Excess fat in the waist and flanks is more important than an excess in the thighs and buttocks.

Obesity: abdominal visceral fat most important

(2) Excess visceral fat in the abdominal cavity has greater significance than excess subcutaneous fat.
• Magnetic resonance imaging is used to access the amount of visceral fat.
2. Pathogenesis
a. Genetic factors account for 50% to 80% of cases.
• Examples—defects in the leptin gene, syndrome X (obesity, hypertension, diabetes)
b. Acquired causes
(1) Endocrine disorders—hypothyroidism, Cushing syndrome
(2) Hypothalamic lesions, menopause
c. Leptin

Leptin: hormone; maintains energy balance (intake and output)

(1) Leptin is a hormone.
(a) Secreted by adipose tissue
(b) Maintains energy balance (intake and output)

TABLE 7-1. CLINICAL FINDINGS ASSOCIATED WITH OBESITY

CLINICAL FINDING	COMMENTS
Cancer	Increased incidence of estrogen-related cancers (e.g., endometrial, breast) because of increased aromatization of androgens to estrogens in adipose tissue
Cholelithiasis	Increased incidence of cholecystitis and cholesterol stones: bile is supersaturated with cholesterol
Diabetes mellitus, type 2	Increased adipose downregulates insulin receptor synthesis Hyperinsulinemia increases adipose stores Weight reduction upregulates insulin receptor synthesis
Hepatomegaly	Fatty change accompanied by liver cell injury and repair by fibrosis
Hypertension	Hyperinsulinemia increases sodium retention, leading to increase in plasma volume Left ventricular hypertrophy and stroke complicate hypertension
Hypertriglyceridemia	Hypertriglyceridemia decreases serum high-density lipoprotein levels, increasing risk of coronary artery disease
Increased low-density lipoprotein levels	Hypercholesterolemia predisposes to coronary artery disease
Obstructive sleep apnea	Weight of adipose tissue compresses upper airways causing respiratory acidosis and hypoxemia Potential for developing cor pulmonale (pulmonary hypertension and right ventricular hypertrophy)
Osteoarthritis	Degenerative arthritis in weight-bearing joints (e.g., femoral heads)

(2) Leptin increases when adipose stores are adequate.
    (a) Decreases food intake (inhibits satiety center)
    (b) Increases energy expenditure (stimulates β-oxidation of fatty acids)
(3) Leptin decreases when adipose stores are inadequate.
    (a) Increases food intake (stimulates the satiety center)
    (b) Decreases energy expenditure (inhibits β-oxidation of fatty acids)
(4) Obesity related to leptin dysfunction may be caused by the following:
    (a) Resistance to leptin effects
    (b) Mutations resulting in inhibition of leptin release
  3. Clinical findings (Table 7-1)

V. Fat-Soluble Vitamins
- Vitamins A, D, E, and K are fat soluble.
  A. Vitamin A
    1. Retinol
      a. Derived from dietary β-carotenes and retinol esters
        (1) Increased β-carotenes in the diet cause the skin to turn yellow.
        (2) The sclera remains white, unlike in jaundice, in which the sclera is yellow.
      b. Main transport and storage form of vitamin A
    2. Retinal
      a. Product of the oxidation of retinol
      b. Component of the visual pigment rhodopsin
    3. Sources of vitamin A
      a. Preformed vitamin A in liver egg yolk, butter, and milk
      b. β-Carotenes in dark-green and yellow vegetables
    4. Functions of vitamin A
      a. Normal vision in reduced light
      b. Potentiating differentiation of mucus-secreting epithelium
      c. Stimulating the immune system
      d. Growth and reproduction
    5. Clinical uses of vitamin A
      a. Treatment of acne (e.g., isotretinoin)
      b. Treatment of acute promyelocytic leukemia (refer to Chapter 12)
    6. Causes of deficiency
      a. Diets lacking sufficient yellow and green vegetables
      b. Fat malabsorption (e.g., celiac disease)
    7. Causes of toxicity
      a. Consumption of bear liver
      b. Megadoses of vitamin A
      c. Treatment with isotretinoin

Margin notes:

3500 calorie excess = 1 pound

Leptin gene: often defective in obesity

Obesity: ↑ adipose causes ↓ synthesis insulin receptors

β-carotenemia: yellow skin, white sclera

Vitamin A: vision, cell differentiation, growth/reproduction

Night blindness: first sign of vitamin A deficiency

Vitamin A in treatment: acne, acute promyelocytic leukemia

Vitamin A toxicity: consumption of bear liver

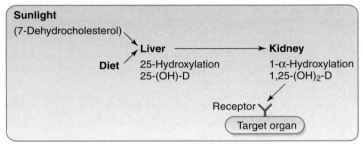

7-3: Vitamin D metabolism. See text for discussion.

B. Vitamin D
1. Sources of vitamin D
   a. Fish oil, egg yolk, liver
   b. Fortified milk
2. Metabolism (Fig. 7-3)
   a. Preformed vitamin D in the diet consists of cholecalciferol (fish) and ergocalciferol (plants).
   b. Endogenous synthesis of vitamin D in the skin occurs by photoconversion of 7-dehydrocholesterol via sunlight.
   c. Reabsorption occurs in the small intestine.
   d. Liver hydroxylation to 25-hydroxyvitamin D (25-OH-D; calcidiol) occurs in the cytochrome P-450 system.
   e. Kidney hydroxylation by 1-α-hydroxylase produces 1,25-(OH)$_2$-D (active form of vitamin D; calcitriol).
   f. Calcitriol attaches to nuclear receptors in target tissues.
3. Functions
   a. Maintenance of serum calcium and phosphorus
      • Increases reabsorption of calcium and phosphorus from the intestine
   b. Required for mineralization of epiphyseal cartilage and osteoid matrix
      (1) Receptor located on osteoblasts
      (2) Stimulates release of alkaline phosphatase
      (3) Alkaline phosphatase dephosphorylates pyrophosphate, which normally inhibits bone mineralization.
   c. Stimulates macrophage stem cell conversion into osteoclasts
4. Causes of deficiency
   a. Renal failure
      • Decrease in 1-α-hydroxylation
   b. Inadequate exposure to sunlight
      • Decreased synthesis from 7-dehydrocholesterol
   c. Fat malabsorption
      • Decreased reabsorption of vitamin D
   d. Chronic liver disease
      • Decreased synthesis of 25-(OH)-D
   e. Enzyme induction of the cytochrome P-450 enzyme system (e.g., alcohol)
      • Increased metabolism of 25-(OH)-D into inactive metabolite
5. Megadoses may cause toxicity.

C. Vitamin E
1. Sources
   • Nuts (almonds, seeds), green leafy vegetables, olives, vegetable oil, wheat germ
2. Serves as an antioxidant
   a. Protects cell membranes from lipid peroxidation from free radicals
   b. Prevents oxidation of low-density lipoprotein to a free radical form
3. Deficiency is uncommon; may occur in a few disorders:
   a. Fat malabsorption in children with cystic fibrosis
   b. Abetalipoproteinemia
4. Megadoses may cause toxicity.

D. Vitamin K
1. Sources
   • Derived from endogenous bacteria (most common source), dark green vegetables

2. Activated by the liver microsomal enzyme epoxide reductase
   - Anticoagulant effect of coumarin derivatives results from the inhibition of epoxide reductase.
3. Function (also refer to Chapter 14)
   a. γ-Carboxylates glutamate residues in vitamin K–dependent procoagulants and anticoagulants (proteins C and S)
      (1) Procoagulants include factors II (prothrombin), VII, IX, X.
      (2) Procoagulants are nonfunctional.
   b. γ-Carboxylation allows vitamin K–dependent procoagulants to bind to calcium in fibrin clot formation.
4. Causes of deficiency
   a. Use of broad-spectrum antibiotics
      - Destroy bacterial synthesis of vitamin K
   b. Newborns
      (1) Lack bacterial colonization of the bowel
      (2) Must receive vitamin K at birth
         (a) Prevents hemorrhagic disease of the newborn
         (b) Breast milk is deficient in vitamin K.
   c. Coumarin derivatives/cirrhosis
      - Decreases epoxide reductase activation of vitamin K
   d. Fat malabsorption
      - Decreased intestinal reabsorption of vitamin K
5. Toxicity caused by excessive intake of vitamin K is uncommon.

E. Summary
   - Table 7-2 summarizes clinical findings and toxicities of all fat-soluble vitamins (Fig. 7-4A–C).

VI. Water-Soluble Vitamins
   A. Thiamine (vitamin B$_1$)
   1. Sources
      a. Liver; eggs; whole grain cereal, rice, wheat
      b. Outer layers of grain and the seed
         - Removal of the outer grain in the refining process (white rice, white bread) significantly lowers thiamine content.
   2. Function
      a. Cofactor in biochemical reactions that produce adenosine triphosphate (ATP)
      b. Example—pyruvate dehydrogenase–catalyzed conversion of pyruvate to acetyl CoA
   3. Causes of deficiency
      a. Chronic alcoholism (in the United States)
      b. Diet of nonenriched rice (in developing countries)

Margin notes:

Vitamin K: majority synthesized by colonic bacteria

Vitamin K: γ-carboxylates II, VII, IX, X

Broad-spectrum antibiotics: most common cause of vitamin K deficiency in a hospital

Newborns: require vitamin K injection

Rat poison contains coumarin derivatives.

Thiamine: present in outer shell and seed of grain

Thiamine: important in ATP synthesis

Chronic alcoholism: most common cause of thiamine deficiency in the United States

TABLE 7-2. FAT-SOLUBLE VITAMINS: CLINICAL FINDINGS IN DEFICIENCY AND TOXICITY

VITAMIN	EFFECTS OF DEFICIENCY	EFFECTS OF TOXICITY
A	Impaired night vision, blindness (squamous metaplasia of corneal epithelium; see Fig. 7-4A) Follicular hyperkeratosis (loss of sebaceous gland function; see Fig. 7-4B), pneumonia, growth retardation, renal calculi	Papilledema and seizures (due to an increase in intracranial pressure), hepatitis, bone pain (due to periosteal proliferation)
D	Pathologic fractures, excess osteoid, bow legs (see Fig. 7-4C) Children: rickets; craniotabes (soft skull bones); rachitic rosary (defective mineralization and overgrowth of epiphyseal cartilage in ribs) Adults: called osteomalacia Continuous muscle contraction (tetany)	Hypercalcemia with metastatic calcification, renal calculi
E	Hemolytic anemia (damage to RBC membrane) Peripheral neuropathy, degeneration of posterior column (poor joint sensation) and spinocerebellar tract (ataxia)	Decreased synthesis of vitamin K–dependent procoagulant factors; synergistic effect with warfarin anticoagulation
K	Newborns: hemorrhagic disease of newborn (CNS bleeding, ecchymoses) Adults: gastrointestinal bleeding, ecchymoses; prolonged prothrombin time and partial thromboplastin time	Hemolytic anemia and jaundice in newborns if mother receives excess vitamin K

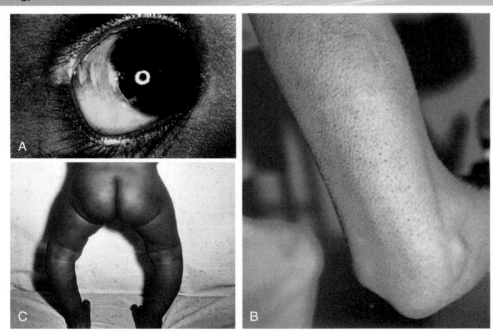

7-4: A, Squamous metaplasia of conjunctiva (Bitot's spot) in vitamin A deficiency. Note the raised white area on the conjunctiva (*arrow*) encroaching on the cornea. **B,** Follicular hyperkeratosis in vitamin A deficiency. Note the "goose-bump" appearance of the raised, hyperkeratotic lesions. **C,** Child with rickets. Note the bow legs. (*A reprinted with permission from Oomen HAPC: Vitamin A deficiency, xerophthalmia and blindness. Nutr Rev 1974;32:161-166, Wiley-Blackwell; **B** from Morgan SL, Weinsier RL: Fundamentals of Clinical Nutrition, 2nd ed. St. Louis, Mosby, 1998; **C** from Kumar V, Fausto N, Abbas A: Robbins and Cotran's Pathologic Basis of Disease, 8th ed. Philadelphia, WB Saunders, 2007, p 455, Fig. 8-21.*)

B. Riboflavin (vitamin B₂)

> Riboflavin: FAD and FMN in citric acid cycle

1. Sources
   - Liver, dairy products, nuts, green leafy vegetables, soybeans
2. Active forms include flavin adenine dinucleotide (FAD) and flavin mononucleotide (FMN).
   - Located in the citric acid cycle
3. Deficiency is caused by severe malnourishment.

C. Niacin (vitamin B₃, nicotinic acid)

1. Sources
   - Most animal products, fruits and vegetables, and seeds

> Niacin: NAD and NADP cofactors

2. Functions
   a. Active forms of niacin
      (1) Oxidized nicotinamide adenine dinucleotide (NAD)
      (2) Oxidized nicotinamide adenine dinucleotide phosphate (NADP)
   b. NAD and NADP are cofactors in oxidation-reduction reactions.

> Corn-based diets: deficient in tryptophan and niacin

3. Causes of deficiency (pellagra)
   a. Diets deficient in niacin
      (1) Corn-based diets
      (2) Corn is deficient in tryptophan and niacin.
   b. Deficiency of tryptophan

> Tryptophan: used to synthesize niacin

> Trytophan deficiency: Hartnup disease, carcinoid syndrome

      (1) Tryptophan is used to synthesize niacin.
      (2) Causes of tryptophan deficiency
         (a) Diets deficient in tryptophan
         (b) Hartnup disease
            - Inborn error of metabolism with inability to reabsorb tryptophan in the small bowel and kidneys
         (c) Carcinoid syndrome
            - Tryptophan is used up in synthesizing serotonin.

> Three Ds of pellagra: dermatitis, diarrhea, dementia

4. Excessive intake of niacin
   a. Leads to flushing caused by vasodilation
      - Adverse effect of nicotinic acid, a lipid-lowering drug
   b. Intrahepatic cholestasis

D. Pyridoxine (vitamin B$_6$)
  1. Sources
     - Meats, fish, seeds, wheat germ, and whole-grain flour
  2. Functions
     - Required for transamination, heme synthesis, and neurotransmitter synthesis
  3. Causes of deficiency
     a. Isoniazid (used in treating tuberculosis)
     b. Goat milk, chronic alcoholism

E. Cobalamin (vitamin B$_{12}$) (refer to Chapter 11)
  1. Present only in animal products (eggs, meat, dairy products)
  2. Requires intrinsic factor for reabsorption in the terminal ileum
  3. Functions
     a. DNA synthesis
     b. Propionate (odd-chain fatty acid) metabolism
  4. Causes of deficiency
     a. Strict vegan diet
     b. Pernicious anemia
     c. Terminal ileal disease (e.g., Crohn's disease), bacterial overgrowth

F. Folic acid (refer to Chapter 11)
  1. Present in most foods
  2. Function
     - DNA synthesis
  3. Causes of deficiency
     a. Dietary deficiency
        - Elderly individuals, goat milk
     b. Drugs
        - Alcohol, methotrexate, phenytoin, oral contraceptives, trimethoprim, 5-fluorouracil
     c. Malabsorption, overutilization (e.g., pregnancy)

G. Biotin
  1. Present in most foods
  2. Function
     a. Cofactor in carboxylase reactions
     b. Example—pyruvate carboxylase–catalyzed conversion of pyruvate to oxaloacetate
  3. Causes of deficiency
     a. Eating raw eggs (avidin binds biotin)
     b. Taking antibiotics

H. Ascorbic acid (vitamin C)
  1. Functions
     a. Hydroxylation of lysine and proline residues in collagen synthesis
        (1) Deficiency leads to collagen with reduced tensile strength.
        (2) Hydroxylation sites are anchors for cross-linking of tropocollagens.
     b. Antioxidant activity
        (1) Regenerates vitamin E and reduces oxidation of low-density lipoprotein
        (2) Best vitamin to neutralize hydroxyl free radicals
     c. Reduces nonheme iron (3 valence) from plants to the ferrous (2 valence) state for reabsorption in the duodenum
        - Deficiency may produce iron deficiency (microcytic anemia).
     d. Keeps tetrahydrofolate (FH$_4$) in its reduced form
        - Deficiency may produce folate deficiency (macrocytic anemia).
     e. Cofactor in the conversion of dopamine to norepinephrine in catecholamine synthesis
  2. Causes of deficiency
     a. Diets lacking fruits and vegetables
     b. Cigarette smoking
        - Used up in neutralizing free radicals in cigarette smoke
  3. Excess intake (hypervitaminosis C) may lead to the formation of renal calculi composed of uric acid.

I. Summary
  - Table 7-3 summarizes the clinical findings in the water-soluble vitamin deficiencies (Fig. 7-5A–D).

Pyridoxine: heme synthesis, transamination, neurotransmitters

Isoniazid therapy: most common cause pyridoxine deficiency

Vitamin B$_{12}$: only in animal products

Vitamin B$_{12}$: DNA synthesis; odd-chain fatty acid synthesis

Pernicious anemia: most common cause of vitamin B$_{12}$ deficiency

Folic acid: DNA synthesis

Goat milk: lacks folate and pyridoxine

Alcohol excess: most common cause folate deficiency

Biotin deficiency: eating raw eggs

Ascorbic acid: collagen synthesis, antioxidant, reducing agent

Ascorbic acid: cofactor conversion dopamine to norepinephrine

Scurvy: deficiency of ascorbic acid

TABLE 7-3. **WATER-SOLUBLE VITAMINS: CLINICAL FINDINGS IN DEFICIENCY**

VITAMIN	EFFECTS OF DEFICIENCY
Thiamine (vitamin B₁)	Dry beriberi: peripheral neuropathy (demyelination) Wernicke's syndrome: ataxia, confusion, nystagmus, mamillary body hemorrhage Korsakoff's syndrome: antegrade and retrograde amnesia; demyelination in limbic system Wet beriberi: congestive cardiomyopathy with biventricular failure
Riboflavin (vitamin B₂)	Corneal neovascularization, glossitis, cheilosis (cracked lips), angular stomatitis (fissuring at angles of mouth)
Niacin (vitamin B₃)	Pellagra: diarrhea, dermatitis (hyperpigmentation in sun-exposed areas; see Fig. 7-5A), dementia
Pyridoxine (vitamin B₆)	Sideroblastic anemia (microcytic anemia with ringed sideroblasts; see Fig. 11-13), convulsions, peripheral neuropathy
Cobalamin (vitamin B₁₂)	Megaloblastic anemia, neurologic disease (posterior column and lateral corticospinal tract demyelination), glossitis
Folic acid	Megaloblastic anemia, with *no* neurologic disease (unlike vitamin B₁₂), glossitis
Biotin	Dermatitis, alopecia, lactic acidosis
Ascorbic acid (vitamin C)	Weak capillaries and venules, skin ecchymoses, perifollicular hemorrhage (ring of hemorrhage around hair follicles; see Fig. 7-5B), corkscrew hairs (see Fig. 7-5C), hemarthrosis, bleeding gums (see Fig. 7-5D), anemia (combined iron and folate deficiency) Loosened teeth, glossitis, poor wound healing

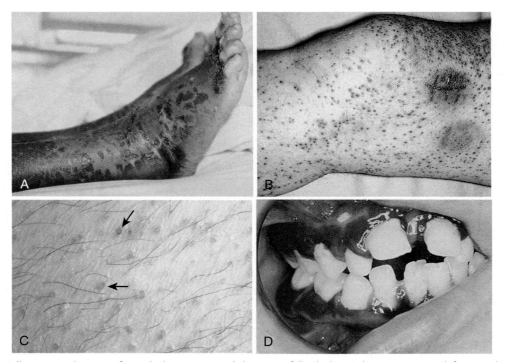

7-5: A, Pellagra. Note the areas of irregular hyperpigmented skin. **B,** Perifollicular hemorrhage in vitamin C deficiency. The areas of hemorrhage surround hair follicles. **C,** Corkscrew hairs in vitamin C deficiency. Note the coiled hairs lying within plugged follicles. **D,** Gums showing the effects of scurvy. The swelling, inflammation, and bleeding of the gingival papillae are prominent. *(**A** and **D** from Morgan SL, Weinsier RL: Fundamentals of Clinical Nutrition, 2nd ed. St. Louis, Mosby, 1998; **B** from Callen JP, Paller AS, Greer KE, Swinyer LJ: Color Atlas of Dermatology, 2nd ed. Philadelphia, WB Saunders, 2000; **C** from Savin JA, Hunter JAA, Hepburn NC: Diagnosis in Color: Skin Signs in Clinical Medicine. London, Mosby-Wolfe, 1997, p 85, Fig. 3-8.)*

VII. Trace Elements
- Trace elements are micronutrients that are required in the normal diet.
  A. Zinc
  1. Functions
     a. Cofactor for metalloenzymes (e.g., collagenase in wound remodeling)
     b. Growth and spermatogenesis in children
  2. Causes of zinc deficiency
     a. Alcoholism, diabetes mellitus, chronic diarrhea

TABLE 7-4. TRACE METALS: CLINICAL FINDINGS IN DEFICIENCY

TRACE METAL	EFFECTS OF DEFICIENCY
Chromium	Metabolic: impaired glucose tolerance, peripheral neuropathy
Copper	Blood: microcytic anemia (cofactor in ferroxidase) Vessels: aortic dissection (weak elastic tissue) Metabolic: poor wound healing (cofactor in lysyl oxidase)
Fluoride	Teeth: dental caries
Iodide	Thyroid: thyroid enlargement (goiter), hypothyroidism
Selenium	Muscle: muscle pain and weakness, dilated cardiomyopathy
Zinc	Metabolic: poor wound healing (cofactor in collagenase) Mouth: dysgeusia (cannot taste), anosmia (cannot smell), perioral rash Children: hypogonadism, growth retardation

  b. Acrodermatitis enteropathica
    (1) Autosomal recessive disease
    (2) Dermatitis, growth retardation, decreased spermatogenesis, poor wound healing
  3. Clinical findings in zinc deficiency (Table 7-4)

B. Copper
  1. Functions as a cofactor
    a. Ferroxidase (binds iron to transferrin)
    b. Lysyl oxidase (cross-linking of collagen and elastic tissue)
    c. Tyrosinase (melanin synthesis)
  2. Copper deficiency
    • Most often due to total parenteral nutrition (TPN)
  3. Clinical findings in copper deficiency (see Table 7-4)
  4. Copper excess, Wilson's disease
    a. Autosomal recessive disease
    b. Defect in eliminating copper into bile
    c. Defect in incorporating copper into ceruloplasmin (binding protein for copper)
    d. Chronic liver disease, Kayser-Fleischer ring in cornea, basal ganglia degeneration

C. Iodine
  1. Function
    • Synthesis of thyroid hormone
  2. Iodine deficiency
    • Most often due to inadequate intake of iodized table salt
  3. Clinical findings in iodide deficiency (see Table 7-4)

D. Chromium
  1. Functions
    a. Component of glucose tolerance factor (maintains a normal glucose)
    b. Cofactor for insulin that facilitates binding of glucose to adipose and muscle
  2. Chromium deficiency
    • Most often due to TPN
  3. Clinical findings in chromium deficiency (see Table 7-4)

E. Selenium
  1. Component of glutathione peroxidase
    • Antioxidant that converts peroxide to water using reduced glutathione (GSH)
  2. Selenium deficiency
    • Most often due to TPN
  3. Clinical findings in selenium deficiency (see Table 7-4)

F. Fluoride
  1. Function
    • Component of calcium hydroxyapatite in bone and teeth
  2. Fluoride deficiency
    • Most often due to inadequate intake of fluoridated water
  3. Fluoride excess
    a. Chalky deposits on the teeth
    b. Calcification of ligaments
    c. Increased risk for bone fractures
  4. Clinical findings in fluoride deficiency (see Table 7-4)

Zinc deficiency: poor wound healing, dysgeusia, perioral rash

Copper excess: Wilson's disease

Iodide deficiency: multinodular goiter

Chromium: useful in diabetics

Selenium: antioxidant

Fluoride: component of calcium hydroxyapatite

Fluoride deficiency: dental caries

VIII. Dietary Fiber

    A. Types/function

Fiber types: insoluble, soluble

        1. Insoluble fiber

           a. Nonfermentable

             • Examples—wheat bran, wheat germ

           b. Absorbs water

           c. Binds potential carcinogens

             (1) Lithocholic acid

                (a) Only bile acid that is *not* reabsorbed in the terminal ileum

                (b) May have causative role in producing colorectal cancer

             (2) Estrogen

                • Unopposed increase in estrogen increases risk for endometrial and breast cancer.

           d. Stool eliminated faster

Soluble fiber: lowers cholesterol

        2. Soluble fiber

           a. Fermentable

             • Examples—oat bran, psyllium seeds, fruits

           b. Decreases serum cholesterol

           c. Increases fecal bacterial mass

        3. Benefits of increased fiber

           a. Reduces deconjugation of estrogen delivered in bile

             • Decreases reabsorption of estrogen, which decreases risk for estrogen-related cancers

           b. Decreases risk for developing diverticulosis by preventing constipation

           c. May reduce the risk for developing colorectal and estrogen-related cancers

Fiber: ↓ risk for sigmoid diverticulosis, certain cancers, heart disease

           d. Decreases risk for developing heart disease

             • Decreases cholesterol

    B. Recommendation for fiber in diet

        • 20 to 30 g of fiber/day

IX. Special Diets

    A. Sodium restriction

        1. Reduces blood pressure

        2. Nonpharmacologic treatment

Sodium restriction: hypertension, heart failure, chronic liver/kidney disease

           a. Essential hypertension

           b. Congestive heart failure

           c. Chronic renal disease

           d. Cirrhosis

    B. Protein-restricted diets

        • Reduces the formation of urea and ammonia

Protein-restricted diet: chronic renal failure, cirrhosis

        1. Chronic renal disease

           • Decreases urea load

         2. Cirrhosis of liver

           a. Dysfunctional urea cycle cannot metabolize ammonia.

           b. Increased ammonia produces hepatic encephalopathy.

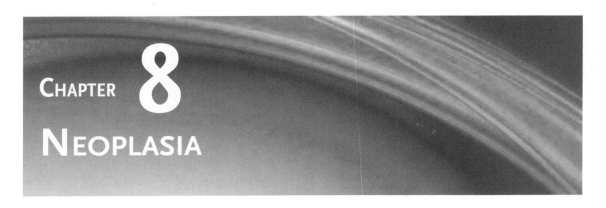

CHAPTER 8

NEOPLASIA

I. Nomenclature
   A. **Benign tumors**
      1. Suffix "oma" generally indicates a benign tumor.
      2. Benign tumors of epithelial origin
         a. Arise from ectoderm or endoderm
         b. Example—tubular adenoma (adenomatous polyp) arising from glands in the colon (Fig. 8-1A; see Fig. 17-37)
      3. Benign tumors of connective tissue origin arise from mesoderm.
         • Example—lipoma from adipose (Fig. 8-1B)
      4. Tumors that are usually benign
         a. Mixed tumors
            (1) Neoplastic cells have two different morphologic patterns but derive from the same germ cell layer.
            (2) Example—pleomorphic adenoma of the parotid gland
         b. Teratomas
            (1) Tumors that derive from more than one germ cell layer
               • Contain tissue derived from ectoderm, endoderm, and mesoderm (Fig. 8-1C)
            (2) Sites
               • Ovaries, testes, anterior mediastinum, and pineal gland
   B. **Malignant tumors (cancer)**
      1. Carcinomas
         a. Derive from epithelial tissue—squamous, glandular, transitional
         b. Sites of squamous cell carcinoma (Fig. 8-1D)
            • Oropharynx, larynx, upper/middle esophagus, lung, cervix, skin
         c. Sites of adenocarcinoma (glandular epithelium; Fig. 8-1E)
            • Lung, distal esophagus to rectum, pancreas, liver, breast, endometrium, ovaries, kidneys, prostate
         d. Sites of transitional cell carcinoma
            • Urinary bladder, ureter, renal pelvis
      2. Sarcomas
         a. Derive from connective tissue
         b. Example—osteogenic sarcoma in bone (Fig. 8-1F)
   C. **Tumor-like conditions**
      1. Hamartoma
         a. Non-neoplastic overgrowth of disorganized tissue indigenous to a particular site
         b. Examples—bronchial hamartoma (contains cartilage), Peutz-Jeghers polyp
      2. Choristoma (heterotopic rest)
         a. Non-neoplastic normal tissue in a foreign location
         b. Examples—pancreatic tissue in the stomach wall; parietal cells in Meckel diverticulum
II. Properties of Benign and Malignant Tumors
   A. **Components of benign and malignant tumors**
      1. Parenchyma
         • Neoplastic component that determines the tumor's biologic behavior
      2. Stroma
         a. Non-neoplastic supportive tissue
         b. Most infiltrating carcinomas induce production of a dense, fibrous stroma

Benign tumors: epithelial or connective tissue origin

Epothelial tissue origin: ectoderm, endoderm

Connective tissue origin: mesoderm

Teratoma: derives from ectoderm, endoderm, mesoderm

Carcinomas: derive from squamous, glandular (adenocarcinoma), transitional epithelium

Sarcomas: derive from connective tissue

Hamartoma: non-neoplastic overgrowth of tissue

Choristoma: normal tissue where it should *not* be

Parenchyma: neoplastic component

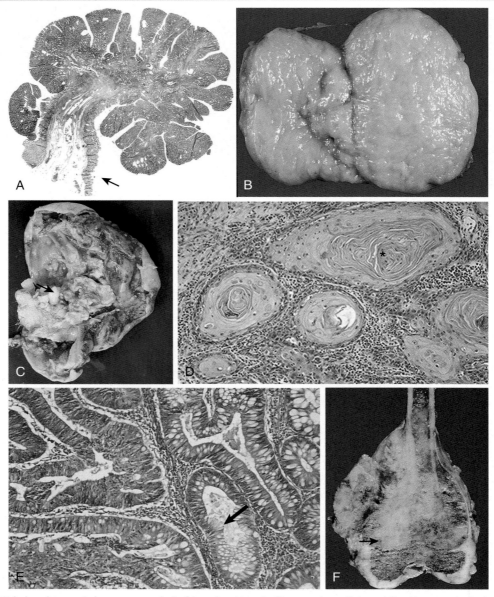

8-1: A, Tubular adenoma (adenomatous polyp) of the colon. Note the fibrovascular stalk (*arrow*) lined by normal colonic mucosa and a branching head surfaced by dysplastic (blue-staining) epithelial glands. **B,** Lipoma showing a well-circumscribed yellow tumor. **C,** Cystic teratoma of the ovary, showing the cystic nature of the tumor. Hair is present, and a tooth is visible (*arrow*). **D,** Squamous cell carcinoma. The many well-differentiated foci of eosinophilic-staining neoplastic cells produce keratin in layers (keratin pearls). **E,** Adenocarcinoma. Irregular glands infiltrate the stroma. The nuclei lining the gland lumens are cuboidal and contain nuclei with hyperchromatic nuclear chromatin. Many of the gland lumens contain secretory material (*arrow*). **F,** Osteogenic sarcoma of the distal femur. The light-colored mass of tumor in the metaphysis abuts the epiphyseal plate (*arrow*) and has spread laterally out through the cortex and into the surrounding tissue. (*A from Kumar V, Fausto N, Abbas A: Robbins and Cotran's Pathologic Basis of Disease, 7th ed. Philadelphia, WB Saunders, 2004, p 860, Fig. 17-57A; B and C from Damjanov I: Pathology for the Health-Related Professions, 2nd ed. Philadelphia, WB Saunders, 2000, pp 77, 79, Figs. 4-7, 4-11, respectively; D from Klatt E: Robbins and Cotran's Atlas of Pathology. Philadelphia, WB Saunders, 2006, p 302, Fig. 13-35; E and F from Damjanov I, Linaer J: Pathology: A Color Atlas. St. Louis, Mosby, 2000, pp 139, 369, Figs. 7-59, 17-35B, respectively.*)

B. Differentiation
1. Benign tumors
   - Usually well differentiated (resemble parent tissue)
2. Malignant tumors
   a. Well differentiated or low grade
      (1) Resemble parent tissue
      (2) Example—produce keratin pearls or glandular lumens with secretions (see Fig. 8-1D and E)

Grade of cancer: does the cancer resemble its parent tissue or not?

b. Poorly differentiated, high grade, or anaplastic
  • No differentiating features
c. Intermediate grade
  • Features are between low- and high-grade cancer.

C. Nuclear features
1. Benign tumors
   a. Nuclear/cytoplasmic ratio is close to normal.
   b. Mitoses have normal mitotic spindles.
   c. Nuclear/cytoplasmic ratio is increased, and nucleoli are prominent.
   d. Mitoses have normal and atypical mitotic spindles.

D. Growth rate
1. Benign tumors usually have a slow growth rate.
2. Malignant tumors have a variable growth rate.
   a. Correlates with the degree of differentiation
   b. Anaplastic (high-grade) cancers have an increased growth rate.
3. Thirty doubling times are required for a tumor to be clinically evident.
   • Equivalent to 10^9 cells, 1 g of tissue, volume of 1 mL
4. Malignant cells in the cell cycle are primarily targeted by chemotherapy.
   a. DNA is exposed and is susceptible to damage by drugs and radiation causing the cells to die.
   b. Loss of the cells causes more cancer cells to go into the cell cycle; hence debulking the tumor as these cells also get destroyed.

E. Monoclonality
1. Benign and malignant tumors derive from a single precursor cell.
2. Non-neoplastic proliferations derive from multiple cells (polyclonal).

The **monoclonal origin** of neoplasms has been shown by studying glucose-6-phosphate dehydrogenase (G6PD) isoenzymes A and B in selected neoplasms (e.g., leiomyoma of the uterus). All the neoplastic smooth muscle cells in uterine leiomyomas have either the A or the B G6PD isoenzyme. Non-neoplastic smooth muscle proliferations in the uterus (e.g., pregnant uterus) have some cells with the A isoenzyme and others with the B isoenzyme, indicating their polyclonal origin.

F. Telomerase activity
1. Telomerase function
   a. Preserves length of telomeres
     • Sequences of nontranscribed DNA at the ends of chromosomes
   b. Prevents gene loss after multiple cell divisions
2. Benign tumors have normal telomerase activity.
3. Malignant tumors have upregulation of telomerase activity.
   • They do *not* lose genetic material after multiple cell divisions.

G. Local invasion
1. Benign tumors
   a. They do *not* invade.
   b. They are usually enclosed by a fibrous capsule.
     • Exception—uterine leiomyomas do *not* have a fibrous tissue capsule.
2. Malignant tumors invade tissue.
3. Some tissues resist invasion.
   • Examples—mature cartilage, elastic tissue in arteries
4. Sequence of invasion by malignant tumors
   a. Loss of intercellular adherence
     • E-cadherin (intercellular adhesion agent) is *not* produced.
   b. Cell invasion occurs.
     (1) Cell receptors attach to laminin (glycoprotein in the basement membrane).
     (2) Cells release type IV collagenase (metalloproteinase containing zinc).
       • Dissolves the basement membrane
     (3) Cell receptors attach to fibronectin in the extracellular matrix.
     (4) Cells produce cytokines (stimulate locomotion) and proteases (dissolve connective tissue).
     (5) Cells produce factors that stimulate angiogenesis.
       • Secrete vascular endothelial growth factor and basic fibroblast growth factor

Malignant tumors: ↑ nuclear/cytoplasmic ratio; abnormal mitotic spindles

Malignant tumors: 30 doubling times before detected

Benign and malignant tumors: monoclonal

Malignant tumors: upregulation telomerase activity

Basal cell carcinomas of the skin: invade tissue but do *not* metastasize

Invasion: second most important criterion for malignancy

Resist invasion: cartilage, elastic tissue

Loss of intercellular aherence → cell invasion

H. Metastasis
1. Benign tumors do *not* metastasize.
2. Malignant tumors metastasize.
3. Pathways of dissemination
   a. Lymphatic spread to lymph nodes
      - Usual mechanism of dissemination of carcinomas

Regional lymph nodes are the first line of defense against the spread of a carcinoma. However, if the nodal architecture is destroyed, malignant cells enter the efferent lymphatics, which empty into the bloodstream. In the bloodstream, malignant cells metastasize to distant organ sites (e.g., liver, lungs, bone).

   b. Hematogenous spread
      (1) Usual mechanism of dissemination for sarcomas
      (2) Cells entering the portal vein metastasize to the liver.
      (3) Cells entering the vena cava metastasize to the lungs.

Some carcinomas have both lymphatic and hematogenous spread. Renal cell carcinomas commonly invade the renal vein, where the tumor has the potential for extending into the vena cava to as far as the right side of the heart. Hepatocellular carcinomas invade the portal and hepatic veins. Tumor obstruction of either vein produces portal hypertension, splenomegaly, and ascites.

   c. Seeding
      - Malignant cells exfoliate from a surface and implant and invade tissue in a body cavity.
      (1) Primary surface-derived ovarian cancers (e.g., serous cystadenocarcinoma) commonly seed the omentum.
      (2) Peripherally located lung cancers commonly seed the parietal and visceral pleurae.
      (3) Glioblastoma multiforme commonly seeds the cerebrospinal fluid causing spread to the brain and spinal cord.
4. Bone metastasis
   a. Vertebral column
      (1) Most common metastatic site in bone (Fig. 8-2A)
      (2) Due to the Batson paravertebral venous plexus
         - It has connections with the vena cava and the vertebral bodies.
   b. Osteoblastic metastases
      (1) Increased serum alkaline phosphatase indicates reactive bone formation (Fig. 8-2B).
      (2) Radiodensities are seen on radiographs (e.g., prostate cancer; Fig. 8-2C).
   c. Osteolytic metastases
      (1) Radiolucencies are seen on radiographs (e.g., lung cancer; Fig. 8-2D).
      (2) Pathogenesis
         (a) Tumor may produce substances that locally activate osteoclasts producing lytic lesions.
            - Example—prostaglandin E_2, interleukin 1
         (b) Tumor produces parathyroid hormone (PTH)–related protein; no lytic lesions due to generalized increase in osteoclast activity
            - Examples—squamous cell carcinoma in the lung, renal cell carcinoma
      (3) Potential consequences of osteolytic metastases
         (a) Pathologic fractures
         (b) Hypercalcemia
   d. Pain in bone metastasis is treated with local radiation therapy.
5. Metastasis is often more common than a primary cancer in:
   a. Lymph nodes (e.g., metastatic breast and lung cancer)
   b. Lungs (e.g., metastatic breast cancer)
   c. Liver (e.g., metastatic lung cancer) (Fig. 8-2E)
   d. Bone (e.g., metastatic breast cancer)
   e. Brain (e.g., metastatic lung cancer)

Margin notes:

Extranodal metastasis (e.g., liver) has greater prognostic significance than nodal metastasis.

Lymph nodes: first line of defense in carcinomas

Routes of metastasis: lymphatic, hematogenous, seeding of body cavities

Seeding: common with surface-derived ovarian cancers

Bone metastasis: vertebra most common site; paravertebral venous plexus

Osteoblastic metastasis: ↑ serum alkaline phosphatase

Osteolytic metastasis: potential for hypercalcemia, pathologic fractures

Bone metastasis: osteoblastic (radiodense) or osteolytic (radiolucent).

Lymph node: most common tissue metastasized to

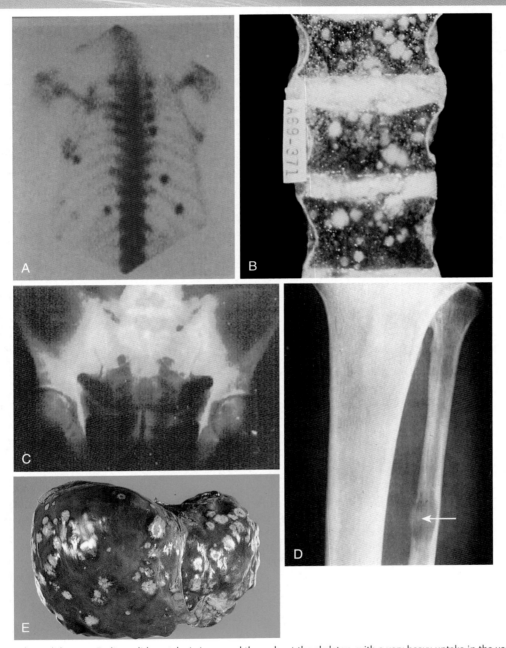

8-2: A, Radionuclide scan. Radionuclide uptake is increased throughout the skeleton, with a very heavy uptake in the vertebral column. The patient had a primary breast cancer, which is the most common cancer metastatic to bone. **B,** Prostate cancer metastatic to the vertebral column. Multiple white foci of metastatic prostate cancer produce an osteoblastic response in the bone. **C,** Radiograph showing osteoblastic metastases. Note the increased density of bone in the lower lumbar vertebra and pelvic bone in metastatic prostate cancer. **D,** Radiograph showing osteolytic lesions. Note the radiolucent areas in the midshaft of the femur (*arrow*) in metastatic breast cancer. **E,** Metastasis to the liver. The liver contains multiple nodules that have a depressed central area ("umbilicated") and stellate-shaped borders. (*A from Bouloux P: Self-Assessment Picture Tests: Medicine, Vol. 1. London, Mosby-Wolfe, 1997, p 70, Fig. 140; B from Kumar V, Fausto N, Abbas A: Robbins and Cotran's Pathologic Basis of Disease, 7th ed. Philadelphia, WB Saunders, 2004, p 1052, Fig. 21-35; C from Bouloux P: Self-Assessment Picture Tests: Medicine, Vol. 3. London, Mosby-Wolfe, 1997, p 11, Fig. 21; D from Rosai J, Ackerman LV: Surgical Pathology, 9th ed. St. Louis, Mosby, 2004, p 2187, Fig. 24-92; E from Damjanov I: Pathology for the Health-Related Professions, 2nd ed. Philadelphia, WB Saunders, 2000, p 303, Fig. 11-18.*)

III. Cancer Epidemiology
A. General
1. Cancer is the second most common cause of death in the United States.
2. Causes
   a. External factors
   - Tobacco, alcohol, chemicals, radiation, pathogens

Cancer: 2nd most common cause death in US

b. Internal factors
  • Hormones, immune conditions, inherited mutations
3. Risk for developing cancer increases with age.
  • More than 75% of cancers are in persons 55 and older.
4. Lifetime risk
  a. Probability that a person will develop or die from cancer
  b. In the United States, men have slightly less than 1 in 2 lifetime risk
  c. In the United States, women have a little more than 1 in 3 lifetime risk

Lifetime risk for cancer: men > women

5. Relative risk
  a. Measure of the strength of a relationship between risk factors and a particular cancer
  b. Compares risk of developing cancer in individuals at risk with those that are not
    (1) Compares risk for cancer in male smokers versus nonsmokers
    (2) Male smokers have 23 times greater risk than male nonsmokers; relative risk is 23.
    (3) Women with a history of breast cancer in a first-degree relative (mother, sister, daughter) have a two times greater risk for developing breast cancer (relative risk is 2).
6. Relative survival rates
  a. Refers to percentage of cancer patients alive after a period of time (usually 5 years) relative to persons without cancer
  b. Should be interpreted with caution, because some cancers commonly recur after 5 years.
    • Examples–breast, kidney

Blacks: greatest overall risk for cancer

7. Blacks
  a. Greatest risk for cancer and cancer-related deaths of any other racial group or ethnicity
  b. Applies to almost all cancers *except* malignant melanoma
8. Hispanics and Asians
  a. Lower incidence rates for all cancers combined than whites
  b. Exceptions are for cancers associated with infections—cervix (human papillomavirus), liver (hepatitis B and C), stomach (*Helicobacter pylori*)
9. Native Americans
  • Highest incidence and cancer-related deaths due to kidney cancer than all racial and ethnic populations.

B. Cancer incidence
1. Cancers in children
  a. Second most common cause of death in children (accidents most common cause)
  b. Acute lymphoblastic leukemia (~33%), central nervous system (CNS) tumors (~21%), neuroblastoma (~7%), Wilms' tumor (~5%)
    • These are *not* common tumors in adults.

Most common cancer in children: acute lymphoblastic leukemia

2. Cancers in men (in decreasing order)
  • Prostate, lung, colorectal
3. Cancers in women (in decreasing order)
  • Breast, lung, colorectal
4. Gynecologic cancers (in descending order)
  a. Endometrium
  b. Ovarian
  c. Cervical
    • Least common due to cervical Pap smears detecting dysplasia

Cancer in men: prostate, lung, colorectal

Cancer in women: breast, lung, colorectal

Gynecologic cancer: endometrium, ovary, cervical

C. Cancer-related deaths
1. Cancer-related deaths in men (in decreasing order)
  • Lung, prostate, colorectal
2. Cancer-related deaths in women (in decreasing order)
  • Lung, breast, colorectal
3. Gynecologic cancer-related deaths (in descending order)
  a. Endometrium
  b. Ovary
  c. Cervix

Most common cause of cancer death in adults: lung cancer

D. Cancer and heredity
1. Inherited predisposition to cancer accounts for 5% of all cancers.
2. Categories of inherited cancers (Table 8-1 and Fig. 8-3)
  a. Autosomal dominant cancer syndromes
  b. Autosomal recessive disorders involving DNA repair
  c. Familial cancers

TABLE 8-1. **SELECTED INHERITED CANCER SYNDROMES**

CATEGORY	CANCER
Autosomal dominant cancer syndromes	**Retinoblastoma:** malignancy of eye in children; 40% are inherited; point mutation inactivates *RB* suppressor gene on chromosome 13; one gene inactivated in germ cells, remaining gene inactivated after birth (two-hit theory); predisposition for osteogenic sarcoma in adolescence **Familial adenomatous polyposis:** development of colorectal cancer from malignant transformation of polyps by age 50; inactivation of *APC* suppressor gene **Li-Fraumeni syndrome:** increased risk for sarcomas, leukemia, carcinomas (e.g., breast) before age 50; inactivation of *TP53* suppressor gene **Hereditary nonpolyposis colon cancer (Lynch syndrome):** increased risk for colorectal cancers *without* previous polyps; inactivation of DNA mismatch repair genes; cannot correct errors in nucleotide pairing; characteristic finding is alteration in microsatellite nucleotide sequences (normally do not change in cells) ***BRCA1* and *BRCA2* genes:** inactivation of genes increases risk for developing breast and ovarian cancer
Autosomal recessive syndromes with defects in DNA repair (see Fig. 8-3)	**Xeroderma pigmentosum:** increased risk for developing skin cancers due to ultraviolet light (cross-links adjacent pyrimidine producing pyrimidine dimers); examples include basal cell carcinoma, squamous cell carcinoma **Chromosome instability syndromes:** chromosomes susceptible to damage by ionizing radiation and drugs; predisposition to cancers (e.g., leukemia, lymphoma); disorders include Fanconi anemia, ataxia telangiectasia, Bloom syndrome
Familial cancer syndromes	No defined pattern of inheritance, but cancers (e.g., breast, ovary, colon) develop with increased frequency in families; sometimes involves *BRCA1* and *BRCA2* genes

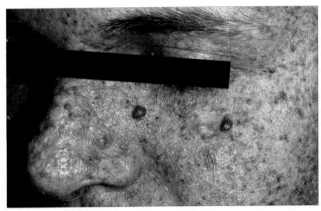

8-3: Xeroderma pigmentosum. Note the numerous hyperpigmented lesions, nodular and scaly growths on the face. Many of these lesions are precancerous or ultraviolet light–related cancers. *(Courtesy of R.A. Marsden, MD, St. George's Hospital, London.)*

E. Cancer and geography
1. Worldwide
   - Malignant melanoma is increasing at the most rapid rate of all cancers.
2. China
   - Nasopharyngeal carcinoma secondary to Epstein-Barr virus (EBV)
3. Japan
   - Stomach adenocarcinoma due to smoked foods
4. Southeast Asia
   - Hepatocellular carcinoma due to hepatitis B virus plus aflatoxins (produced by *Aspergillus*) in food
5. Africa
   - Burkitt's lymphoma due to EBV and Kaposi's sarcoma due to human herpesvirus 8

F. Acquired preneoplastic disorders (Table 8-2)
G. Prevention modalities in cancer
1. Lifestyle modifications
   a. Stop smoking cigarettes—the most important factor (refer to Chapter 6)
   b. Increase fiber/decrease dietary saturated animal fat
      - Decreases risk for colorectal cancer
   c. Reduce alcohol intake (refer to Chapter 6)
   d. Reduce weight

Malignant melanoma: most rapidly increasing cancer

Actinic (solar) keratosis: precursor of squamous cell carcinoma

Cessation of smoking is most important factor in decreasing risk for cancer.

TABLE 8-2. **ACQUIRED PRENEOPLASTIC DISORDERS***

PRECURSOR LESION	CANCER
Actinic (solar) keratosis	Squamous cell carcinoma
Atypical hyperplasia of ductal epithelium of breast	Adenocarcinoma
Chronic irritation at sinus orifice, third-degree burn scars	Squamous cell carcinoma
Chronic ulcerative colitis	Adenocarcinoma
Complete hydatidiform mole	Choriocarcinoma
Dysplastic nevus	Malignant melanoma
Endometrial hyperplasia	Adenocarcinoma
Glandular metaplasia of esophagus (Barrett's esophagus)	Adenocarcinoma
Glandular metaplasia of stomach (*Helicobacter pylori*)	Adenocarcinoma
Myelodysplastic syndrome	Acute leukemia
Regenerative nodules in cirrhosis	Adenocarcinoma
Scar tissue in lung	Adenocarcinoma
Squamous dysplasia of oropharynx, larynx, bronchus, cervix	Squamous cell carcinoma
Tubular adenoma of colon	Adenocarcinoma
Vaginal adenosis (diethylstilbestrol exposure)	Adenocarcinoma
Villous adenoma of rectum	Adenocarcinoma

*Metaplastic and hyperplastic cells become dysplastic *before* progressing to cancer.

(1) Increased adipose tissue increases aromatase conversion of androgens to estrogen.
(2) Increased estrogen increases risk for endometrial and breast cancer.
2. Immunization
a. Hepatitis B (HBV) vaccination
• Immunization decreases the risk for hepatocellular carcinoma due to hepatitis B–induced postnecrotic cirrhosis.
b. Human papillomavirus (HPV) immunization
• Decreases the risk for developing cervical squamous cancer
3. Screening procedures
a. Cervical Papanicolaou (Pap) smears
(1) Decreases risk for cervical cancer
(2) Pap smear detects cervical dysplasia, which can be surgically removed.
(a) Detection of low-grade dysplasia—sensitivity ~70%, specificity 75%
(b) Detection of high-grade dysplasia—sensitivity 75%, specificity 95%
b. Colonoscopy
• Detects and removes polyps that are precancerous
c. Mammography
• Detects nonpalpable breast masses
d. Prostate-specific antigen (PSA)
(1) Detects prostate cancer
(2) Lacks specificity (increased false positive results)
• PSA may be increased in prostate hyperplasia
4. Treatment of conditions that predispose to cancer
a. Treatment of *Helicobacter pylori* infections
• Decreases risk for developing malignant lymphoma and adenocarcinoma of the stomach
b. Treatment of gastroesophageal reflux disease (GERD)
• Decreases the risk for developing distal adenocarcinoma arising from Barrett's esophagus

IV. **Carcinogenesis**
• Cancer is a multistep process involving gene mutations, telomerase activation, angiogenesis, invasion, and metastasis.
A. **Types of gene mutations**
1. Point mutations are the most common type of mutation.
2. Balanced translocations
3. Other mutations
• Deletion, gene amplification (multiple copies of a gene), overexpression (increase in baseline gene activity)

Margin notes:

HBV immunization: ↓ risk for hepatocellular carcinoma

Human papillomavirus immunization: ↓ risk for cervical cancer

Cervical cancer is the least common gynecologic cancer in the United States.

Cervical Pap smear: most responsible for ↓ incidence/mortality rate for cervical cancer

PSA: more sensitive than specific

Rx *H. pylori* infection: ↓ risk for developing gastric lymphoma/adenocarcinoma

Rx GERD: ↓ risk for distal adenocarcinoma of esophagus

Point mutations: most common type of mutation in cancer

B. Genes involved in cancer

1. Proto-oncogenes
   a. Involved in normal growth and repair
   b. Functions of proto-oncogene protein products
      - Growth factors, growth factor receptors, signal transducers, nuclear transcribers
   c. Mutations cause sustained activity of the genes (Table 8-3)
2. Suppressor genes (anti-oncogenes)
   a. Protect against unregulated cell growth
   b. Control G_1 to S phase of the cell cycle and nuclear transcription
   c. Mutations cause unregulated cell proliferation (Table 8-4).
3. Antiapoptosis genes; *BCL2* family of genes
   a. Protein products prevent cytochrome *c* from leaving mitochondria.
      - Cytochrome *c* in the cytosol activates caspases initiating apoptosis.
   b. Mutation causes increased gene activity (e.g., overexpression), which prevents apoptosis; e.g., B-cell follicular lymphoma.
      (1) *BCL2* gene family (chromosome 18) produces gene products that prevent mitochondrial leakage of cytochrome *c* (signal for apoptosis).
      (2) Translocation t(14;18) causes overexpression of the BCL2 protein product.
         - Prevents apoptosis of B lymphocytes causing B-cell follicular lymphoma
4. Apoptosis genes
   a. Regulate programmed cell death
   b. Example—*BAX* apoptosis gene
      (1) Activated by a *TP53* suppressor gene product if DNA damage is excessive
      (2) BAX protein product inactivates the *BCL2* antiapoptosis gene.
      (3) Mutation inactivating *TP53* suppressor gene renders the *BAX* gene inoperative, which prevents apoptosis.

Proto-oncogenes: involved in normal growth and repair

Suppressor genes: protect against unregulated cell growth

BCL2 gene family: antiapoptosis genes

BAX gene: apoptosis gene

TABLE 8-3. SOME PROTO-ONCOGENES AND THEIR FUNCTIONS, MUTATIONS, AND ASSOCIATED CANCERS

PROTO-ONCOGENE	FUNCTION	MUTATION	CANCER
ABL	Nonreceptor tyrosine kinase activity	Translocation t(9;22)	Chronic myelogenous leukemia (chromosome 22 is Philadelphia chromosome)
HER (ERBB2)	Receptor synthesis	Amplification	Breast carcinoma (marker of aggressiveness)
MYC	Nuclear transcription	Translocation t(8;14)	Burkitt's lymphoma
N-MYC	Nuclear transcription	Amplification	Neuroblastoma
RAS	Guanosine triphosphate signal transduction	Point mutation	Leukemia; lung, colon, pancreatic carcinomas
RET	Receptor synthesis	Point mutation	Multiple endocrine neoplasia IIa/IIb syndromes
SIS	Growth factor synthesis	Overexpression	Osteogenic sarcoma, astrocytoma

TABLE 8-4. SOME TUMOR SUPPRESSOR GENES, THEIR FUNCTIONS, AND ASSOCIATED CANCERS

GENE	FUNCTION	ASSOCIATED CANCERS
APC	Prevents nuclear transcription (degrades catenin, an activator of nuclear transcription)	Familial polyposis (colorectal carcinoma)
BRCA1/BRCA2	Regulates DNA repair	Breast, ovary, prostate carcinomas
RB	Inhibits G_1 to S phase	Retinoblastoma, osteogenic sarcoma, breast carcinoma
TGF-β	Inhibits G_1 to S phase	Pancreatic and colorectal carcinomas
TP53	Inhibits G_1 to S phase Repairs DNA, activates *BAX* gene (initiates apoptosis)	Lung, colon, breast carcinomas Li-Fraumeni syndrome: breast carcinoma, brain tumors, leukemia, sarcomas
VHL	Regulates nuclear transcription	Von Hippel–Lindau syndrome: cerebellar hemangioblastoma, retinal angioma, renal cell carcinoma (bilateral), pheochromocytoma (bilateral)
WT1	Regulates nuclear transcription	Wilms' tumor

APC, adenomatous polyposis coli; *BRCA*, breast cancer; *RB*, retinoblastoma; *TGF-β*, transforming growth factor β; *VHL*, von Hippel–Lindau; *WT*, Wilms' tumor.

Repair genes: correct errors in nucleotide pairing; excise pyrimidine dimers

Enzymes involved in dimer excision: endonuclease, exonuclease, ligase

Tobacco is the agent most responsible for cancer and cancer deaths in the United States.

Chemical carcinogenesis: initiation → promotion → progression

5. DNA repair genes (see Tables 8-1 and 8-4)
   a. Examples of DNA repair
      (1) Mismatch repair genes produce proteins that correct errors in nucleotide pairing.
      (2) Nucleotide excision repair pathway excises pyrimidine dimers in ultraviolet light (UV)–damaged skin (Fig. 8-4).
   b. Effect of mutations involving DNA repair genes
      • Allows cells with nonlethal damage to proliferate, which increases the risk for cancer

V. **Carcinogenic Agents**
   A. **Chemical carcinogens** (Table 8-5)
      1. Polycyclic hydrocarbons in tobacco smoke
         • Most common group of carcinogens in the United States
      2. Mechanisms
         a. Direct-acting carcinogens
            • Contain electron-deficient atoms that react with electron-rich atoms in DNA (e.g., alkylating agents)
         b. Indirect-acting carcinogens
            • Activated by the liver cytochrome P-450 system (e.g., polycyclic hydrocarbons)
      3. Sequence of chemical carcinogenesis
         a. Initiation
            • Irreversible mutation

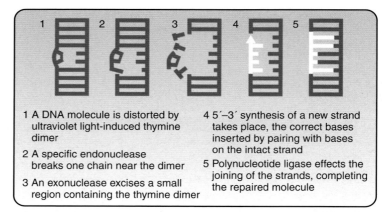

1 A DNA molecule is distorted by ultraviolet light-induced thymine dimer

2 A specific endonuclease breaks one chain near the dimer

3 An exonuclease excises a small region containing the thymine dimer

4 5´–3´ synthesis of a new strand takes place, the correct bases inserted by pairing with bases on the intact strand

5 Polynucleotide ligase effects the joining of the strands, completing the repaired molecule

8-4: Excision-repair mechanism. *(From McKee PH, Calonje E, Granter SR: Pathology of the Skin with Clinical Correlations, 3rd ed. St. Louis, Elsevier Mosby, 2005, p 1228, Fig. 22.193.)*

TABLE 8-5. **CHEMICAL CARCINOGENS**

CARCINOGEN	ASSOCIATED CANCER
Aflatoxin (from *Aspergillus*)	Hepatocellular carcinoma in association with hepatitis B virus
Alcohol	Squamous cell carcinoma of oropharynx and upper/middle esophagus; pancreatic and hepatocellular carcinomas
Alkylating agents	Malignant lymphoma
Arsenic	Squamous cell carcinoma of skin, lung cancer, liver angiosarcoma
Asbestos	Bronchogenic carcinoma, pleural mesothelioma
Benzene	Acute leukemia
Beryllium	Bronchogenic carcinoma
Chromium	Bronchogenic carcinoma
Cyclophosphamide	Transitional cell carcinoma of urinary bladder
Diethylstilbestrol	Clear cell carcinoma of vagina/cervix
β-Naphthylamine (aniline dyes)	Transitional cell carcinoma of urinary bladder
Nickel	Bronchogenic carcinoma
Oral contraceptives	Breast, cervical carcinomas
Polycyclic hydrocarbons	Squamous cell carcinoma: oral cavity, midesophagus, larynx, lung Adenocarcinoma: distal esophagus, pancreas Transitional cell carcinoma: urinary bladder, renal pelvis
Polyvinyl chloride	Liver angiosarcoma
Silica	Bronchogenic carcinoma

TABLE 8-6. ONCOGENIC RNA AND DNA VIRUSES

VIRUS	MECHANISM	ASSOCIATED CANCER
RNA Viruses		
HCV	Produces postnecrotic cirrhosis	Hepatocellular carcinoma
HTLV-1	Activates *TAX* gene, stimulates polyclonal T-cell proliferation, inhibits *TP53* suppressor gene	T-cell leukemia and lymphoma
DNA Viruses		
EBV	Promotes polyclonal B-cell proliferation, which increases risk for t(8;14) translocation	Burkitt's lymphoma, CNS lymphoma in AIDS, mixed cellularity Hodgkin's lymphoma, nasopharyngeal carcinoma
HBV	Activates proto-oncogenes, inactivates *TP53* suppressor gene	Hepatocellular carcinoma
HHV-8	Acts via cytokines released from HIV and HSV	Kaposi's sarcoma in AIDS
HPV types 16 and 18	Type 16 (~50% of cancers): E6 gene product inhibits *TP53* suppressor gene Type 18 (~10% of cancers): E7 gene product inhibits *RB* suppressor gene	Squamous cell carcinoma of vulva, vagina, cervix, anus (associated with anal intercourse), larynx, oropharynx

EBV, Epstein-Barr virus; HBV, hepatitis B virus; HCV, hepatitis C virus; HHV, human herpesvirus; HPV, human papillomavirus; HSV, herpes simplex virus; HTLV, human T-cell lymphotropic virus.

  b. Promotion
   • Promoters (e.g., estrogen) stimulate mutated cells to enter the cell cycle.
  c. Progression
   (1) Development of tumor heterogeneity
   (2) Examples—production of cells that invade or metastasize
 B. Microbes
  1. Viruses (Table 8-6)
  2. Bacteria
   • Examples—stomach cancer and low-grade malignant lymphoma due to *Helicobacter pylori*
  3. Parasites
   a. *Schistosoma hematobium*
    • Squamous cell carcinoma of the urinary bladder
   b. *Clonorchis sinensis* and *Opisthorchis viverrini*
    • Cholangiocarcinoma of the bile ducts

Pathogens and cancer: viruses > bacteria > parasites

 C. Radiation
  1. Ionizing radiation–induced cancers
   a. Mechanism
    • Hydroxyl free radical injury to DNA
   b. Examples
    (1) Acute myelogenous or chronic myelogenous leukemia
     • Increased risk of leukemia in radiologists and individuals exposed to radiation in nuclear reactors
    (2) Papillary thyroid carcinoma
    (3) Lung, breast, and bone cancers
    (4) Liver angiosarcoma
     • Due to radioactive thorium dioxide used to visualize the arterial tree

Leukemia: most common cancer due to ionizing radiation

  2. UV light–induced cancers
   a. Mechanism
    • Formation of pyrimidine dimers, which distort DNA (see Fig. 8-4)
   b. Basal cell carcinoma (see Fig. 24-7B), squamous cell carcinoma (see Fig. 24-7D), malignant melanoma (see Fig. 24-5H)

Basal cell carcinoma: most common cancer due to excessive UV light exposure

 D. Physical injury
  1. Squamous cell carcinoma may develop in third-degree burn scars.
  2. Squamous cell carcinoma may develop at the orifices of chronically draining sinuses (e.g., chronic osteomyelitis).
VI. Clinical Oncology
 A. Host defense against cancer
  1. Humoral immunity
   • Involves antibodies and complement

2. Type IV cellular immunity
   a. Efficient mechanism for killing cancer cells
   b. Cytotoxic CD8 T cells
      • Recognize altered class I antigens on neoplastic cells and destroy them

3. Natural killer cells
   • Direct killing and indirect killing through type II hypersensitivity
4. Macrophages
   • Activated by γ-interferon

B. Grading and staging of cancer
   1. Grading criteria
      a. Degree of differentiation (e.g., low, intermediate, or high grade)
      b. Nuclear features, invasiveness

   2. Staging criteria
      a. Most important prognostic factor
      b. TNM system
         (1) Progresses from the least to the most important prognostic factor
         (2) T refers to tumor size.
            • ≥ 2 cm correlates with metastatic ability.
         (3) N refers to whether lymph nodes are involved.
         (4) M refers to extranodal metastases (e.g., liver, lung).

C. Cancer effects on the host
   1. Cachexia (wasting disease)
      a. Generalized catabolic reaction
         • Anorexia, muscle wasting, loss of subcutaneous fat, fatigue

      b. Mechanism
         (1) Chronic low levels of tumor necrosis factor-α (called cachectin)
         (2) Secreted from host macrophages and cancer cells
         (3) Suppresses appetite center in hypothalamus
         (4) Stimulus for apoptosis of cells
   2. Anemia
      a. Anemia of chronic disease
      b. Iron deficiency

         • Due to gastrointestinal blood loss (e.g., colorectal cancer)
      c. Macrocytic anemia
         • Due to folate deficiency from rapid tumor growth
      d. Myelophthisic anemia
         (1) Anemia related to metastasis to bone
         (2) Immature hematopoietic elements in peripheral blood (i.e., leukoerythroblastic smear) (see Fig. 12-1)
            (a) Nucleated red blood cells, immature neutrophils (e.g., myeloblasts, metamyelocytes) in peripheral blood
            (b) Tear drop red blood cells indicate myelofibrosis secondary to bone metastasis

   3. Hemostasis abnormalities
      a. Increased risk for vessel thrombosis
         (1) Due to thrombocytosis, increased synthesis of coagulation factors (e.g., fibrinogen, factors V and VIII)
         (2) Release of procoagulants from cancer cells (e.g., pancreatic carcinoma)
      b. Disseminated intravascular coagulation
         • Due to release of tissue thromboplastin from cancer cells

   4. Fever
      a. Usually due to infection
      b. Example—gram-negative sepsis from *Escherichia coli* or *Pseudomonas aeruginosa*

   5. Paraneoplastic syndromes
      a. Distant effects of a tumor that are unrelated to metastasis
         • May predate the onset of metastasis
      b. Occur in 10% to 15% of cancer patients
      c. Involve multiple organ systems and mimic metastatic disease (Table 8-7; Fig. 8-5)
      d. May involve ectopic secretion of hormone (Table 8-8)

TABLE 8-7. PARANEOPLASTIC SYNDROMES

SYNDROME	ASSOCIATED CANCER	COMMENT
Acanthosis nigricans (see Fig. 24-6B)	Stomach carcinoma	Black, verrucoid-appearing lesion
Eaton-Lambert syndrome	Small cell carcinoma of lung	Myasthenia gravis–like symptoms (e.g., muscle weakness); antibody directed against calcium channel
Hypertrophic osteoarthropathy (see Fig. 8-5)	Bronchogenic carcinoma	Periosteal reaction of distal phalanx (often associated with clubbing of nail)
Nonbacterial thrombotic endocarditis	Mucus-secreting pancreatic and colorectal carcinomas	Sterile vegetations on mitral valve
Seborrheic keratosis (see Fig. 24-6A)	Stomach carcinoma	Sudden appearance of numerous pigmented seborrheic keratoses (Leser-Trélat sign)
Superficial migratory thrombophlebitis	Pancreatic carcinoma	Release of procoagulants (Trousseau's sign)
Nephrotic syndrome	Lung, breast, stomach carcinomas	Diffuse membranous glomerulopathy

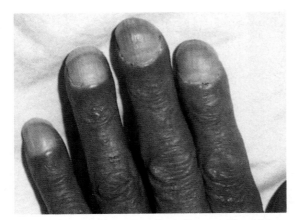

8-5: Hypertrophic osteoarthropathy with finger clubbing. Note the bulbous swelling of the connective tissue in the terminal phalanxes. *(From Grieg JD: Color Atlas of Surgical Diagnosis. London, Mosby-Wolfe, 1996, p 57, Fig. 8.33.)*

TABLE 8-8. PARANEOPLASTIC SYNDROME ENDOCRINOPATHIES

DISORDER	ASSOCIATED CANCER	ECTOPIC HORMONE
Cushing syndrome	Small cell carcinoma of lung, medullary carcinoma of thyroid	ACTH
Gynecomastia	Choriocarcinoma (testis)	hCG
Hypercalcemia	Renal cell carcinoma, primary squamous cell carcinoma of lung, breast carcinoma Malignant lymphomas (contain 1α-hydroxylase)	PTH-related protein Calcitriol (vitamin D)
Hypocalcemia	Medullary carcinoma of thyroid	Calcitonin
Hypoglycemia	Hepatocellular carcinoma	Insulin-like factor
Hyponatremia	Small cell carcinoma of lung	Antidiuretic hormone
Secondary polycythemia	Renal cell and hepatocellular carcinomas	Erythropoietin

ACTH, adrenocorticotropic hormone; hCG, human chorionic gonadotropin; PTH, parathyroid hormone.

TABLE 8-9. TUMOR MARKERS AND ASSOCIATED CANCERS

TUMOR MARKER	ASSOCIATED CANCER
AFP	Hepatocellular carcinoma, yolk sac tumor (endodermal sinus tumor) of ovary or testis
Bence Jones protein	Multiple myeloma, Waldenström's macroglobulinemia (represent light chains in urine)
CA 15-3	Breast carcinoma
CA 19-9	Pancreatic, colorectal carcinomas
CA 125	Surface-derived ovarian cancer (e.g., serous cystadenocarcinoma; helpful in distinguishing benign from malignant tumors)
CEA	Colorectal and pancreatic carcinomas (monitor for recurrences)
LDH	Malignant lymphoma (prognostic factor for response to standard therapy)
PSA	Prostate carcinoma (also increased in prostate hyperplasia)

AFP, α-fetoprotein; CEA, carcinoembryonic antigen; LDH, lactate dehydrogenase; PSA, prostate-specific antigen.

Hormone tumor marker: calcitonin (medullary carcinoma of thyroid)

D. Tumor markers (biomarkers)
1. Biologic markers (Table 8-9)
   • Include hormones, enzymes, oncofetal antigens, glycoproteins
2. Identify tumors
3. Estimate tumor burden
4. Detect recurrence
5. Indicator of tumor response to treatment

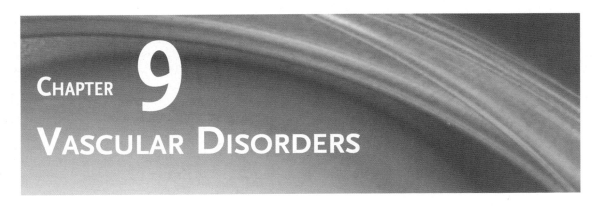

VASCULAR DISORDERS

I. **Lipoprotein Disorders**
   A. **Lipoprotein fractions**
      1. Chylomicron (Fig. 9-1A)
         a. Transports diet-derived triglyceride (TG) in the blood
         b. Composition
            (1) Protein (2%)
            (2) TG (87%)
            (3) Cholesterol (CH; 3%)
            (4) Phospholipid (8%)
         c. Synthesized in intestinal epithelium
            (1) Requires apolipoprotein (apo) B-48 for assembly and secretion
            (2) Nascent chylomicrons in the circulation obtain apo CII and apo E from high density lipoprotein (HDL)
         d. Absent during fasting
         e. If increased, it forms a creamy supranate.
            (1) Test tube must be left upright in a refrigerator overnight.
            (2) Chylomicron floats on top of plasma because it has very little protein (low density).
         f. Source of fatty acids and glycerol
            • Used to synthesize TG in the liver and adipose
         g. Hydrolysis by capillary lipoprotein lipase (CPL) leaves a chylomicron remnant.
            • Chylomicron remnants are removed by apo E receptors in the liver.
      2. Very low density lipoprotein (VLDL) (Fig. 9-1B)
         a. Transports liver-synthesized TG in the blood
            • Requires apolipoprotein B-100 for assembly and secretion
         b. Composition
            (1) Protein (9%)
            (2) TG (55%)
            (3) CH (17%)
            (4) Phospholipid (19%)
         c. Source of fatty acids and glycerol
            (1) Used to synthesize TG in the adipose tissue
            (2) Hydrolysis by CPL produces intermediate-density lipoprotein (IDL) and low-density lipoprotein (LDL).
            (3) Some of the IDL is removed from blood by apo E receptors in the liver.
         d. Cholesterol ester transport protein (CETP)
            (1) Transfers CH from HDL to VLDL
            (2) Transfers TG from VLDL to HDL
            (3) An increase in VLDL always causes a decrease in HDL-CH.
         e. If increased, it forms a creamy infranate.
            • Note that the protein is greater in VLDL than in chylomicrons, so it sinks rather than floats in plasma.
         f. TG levels
            (1) Optimal level < 150 mg/dL
            (2) Borderline high level 150 to 199 mg/dL
            (3) High level 200 to 499 mg/dL
            (4) Very high level > 500 mg/dL

Chylomicron: diet-derived triglyceride

Chylomicrons: absent during fasting

Chylomicrons: turbid supranate

VLDL: liver-derived triglyceride

Hypertriglyceridemia: causes turbidity in plasma

VLDL → IDL → LDL

9-1: Schematics of lipid metabolism and hyperlipoproteinemias. **A,** Chylomicron metabolism. See text for discussion. **B,** VLDL, IDL, LDL, HDL metabolism. See text for discussion. CETP, cholesterol ester transport protein; CH, cholesterol; CPL, capillary lipoprotein lipase; HDL, high density lipoprotein; IDL, intermediate density lipoprotein; LDL, low density lipoprotein; TG, triglyceride; VLDL, very low density lipoprotein. *(From Pelley J, Coljan E: Rapid Review Biochemistry, 2nd ed. Philadelphia, Mosby, 2007, pp 126, 127, Figs. 7-8, 7-9, respectively.)*

3. Low-density lipoprotein (LDL) (see Fig. 9-1B)
   a. Transports cholesterol in the blood
   b. Derives from continued hydrolysis of IDL by CPL
   c. Removed from blood by LDL receptors in peripheral tissue
   d. Composition
      (1) Protein (22%)
      (2) TG (10%)
      (3) CH (47%)
      (4) Phospholipid (21%)
   e. Calculated LDL = CH – HDL – TG/5
      (1) Presence of chylomicrons falsely lowers calculated LDL by increasing diet-derived triglyceride; hence, fasting is required for an accurate calculated LDL.
      (2) To reduce the chance for a falsely low calculated LDL, LDL is directly measured if the serum TG > 400 mg/dL.
   f. Functions of cholesterol
      (1) Component of the cell membrane
      (2) Synthesis of vitamin D, adrenal cortex hormones, bile salts and acids
   g. Ranges of LDL
      (1) Optimal level < 100 mg/dL.
         • Risk for coronary heart disease (CHD) markedly reduced
      (2) Near optimal level is 100 to 129 mg/dL.
      (3) Borderline high level is 130 to 159 mg/dL.
      (4) High level is 160 to 189 mg/dL.
      (5) Very high level > 190 mg/dL.
         • Greatest risk for CHD
   h. Fasting is *not* required for an accurate serum CH.
      • Note that the CH content in chylomicrons is <3%; hence, fasting does *not* have a medically significant effect on the serum level.

LDL: transports cholesterol

LDL = CH – HDL – TG/5

Serum CH: fasting not required

The intensity of **treatment to lower cholesterol** is directly related to the degree of risk for CHD. The LDL cholesterol goal < 100 mg/dL (some studies suggest <70 mg/dL) if the patient has known coronary heart disease, which invariably requires the use of hydroxy-3-methylglutaryl (HMG) CoA reductase inhibitors. For persons without CHD, the LDL cholesterol goal is subdivided into those with a 0–1 risk factor (goal < 160 mg/dL) or those with multiple (2+) risk factors (goal < 130 mg/dL). The risk factors include age (male ≥ 45 years, female ≥ 55 years); family history of premature CHD (e.g., family member with myocardial infarction before 55 years of age); LDL > 160 mg/dL; current cigarette smoking; blood pressure ≥ 140/90 mg/dL (or on antihypertensive medicine); and HDL < 40 mg/dL (if ≥60 mg/dL, subtract 1).

4. High-density lipoprotein (HDL) (see Fig. 9-1B)
   a. "Good cholesterol"
      • Increased by exercise, wine, estrogen
   b. Composition
      (1) Protein (50%)
      (2) TG (3%; unless VLDL is increased)
      (3) CH (20%)
      (4) Phospholipid (27%)
   c. Synthesized by the liver and small intestine
   d. Functions of HDL
      (1) Source of apolipoproteins for other lipoprotein fractions
      (2) Removes cholesterol from atherosclerotic plaques
         (a) Delivers CH from peripheral tissue to the liver
         (b) CH is either excreted into bile or converted into bile acids/salts.
   e. Measured in the laboratory as HDL-CH
      (1) Inverse association of levels of HDL-CH and incidence and prevalence of CHD
      (2) Decreased if VLDL is increased (see earlier)
      (3) Ranges of HDL-CH
         (a) High level (optimal) ≥ 60 g/dL
         (b) Low level (suboptimal) < 40 mg/dL
      (4) Fasting is *not* required for an accurate serum HDL-CH.
         • Same reason as for serum CH.

B. **Lipoprotein disorders**
   1. Type I hyperlipoproteinemia
      a. Epidemiology
         (1) Autosomal recessive
         (2) Rare childhood disease
      b. Pathogenesis (see Fig. 9-1A and B)
         (1) Deficiency of CPL *or*
         (2) Deficiency of apo CII
      c. Clinical findings
         (1) Chylomicrons are primarily increased in early childhood.
         (2) VLDL increases later in life.
         (3) Presents with acute pancreatitis
            • Pancreatic vessels filled with chylomicrons rupture.
      d. Laboratory findings
         (1) Increase in serum TG > 1000 mg/dL (primarily chylomicrons)
         (2) Turbid supranate (chylomicrons) and clear infranate (early childhood)
         (3) Normal (usual case) to moderately increased serum CH
   2. Type II hyperlipoproteinemia
      a. Laboratory findings
         (1) Serum LDL > 190 mg/dL
         (2) Serum CH > 260 mg/dL
            (a) Serum TG < 300 mg/dL (called type IIa)
            (b) Serum TG > 300 mg/dL (called type IIb)
      b. Pathogenesis
         • Decreased synthesis of LDL receptors (see Fig. 9-1B)
      c. Acquired causes of hypercholesterolemia
         (1) Primary hypothyroidism
            • Decrease in LDL receptor synthesis or function

HDL: "good CH"

HDL: source of apolipoproteins

HDL: removes cholesterol from plaques for disposal in the liver

↑ VLDL causes ↓ HDL

Type I: ↓ CPL or ↓ apo CII

Type II hyperlipoproteinemia: ↑ LDL due to ↓ LDL receptors

(2) Nephrotic syndrome
- Increase in LDL correlates with the degree of hypoalbuminemia

(3) Extrahepatic cholestasis (obstruction of bile)
- Bile contains CH for excretion

d. Familial hypercholesterolemia
(1) Autosomal dominant (AD) disorder
(2) Deficiency of LDL receptors
(3) Clinical findings
  (a) Premature coronary artery disease and stroke
  (b) Tendon xanthomas (Fig. 9-2A)
    - Cholesterol deposit located over tendons (e.g., Achilles) and extensor surfaces of joints
  (c) Xanthelasma (Fig. 9-2B)
    - Yellow, raised plaque on the eyelid

e. Polygenic hypercholesterolemia (type IIa)
(1) Most common hereditary cause (85% of cases)
(2) Multifactorial (polygenic) inheritance
(3) Alteration in regulation of LDL levels
(4) Normal serum TG

f. Familial combined hypercholesterolemia (type IIb)
(1) AD inheritance.
(2) Serum CH and TG begin to increase around puberty.
(3) Associated with metabolic syndrome (refer to Chapter 22)
(4) Increase in CH and TG and decrease in HDL

> **Nonpharmacologic treatment** includes dietary modification, increasing activity with aerobic exercises, and cessation of smoking. Dietary modification consists of a low CH, low fat diet (fat intake < 30% of total caloric intake); polyunsaturated fat up to 10% of total calories; monounsaturated fat up to 20% of total calories; saturated fat < 7% of total calories; no more than 200 mg/day of CH; and dietary fiber 20 to 30 g/day. Pharmacologic treatment consists of the use of HMG-CoA reductase inhibitors ("statins"; most effective); nicotinic acid (least expensive lipid-lowering agent; also decreases TG, and increases HDL greater than other drugs); bile salt sequestrants; and cholesterol absorption inhibitors.

Achilles tendon xanthoma: pathognomonic for familial hypercholesterolemia

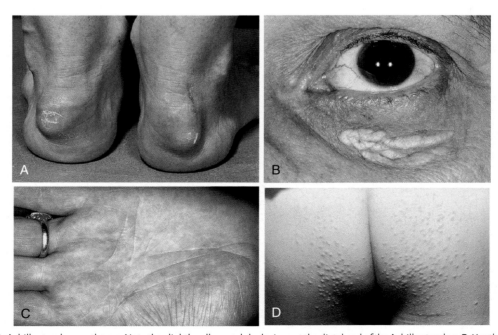

9-2: A, Achilles tendon xanthoma. Note the slightly yellow nodular lesions at the distal end of the Achilles tendon. **B,** Xanthelasma. Yellow, raised lesions are noted on the lower left eyelid. **C,** Palmar xanthomas. Note the yellow macules on the palm that are accentuated in the creases. **D,** Eruptive xanthomas. Note the numerous small yellow papular lesions distributed over the buttocks. *(A courtesy of A.F. Lant, MD, and J. Dequeker, MD, London; B from Yanoff M, Duker J: Ophthalmology, 3rd ed. St. Louis, Mosby, 2009, Fig. 12-9-18; C and D courtesy of R.A. Marsden, MD, St George's Hospital, London.)*

3. Type III hyperlipoproteinemia
   a. Laboratory findings
      (1) Serum CH and TG > 300 mg/dL
      (2) Serum CH 250 to 500 mg/dL
      (3) LDL < 190 mg/dL
   b. Familial dysbetalipoproteinemia ("remnant disease")
      (1) AD inheritance
      (2) Deficiency of apo E (see Fig. 9-1B)
      (3) Decreased liver uptake of chylomicron remnants and IDL
   c. Clinical findings
      (1) Palmar xanthomas in flexor creases (Fig. 9-2C)
      (2) Increased risk for coronary artery disease
      (3) Increased risk for peripheral vascular disease (unlike type II disorders)
   d. Laboratory findings
      (1) Serum CH and TG > 300 mg/dL
      (2) Serum CH 250 to 500 mg/dL
      (3) LDL < 190 mg/dL
      (4) Confirm diagnosis with ultracentrifugation to identify remnants
         • Lipoprotein electrophoresis and identification of apo E gene defect are other studies that can be used.
   e. Treatment
      • Fibric acid derivatives
4. Type IV hyperlipoproteinemia
   a. Laboratory findings
      (1) Serum TG > 300 mg/dL
      (2) Serum CH 250 to 500 mg/dL
      (3) Serum LDL < 190 mg/dL
      (4) Turbid infranate after refrigeration
   b. Increase in VLDL
      • Due to increase in synthesis or decrease in catabolism (see Fig. 9-1B)
   c. Acquired causes of hypertriglyceridemia
      (1) Excess alcohol intake
      (2) Oral contraceptives
         • Estrogen increases synthesis of VLDL
      (3) Diabetes mellitus
         • Decreased muscle and adipose CLP
      (4) Chronic renal failure
         • Increased synthesis of VLDL
      (5) Thiazides, β-blockers
         • Possible inhibition of CPL
   d. Familial hypertriglyceridemia
      (1) Autosomal dominant disorder
      (2) Clinical findings
         (a) Eruptive xanthomas (Fig. 9-2D)
            • Yellow, papular lesions
         (b) Increased risk for coronary artery and peripheral vascular disease

Nonpharmacologic treatment is to reduce alcohol intake and carbohydrate intake. Increase intake of omega-3 fatty acids from fish, flaxseed oil, or other sources (up to 3 g/day). **Pharmacologic therapy** consists of nicotinic acid or fibric acid derivatives.

5. Type V hyperlipoproteinemia
   a. Pathogenesis
      (1) Increase in chylomicrons and VLDL
      (2) Due to decreased activation and release of CPL (see Fig. 9-1A and B)
   b. Familial hypercholesterolemia (type IV) + exacerbating disorder
      • Exacerbating disorders—diabetic ketoacidosis (DKA; most common), alcohol
   c. Increased serum TG > 1000 mg/dL; normal CH and LDL
   d. Turbid plasma
      (1) Supranate after refrigeration, due to increased chylomicrons
      (2) Infranate after refrigeration, due to increased VLDL

Marginal notes:

Type III hyperlipoproteinemia: deficiency apo E; ↑ remnants

Type III: palmar xanthomas

Type IV hyperlipoproteinemia: ↑ VLDL; most common lipid disorder

Type IV hyperlipoproteinemia: most common cause is alcohol excess

Type IV: eruptive xanthomas

Type IV Rx: ↓ carbohydrate and alcohol intake

Type V hyperlipoproteinemia: ↑ VLDL + chylomicrons

e. Hyperchylomicronemia syndrome
   (1) Eruptive xanthomas
   (2) Increased incidence of acute pancreatitis
   (3) Lipemia retinalis
      • Retinal vessels look like milk; blurry vision
   (4) Dyspnea and hypoxemia
      • Impaired gas exchange in pulmonary capillaries
   (5) Hepatosplenomegaly
   (6) Increase in serum TG (usually >1000 mg/dL)
   (7) Normal serum CH and LDL
   (8) Turbid supranate and infranate after refrigeration
f. Treatment
   (1) Treat exacerbating disorder (e.g., DKA)
   (2) Nicotinic acid or fibric acid derivatives
6. Apolipoprotein B deficiency (abetalipoproteinemia)
   a. Autosomal recessive

   b. Deficiency of apolipoprotein B-48 and B-100
      (1) Deficiency of chylomicrons, VLDL, and LDL
      (2) Decrease in serum CH and TG
   c. Clinical findings
      (1) Malabsorption
         (a) Chylomicrons accumulate in villi and prevent reabsorption of micelles.
         (b) Marked decrease in vitamin E
      (2) Ataxia (spinocerebellar degeneration), hemolytic anemia with thorny RBCs (acanthocytes) related to vitamin E deficiency.
   d. Treatment
      • Vitamin E

II. Arteriosclerosis
   • Arteriosclerosis is thickening and loss of elasticity of arterial walls.

A. Medial calcification

   1. Dystrophic calcification in the wall of muscular arteries
      • Examples—calcification in uterine and radial arteries
   2. No clinical consequence unless associated with atherosclerosis

B. Atherosclerosis
   1. Pathogenesis

      a. Endothelial cell damage of muscular and elastic arteries
      b. Causes of endothelial cell injury
         • Hypertension, smoking tobacco, homocysteine, LDL
      c. Cell response to endothelial injury
         (1) Macrophages and platelets adhere to damaged endothelium.
         (2) Released cytokines cause hyperplasia of medial smooth muscle cells.
         (3) Smooth muscle cells migrate to the tunica intima.
         (4) Cholesterol enters smooth muscle cells and macrophages (called foam cells).
         (5) Smooth muscle cells release cytokines that produce extracellular matrix.
            • Matrix components include collagen, proteoglycans, and elastin.

      d. Development of fibrous cap (plaque)
         (1) Components of fibrous cap
            • Smooth muscle, foam cells, inflammatory cells, extracellular matrix
         (2) Fibrous cap overlies a necrotic center.
            • Cellular debris, cholesterol crystals (slit-like spaces), foam cells

         (3) Disrupted plaques may extrude underlying necrotic material leading to vessel thrombosis (see Fig. 4-13).

> **Serum C–reactive peptide** (CRP) is increased in patients with disrupted (inflammatory) plaques. Plaques may rupture and produce vessel thrombosis, which leads to acute myocardial infarction (MI). CRP may be a stronger predictor of cardiovascular events than LDL.

         (4) Fibrous plaque becomes dystrophically calcified and ulcerated.
   2. Sites for atherosclerosis (descending order)
      a. Abdominal aorta
      b. Coronary artery

        c. Popliteal artery
        d. Internal carotid artery
    3. Complications of atherosclerosis
        a. Vessel weakness (e.g., abdominal aortic aneurysm)
        b. Vessel thrombosis
            (1) Acute MI (coronary artery)
            (2) Stroke (internal carotid artery, middle cerebral artery)
            (3) Small bowel infarction (superior mesenteric artery)
        c. Hypertension
            • Renal artery atherosclerosis may activate the renin-angiotensin-aldosterone system.
        d. Peripheral vascular disease
            (1) Increased risk of gangrene
            (2) Pain in the buttocks and when walking (claudication)
        e. Cerebral atrophy
            • Atherosclerosis may involve circle of Willis vessels or internal carotid artery.

C. Arteriolosclerosis
    • Hardening of arterioles
    1. Hyaline arteriolosclerosis
        a. Pathogenesis
            • Increased protein is deposited in the vessel wall and occludes the lumen (Fig. 9-3).
        b. Associated conditions
            (1) Diabetes mellitus
                (a) Due to nonenzymatic glycosylation of proteins in the basement membrane
                (b) Basement membrane leaks protein into the vessel wall.
            (2) Hypertension
                • Increased intraluminal pressure pushes plasma proteins into the vessel wall.
    2. Hyperplastic arteriolosclerosis
        a. Pathogenesis
            (1) Renal arteriole effect caused by an acute increase in blood pressure.
                • Example—malignant hypertension
            (2) Smooth muscle cell hyperplasia and basement membrane duplication
        b. Arterioles have an "onion skin" appearance (see Fig. 19-13).

III. Vessel Aneurysms
    • Vessel aneurysms are due to weakening of the vessel wall, followed by dilation and a tendency to rupture.

A. Abdominal aortic aneurysm
    1. Usually located below the renal artery orifices
    2. Pathogenesis
        a. Atherosclerosis weakens vessel wall
            (1) Vessel wall stress increases with vessel diameter.
            (2) Lumen fills with atheromatous debris and blood clots (Fig. 9-4).
        b. Familial factors, structural defects in connective tissue, no vasa vasorum
    3. Clinical findings
        a. Usually asymptomatic
        b. Rupture is the most common complication.

Complications of atherosclerosis: aneurysms, thrombosis, ischemia

Hyaline arteriolosclerosis: diabetes mellitus, hypertension

Abdominal aortic aneurysm: most common aneurysm in men > 55 years of age

Rupture triad: left flank pain, hypotension, pulsatile mass

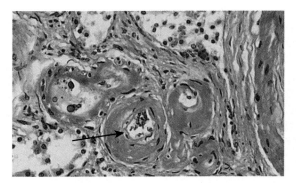

9-3: Hyaline arteriolosclerosis. The arrow depicts eosinophilic material representing protein that has leaked through the basement membrane and deposited in the wall of an arteriole. Other neighboring arterioles demonstrate similar changes. *(From Damjanov I, Linder J: Pathology: A Color Atlas. St. Louis, Mosby, 2000, p 32, Fig. 2-1A.)*

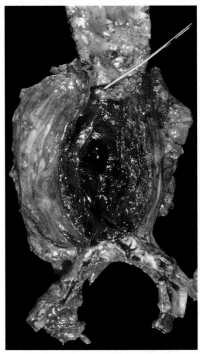

9-4: Abdominal aortic aneurysm. The aneurysmal dilation of the aorta is just above the bifurcation of the aorta. The probe is located at the rupture site. The lumen is filled with atherosclerotic debris and clot material. Ulcerated atheromatous plaques are proximal and distal to the aneurysm. *(From Kumar V, Fausto N, Abbas A: Robbins and Cotran's Pathologic Basis of Disease, 7th ed. Philadelphia, WB Saunders, 2004, p 531, Fig. 11-19B.)*

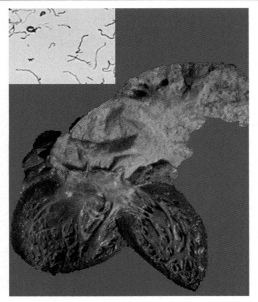

9-5: Syphilitic aortitis. Note the dilated aortic valve root and the irregular intimal wrinkling ("tree barking") due to scarring in the wall of the aorta. The inset shows a silver stain with spirochetes. *(From Klatt E: Robbins and Cotran's Atlas of Pathology. Philadelphia, WB Saunders, 2006, p 9, Figs. 1-22 [gross picture] and 1-24 [spirochete inset].)*

(1) Severe left flank pain is followed by hypotension from blood loss in the retroperitoneum.

(2) A pulsatile mass can be palpated.

B. Mycotic aneurysm

　1. Pathogenesis

　　a. Vessel wall weakening due to an infection

　　　• Does *not* have to be fungal

Fungal vessel invaders: *Aspergillus, Candida, Mucor*

　　b. Fungi that invade vessels

　　　• *Aspergillus, Candida, Mucor*

　　c. Bacteria that invade vessels

　　　• *Bacteroides fragilis, Pseudomonas aeruginosa, Salmonella* species

Bacterial vessel invaders: *B. fragilis, P. aeruginosa, Salmonella*

　2. Clinical findings

　　a. Thrombosis with or without infarction

　　b. Rupture

C. Berry aneurysm of cerebral arteries

　1. Pathogenesis

　　a. Defect at the junction of communicating branches with main cerebral vessels (see Fig. 25-19)

　　　• Vessel lacks an internal elastic lamina and smooth muscle.

　　b. Risk factors for developing the aneurysm

　　　(1) Normal hemodynamic stress

　　　(2) Presence of hypertension of any cause

　　　(3) Coarctation of the aorta

CNS berry aneurysms: junction communicating branch with main vessel

　　c. Rupture releases blood into the subarachnoid space.

　2. Clinical findings

　　a. Sudden onset of severe occipital headache

　　　• Described as the "worst headache I have ever had"

b. Nuchal rigidity from irritation of the meninges
c. Complications
(1) Death may occur shortly after the bleed.
(2) Rebleed, hydrocephalus, neurologic deficits

D. Syphilitic aneurysm
1. Complication of tertiary syphilis due to *Treponema pallidum* (spirochete)
   • Usually occurs in men 40 to 55 years of age
2. Pathogenesis
   a. *T. pallidum* infects the vasa vasorum of the ascending and transverse portions of aortic arch (Fig. 9-5).
      (1) Vasculitis is called endarteritis obliterans.
      (2) Characteristic plasma cell infiltrate is present in the vessel wall.
   b. Vessel ischemia of the medial tissue leads to dilation of the aorta and aortic valve ring.
3. Clinical findings
   a. Aortic valve regurgitation

> **Aortic regurgitation** is a problem in closing the aortic valve. Because the aortic valve closes in diastole, the murmur occurs in early diastole as blood leaks back into the ventricle. The increase in left ventricular end-diastolic volume results in an increase in stroke volume (increased systolic pressure). Blood rapidly draining back into the left ventricle produces a drop in the diastolic pressure. The wide pulse pressure (difference between the systolic and diastolic pressure) is manifested by a hyperdynamic circulation (e.g., pulsating uvula, bounding pulses). Excessive blood dripping back onto the anterior mitral valve leaflet produces another diastolic murmur called the Austin Flint murmur. This finding indicates the need for aortic valve replacement.

   b. Brassy cough
      • Left recurrent laryngeal nerve is stretched by the aneurysm.

E. Aortic dissection
1. Epidemiology
   a. Men with a mean age of 40 to 60 years with antecedent hypertension
      • Most common group
   b. Young patients with a connective tissue disorder
      • Examples—Marfan syndrome, Ehlers-Danlos syndrome (EDS)

> **Marfan syndrome** is an autosomal dominant disorder resulting in the production of weak elastic tissue due to a defect in synthesizing fibrillin (missense mutation). Cardiovascular abnormalities dominate. Dilation of the ascending aorta may progress to aortic dissection or aortic regurgitation. Mitral valve prolapse is the most common valvular defect and is often associated with conduction defects causing sudden death. Skeletal defects include hypermobile joints, eunuchoid proportions (lower body length > upper body length, arm span > height), and arachnodactyly (spider hands; Fig. 9-6A). Dislocation of the lens is another finding, because the suspensory ligament holding the lens is composed of elastic tissue.

2. Pathogenesis
   a. Cystic medial degeneration (CMD)
      (1) Elastic tissue fragmentation
      (2) Matrix material collects in areas of fragmentation in the tunica media.
   b. Risk factors for CMD
      (1) Increase in wall stress
         • Hypertension, pregnancy (increased plasma volume), coarctation
      (2) Defects in connective tissue
         • Marfan syndrome (defect in elastic tissue), EDS (defect in collagen)
   c. Intimal tear
      (1) Due to hypertension or underlying structural weakness in the media
      (2) Usually occurs within 10 cm of the aortic valve (Fig. 9-6B)
      (3) Blood dissects under arterial pressure through areas of weakness.
      (4) Blood dissects proximally and/or distally (Fig. 9-6C).
3. Clinical findings
   a. Acute onset of severe retrosternal chest pain radiating to the back

---

Margin notes:

Aortic arch aneurysm: tertiary syphilis; vasa vasorum vasculitis

Syphilitic aneurysm: produces aortic regurgitation; bounding pulses

Most common cause of death in Marfan syndrome and EDS: aortic dissection

Aortic dissection: cystic medial degeneration

Aortic dissection: pain radiates into the back; absent pulse

9-6: A, Marfan syndrome. Note the arachnodactyly ("spider" fingers) in both hands. **B,** Aortic dissection. The aortic valve (AV) is bicuspid. A large, irregular tear in the intima (AD) of the aorta shows clot material beneath the surface. **C,** Type A (proximal) and type B (distal) aortic dissection. Note that the proximal type can be limited to the arch or involve the arch and distal aorta, while type B (distal) spares the proximal aorta and primarily involves the distal aorta. **D,** Radiograph of an aortic dissection. The *arrows* show widening of the aortic valve root. (*A from Bouloux P: Self-Assessment Picture Tests: Medicine, Vol. 1. London, Mosby-Wolfe, 1997, p 1, Fig. 2; B from Grieg JD, Garden JO: Color Atlas of Surgical Diagnosis. London, Mosby-Wolfe, 1996, p 102, Fig. 15-4; C from Braunwald E, Zipes DP, Libby P, Bonow RO [eds]: Braunwald's Heart Disease: A Textbook of Cardiovascular Medicine, 7th ed. Philadelphia, Saunders, 2004, p 1416; D from Herring W: Learning Radiology: Recognizing the Basics. St. Louis, Mosby Elsevier, 2007, Fig. 13-11.)*

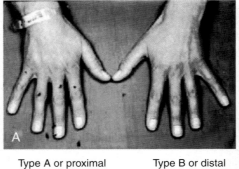

Type A or proximal Type B or distal

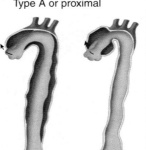
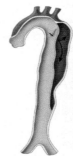
C

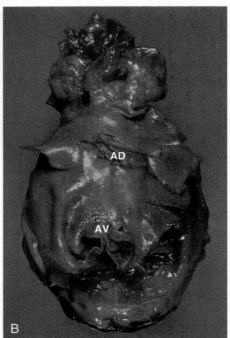

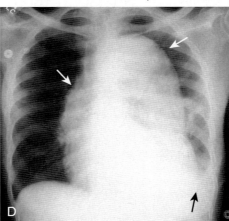

b. Aortic valve regurgitation
   (1) Due to aortic valve ring dilation
   (2) A radiograph or echocardiogram shows widening of the aortic valve root (Fig. 9-6D).
c. Loss of the upper extremity pulse
   • Due to compression of the subclavian artery
d. Rupture
   • Usually into the pericardial sac, pleural cavity, or peritoneal cavity

IV. **Venous System Disorders**
   A. Saphenous venous system
      1. Superficial veins drain blood into the deep veins via penetrating branches.
      2. Valves prevent reversal of blood flow into the superficial system.
      3. Deep veins direct blood back to the heart.
   B. Varicose veins
      1. Abnormally distended, lengthened, and tortuous veins
      2. Locations
         a. Superficial saphenous veins (most common site)
         b. Distal esophagus (due to portal hypertension)
         c. Anorectal region (e.g., hemorrhoids)
         d. Left scrotal sac (e.g., varicocele)

Aortic dissection: cardiac tamponade most common cause of death

3. Superficial varicosities; causes:
   a. Valve incompetence of perforator branches with reversal of blood flow from high-pressure deep venous system into superficial system
      - Exacerbated by pregnancy, prolonged standing, obesity, oral contraceptives, advanced age
   b. Familial tendency
   c. Secondary to deep venous thrombosis
      - Retrograde blood flow through perforating branches into the superficial system
   d. Treatment
      (1) Nonpharmacologic
         - Graded compression stockings
      (2) Chronic treatment
         (a) Compression sclerotherapy
         (b) Ligation and stripping
         (c) Endovenous obliteration using radiofrequency (diathermy) or laser

C. Phlebothrombosis

1. Thrombosis of a vein *without* inflammation
2. Causes
   a. Stasis of blood flow
   b. Hypercoagulability (e.g., antithrombin III deficiency)
3. Location
   a. Most often occurs in the deep vein of the calf
   b. Less common sites include portal vein, hepatic vein, dural sinuses.
4. Clinical findings associated with deep vein thrombosis
   a. General findings
      (1) Swelling
      (2) Pain on dorsiflexion of foot (Homans' sign) and compression of the calf
      (3) Pitting edema distal to the thrombosis (increased hydrostatic pressure)
   b. Pulmonary thromboembolism
      - Occurs when the thrombus extends into the femoral vein
   c. Deep venous insufficiency
      (1) Stasis dermatitis (Fig. 9-7)
         (a) Orange discoloration (hemosiderin) and ischemic ulcers (poor O_2 perfusion) around the ankles
         (b) Caused by rupture of the penetrating branches
            - Due to back-up of pressure (retrograde blood flow) from chronic deep vein insufficiency (related to deep vein thromboses [DVTs], trauma, pregnancy)
         (c) Treatment
            - Topical high potency corticosteroids; antibiotics if infection is present
      (2) Varicosities develop in the superficial system
         - Due to retrograde blood flow into the superficial system from the blocked deep vein thrombosis
   d. Diagnosis of DVT
      - Compression venous ultrasonography + serum D-dimer assay (refer to Chapter 14)
   e. Treatment of DVT
      (1) Low-molecular-weight heparin

Superficial varicosities: valve incompetence

Phlebothrombosis: stasis of blood flow most common cause

Stasis dermatitis: sign of DVT

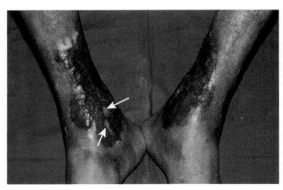

9-7: Stasis dermatitis. Note bilateral hemorrhage and ulceration of the skin over the medial malleoli (*arrows*). (*From Swartz MH: Textbook of Physical Diagnosis, 5th ed. Philadelphia, Saunders Elsevier, 2006, p 442, Fig. 15-1.*)

(2) Compression stockings

(3) Long-term treatment (3–6 months) to prevent recurrent DVTs—warfarin therapy

D. Thrombophlebitis

1. Pain and tenderness along the course of a superficial vein

2. Association with occult DVT in 20% of cases

3. Pathogenesis

   a. Intravenous cannulation of veins

   b. Infection (*Staphylococcus aureus*)

   c. Carcinoma of the pancreatic head

     (1) Produces superficial migratory thrombophlebitis

     (2) Due to the release of thrombogenic substances by the cancer

4. Clinical findings

   a. Tender and palpable cord

   b. Erythema and edema of the overlying skin and subcutaneous tissue

5. Treatment

   a. Warm, moist compresses

   b. NSAIDs

E. Superior vena cava (SVC) syndrome

1. Pathogenesis

   a. Extrinsic compression of the superior vena cava

   b. Due to a primary lung cancer (90% of cases)

     • Usually a small cell carcinoma of the lung

2. Clinical findings

   a. "Puffiness" and blue to purple discoloration of the face, arms, and shoulders (see Fig. 16-34)

   b. Retinal hemorrhage, stroke

3. Treatment

   • Radiation; stent to bypass obstruction

F. Thoracic outlet syndrome

1. Pathogenesis

   a. Compression of the neurovascular compartment in the neck

   b. Causes

     • Cervical rib, spastic anterior scalene muscles, or positional change in the neck and arms

2. Clinical findings

   a. Vascular signs (e.g., arm "falls asleep" while person is sleeping)

   b. Nerve root signs (e.g., numbness, paresthesias)

   c. Positive Adson test

     • Pulse disappears when the arm is outstretched and the patient looks to the side of the outstretched arm.

3. Treatment

   • Manipulation therapy; home exercise

V. Lymphatic Disorders

A. Structure of lymphatic vessels

   • Lymphatic vessels have incomplete basement membranes, which predisposes them to infection and tumor invasion.

B. Acute lymphangitis

1. Inflammation of lymphatics ("red streak")

2. Usually due to cellulitis caused by *Streptococcus pyogenes*

C. Nodular lymphangitis

   • Sporotrichosis (refer to Chapter 24)

D. Lymphedema

1. Collection of lymphatic fluid in interstitial tissue or body cavities

2. Obstructive lymphedema

   a. Radiation damage following radical mastectomy (Fig. 9-8)

   b. Complex decongestive therapy

     • Leg elevation, limb massage, pneumatic leg compression

3. Turner's syndrome (refer to Chapter 5)

   a. Lymphedema of hands and feet in newborns caused by defective lymphatics

   b. Dilated lymphatic channels in the neck (cystic hygroma) produce webbed neck (see Fig. 5-16).

Thrombophlebitis: pain and tenderness overlying the vein

SVC syndrome: compression of SVC by primary lung cancer

Thoracic outlet syndrome: common among weight lifters; tight scalenus muscles

Acute lymphangitis: *Streptococcus pyogenes* cellulitis

Turner's webbed neck: lymphatic abnormality

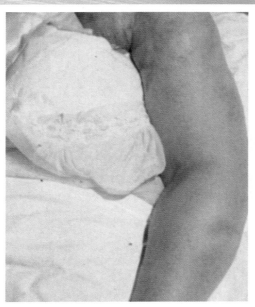

9-8: Lymphedema. Note the swelling of the entire arm. The patient had a modified radical mastectomy followed by radiation. *(From Grieg JD, Garden JO: Color Atlas of Surgical Diagnosis. London, Mosby-Wolfe, 1996, p 36, Fig. 6-29.)*

4. Chylous effusions (e.g., pleural cavity)
   a. Contain chylomicrons with triglyceride plus mature lymphocytes
   b. Damage to thoracic duct
      • Causes include malignant lymphoma, trauma

VI. **Vascular Tumors and Tumor-like Conditions**
   A. **Tumors**
      • Most tumors derive from small vessels or arteriovenous anastomoses in glomus bodies.
   B. **Vessel tumors and tumor-like conditions** (Table 9-1 and Fig. 9-9)

VII. **Vasculitic Disorders**
   • Inflammation of small vessels (arterioles, venules, capillaries), medium-sized vessels (muscular arteries), large vessels (elastic arteries), or combinations of these vessel types
   A. **Pathogenesis**
      1. Type III hypersensitivity (immunocomplex)
         • Example—Henoch-Schönlein purpura
      2. Type II hypersensitivity (antigen-antibody)
         • Example—Goodpasture syndrome (anti–basement membrane antibodies)
      3. Antineutrophil cytoplasmic antibodies (ANCA)
         a. Activate neutrophils causing release of their enzymes and free radicals resulting in vessel damage

Bacillary angiomatosis: *Bartonella henselae;* common in AIDS

ANCA: antibodies against components of neutrophils

TABLE 9-1. VASCULAR TUMORS AND TUMOR-LIKE CONDITIONS

TUMOR/CONDITION	CLINICAL FINDINGS
Angiomyolipoma	Kidney hamartoma, composed of blood vessels, muscle, and mature adipose tissue Association with tuberous sclerosis
Angiosarcoma	Liver angiosarcoma associated with exposure to polyvinyl chloride, arsenic, thorium dioxide
Bacillary angiomatosis (see Fig. 9-9A)	Benign capillary proliferation involving skin and visceral organs in AIDS patients Simulates Kaposi's sarcoma in AIDS Caused by *Bartonella henselae*, a gram-negative bacillus
Capillary hemangioma (see Fig. 9-9B)	Facial lesion in newborns that regresses with age
Cavernous hemangioma	Most common benign tumor of liver and spleen May rupture if large

Continued

TABLE 9-1. **VASCULAR TUMORS AND TUMOR-LIKE CONDITIONS—cont'd**

TUMOR/CONDITION	CLINICAL FINDINGS
Cystic hygroma	Lymphangioma in the neck associated with Turner's syndrome
Glomus tumor	Derive from arteriovenous shunts in glomus bodies Painful red subungual nodule in a digit
Hereditary telangiectasia (AD) (see Fig. 9-9C)	Dilated vessels on skin and mucous membranes in mouth and gastrointestinal tract Chronic iron deficiency anemia
Kaposi's sarcoma (see Fig. 3-4)	Malignant tumor arising from endothelial cells or primitive mesenchymal cells Associated with human herpesvirus type 8 Raised, red-purple discoloration that progresses from a flat lesion to a plaque to a nodule that ulcerates Common sites include skin (most common site), mouth, and gastrointestinal tract
Lymphangiosarcoma (see Fig. 9-8)	Malignancy of lymphatic vessels Arises out of long-standing chronic lymphedema (e.g., after modified radical mastectomy)
Pyogenic granuloma	Vascular, red pedunculated mass that ulcerates and bleeds easily Post-traumatic or associated with pregnancy (relation to estrogen); usually regress postpartum
Spider telangiectasia (see Fig. 18-10)	Arteriovenous fistula (disappears when compressed) Associated with hyperestrinism (e.g., cirrhosis, pregnancy)
Sturge-Weber syndrome (see Fig. 9-9D)	Nevus flammeus ("birthmark") on the face in distribution of ophthalmic branch of cranial nerve V (trigeminal) Some cases show ipsilateral malformation of pia mater vessels overlying occipital and parietal lobes
Von Hippel–Lindau syndrome (AD)	Cavernous hemangiomas in cerebellum and retina Increased incidence of pheochromocytoma and bilateral renal cell carcinomas

AD, autosomal dominant.

9-9: **A,** Bacillary angiomatosis. Note the nodular red mass and satellite lesions at the periphery. **B,** Capillary hemangioma. Note the raised, red lesion above the right eyelid in this child. **C,** Hereditary telangiectasia. Note the telangiectasias scattered over the dorsal surface of the tongue. **D,** Sturge-Weber syndrome. Note the nevus flammeus ("birthmark") on the left side of the face in the distribution of cranial nerve V (trigeminal). (*A courtesy of Richard Johnson, MD, Beth Isreal Deaconess Medical Center, Boston; B from Habif T: Clinical Dermatology, 4th ed. St. Louis, Mosby, 2004; C and D from Swartz MH: Textbook of Physical Diagnosis, 5th ed. Philadelphia, Saunders Elsevier, 2006, pp 333, 770, Figs. 12-11, 24-8, respectively.*)

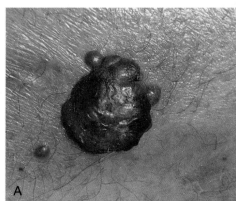
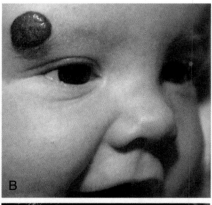
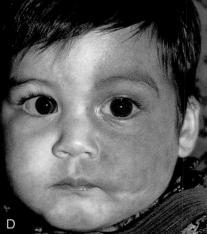
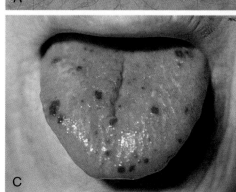

b. c-ANCA type
  (1) Antibodies are directed against proteinase 3 in cytoplasmic granules.
  (2) Example—Wegener's granulomatosis
c. p-ANCA type
  (1) Antibodies are directed against myeloperoxidase.
  (2) Examples—microscopic polyangiitis, Churg-Strauss syndrome
4. Direct invasion by all classes of microbial pathogens
B. Clinical findings
  1. Small vessel vasculitis
    a. Called leukocytoclastic venulitis or hypersensitivity vasculitis
    b. Gross appearance
      (1) Skin overlying the vasculitis is hemorrhagic, raised, and painful to palpation.
        • Called palpable purpura ("tumor" of acute inflammation)
      (2) Examples—Henoch-Schönlein purpura, microscopic polyangiitis

Small vessel vasculitis: palpable purpura

Purpura due to thrombocytopenia or vessel instability (e.g., scurvy) is *not* palpable, because acute inflammation is *not* involved.

c. Microscopic appearance
      • Vessel is disrupted and contains a neutrophilic infiltrate associated with nuclear debris and fibrinoid necrosis.
  2. Medium-sized vessel vasculitis
    a. Muscular artery vasculitis
    b. Presents with vessel thrombosis and infarction or aneurysms
    c. Examples—polyarteritis nodosa, Kawasaki disease
  3. Large vessel vasculitis
    a. Elastic artery vasculitis
    b. Presents with loss of a pulse or stroke
    c. Examples—Takayasu arteritis, giant cell (temporal arteritis)
  4. Summary table of vasculitides (Table 9-2 and Fig. 9-10)

Medium-sized vessel vasculitis: thrombosis, aneurysm formation

Large vessel vasculitis: absent pulse, stroke

VIII. Hypertension
  A. Classification
    1. Normal
      • <120 mm Hg systolic and <80 mm Hg diastolic
    2. Pre-hypertension
      • 120 to 139 mm Hg systolic or 80 to 89 mm Hg diastolic
    3. Stage 1 hypertension
      • 140 to 159 mm Hg systolic or 90 to 99 mm Hg diastolic
    4. Stage 2 hypertension
      • ≥160 mm Hg systolic or ≥100 mm Hg
  B. Pathophysiology of hypertension
    1. Systolic blood pressure
      a. Correlates with stroke volume
      b. Determination of stroke volume:
        (1) Blood volume (equates with sodium homeostasis)
        (2) Force of contraction
        (3) Heart rate
    2. Diastolic blood pressure
      a. Determination of diastolic blood pressure
        (1) Volume of blood in the arteries while the heart is filling in diastole
          • Depends on the vascular tone of the peripheral resistance arterioles
        (2) Elastic recoil of the aorta
      b. Role of the total peripheral resistance (TPR) arterioles
        (1) Abbreviated Poiseuille's equation
          • TPR = viscosity of blood/(radius of arteriole)^4
        (2) Vasodilation decreases TPR
          (a) Decreases diastolic blood pressure
          (b) Increases venous return to the heart
          (c) Vasodilators
            • Nitric oxide, prostaglandin I$_2$, histamine, β-blockers, and calcium-channel blockers

Systolic blood pressure: correlates with stroke volume

Diastolic blood pressure: correlates with tonicity of TPR arterioles

TABLE 9-2. **VASCULITIC DISORDERS: ELASTIC ARTERY, MUSCULAR ARTERY, AND SMALL VESSEL**

DISORDER	VASCULITIS	EPIDEMIOLOGY/ETIOLOGY	CLINICAL/LABORATORY FINDINGS/ TREATMENT
Takayasu arteritis ("pulseless disease")	Granulomatous large vessel vasculitis involving aortic arch vessels	Young Asian women and children	Absent upper extremity pulse Discrepancy in blood pressure between arms > 10 mm Hg Visual defects, stroke *Treatment*: corticosteroids
Giant cell (temporal) arteritis	Granulomatous large vessel vasculitis involving superficial temporal and ophthalmic arteries.	Adults > 50 years of age	Temporal headache, jaw claudication (pain when chewing stretches inflamed artery) Blindness on ipsilateral side Polymyalgia rheumatica (muscle and joint pain; normal serum creatine kinase) Increased ESR *Treatment*: corticosteroids
Polyarteritis nodosa (see Fig. 9-10A)	Necrotizing medium- sized vessel vasculitis involving renal, coronary, mesenteric arteries (spares pulmonary arteries)	Middle-aged men Association with HBsAg (30%)	Vessels at all stages of acute and chronic inflammation Focal vasculitis produces aneurysms (detected with angiography) Organ infarction in kidneys (renal failure), heart (acute MI), bowels (bloody diarrhea), skin (ischemic ulcer), testicle (testicular pain) Angiography and biopsy of lesions confirm the diagnosis. *Treatment*: corticosteroids
Kawasaki disease (see Fig. 9-10B)	Necrotizing medium- sized vessel vasculitis involving coronary arteries (e.g., thrombosis, aneurysms)	Children < 5 years of age Boys > girls Cause unknown (probably infectious) Children of Asian descent have highest incidence Surpassed acute rheumatic heart disease as most common acquired heart disease in children	Fever, erythema and edema of hands and feet convalescing with desquamated rash; cervical adenopathy; oral erythema and cracking of the lips Abnormal ECG (e.g., acute MI) *Treatment*: intravenous immunoglobulin; aspirin; corticosteroids contraindicated (danger of vessel rupture)
Thromboangiitis obliterans (Buerger's disease)	Medium-sized vessel vasculitis with digital vessel thrombosis and damage to neurovascular compartment	Men 25–50 years of age who smoke cigarettes Middle East, Far East, Asia has highest prevalence	Resting pain on the forefoot is characteristic, with possible ischemic ulcers or gangrene of foot/toes; upper limb ischemia (40% to 50% of patients) with ulceration and gangrene; Raynaud's phenomenon. *Treatment*: smoking cessation essential; intravenous iloprost (prostaglandin analogue)
Raynaud's disease	Medium-sized vessel vasculitis involving digital vessels in fingers and toes; also tip of nose and ears in some cases	Young women Exaggerated vasomotor response to cold or stress	Paroxysmal digital color changes (white-blue-red sequence) Ulceration and gangrene in chronic cases *Treatment*: avoid cold temperatures (gloves); calcium channel blockers (e.g., nifedipine)
Raynaud's phenomenon (see Fig. 9-10C)	Medium-sized vessel vasculitis involving digital vessels in fingers and toes; also tip of nose and ears in some cases	Adult men and women Secondary to other diseases (e.g., systemic sclerosis, CREST syndrome, SLE)	Systemic sclerosis and CREST syndrome (see page 47): digital vasculitis with vessel fibrosis, dystrophic calcification, ulceration, gangrene *Treatment*: see above
Wegener's granulomatosis (see Fig. 9-10D)	Necrotizing medium and small-sized vessel vasculitis involving lung (infarctions, renal vessels)	Childhood to middle age	Necrotizing granulomas in skin, upper respiratory tract (nasopharynx—saddle nose deformity, chronic sinusitis, collapse of trachea), lower respiratory tract (cavitating nodular lesions) Necrotizing vasculitis in lungs (infarction, hemoptysis), kidneys (crescentic glomerulonephritis) c-ANCA antibodies (>90% of cases) correlate erratically with therapy *Treatment*: corticosteroids, cyclo- phosphamide 3 Cs: c-ANCA, corticosteroids, cyclophosphamide

TABLE 9-2. VASCULITIC DISORDERS: ELASTIC ARTERY, MUSCULAR ARTERY, AND SMALL VESSEL—cont'd

DISORDER	VASCULITIS	EPIDEMIOLOGY/ETIOLOGY	CLINICAL/LABORATORY FINDINGS/TREATMENT
Microscopic polyangiitis	Small vessel vasculitis involving skin, lung, brain, GI tract, and postcapillary venules and glomerular capillaries	Children and adults Precipitated by drugs (e.g., penicillin), infections (e.g., streptococci), immune disorders (e.g., SLE)	Vessels at same stage of inflammation Palpable purpura, glomerulonephritis p-ANCA antibodies (>80% of cases)
Churg-Strauss syndrome	Small vessel vasculitis involving skin, lung, heart vessels	Children and adults	Allergic rhinitis, asthma p-ANCA antibodies (70% of cases), eosinophilia
Henoch-Schönlein purpura (see Fig. 9-10E)	Small vessel vasculitis involving skin, GI, renal, joint vessels	Children and young adults Males > females Most common vasculitis in children IgA–anti-IgA immunocomplexes	Often follows a viral URI, group A streptococcal pharyngeal infection–pathogens may act as an antigen trigger that causes antibody formation leading to immunocomplex formation Palpable purpura of buttocks and lower extremities Polyarthritis (80%), nephropathy (80%), GI bleeding Recurrence may occur in one third of cases Most have spontaneous recovery in 4 months without therapy. *Treatment:* corticosteroids mainly used if severe GI disease or renal disease
Cryoglobulinemia	Small vessel vasculitis involving skin, GI tract, renal vessels Different types of cryoglobulinemia (mixed, monoclonal, polyclonal)	Adults Association with HCV, type I MPGN, multiple myeloma (monoclonal type)	Cryoglobulins: immunoglobulins that gel at cold temperatures Palpable purpura, acral cyanosis of nose and ears and Raynaud's phenomenon (reverses when in warm room); glomerulonephritis; arthritis; abdominal pain
Infectious vasculitis (see Fig. 9-10F)	Small vessel vasculitis involving skin vessels	Children and adults Involves all microbial pathogens	Rocky Mountain spotted fever: tick transmission of *Rickettsia rickettsiae* Organisms invade endothelial cells producing vasculitis Petechiae on palms spread to trunk Disseminated meningococcemia due to *Neisseria meningitides* Capillary thrombosis produces hemorrhage into skin and confluent ecchymoses

c-ANCA, cytoplasmic antineutrophil cytoplasmic antibodies; ECG, electrocardiogram; ESR, erythrocyte sedimentation rate; GI, gastrointestinal; HBsAg, hepatitis B surface antigen; HCV, hepatitis C virus; MI, myocardial infarction; MPGN, membranoproliferative glomerulonephritis; p-ANCA, perinuclear antineutrophil cytoplasmic antibodies; SLE, systemic lupus erythematosus; URI, upper respiratory infection.

    (3) Vasoconstriction increases TPR.
       • Increases diastolic blood pressure

Factors that contract arteriole smooth muscle cells causing vasoconstriction include α-adrenergic stimuli, catecholamines, angiotensin II, vasopressin, and increased total body sodium.

    3. Role of sodium in hypertension
      a. Excess sodium increases plasma volume.
        • Increases stroke volume and systolic blood pressure
      b. Excess sodium produces vasoconstriction of TPR arterioles
        (1) Sodium enters arteriole smooth muscle cells and opens calcium channels, causing vasoconstriction.
        (2) Increases diastolic blood pressure
  C. Essential hypertension
    1. Accounts for 95% of cases of hypertension
    2. Pathogenesis
      a. Genetic factors reduce renal sodium excretion.
      b. Unknown factors cause vasoconstriction of arterioles.
      c. Obesity, stress

Pathogenesis hypertension: renal retention of sodium commonly involved

Most common type of hypertension: essential hypertension

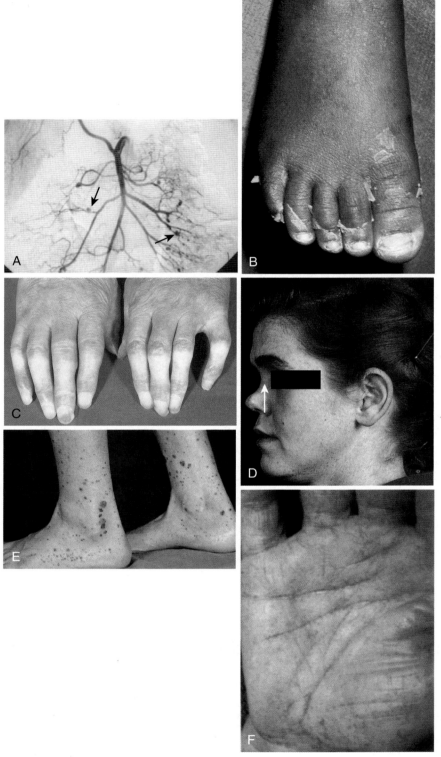

9-10: A, Mesenteric angiogram in polyarteritis nodosa. Note the numerous small aneurysms (arrows) in the medium-sized vessels. **B,** Kawasaki disease: Note the desquamation of the skin of the toes, which is a characteristic skin finding in this disease. **C,** Raynaud's phenomenon. Note the extreme pallor of the digits in both hands in this patient with systemic lupus erythematosus. **D,** Saddle nose deformity in Wegener's granulomatosis. Note the concavity (arrow) below the bridge of the nose having the appearance of a saddle. **E,** Henoch-Schönlein purpura. Multiple erythematous, raised, palpable lesions around the ankles show areas of hemorrhage into the skin overlying areas of immunocomplex vasculitis involving small vessels. **F,** Rocky Mountain spotted fever. The palm shows a few petechial lesions in this patient with a history of a tick bite. (**A** from Goldman L, Ausiello D: Cecil's Textbook of Medicine, 23rd ed. Philadelphia, Saunders Elsevier, 2008, p 2054, Fig. 291-2A; **B** courtesy of J. Ross, MD, Lewisham Hospital, London; **C** from Savin JA, Hunter JAA, Hepburn NC: Diagnosis in Color: Skin Signs in Clinical Medicine. London, Mosby-Wolfe, 1997, p 205, Fig. 8.43; **D** and **E** from Bouloux P-M: Self-Assessment Picture Tests: Medicine, Vol. 3. London, Mosby-Wolfe, 1996, pp 47 and 66, Figs. 92 and 75, respectively; **F** courtesy of Department of Dermatology, University of North Carolina at Chapel Hill, Chapel Hill, NC.)

Reduced renal sodium excretion is the primary mechanism of essential hypertension in blacks and the elderly. Increased plasma volume suppresses renin release from the juxtaglomerular apparatus (low renin hypertension).

D. Secondary hypertension
1. Accounts for 5% of cases of hypertension
2. Renovascular hypertension
   a. Causes
      (1) Elderly men
         • Atherosclerotic plaque partially blocks blood flow at the renal artery orifice (Fig. 9-11).
      (2) Young to middle-aged women
         • Fibromuscular hyperplasia occurs in multifocal areas of the renal artery (Fig. 9-12).
   b. Pathogenesis
      (1) Decreased renal arterial blood flow activates the renin-angiotensin-aldosterone (RAA) system.
      (2) Angiotensin II vasoconstricts TPR arterioles.
      (3) Aldosterone increases sodium retention.
   c. Clinical findings
      (1) Severe, uncontrollable hypertension
      (2) Increased plasma renin activity (PRA)
      (3) Involved kidney has increased PRA in the renal vein.
      (4) Uninvolved kidney has decreased PRA.
         • Increased plasma volume due to aldosterone excess suppresses RAA system in normal kidney.
      (5) Epigastric bruit
         • Sound is due to turbulence of blood flow through the narrow renal artery.
      (6) Angiography
         (a) Involved kidney shows diminished size (atrophy) and delayed emptying.
         (b) Renal artery has "beaded" appearance in fibromuscular hyperplasia.
   d. Other causes of secondary hypertension (Table 9-3)
E. Complications of hypertension (Table 9-4 and Box 9-1)

Renovascular hypertension: most common cause of secondary hypertension

Renovascular hypertension: atherosclerosis in men; fibromuscular hyperplasia in women

Renovascular hypertension: activation of RAA system

PRA: ↑ in involved kidney; ↓ in unaffected kidney

Fibromuscular hyperplasia: "beaded" appearance of renal artery

Complications descending order: acute MI, stroke, renal failure

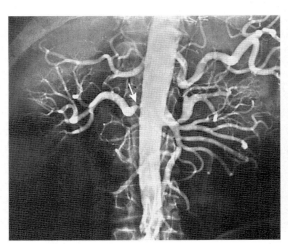

9-11: Angiogram showing right renal artery stenosis with post-stenotic dilation (*arrow*). (*From Katz D, Math K, Groskin S: Radiology Secrets. Philadelphia, Hanley & Belfus, 1998, p 184, Fig. 7.*)

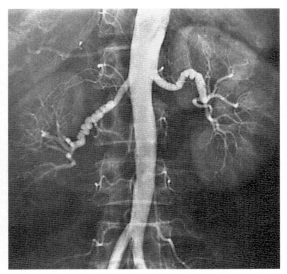

9-12: Angiogram showing bilateral renal artery fibromuscular hyperplasia. Note the beading effect in both vessels. (*From Katz D, Math K, Groskin S: Radiology Secrets. Philadelphia, Hanley & Belfus, 1998, p 180, Fig. 27.*)

Nonpharmacologic treatment of hypertension includes weight loss (most important), limited alcohol intake, aerobic exercise (30 min/day), reduced sodium intake (<1 mmol/day or <2.3 g/day), adequate potassium intake (>3500 mg/day), cessation of smoking, and a cholesterol lowering diet. For pre-hypertension, the lifestyle modifications listed above are recommended to bring the blood pressure under 130/80 mm Hg. For stage 1 hypertension, diuretics are preferred for initial therapy. More selective therapy is used if different disorders are present (e.g., congestive heart failure or diabetes—ACE inhibitor). For stage 2 hypertension, two drug combinations are required (e.g., diuretic + angiotensin II inhibitor). For pregnant women with hypertension (>130/80 mm Hg), the following drugs can be used: methyldopa, hydralazine, labetalol, or atenolol.

Control of hypertension has its greatest benefit in reducing the incidence of strokes; however, it also significantly reduces the risk for developing CHD and renal disease.

TABLE 9-3. **CAUSES OF SECONDARY HYPERTENSION**

SYSTEM OR SOURCE	DESCRIPTION
Adrenal	Cushing syndrome: increased mineralocorticoids Pheochromocytoma: increased catecholamines Neuroblastoma: increased catecholamines 11-Hydroxylase deficiency: increased mineralocorticoids (i.e., deoxycorticosterone) Primary aldosteronism (Conn's syndrome): increased aldosterone
Aorta	Postductal coarctation: activation of RAA system Elderly: systolic hypertension due to decreased elasticity of the aorta
CNS	Intracranial hypertension: release of catecholamines
Drugs	Oral contraceptive: increased synthesis of angiotensinogen; most common cause of hypertension in young women Cocaine: increased sympathetic activity
Parathyroid	Primary hyperparathyroidism: calcium increases peripheral resistance arteriole smooth muscle cell contraction
Pregnancy	Preeclampsia: increased angiotensin II
Renal	Renovascular disease: atherosclerosis (elderly men), fibromuscular hyperplasia (women) Renal parenchymal disease: e.g., diabetic nephropathy, adult polycystic kidney disease, glomerulonephritis; retention of sodium
Thyroid	Graves' disease: systolic hypertension from increased cardiac contraction Hypothyroidism: diastolic hypertension due to retention of sodium

RAA, renin-angiotensin-aldosterone.

TABLE 9-4. **COMPLICATIONS OF HYPERTENSION**

SYSTEM	COMPLICATIONS
Cardiovascular	Left ventricular hypertrophy: most common overall complication Acute myocardial infarction: most common cause of death Atherosclerosis
Central nervous	Intracerebral hematoma: due to rupture of Charcot-Bouchard aneurysms Berry aneurysm: rupture produces a subarachnoid hemorrhage Lacunar infarcts: small infarcts due to hyaline arteriolosclerosis
Renal	Benign nephrosclerosis: kidney disease of hypertension; due to hyaline arteriolosclerosis; atrophy of tubules and sclerosis of glomeruli; progresses to renal failure Malignant hypertension: rapid increase in blood pressure accompanied by renal failure and cerebral edema
Eyes	Hypertensive retinopathy: arteriovenous nicking, hemorrhage of retinal vessels, exudates (increased vessel permeability, retinal infarction), papilledema

BOX 9-1   HYPERTENSIVE RETINOPATHY

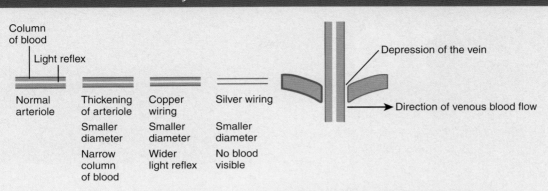

The sequence of events in hypertensive retinopathy involves focal spasm of the arterioles followed by progressive sclerosis and narrowing of the arterioles, leading eventually to flame hemorrhages from rupture of the vessels, formation of exudates (soft and hard), and papilledema (swelling of the optic disk). Normal arteriole walls are transparent; hence, the column of blood is visible and the light reflex is narrow. Sclerotic changes in the vessels are first described as "copper wiring," since blood is still visible through the vessel wall. The light reflex becomes wider. When the vessel wall is thickened enough to prevent visualization of the blood, the light reflects back from the vessel wall to produce a "silver wiring" effect. In some cases, no blood is visible in portions of the vessel. Because arterioles cross over the veins (normal ratio of arteriole to venous diameters is 3:4), as arterioles thicken they create a depression in the wall of the venule, which is called an arteriovenous (AV) nicking defect. The distal vein becomes slightly distended owing to the backup of blood. More advanced nicking literally cuts off the blood flow, and the veins appear to end abruptly. Hemorrhages in the retina are usually the result of rupture of microaneurysms that develop from increased pressure on the arterioles. Grayish-white exudates that are soft, like cotton wool, are due to microinfarctions, whereas exudates that have clear margins (hard exudates) are due to leakage of protein from increased vessel permeability. A brief summary of the Keith-Wagener-Barker classification of hypertensive retinopathy follows:

Grade I: focal narrowing of the arterioles, mild AV nicking
Grade II: arteriole narrowing, copper wiring present, AV nicking more accentuated
Grade III: arteriole narrowing, silver wiring present, hemorrhages, soft and hard exudates, disappearance of the vein under the arteriole, disk normal
Grade IV: arterioles are fine fibrous cords; same as grade III except papilledema is present

CHAPTER 10

HEART DISORDERS

I. **Cardiac Physical Diagnosis** (Box 10-1)
II. **Ventricular Hypertrophy**
   - Compensatory change related to changes in pressure in the wall of the ventricle

   A. Pathogenesis of left and right ventricular hypertrophy
   1. Sustained pressure in the ventricles increases wall stress.
   2. Changes in wall stress produce changes in gene expression.
   3. Changes in gene expression lead to duplication of sarcomeres.
      - Sarcomeres are the contractile element of muscle.
   4. Changes in wall stress related to an increase in afterload
      a. Afterload is the resistance the ventricle contracts against to eject blood in systole.
      b. Increased afterload produces concentric thickening of the ventricular wall (Fig. 10-1A).
         - Sarcomeres duplicate parallel to the long axes of the cells; muscles are thicker.
      c. Causes of concentric left ventricular hypertrophy (LVH)
         (1) Essential hypertension (most common)
         (2) Aortic stenosis
         (3) Hypertrophic cardiomyopathy
      d. Causes of concentric right ventricular hypertrophy (RVH)
         (1) Pulmonary hypertension
         (2) Pulmonary artery stenosis
   5. Changes in wall stress related to increased preload
      a. Preload correlates with left ventricular end-diastolic volume (LVEDV).
      b. Increased preload invokes the Frank-Starling pressure relationship to increase stroke volume.
      c. Increased preload causes dilation and hypertrophy (eccentric hypertrophy) of ventricular wall (Fig. 10-1B).
         - Sarcomeres duplicate in series; muscle length and width are increased.
      d. Causes of eccentric hypertrophy of the left ventricle
         (1) Mitral valve or aortic valve regurgitation
         (2) Left-to-right shunting of blood (e.g., ventricular septal defect)
            - More blood returns to the left side of the heart.
      e. Causes of eccentric hypertrophy of the right ventricle
         - Tricuspid valve or pulmonary valve regurgitation

   B. Consequences of ventricular hypertrophy
   1. Left- and right-sided heart failure
   2. Angina (primarily LVH)
   3. S_4 heart sound (see Box 10-1)
      a. Correlates with atrial contraction in late diastole; atrial gallop (see Box 10-1)
      b. Caused by blood entering a noncompliant ventricle
      c. Examples
         (1) Concentric LVH in essential hypertension or aortic stenosis
         (2) Concentric RVH in pulmonary hypertension or pulmonary stenosis
         (3) Volume overload in mitral regurgitation or tricuspid regurgitation
         (4) Volume overload in aortic regurgitation or pulmonary regurgitation

III. **Congestive Heart Failure (CHF)**
   - The heart fails when it is unable to eject blood delivered to it by the venous system.

   A. Epidemiology
   1. Most common hospital admission diagnosis in elderly patients

---

Wall stress increases gene-controlled sarcomere duplication.

Afterload: resistance ventricle contracts against to eject blood in systole

Ventricular hypertrophy: increased afterload causes concentric hypertrophy

Preload: equivalent to LVEDV

Ventricular hypertrophy: increased preload causes eccentric hypertrophy

Consequences of hypertrophy: heart failure, S_4, angina (LVH)

S_4: blood entering noncompliant ventricle

BOX 10-1   CARDIAC PHYSICAL DIAGNOSIS

Valve Locations for Auscultation

Locations where heart sounds are best heard do *not* always correlate with their anatomic location. The mitral valve (MV) is best heard at the apex; the tricuspid valve (TV) at the left parasternal border; the pulmonary valve (PV) at the left second and third intercostal spaces (ICS); and the aortic valve (AV) at the left sternal border for regurgitation murmurs and right second ICS for ejection murmurs.

Cardiac Cycle Relationships with Heart Sounds

The P wave represents atrial depolarization; the PR interval atrioventricular conduction time; the QRS ventricular depolarization; and the T wave ventricular repolarization, or recovery. The S_1 heart sound occurs at the same time as the QRS complex and marks the beginning of systole, while the S_2 heart sound occurs after the T wave and marks the beginning of diastole.

Heart Sounds

The **S_1 heart sound** corresponds with closure of the MV and TV during systole. The MV closes *before* the TV. It is best heard at the apex and corresponds with the carotid/radial pulse. The **S_2 heart sound** is caused by closure of the AV and PV and marks the beginning of diastole. It is best heard at the left second or third ICS. The aortic component (A_2) normally precedes the pulmonary component (P_2). Unlike the S_1 heart sound, the S_2 splits on inspiration. As the diaphragm descends, it causes a further decrease in negative intrathoracic pressure, which increases the flow of blood out of the vena cava into the right side of the heart. This causes flattening of the jugular neck veins. The excess amount of blood in the right side of the heart delays closure of the PV causing P_2 to separate away from A_2 (see schematic). This physiologic split is best heard over the PV area. A_2 and P_2 become a single sound on expiration as intrathoracic pressure becomes less negative. An **accentuated A_2** is heard in essential hypertension (increased pressure causes it to snap shut), while an **accentuated P_2** is heard in pulmonary hypertension.

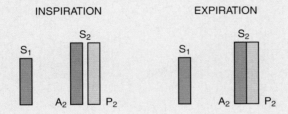

An **S_3 heart sound** (see schematic) is the most clinically significant extra heart sound. It is a normal finding in children and young adults, where it reflects a more energetic expansion and filling of the left ventricle. However, it is considered a pathologic finding after 40 years of age. It is thought to be due to a sudden rush of blood entering a volume overloaded left or right ventricle. It is best heard at the apex with the patient in the left lateral decubitus position. It commonly occurs with regurgitant types of murmurs involving any of the valves. It is the first cardiac sign of congestive heart failure, where increased ventricular volume stretches the MV or TV ring causing volume overload from mitral/tricuspid regurgitation. An S_3 heart sound produces a ventricular gallop. An **S_4 heart sound** (see schematic) coincides with atrial contraction in late diastole and the a wave in the jugular venous pulse (JVP; see below). It is *never* a normal finding and is due to increased resistance to ventricular filling (decreased compliance) following a vigorous atrial contraction. It is heard best at the apex. Causes of decreased ventricular compliance include concentric ventricular hypertrophy (left/right) and a volume overloaded ventricle (no more room to expand). An S_4 heart sound and the a wave of a JVP are absent in atrial fibrillation. Presence of an S_4 heart sound produces an atrial gallop. Presence of an S_3 and S_4 heart sound is called a summation gallop (see schematic) and sounds like a galloping horse.

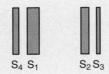

Heart Murmurs

Heart murmurs may occur in systole and diastole. They may be caused by structural valve disease (e.g., damage due to rheumatic fever) or stretching of the valve ring (e.g., volume overload in left- or right-sided heart failure). Murmurs due to stretching of valve rings are often called functional murmurs. Murmurs often radiate.

Continued

BOX 10-1 CARDIAC PHYSICAL DIAGNOSIS—cont'd

For example, AV stenosis radiates into the neck and MV regurgitation radiates into the axilla. They are graded 1 to 6 in terms of their intensity. Grade 1 and 2 murmurs are very hard to hear, while grade 3 murmurs are easy to hear. Grade 4 to 6 murmurs are often accompanied by a palpable precordial thrill. Grade 6 murmurs are audible without a stethoscope. Murmurs and abnormal heart sounds (e.g., S_3 and S_4 heart sounds) change their intensity with respirations. Right-sided murmurs and abnormal heart sounds have increased intensity when the patient takes a deep inspiration and holds the breath for 3 to 5 seconds. This is due to the increase in negative intrathoracic pressure drawing blood out of the venous system into the right side of the heart, hence accentuating the murmur and abnormal heart sound. In contradistinction, left-sided heart murmurs and abnormal heart sounds do *not* change their intensity with deep inspiration. **Continuous murmurs** occur through systole and diastole. The most common cause of a continuous murmur in children is a cervical venous hum. A patent ductus arteriosus also produces a continuous murmur. **Innocent murmurs** occur in children from 3 to 7 years old. They are usually grade 2 systolic murmurs that are caused by increased blood flow through the PV. They are best heard in the PV area, and as expected, their intensity increases with deep, held inspiration. **Stenosis murmurs** occur when there is a problem in opening the valves. Because the AV and PV normally open in systole, AV and PV stenosis occur in systole. They produce an ejection type murmur (schematic A), which has a diamond-shaped configuration. The MV and TV normally open in diastole; hence, the murmurs of MV and TV stenosis are heard in diastole. MV stenosis is accompanied by an opening snap (schematic B), which occurs when the thickened valve is forced open by a forceful atrial contraction. An opening snap is usually absent in TV stenosis. **Regurgitant (insufficiency) murmurs** occur when there is a problem in closing a valve. Because the MV and TV normally close in systole, these murmurs occur in systole. They are even-intensity pansystolic murmurs (schematic C) that often obliterate the S_1 and S_2 heart sounds. AV and PV regurgitant murmurs occur in diastole immediately after the S_2 heart sound (schematic D).

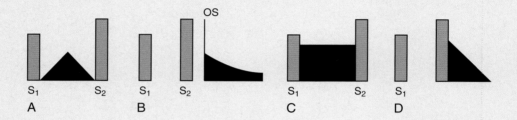

Jugular Venous Pulses (JVPs)
Normal JVPs (see schematic) have three positive waves (a, c, v) and two negative waves (x, y). The **a wave** is a positive wave due to atrial contraction in late diastole. It occurs after the P wave in an electrocardiogram. It disappears in atrial fibrillation. A **giant a wave** occurs when there is restricted filling of the right side of the heart (e.g., TV stenosis, pulmonary hypertension, right ventricular hypertrophy). The **c wave** is a positive wave due to right ventricular contraction in systole causing bulging of the TV into the right atrium producing increased pressure in the atrium and jugular vein. It correlates with the S_1 heart sound and the upstroke of the carotid pulse. The **x wave** is a large negative wave occupying most of systole. It is due to downward displacement of the TV when blood is ejected out of the RV into the pulmonary artery. The **v wave** is a positive wave that correlates with right atrial filling in systole when the TV is closed. The peak of the v wave marks the end of systole and beginning of diastole. A **giant c-v wave** occurs in TV regurgitation as blood refluxes back into the right atrium during systole. The **y wave** is a negative wave occupying most of diastole. It is due to opening of the TV with rapid flow of blood into the right ventricle in diastole.

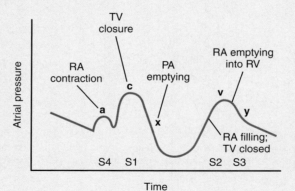

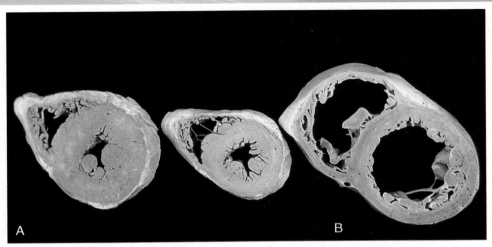

10-1: Left ventricular hypertrophy. The heart in the middle has a normal thickness of the left ventricle (LV). The heart on the left (**A**) has concentric hypertrophy of the LV, while the heart on the right (**B**) has eccentric hypertrophy of the LV. *(Reproduced with permission from Edwards WD: Cardiac anatomy and examination of cardiac specimens. In Emmanouilides GC, Riemenschneider TA, Allen HD, Gutgesell HP [eds]: Moss and Adams Heart Disease in Infants, Children, and Adolescents: Including the Fetus and Young Adults, 5th ed. Philadelphia, Williams & Wilkins, 1995, p 86.)*

    2. Types of CHF
        a. Left-sided heart failure (most common type)
        b. Right-sided heart failure
        c. Biventricular heart failure (left- and right-sided heart failure)
        d. High-output heart failure (least common type)

B. Left-sided heart failure (LHF)
    1. Forward failure
        a. Left ventricle cannot efficiently eject blood into the aorta.
        b. Causes an increase in left ventricular end-diastolic volume (LVEDV) and pressure (LVEDP).
        c. Increased volume and pressure causes backup of blood into the lungs producing pulmonary edema.
          • In LHF blood builds up behind the failed heart.

> *Left-sided heart failure = forward failure → pulmonary edema*

    2. Pathogenesis
        a. Decreased ventricular contraction (systolic dysfunction)
          (1) Most common type of LHF
          (2) Causes of systolic dysfunction
             (a) Ischemia due to coronary artery atherosclerosis (most common cause)
             (b) Post-myocardial infarction, myocardial fibrosis, myocarditis, dilated cardiomyopathy

> *Systolic dysfunction: most common type of LHF*

        b. Noncompliant ventricle (diastolic dysfunction)
          (1) Restricted filling of the left ventricle in diastole
          (2) Causes of diastolic dysfunction
             (a) Concentric LVH due to essential hypertension is the most common cause.
               • Other causes include aortic stenosis, hypertrophic cardiomyopathy.
             (b) Infiltration of muscle with amyloid, glycogen (restrictive cardiomyopathies)
             (c) Left ventricular volume overload due to aortic/mitral regurgitation
               • Ventricular distention restricts filling in diastole.

> *Diastolic dysfunction: most common cause is hypertension*

Systolic dysfunction is characterized by a low ejection fraction (EF) (<40%). The EF equals the stroke volume divided by the left ventricular end-diastolic volume. The normal value ranges from 55% to 80%. **Diastolic dysfunction** is characterized by normal to high EF (stiff ventricle) and an S_4 atrial gallop due to increased resistance to filling in late diastole. There is an increase in left atrial pressure and pulmonary congestion. If left ventricular filling is significantly impaired, cardiac output is decreased.

> *Systolic dysfunction: ↓ ventricular contraction; ↓ EF*
>
> *Diastolic dysfunction: ↑ resistance to filling the ventricle; normal EF*

    3. Gross and microscopic findings
        a. Lungs are heavy, congested, and exude a frothy pink transudate (edema).
        b. Alveolar macrophages contain hemosiderin ("heart failure" cells).

4. Clinical and laboratory findings
   a. Difficulty with breathing (dyspnea)

Dyspnea: cannot take full inspiration

   (1) Patient cannot take a full inspiration.
   (2) Caused by interstitial fluid stimulating juxtacapillary J receptors innervated by the vagus nerve
   b. Pulmonary edema

Pulmonary edema: hydrostatic pressure > oncotic pressure

   (1) Increase in LVEDV increases hydrostatic pressure in the left ventricle, left atrium, pulmonary vein, and pulmonary capillaries which overrides the pulmonary capillary oncotic pressure (refer to Chapter 4).
      (a) A transudate initially leaks into the interstitial space producing dyspnea and then moves into the alveoli producing pulmonary edema.

Kerley's lines: septal edema

      (b) Septal edema produces Kerley's lines in a chest radiograph.
      (c) Peribronchiolar edema produces expiratory wheezing (called cardiac asthma).
   (2) Bibasilar inspiratory crackles
      • Crackles are due to air expanding alveoli filled with fluid.
   (3) Rupture of pulmonary capillaries may occur from increased hydrostatic pressure.

Heart failure cells: alveolar macrophages with hemosiderin

      (a) Blood is phagocytosed by alveolar macrophages.
      (b) Hemosiderin accumulates in alveolar macrophages (called heart failure cells).
         • Sputum has a rusty color.
   (4) Chest radiograph findings in pulmonary edema
      (a) Congestion in upper lobes (early finding)
      (b) Perihilar congestion ("bat wing configuration")
      (c) Alveolar infiltrates (Fig. 10-2)

S_3 heart sound: first cardiac sign of LHF

   c. Left-sided S_3 heart sound (see Box 10-1)
   d. Functional mitral valve (MV) regurgitation
      • Caused by stretching of the MV ring
   e. Paroxysmal nocturnal dyspnea (PND)
      (1) PND refers to a choking sensation that occurs at night when the patient is supine.
      (2) Without the effect of gravity, fluid from the interstitial space moves into the vascular compartment.
      (3) This increases venous return to the right side of the heart and then to the failed left side of the heart.

PND/orthopnea: ↑ venous return to right side of the heart at night

      (4) The failed left side of the heart cannot handle the excess load and blood backs up into the lungs, producing pulmonary edema.
      (5) Dyspnea is relieved by standing or placing pillows under the head (pillow orthopnea).
         • Raising the head on pillows increases the effect of gravity on reducing venous return to the heart.

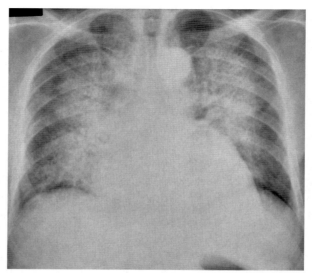

10-2: Chest frontal radiograph showing pulmonary edema. Note the fluffy alveolar infiltrates throughout both lung fields. *(From Goldman L, Ausiello D: Cecil's Textbook of Medicine, 23rd ed. Philadelphia, Saunders Elsevier, 2008, p 596, Fig. 84-2.)*

f. Increased serum brain natriuretic peptide (BNP)
   (1) Cardiac neurohormone secreted from the ventricles (refer to Chapter 4)
   (2) Secreted in response to volume expansion and pressure overload in the ventricle
   (3) Clinical usefulness
      (a) Diagnosing LHF (increased)
      (b) Excluding LHF (normal)
      (c) Predictor of survival

BNP: useful in confirming/excluding LHF

C. Right-sided heart failure (RHF)
   1. Backward failure
      a. Right side of the heart cannot pump blood from the venous system into the lungs.
      b. Blood accumulates under pressure in the venous system.
         • In RHF, blood builds up behind the failed heart.
   2. Pathogenesis
      a. Decreased contraction
         • Example—right ventricular infarction
      b. Noncompliant right ventricle
         • Example—right ventricular hypertrophy
      c. Increased afterload
         • Examples—LHF (most common cause), pulmonary hypertension
      d. Increased preload
         • Examples—tricuspid valve regurgitation, left-to-right shunt
   3. Clinical findings
      a. Prominence of the jugular veins (Fig. 10-3)
         • Due to increased venous hydrostatic pressure
      b. Functional tricuspid valve (TV) regurgitation
         • Caused by stretching of the TV ring from volume overload
      c. Right-sided S_3 and S_4 heart sounds
         • Both are due to volume overload in the ventricle.
      d. Painful hepatomegaly
         (1) Due to passive liver congestion
            • Backup of venous blood into the hepatic veins and then into the central veins (see Fig. 18-5)
         (2) Increase in portal vein pressure may lead to ascites.
         (3) Compression of the congested liver produces jugular neck vein distention (hepatojugular reflux).
      e. Dependent pitting edema (see Fig. 4-4)
         • Due to an increase in venous hydrostatic pressure
      f. Cyanosis of mucous membranes

RHF = backward failure → increase in venous hydrostatic pressure

RHF: most common cause of LHF

RHF: ↑ venous hydrostatic pressure

RHF: neck vein distention, hepatomegaly, dependent pitting edema, ascites

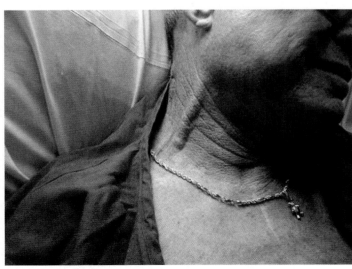

10-3: Distention of internal jugular vein: The patient has right-sided heart failure. *(From http://courses.cvcc.vccs.edu/ WisemanDIjugular_vein_distention.htm.)*

(1) More likely to occur in RHF than LHF
(2) Increased time for peripheral tissue to extract O_2; hence, decreasing O_2 saturation (refer to Chapter 1)

> **Nonpharmacologic therapy** in congestive heart failure involves restricting sodium (<2 g/day) and water (<2 L/day), both of which are increased due to the decreased cardiac output and renal retention of sodium and water (refer to Chapter 4). Systolic dysfunction is treated with drugs that reduce the workload of the left ventricle. This is accomplished by decreasing afterload and preload. A mainstay of treatment for systolic dysfunction are the angiotensin-converting enzyme (ACE) inhibitors or receptor inhibitors if patients develop chronic cough. ACE inhibitors decrease afterload by decreasing angiotensin II and decrease preload by decreasing aldosterone. Diuretics (e.g., loop diuretics, aldosterone blockers) complement ACE inhibitors by decreasing preload. β-Blockers decrease sympathetic tone, which reduces myocardial O_2 consumption. Digitalis may be useful because of its inotropic and vagotonic effects particularly in severe heart failure or those with atrial arrhythmias. Direct vasodilating drugs (e.g., hydralazine) reduce systemic vascular resistance and pulmonary venous pressure. Therapeutic options for treating diastolic dysfunction are based on the cause of diastolic dysfunction. If hypertension is the primary cause, calcium channel blockers, ACE inhibitors, and β-blockers are used, the latter decreasing heart rate, which prolongs diastolic filling. Diuretics must be used with caution, because excessive diuresis may produce volume depletion and decrease the cardiac output.

ACE inhibitors: ↓ afterload, ↓ preload

β-Blockers: ↓ myocardial O_2 consumption; ↓ heart rate

D. High-output heart failure
1. Definition
   - Form of heart failure in which cardiac output is increased compared with values for the normal resting state
2. Pathogenesis
   a. Increase in stroke volume (SV)
      - Example—hyperthyroidism
   b. Decrease in blood viscosity
      (1) Decreases total peripheral resistance (TPR)
      (2) Increases venous return to the heart.
      (3) Example—severe anemia
   c. Vasodilation of peripheral resistance arterioles
      (1) Increases venous return to the heart
      (2) Examples—thiamine deficiency (refer to Chapter 7), early phase of endotoxic shock (refer to Chapter 4)
   d. Arteriovenous fistula
      (1) Arteriovenous communications bypass the microcirculation.
      (2) Increases venous return to the heart
      (3) Causes of arteriovenous fistulas
         (a) Trauma from a knife wound (most common cause)
         (b) Surgical shunt for hemodialysis
         (c) Mosaic bone in Paget's disease (refer to Chapter 23)

High output failure: ↑ SV, ↓ TPR, arteriovenous fistula

IV. Ischemic Heart Disease
- Imbalance between myocardial O_2 demand and supply from the coronary arteries
A. Coronary artery blood flow
1. Provides oxygen to cardiac muscle
   a. Coronary vessels fill in diastole.
   b. Tachycardia (>180 bpm) decreases filling time, leading to ischemia.
2. Left anterior descending (LAD) coronary artery
   a. Distribution
      (1) Anterior portion of the left ventricle
      (2) Anterior two thirds of the interventricular septum
   b. Site for 40% to 50% of coronary artery thromboses
3. Right coronary artery (RCA)
   a. Distribution
      (1) Posteroinferior part of the left ventricle
      (2) Posterior one third of the interventricular septum
      (3) Right ventricle
      (4) Posteromedial papillary muscle in left ventricle
      (5) Primary supply for atrioventricular and sinoatrial nodes
   b. Site for 30% to 40% of coronary artery thromboses

Tachycardia: decreases diastole and filling of coronary arteries

LAD: most common site of coronary artery thrombosis

4. Left circumflex coronary artery
    a. Supplies the lateral wall of the left ventricle
    b. Site for 15% to 20% of coronary artery thromboses

B. Epidemiology
1. Ischemic heart disease is the major cause of death in the United States.
    a. It is more common in men.
    b. Incidence peaks in men after age 60 and in women after age 70.
2. Types of ischemic heart disease
    a. Angina pectoris (most common type)
    b. Chronic ischemic heart disease
    c. Sudden cardiac death
    d. Myocardial infarction
3. Risk factors
    a. Age
       • Men ≥ 45 years old, women ≥ 55 years old
    b. Family history of premature coronary artery disease or stroke
    c. Lipid abnormalities
       (1) Low-density lipoprotein > 160 mg/dL
       (2) High-density lipoprotein (HDL) < 40 mg/dL
    d. Smoking tobacco, hypertension, diabetes mellitus
    e. Subtract 1 from the total number of risk factors if HDL > 60 mg/dL.

C. Angina pectoris
1. Epidemiology
    a. Most common in middle-aged males and elderly males
    b. Females usually affected after menopause
    c. Within 1 year of a diagnosis of stable angina, 10% to 20% will develop an acute myocardial infarction or unstable angina.
2. Chronic (stable) angina
    a. Most common variant
    b. Causes of stable angina
       (1) Fixed, atherosclerotic coronary artery disease (most common)
          (a) One or more vessel obstructions is likely.
          (b) Severity of stenosis is usually >70%.
       (2) Aortic stenosis or hypertension with concentric LVH
          • O_2 supply is *not* adequate for the thickened muscle wall.
       (3) Hypertrophic cardiomyopathy
       (4) Cocaine-induced coronary artery vasoconstriction
    c. Pathogenesis
       • Subendocardial ischemia due to decreased coronary artery blood flow or thick muscle wall
    d. Clinical findings
       (1) Exercise-induced substernal chest pain lasting 30 seconds to 30 minutes
       (2) Often accompanied by shortness of breath, diaphoresis, numbness and pain in left arm, shoulder, or jaw
       (3) Relieved by resting or nitroglycerin
       (4) Stress test shows ST-segment depression > 1 mm (Fig. 10-4).

Margin notes:
Angina pectoris: most common manifestation of coronary artery disease

Angina pectoris: age most important risk factor

Angina pectoris: males > females

Stable angina: most common type of angina

Stable angina: exercise-induced substernal chest pain

Stable angina: subendocardial ischemia with ST-segment depression

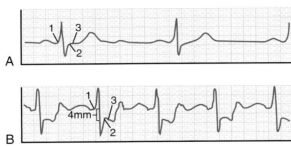

10-4: Electrocardiogram with ST segment depression. Tracing A is the patient at rest with 1 representing the PQ junction (baseline reference); 2, the J point, where the QRS complex joins the ST segment; and 3, the ST segment 80 msec from the PQ point. Tracing B shows the amount of ST segment depression measured 80 msec past the J point is 4 mm. *(From Goldman L, Ausiello D: Cecil's Textbook of Medicine, 23rd ed. Philadelphia, Saunders Elsevier, 2008, p 481, Fig. 70-2.)*

3. Prinzmetal's angina
   a. Pathogenesis
      (1) Intermittent coronary artery vasospasm at rest with or without superimposed coronary artery atherosclerotic disease
      (2) Vasoconstriction is due to platelet thromboxane A_2 or an increase in endothelin.
   b. Clinical findings
      • Stress test shows ST-segment elevation (transmural ischemia).
4. Unstable angina
   a. Pathogenesis
      (1) Severe, fixed, multivessel atherosclerotic disease
      (2) Disrupted plaques with or without platelet nonocclusive thrombi (refer to Chapters 4 and 9)
   b. Clinical findings
      (1) Frequent bouts of chest pain at rest or with minimal exertion
      (2) May progress to acute myocardial infarction (MI)

Nonpharmacologic therapy of angina includes losing weight, cessation of smoking, placing the patient on a low cholesterol diet, and encouraging daily aerobic exercise. **Pharmacologic therapy** for angina involves the use of anti-ischemic agents. Nitrates (release nitric oxide) cause venodilation (reduces preload and wall tension in the ventricles), vasodilation of the coronary arteries, and vasodilation of peripheral resistance arterioles (reduces afterload). β-Blockers decrease myocardial O_2 consumption by reducing heart rate and systolic blood pressure. Calcium channel blockers cause vasodilation of the coronary arteries and peripheral resistance arteries. They are the drug of choice for treating Prinzmetal's angina. Aspirin inhibits platelet aggregation, which decreases the risk for developing a platelet thrombus (refer to Chapters 4 and 14). Heparin plus aspirin is used for patients with unstable angina and reduces the risk for developing a myocardial infarction and refractory angina. If homocysteine levels are increased, the patient should be placed on pharmacologic doses of folate. If C-reactive protein is increased, the patient should be placed on "statin" drugs to lower the LDL levels to 70 mg/dL or less. This stabilizes disrupted plaques and reduces the risk for thrombosis. Revascularization procedures include percutaneous transluminal coronary angioplasty (PTCA) and stenting. Balloon angioplasty dilates and ruptures the atheromatous plaque to improve blood flow (restenosis commonly occurs) and intracoronary stents (the most common procedure) bypass the obstruction (restenosis less common). Complications are associated with either procedure (e.g., thrombosis, localized dissection). In order to prevent platelet thrombosis in these revascularization procedures, abciximab (inhibits the GpIIb-IIIa fibrinogen receptor in platelets; refer to Chapter 14) is used. Coronary artery bypass graft (CABG) is reserved for patients with left main coronary artery disease and for those patients with symptomatic three-vessel disease. Internal mammary artery grafts have the best graft patency after 10 years, while saphenous vein grafts commonly show "arterialization" of the vessels with fibrosis after 10 years.

D. Chronic ischemic heart disease
   1. Progressive CHF resulting from long-term ischemic damage to myocardial tissue
   2. Replacement of myocardial tissue with noncontractile scar tissue
   3. Clinical findings
      a. Biventricular CHF
      b. Angina pectoris
      c. May develop dilated cardiomyopathy
E. Sudden cardiac death (SCD)
   1. Unexpected death within 1 hour after the onset of symptoms
   2. Risk factors
      a. Obesity
      b. Glucose intolerance
      c. Hypertension
      d. Recent non–Q wave myocardial infarction
      e. Smoking
   3. Occurs more frequently in the morning hours when hypercoagulability is at its peak
   4. Pathogenesis
      a. Severe atherosclerotic coronary artery disease
      b. Disrupted fibrous plaques
      c. Absence of occlusive vessel thrombus (>80% of cases)
      d. Cause of death is ventricular fibrillation.

Prinzmetal's angina: vasospasm with transmural ischemia and ST-segment elevation

Unstable angina: angina at rest; multivessel disease; disrupted plaques

Prinzmetal's angina: calcium channel blockers vasodilate coronary arteries

Chronic ischemic heart disease: replacement of muscle by fibrous tissue

Sudden cardiac death: unexpected death within 1 hour after symptoms

Sudden cardiac death: coronary artery thrombosis *not* usually present

5. Diagnosis of exclusion after the following causes are ruled out
   a. Mitral valve prolapse (MVP)
   b. Hypertrophic cardiomyopathy
   c. Calcific aortic stenosis
   d. Conduction system abnormalities
   e. Cocaine abuse

F. Acute myocardial infarction (AMI)
   1. Epidemiology
      a. Most common cause of death in adults in the United States.
      b. Prominent in males between 40 and 65 years old
      c. No predominant sex predilection after 65 years old
      d. At least 25% of AMIs are clinically unrecognized.
   2. Pathogenesis
      a. Sequence
         (1) Sudden disruption of an atheromatous plaque (see Fig. 4-13)
         (2) Subendothelial collagen and thrombogenic necrotic material are exposed.
         (3) Platelets adhere to the exposed material and eventually form an occlusive platelet thrombus.
      b. Role of thromboxane A_2 (refer to Chapter 14)
         (1) Contributes to formation of the platelet thrombus
         (2) Causes vasospasm of the artery to reduce blood flow
   3. Less common causes of AMI
      a. Vasculitis (e.g., polyarteritis nodosa, Kawasaki disease)
      b. Cocaine use
         • AMI with normal coronary arteries
      c. Embolization of plaque material
         • From atheromatous plaques in the aorta or coronary artery
      d. Thrombosis syndromes
         • Examples—antithrombin III deficiency, polycythemia
      e. Dissection into the wall of coronary arteries
         • Examples—revascularization procedure, aortic dissection
   4. Types of myocardial infarction
      a. Transmural infarction (Q wave infarction)
         (1) Involves the full thickness of the myocardium
         (2) New Q waves develop in an electrocardiogram (ECG).
      b. Subendocardial infarction (non–Q wave infarction)
         (1) Involves the inner third of the myocardium
         (2) Q waves are absent.
   5. Reperfusion injury
      a. Follows thrombolytic (fibrinolytic) therapy
      b. Early reperfusion salvages some injured but viable myocytes but destroys myocytes that are irreversibly damaged.
         (1) Removal of irreversibly damaged myocytes improves short- and long-term function and survival.
         (2) Prevents any further damage to myocardial cells
         (3) Limits the size of the infarction
      c. Reperfusion histologically alters irreversibly damaged cells.
         (1) Produces contraction band necrosis
         (2) Caused by hypercontraction of myofibrils in dying cells
            • Due to the influx of Ca^{2+} into the cytosol
   6. Gross and microscopic findings of AMI
      a. During 0 to 24 hours
         (1) No gross changes are evident until 24 hours.
         (2) Coagulation necrosis is present within 12 to 24 hours.
         (3) Neutrophils begin to enter the area of infarction from the periphery.
      b. During 1 to 3 days
         (1) Pallor of the infarcted tissue
         (2) Myocyte nuclei and striations disappear (see Fig. 1-11A).
         (3) Neutrophils are abundant and lyse dead myocardial cells.
      c. During 3 to 7 days
         (1) Red granulation tissue surrounds the area of infarction.
         (2) Macrophages begin to remove necrotic debris.

MVP sudden death: arrhythmias from mitral regurgitation or CHF

AMI: most common cause of death in United States

Rupture of disrupted plaque → platelet thrombus → AMI

Cocaine: AMI with normal coronary arteries

AMI: Q wave type transmural, non–Q wave type subendocardial

Reperfusion: ↑ short/long-term survival

Contraction band necrosis: reperfusion; hypercontraction myofibrils due to Ca^{2+}

AMI: coagulation necrosis within 24 hours

AMI: heart softest 3–7 days; danger of rupture

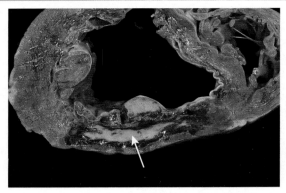

10-5: Acute myocardial infarction (day 7) in the posterior wall of the left ventricle. The yellow area (*arrow*) is surrounded by a rim of dark, red granulation tissue. *(From Damjanov I, Linder J: Pathology: A Color Atlas. St. Louis, Mosby, 2000, p 22, Fig. 1-47.)*

<table>
<tr><td>

AMI: retrosternal pain, radiation to left arm/ shoulder, diaphoresis

</td><td>

   d. During 7 to 10 days
      (1) The necrotic area is bright yellow (Fig. 10-5; see also Fig. 1-11B).
      (2) Granulation tissue and collagen formation are well developed.
   e. During 2 months
      • Infarcted tissue replaced by white, patchy, noncontractile scar tissue
  7. Clinical findings
   a. Sudden onset of severe, crushing retrosternal pain
      (1) Lasts >30 minutes
      (2) *Not* relieved by nitroglycerin
      (3) Usually radiates down the left arm into the shoulders or into the jaw or epigastrium
      (4) Associated with sweating (diaphoresis), anxiety, and hypotension

</td></tr>
</table>

d. During 7 to 10 days
   (1) The necrotic area is bright yellow (Fig. 10-5; see also Fig. 1-11B).
   (2) Granulation tissue and collagen formation are well developed.
e. During 2 months
   • Infarcted tissue replaced by white, patchy, noncontractile scar tissue
7. Clinical findings
  a. Sudden onset of severe, crushing retrosternal pain
   (1) Lasts >30 minutes
   (2) *Not* relieved by nitroglycerin
   (3) Usually radiates down the left arm into the shoulders or into the jaw or epigastrium
   (4) Associated with sweating (diaphoresis), anxiety, and hypotension
  b. "Silent" AMIs in ~20% of cases
   (1) May occur in the elderly and in individuals with diabetes mellitus
   (2) Due to high pain threshold or problems with nervous system

Q wave AMI: ↑ early mortality rate

  c. Q wave AMI has increased early mortality rate compared to non–Q wave AMI.
  d. Non–Q wave AMI

Non–Q wave AMI: ↑ risk for SCD

   (1) Increased risk of reinfarction
   (2) Increased risk for sudden cardiac death post-MI
8. Complications
  a. Cardiogenic shock occurs in ~7% of cases.
   • Revascularization improves survival.
  b. Arrhythmias
   (1) Ventricular premature contractions (most common)

Ventricular fibrillation: most common cause of death in acute MI

   (2) Most common cause of death is ventricular fibrillation.
     • Frequently associated with cardiogenic shock
   (3) Heart block
     (a) Occurs in 5% of inferior AMIs
     (b) Occurs in 3% of anterior AMIs
  c. Congestive heart failure
   • Usually occurs within the first 24 hours
  d. Rupture

Myocardial rupture: most common at 3–7 days

   (1) Most commonly occurs between days 3 and 7 (range, 1–10 days)
   (2) Anterior wall rupture (Fig. 10-6)
     (a) Causes cardiac tamponade
     (b) Associated with thrombosis of the LAD coronary artery

Posteromedial papillary muscle rupture: RCA thrombosis; mitral regurgitation

   (3) Posteromedial papillary muscle rupture or dysfunction
     (a) Most often associated with RCA thrombosis
       • Most often with inferior AMIs
     (b) Acute onset of mitral valve regurgitation and LHF
   (4) Interventricular septum rupture
     (a) Most often associated with LAD coronary artery thrombosis
     (b) Produces a left-to-right shunt causing RHF
       • Increased O_2 saturation and pressure in right ventricle

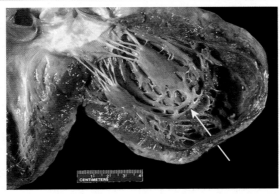

10-6: Acute myocardial infarction with rupture of the free wall of the left ventricle *(arrow)*. This rupture is unusual in that it occurred 3 weeks after an acute myocardial infarction. *(From Klatt E: Robbins and Cotran's Atlas of Pathology. Philadelphia, WB Saunders, 2006, p 35, Fig. 2-30.)*

e. Mural thrombus
  (1) Occurs in ~10% of AMIs
  (2) Most often associated with LAD coronary artery thrombosis
  (3) Danger of embolization
f. Fibrinous pericarditis with or without effusion (see Fig. 2-7)
  (1) Days 1 to 7 of a Q wave AMI
    (a) Substernal chest pain is relieved by leaning forward and aggravated by leaning backward.
    (b) A precordial friction rub is present (see later).
      • Due to increased vessel permeability in the pericardium; exudate of acute inflammation
  (2) Autoimmune pericarditis
    (a) Develops 6 to 8 weeks after an acute MI
    (b) Autoantibodies are directed against damaged pericardial antigens.
    (c) Fever and a precordial friction rub are present.
g. Ventricular aneurysm (Fig. 10-7)
  (1) Clinically recognized within 4 to 8 weeks
    • Begins developing in the first 48 hours.

Mural thrombus: danger of embolization

Fibrinous pericarditis: early (acute inflammation) and late complication (autoimmune)

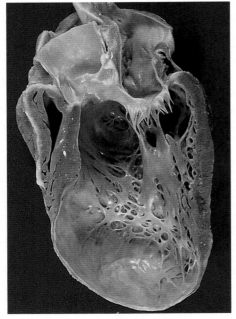

10-7: Left ventricular aneurysm. The bulging aneurysm has a thin wall of scar tissue. *(From Damjanov I, Linder J: Pathology: A Color Atlas. St. Louis, Mosby, 2000, p 24, Fig. 1-58.)*

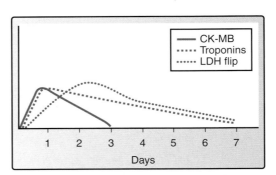

10-8: Cardiac enzymes used in the diagnosis of an acute myocardial infarction. CK-MB, creatine kinase MB; LDH, lactate dehydrogenase. See text for discussion.

(2) Precordial bulge occurs during systole.
- Blood enters the aneurysm causing anterior chest wall movement.

(3) Complications
(a) CHF occurs due to the lack of contractile tissue.
(b) Danger of embolization of clot material
(c) Rupture is uncommon.
- Scar tissue has good tensile strength.

h. Right ventricular AMI
(1) Associated with RCA thrombosis
(2) Occurs in one third of inferior AMIs
- Clinically significant in 30% of cases
(3) Clinical findings
- Hypotension, RHF, and preserved left ventricle function

9. Laboratory diagnosis of AMI (Fig. 10-8)
a. Serial testing for creatine kinase isoenzyme MB (CK-MB)
(1) CK-MB appears within 4 to 8 hours; peaks at 24 hours; disappears within 1.5 to 3 days.
- Sensitivity and specificity 95%.
(2) Reinfarction
(a) Occurs in 10% of AMIs
(b) Reappearance of CK-MB after 3 days

b. Serial testing for cardiac troponins I (cTnI) and T (cTnT)
(1) Normally regulate calcium-mediated contraction
(2) cTnI and cTnT appear within 3 to 12 hours; peak at 24 hours; disappear within 7 to 10 days.
(a) Sensitivity 84% to 96%, specificity 80% to 95%
(b) False positive results are usually related to ischemia (e.g., unstable angina).
(3) CK-MB is used in conjunction with troponins to diagnose an AMI.
(a) Detects reinfarction (troponins cannot)
(b) Improves overall sensitivity and specificity in diagnosing an AMI

c. Lactate dehydrogenase $(LDH)_{1-2}$ "flip"
(1) Normally, LDH_2 is higher than LDH_1.
- In AMI, LDH_1 in cardiac muscle is released, causing the "flip."
(2) LDH_{1-2}
- Appears within 10 hours; peaks at 2 to 3 days; disappears within 7 days
(3) This test has been replaced by troponins I and T.

10. Correlation of ECG changes with microscopic changes (Fig. 10-9)
a. Inverted T waves
- Correlate with areas of ischemia at the periphery of the infarct
b. Elevated ST segment
- Correlates with injured myocardial cells surrounding the area of necrosis
c. New Q waves
- Correlate with the area of coagulation necrosis

11. Classic ECG patterns in AMI
a. LAD coronary artery anterior wall infarction
- Q waves in leads V_1–V_4
b. Anteroseptal infarction due to proximal LAD occlusion
- Q waves in leads V_1–V_2

Margin notes:

Ventricular aneurysm: CHF most common cause of death

RV AMI: hypotension, RHF, preserved LV function

Reinfarction: reappearance of CK-MB after 3 days

cTnI, cTnT: cannot diagnose reinfarction

cTnI, cTnT: gold standard for diagnosis of AMI

ECG findings in AMI: inverted T waves, elevated ST segment, Q waves

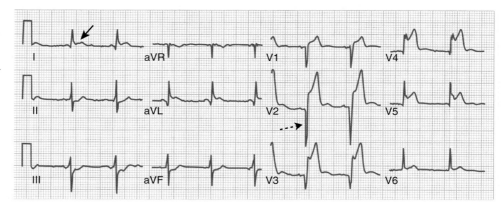

10-9: Electrocardiogram showing an acute anterior myocardial infarction. There is ST segment elevation in lead 1 (*solid arrow*), aVL, and V_1 to V_6 and Q waves (*interrupted arrow*) in leads V_1 to V_4. *(From Goldman L, Ausiello D: Cecil's Textbook of Medicine, 23rd ed. Philadelphia, Saunders Elsevier, 2008, p 502, Fig. 72-1.)*

   c. Anterolateral infarction due to mid-LAD or circumflex coronary arteries
- Q waves in leads V_4–V_6, I, aVL

   d. Lateral wall infarction due to left circumflex artery
- Q waves in leads I, aVL

   e. RCA inferior wall infarction
- Q waves in leads II, III, aVF

   f. Posterior wall infarction due to posterior descending artery occlusion
    (1) Q wave in lead V_6
    (2) R wave > S wave in lead V_1

Nonpharmacologic therapy of an acute MI includes limiting patient activity, cessation of smoking, low salt diet, and placing the patient on a low cholesterol diet. **Pharmacologic therapy** includes anti-platelet therapy (aspirin, clopidogrel if allergic to aspirin); nitrates (reduce coronary artery spasm; venodilation decreases ventricular preload, hence reducing myocardial O_2 consumption); pain medication (morphine); nasal O_2 (2–4 liters/minute); β-blockers (decrease sympathetic tone, hence decreasing myocardial O_2 consumption; also prevent tachyarrhythmias); ACE inhibitors (reduce left ventricular dysfunction and dilation, hence slowing the progression of congestive heart failure); warfarin (often used along with aspirin); and myocardial reperfusion, which markedly improves survival. Reperfusion can be accomplished using fibrinolytic therapy (if duration of pain is <6 hours); percutaneous coronary intervention; or CABG. It is important to measure the ejection fraction prior to discharge to evaluate the severity of damage and to provide an index of prognosis.

V. Congenital Heart Disease (CHD)
   A. Fetal circulation (Fig. 10-10)
    1. Chorionic villus in the placenta (refer to Chapter 21)
     a. Derived from the fetus
     b. Primary site for O_2 exchange
     c. Chorionic villus vessels become the umbilical vein.

> Chorionic villus: primary site for O_2 exchange

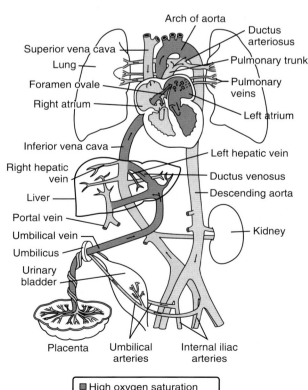

10-10: Fetal circulation. See text for discussion. (*From Moore NA, Roy WA: Rapid Review Gross and Developmental Anatomy, 2nd ed. St. Louis, Mosby Elsevier, 2007, p 56, Fig. 2-23.*)

2. Umbilical vein
  • Vessel with the highest Po$_2$ in the fetal circulation
3. Inferior vena cava blood drains into the right atrium.
  • Most blood is directly shunted into the left atrium through the foramen ovale.
4. Superior vena cava blood
  • Most blood is directed from the right atrium into the right ventricle.
5. Pulmonary artery blood
  a. Blood is shunted through a patent ductus arteriosus into the aorta.
    • Ductus arteriosus is kept open by prostaglandin E$_2$, a vasodilator synthesized by the placenta.

  b. Fetal pulmonary arteries
    (1) Hypertrophied from chronic vasoconstriction due to decreased Po$_2$
    (2) Prevents blood from entering the pulmonary capillaries and left atrium
6. Descending aorta
  a. Blood flows toward the placenta via two umbilical arteries.
    • Increased risk for congenital abnormalities with single umbilical artery

  b. Umbilical arteries have the lowest O$_2$ concentration.
7. Changes at birth

  a. Ductus arteriosus (DA) closes
    (1) Anatomic closure within 2 to 8 weeks in most cases
    (2) Becomes the ligamentum arteriosum
  b. Gas exchange occurs in the lungs.
    • Pulmonary artery opens up due to the increase in Pao$_2$.

  c. Foramen ovale functionally closes in 24 hours.
B. Features of congenital heart disease
  1. Epidemiology
    a. Most common heart disease in children
    b. Incidence is higher in premature than full-term newborns.
    c. No identifiable cause for CHD in ~90% of cases.

    d. Risk factors for CHD
      (1) Previous child with CHD (1:50 chance second child with CHD)
      (2) Down syndrome and other trisomy syndromes (refer to Chapter 5)
      (3) Maternal risk factors
        (a) Increased age
        (b) Poorly controlled diabetes mellitus
        (c) Alcohol intake
        (d) Congenital infection (e.g., rubella; refer to Chapter 5)
    e. Spectrum of CHD
      (1) Valvular diseases (e.g., pulmonary stenosis)
      (2) Shunts (noncyanotic and cyanotic)
    f. Systemic complications
      (1) Secondary polycythemia with clubbing of the fingers in cyanotic CHD
        • Decreased Pao$_2$ stimulates the release of erythropoietin.
      (2) Increased risk for developing infective endocarditis
      (3) Metastatic abscesses (particularly in cyanotic CHD)

  2. O$_2$ saturation (Sao$_2$) in shunts
    a. Left-sided to right-sided heart shunts
      • There is an increased Sao$_2$ (step up) from 75% to ~80% in affected chambers and vessels.
    b. Right-sided to left-sided heart shunts
      (1) Decreased Sao$_2$ (step down) from 95% to ~80% in affected chambers and vessels
      (2) Cyanosis depends on how low Sao$_2$ percentage is in the left side of the heart.
  3. Left-sided to right-sided heart shunts

    a. Volume overload occurs in the right side of the heart; may have several complications:
      (1) Pulmonary hypertension (PH)
      (2) RVH due to PH
        • PH increases afterload the right ventricle must contract against to eject blood.
      (3) LVH due to excess blood originating from the right side of the heart
        • Eccentric hypertrophy due to volume overload (see section II)
      (4) Reversal of the shunt

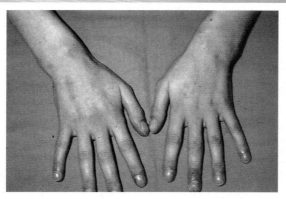

10-11: Cyanotic congenital heart disease. This patient with a ventricular septal defect that eventually showed reversed shunting (Eisenmenger syndrome) has cyanosis and clubbing of the nails. *(From Grieg JD: Color Atlas of Surgical Diagnosis. London, Mosby-Wolfe, 1996, p 93, Fig. 14-1.)*

        (a) Occurs when pressure in the right ventricle overrides the left ventricular pressure
        (b) Cyanosis (Eisenmenger syndrome) and clubbing develop (Fig. 10-11).
           • Another term is cyanosis tardive (late-onset cyanosis).
  b. Ventricular septal defect (VSD; Fig. 10-12A)
    (1) Most common CHD (20% of cases)
    (2) Defect in the membranous interventricular septum
    (3) Harsh pansystolic murmur at lower left sternal border
    (4) Associations
        (a) Corrected transposition
        (b) Tetralogy of Fallot
        (c) Cri du chat syndrome (refer to Chapter 5)
        (d) Fetal alcohol syndrome (refer to Chapter 5)
    (5) Increased Sao_2 in right ventricle and pulmonary artery
    (6) Spontaneously close in 30% to 50% of cases
    (7) Lifetime risk for infective endocarditis ranges from 5% to 30%.
  c. Atrial septal defect (ASD; Fig. 10-12B)
    (1) Patent foramen ovale (secundum type; most common type)
        (a) Accounts for 10% to 15% of all CHD
        (b) Most common adult CHD
    (2) Associations
        (a) Fetal alcohol syndrome
        (b) Down syndrome (primum type in 25%)
        (c) Paradoxic embolism (refer to Chapter 4)
    (3) Mild systolic murmur at upper sternal border in secundum type
    (4) Fixed splitting of S_2
        • Excess blood in right atrium causes delay in closure of pulmonary valve.
    (5) Increased Sao_2 in right atrium, right ventricle and pulmonary artery
  d. Patent ductus arteriosus (PDA; Fig. 10-12C)
    (1) Accounts for 10% of all CHD
    (2) Ductus arteriosus remains open.
        • Isolated defect in 75% of cases
    (3) Associations
        (a) Congenital rubella
        (b) Respiratory distress syndrome
           • Due to decreased Pao_2
        (c) Complete transposition
    (4) Increased Sao_2 in the pulmonary artery
    (5) Reversal of the shunt due to pulmonary hypertension
        (a) Unoxygenated blood enters the aorta *below* the subclavian artery
        (b) Produces a pink upper body and cyanotic lower body
           • Called differential cyanosis
    (6) Machinery murmur is heard during systole and diastole.

Margin notes:

VSD: most common congenital heart disease in children

VSD: defect in membranous septum

ASD: most common CHD in adults

ASD: patent foramen ovale

ASD: fixed splitting of S_2; most common adult CHD

PDA: closed with indomethacin; machinery murmur

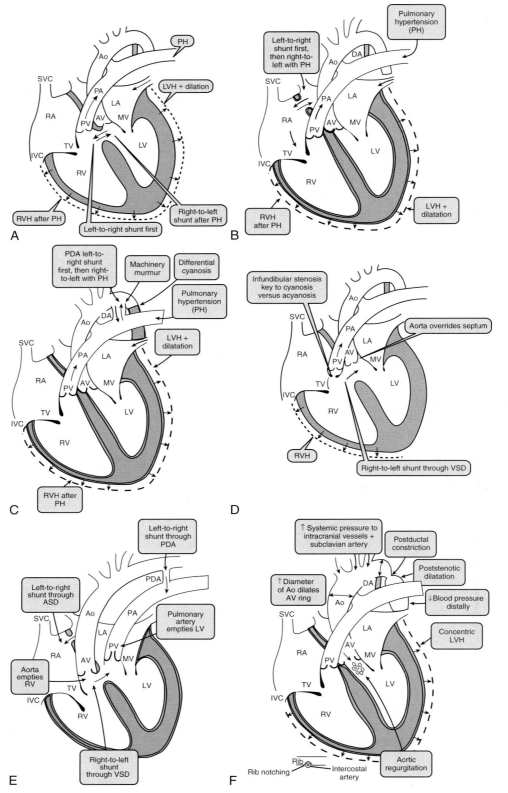

10-12: A, Ventricular septal defect (VSD). Refer to the text for discussion. **B,** Atrial septal defect (ASD). See text for discussion. **C,** Patent ductus arteriosus (PDA). See text for discussion. **D,** Tetralogy of Fallot. Refer to the text for discussion. **E,** Complete transposition of the great vessels. See text for discussion. **F,** Postductal coarctation. See text for discussion. Ao, aorta; AV, aortic valve; DA, ductus arteriosus; IVC, inferior vena cava; LA, left atrium; LV, left ventricle; LVH, left ventricular hypertrophy; MV, mitral valve; PA, pulmonary artery; PH, pulmonary hypertension; PV, pulmonary valve; RA, right atrium; RV, right ventricle; RVH, right ventricular hypertrophy; SVC, superior vena cava; TV, tricuspid valve. (**B, C, E,** and **F** from Goljan EF: *Star Series: Pathology.* Philadelphia, WB Saunders, 1998.)

(7) Treatment
    (a) Intravenous indomethacin inhibits prostaglandin E_2 (vasodilator)
    (b) Surgical closure (e.g., banding)
4. Right-sided to left-sided heart shunts
  a. Cyanotic CHD
  b. Complications (see above)
  c. Tetralogy of Fallot
    (1) Most common cyanotic CHD (Fig. 10-12D)
      (a) Accounts for 10% of all cases of CHD
      (b) Accounts for 50% to 70% of cyanotic CHD
      (c) Accounts for 85% of adults with cyanotic CHD
    (2) Defects
      (a) Ventricular septal defect
      (b) Infundibular or valvular pulmonary stenosis
      (c) Right ventricular hypertrophy
      (d) Dextrorotated aorta with right-sided aortic arch (25% of cases)
    (3) Onset of cyanosis usually after 3 months of age
    (4) Systolic murmur is heard along the left sternal border.
    (5) Minimal pulmonary valve (PV) stenosis
      (a) Leads to increased oxygenation of blood in the lungs
      (b) Less right-to-left shunting through the VSD
      (c) Absence of cyanosis ($Sao_2 > 80\%$)
    (6) Severe PV stenosis
      (a) Less oxygenation of blood in the lungs
      (b) Increased right-to-left shunting through the VSD
      (c) Cyanosis ($Sao_2 < 80\%$)
    (7) Decreased Sao_2 in the left ventricle and aorta
    (8) Cardioprotective shunts increase oxygenation.
      (a) ASD steps up Sao_2 in the right atrium.
      (b) PDA shunts blood from the aorta to the pulmonary artery.
    (9) Tet spells (hypoxic spells)
      (a) Caused by a sudden increase in hypoxemia and cyanosis
      (b) Squatting increases systemic vascular resistance, causing temporary reversal of the shunt.
      (c) Unoxygenated blood is forced back into the pulmonary artery for oxygenation.
  d. Complete transposition of the great vessels (Fig. 10-12E)
    (1) Defects
      (a) Aorta arises from the right ventricle.
      (b) Pulmonary artery arises from the left ventricle.
      (c) Left and right atria are normal.
    (2) Cardioprotective shunts
      (a) ASD steps up Sao_2 in the right atrium.
        • Increases Sao_2 in the right ventricle for delivery to tissue via the aorta
      (b) VSD shunts blood into the left ventricle for oxygenation in the lungs via the pulmonary artery.
      (c) PDA shunts blood into the pulmonary artery for oxygenation in the lungs.
  e. Other types of cyanotic CHD
    (1) Total anomalous pulmonary venous return
      • Pulmonary vein empties oxygenated blood into the right atrium.
    (2) Truncus arteriosus
      • Aorta and pulmonary artery share a common trunk and intermix blood.
    (3) Tricuspid atresia
      • Usually have an ASD with a right-to-left shunt

C. Coarctation of the aorta (Fig. 10-12F)
1. Accounts for 10% of all CHD
2. Infantile (preductal) coarctation
  a. Accounts for 70% of coarctations
  b. Constriction of aorta between the subclavian artery and ductus arteriosus
  c. Associated with Turner's syndrome
3. Adult coarctation
  a. Accounts for 30% of coarctations
  b. Develops during adult life

Margin notes:

Tetralogy of Fallot: most common cyanotic CHD

Tetralogy of Fallot: degree of PV stenosis correlates with presence or absence of cyanosis

Cardioprotective shunts: ASD, PDA

Tet spells: squatting ↑ systemic vascular resistance; ↑ Pao_2

Transposition: aorta empties RV, pulmonary artery empties LV, atria normal

Infantile coarctation: associated with Turner's syndrome

c. Constriction of the aorta distal to the ligamentum arteriosum
   (1) Blood flow into the proximally located branch vessels is increased.
   (2) Blood flow below the constriction is decreased.
   (3) Produces a systolic murmur
   (4) Additional defect is a bicuspid aortic valve (50% of cases)

Adult coarctation: disparity between upper/lower extremity blood pressure > 10 mm Hg

d. Clinical findings proximal to the constriction
   (1) Increased upper extremity blood pressure
   (2) Dilation of aorta and aortic valve ring (regurgitation)
      • Increased risk for developing an aortic dissection
   (3) Increased cerebral blood flow (increased risk for berry aneurysms)

e. Clinical findings distal to the constriction
   (1) Decreased blood pressure in the lower extremity
   (2) Leg claudication (pain in calf or buttocks when walking)
   (3) Decreased renal blood flow

Hypertension: due to activation RAA system

      • Activates the renin-angiotensin-aldosterone (RAA) system, causing hypertension

f. Development of collateral circulation
   (1) Collaterals develop between intercostal arteries above and below the constriction.
      (a) Anterior intercostal arteries (AIAs) arise from internal thoracic artery.
      (b) Posterior intercostal arteries (PIAs) arise from aorta.
      (c) Increased pressure in the aorta extends into the subclavian artery → into the internal thoracic artery → into the AIAs, which stimulates the formation of a collateral circulation with the PIAs causing reversal of the blood flow into the aorta.

Coarctation collaterals: AIA-PIA to aorta; SEA-IEA to external iliac artery

   (2) Collateral circulation between the superior epigastric artery (SEA) and the inferior epigastric artery (IEA)
      (a) Internal thoracic artery becomes the SEA.
      (b) SEA forms collaterals with the IEA (branch of the external iliac artery).
      (c) Reversal of flood flow in the IEA forces blood into the external iliac artery.
   (3) Chest radiograph shows rib notching on the undersurface of the ribs.
      • Increased blood flow through enlarged, pulsating intercostal arteries wears the bone away.

g. Surgical removal of a coarctation corrects the hypertension.

VI. Acquired Valvular Heart Disease
  A. Rheumatic fever (RF)
    1. Epidemiology
      a. Occurs at 5 to 15 years of age

Acute RF: after group A streptococcal pharyngitis

      b. Develops over 1 to 5 weeks (average 20 days) after group A streptococcal (*Streptococcus pyogenes*) pharyngitis
        • Only site for infection leading to RF
      c. Risk factors for streptococcal pharyngitis
        (1) Crowding
        (2) Poverty
        (3) Young age
      d. Recurrent RF produces chronic valvular disease.
    2. Pathogenesis
      a. Immune-mediated disease that follows group A streptococcal infection
      b. Antibodies develop against group A streptococcal M proteins.

Acute RF: immune-mediated type II hypersensitivity reaction; cell-mediated immunity type IV

        (1) Antibodies cross-react with similar proteins in human tissue (called mimicry).
          • Type II hypersensitivity reaction
        (2) Cell-mediated immunity has also been implicated.
          • Type IV hypersensitivity reaction
      c. Nephrogenic strains of group A streptococcus lack M protein.
        • Never associated with RF
    3. Clinical findings

Acute RF: migratory polyarthritis most common initial presentation

      a. Migratory polyarthritis (~75%)
        (1) Most common initial presentation of acute rheumatic fever
        (2) Occurs in large joints (knees), ankles, and wrists
        (3) *No* permanent joint damage
      b. Carditis (~35%)
        (1) Most serious complication

(2) Fibrinous pericarditis
  • Precordial chest pain with friction rub
(3) Myocarditis
  (a) Most common cause of death in acute disease
  (b) Aschoff bodies are present.
    • Central area of fibrinoid necrosis surrounded by Anitschkow cells (reactive histiocytes)
(4) Endocarditis
  (a) Most commonly involves the MV (then aortic valve)
  (b) Sterile, verrucoid-appearing vegetations develop along the line of closure of the valve (Fig. 10-13).
    • Embolism is uncommon.
  (c) MV regurgitation or aortic valve (AV) regurgitation
    • May result in congestive heart failure
  (d) Recurrent infection of the MV and AV leads to MV stenosis or AV stenosis.
  c. Subcutaneous nodules (~10%) occur on extensor surfaces.
  d. Erythema marginatum (~10%)
    • Evanescent circular ring of erythema that develops around normal skin
  e. Sydenham's chorea (~10%)
    (1) Reversible rapid, involuntary movements affecting all muscles
    (2) Late manifestation of acute RF
4. Diagnosis of acute RF (revised Jones criteria)
  a. One major and two minor criteria if supported by evidence of an antecedent group A streptococcal pharyngitis
  b. Major criteria
    (1) Carditis
    (2) Migratory polyarthritis
    (3) Chorea
    (4) Erythema marginatum
    (5) Subcutaneous nodules
  c. Minor criteria
    (1) Previous RF or rheumatic heart disease
    (2) Arthralgia (pain without joint swelling)
    (3) Fever
    (4) Increased acute phase reactants (refer to Chapter 2)
      (a) Increased erythrocyte sedimentation rate (ESR; refer to Chapter 2)
      (b) Increased C-reactive protein
      (c) Absolute neutrophilic leukocytosis

Acute RF: myocarditis most common cause of death

Acute RF: MV most often involved followed by AV

Rheumatic fever: mitral regurgitation in acute attack; mitral stenosis in chronic disease

Acute RF: diagnose with Jones criteria

Acute RF: carditis, arthritis, chorea, erythema marginatum subcutaneous nodules

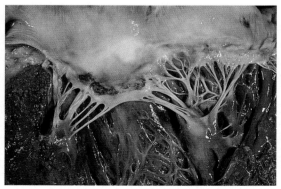

10-13: Acute rheumatic fever. Uniform, verrucoid-appearing sterile vegetations appear along the line of closure of the mitral valve. *(From Damjanov I, Linder J: Pathology: A Color Atlas. St. Louis, Mosby, 2000, p 13, Fig. 1-22.)*

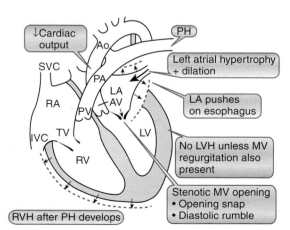

10-14: Mitral stenosis. Refer to the text for discussion. Ao, aorta; AV, aortic valve; IVC, inferior vena cava; LA, left atrium; LV, left ventricle; LVH, left ventricular hypertrophy; MV, mitral valve; PA, pulmonary artery; PH, pulmonary hypertension; PV, pulmonary valve; RA, right atrium; RV, right ventricle; RVH, right ventricular hypertrophy; SVC, superior vena cava; TV, tricuspid valve.

(5) Prolonged PR interval (first-degree heart block)

d. Laboratory tests

(1) Increased antistreptolysin O (ASO) titers > 400 Todd units

(a) Peak at 4 to 5 weeks after streptococcal pharyngitis

(b) High titers are supportive, but *not* diagnostic for RF.

(2) Increased anti-DNase B titers (less reliable than ASO titers)

(3) Throat cultures may or may not be positive.

e. Treatment for acute RF

(1) Bed rest

(2) Course of penicillin to eradicate throat carriage of group A streptococcus

• Continue penicillin for years if severe carditis

(3) Aspirin with or without presence of a murmur

(4) Carditis and heart failure

• Corticosteroids if murmur is present

f. Chronic RF

• Monthly treatment with benzathine penicillin IM to prevent recurrences

B. Mitral valve stenosis

1. Etiology

• Most often caused by recurrent attacks of rheumatic fever

2. Pathophysiology

a. Narrowing of the mitral valve orifice (Fig. 10-14)

b. Left atrium becomes dilated and hypertrophied

• Due to increased work in filling the ventricle in diastole

3. Clinical findings

a. Dyspnea and hemoptysis with rust-colored sputum (heart failure cells)

• Due to pulmonary capillary congestion and hemorrhage into the alveoli

b. Atrial fibrillation

(1) Due to left atrial dilation and hypertrophy

(2) Intra-atrial thrombus develops due to stasis (refer to Chapter 4).

• Danger of systemic embolization

c. Pulmonary venous hypertension

(1) Due to chronic backup of atrial blood into the pulmonary vein

(2) Right-sided heart failure and right ventricular hypertrophy may occur.

d. Dysphagia for solids

(1) Left atrium is the most posteriorly located chamber in the heart.

(2) Dilation of the left atrium compresses the esophagus.

e. Opening snap followed by an early to mid-diastolic rumble (see Box 10-1)

C. Mitral valve regurgitation

1. Etiology

a. Mitral valve prolapse (most common cause)

b. Functional MV regurgitation (stretching of the MV ring)

• Example—left-sided heart failure

c. Infective endocarditis

d. Rupture or dysfunction of the papillary muscle in acute MI

e. Acute rheumatic fever, Libman-Sacks endocarditis in systemic lupus erythematosus

2. Pathophysiology (Fig. 10-15)

a. Retrograde blood flow into the left atrium during systole

(1) Due to an incompetent MV or dilated MV ring

(2) Left atrium becomes dilated and hypertrophied

b. Volume overload in the left ventricle and left atrium leads to LHF.

3. Clinical findings

a. Dyspnea, inspiratory crackles, and cough from LHF

b. Pansystolic murmur; S_3 and S_4 heart sounds (see Box 10-1)

D. Mitral valve prolapse

1. Epidemiology

a. Autosomal dominant inheritance in some cases

b. More common in women

c. Associated with Marfan and Ehlers-Danlos syndromes

2. Pathophysiology

a. Posterior bulging of the anterior and/or posterior leaflets into the left atrium during systole (Fig. 10-16)

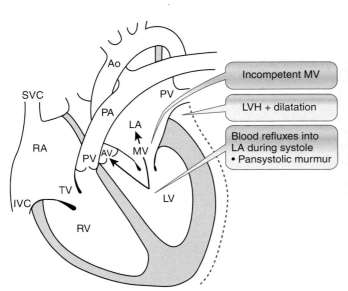

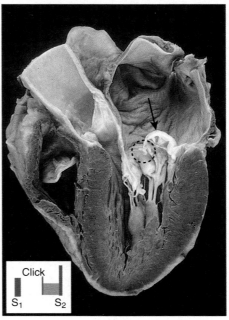

10-15: Mitral regurgitation. See text for discussion. Ao, aorta; AV, aortic valve; IVC, inferior vena cava; LA, left atrium; LV, left ventricle; LVH, left ventricular hypertrophy; MV, mitral valve; PA, pulmonary artery; PH, pulmonary hypertension; PV, pulmonary valve; RA, right atrium; RV, right ventricle; SVC, superior vena cava; TV, tricuspid valve. *(From Goljan EF: Star Series: Pathology. Philadelphia, WB Saunders, 1998.)*

10-16: Mitral valve prolapse. The *arrow* shows prolapse of the posterior mitral leaflet into the left atrium. *(From Kumar V, Fausto N, Abbas A: Robbins and Cotran's Pathologic Basis of Disease, 7th ed. Philadelphia, WB Saunders, 2004, p 592, Fig. 12-23.)*

    b. Redundancy of valve tissue
       (1) Myxomatous degeneration of the mitral valve leaflets
       (2) Due to excess production of dermatan sulfate
   3. Clinical findings
    a. Most patients are asymptomatic.
    b. Heart murmur
       (1) Mid-systolic click
          • Due to sudden restraint by the chordae of the prolapsed valve
       (2) Mid to late systolic regurgitant murmur follows the click.
       (3) Decreased preload causes the click and murmur to move closer to the S_1 heart sound; examples:
         (a) Anxiety
            • Increased heart rate decreases diastolic filling of left ventricle.
         (b) Standing
            • Decreases venous return to the right side of the heart
         (c) Valsalva maneuver (holding breath with epiglottis closed)
            • Positive intrathoracic pressure decreases venous return to the heart.
       (4) Increased preload causes the click and murmur to move closer to the S_2 heart sound; examples:
         (a) Reclining
            • Increases venous return to the right side of the heart
         (b) Squatting or sustained hand grip
            • Increases systemic vascular resistance, which impedes emptying of the left ventricle
    c. Palpitations, chest pain, rupture of chordae producing acute MV regurgitation
   4. Treatment in symptomatic patients
      • β-Blocker decreases heart rate and force of contraction leading to less stretch and trauma to the prolapsed leaflets.
E. Aortic valve (AV) stenosis
   1. AV orifice is normally 3 cm².
    a. Symptoms appear when the orifice < 1 cm².
    b. Severe AV stenosis is present when the orifice < 0.5 cm².

MVP: systolic click followed by murmur

MVP: preload alters click and murmur relationship to S_1/S_2

Symptomatic MVP: β-blockers

2. Etiology

Calcific AV stenosis: most common cause in patients > 60 years old

   a. Calcific AV stenosis of normal or bicuspid aortic valve (Fig. 10-17)
   - Most common cause of AV stenosis in patients > 60 years old
   b. Congenital AV stenosis
   - Most common cause in patients < 30 years old
   c. Age-related sclerosis of the aortic valve
   d. Chronic rheumatic fever

3. Pathophysiology (Fig. 10-18)
   a. Obstruction to left ventricular outflow during systole
   b. Reduction in the aortic valve orifice area produces concentric LVH.

4. Clinical findings
   a. Systolic ejection murmur; S_4 heart sound (see Box 10-1)
   b. Decreasing preload lessens the volume the left ventricle must eject.
   - Murmur intensity decreases.

AV stenosis: ejection murmur; S_4; ↓ intensity with ↓ preload; ↑ intensity with ↑ preload

   c. Increasing preload increases the volume the left ventricle must eject.
   - Murmur intensity increases.
   d. Opposite effect occurs in hypertrophic cardiomyopathy (see later).
   e. Angina with exercise
   (1) Decreased blood flow through the stenotic valve leads to less filling of the coronary arteries during diastole.
   (2) Subendocardium of concentrically hypertrophied heart receives less blood.

AV stenosis: most common valvular lesion causing syncope and angina with exercise

   f. Syncope with exercise
   - Decreased blood flow through the stenotic valve leads to decreased blood flow to the brain.

AV stenosis: microangiopathic hemolytic anemia with schistocytes, hemoglobinuria

   g. Hemolytic anemia with schistocytes (refer to Chapter 11)
   - Indication for AV replacement

F. Aortic valve regurgitation

1. Etiology
   a. Isolated AV root dilation
   b. Infective endocarditis
   - Most common infectious cause of acute AV regurgitation

Isolated AV root dilation: most common cause of aortic regurgitation

   c. Long-standing essential hypertension
   d. Chronic rheumatic fever
   e. Aortic dissection (refer to Chapter 9)
   f. Coarctation
   g. Syphilitic aortitis (refer to Chapter 9)
   h. Aortitis in ankylosing spondylitis (refer to Chapter 23)
   i. Takayasu arteritis (refer to Chapter 9)

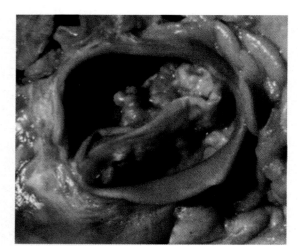

10-17: Aortic stenosis. The superior view shows a bicuspid aortic valve with severe stenosis due to fibrocalcific involvement of the two valve cusps. *(From Silver MD, Gotlieb AI, Schoen FJ: Cardiovascular Pathology, 3rd ed. London, Churchill Livingstone, 2001, p 424, Fig. 13.26B.)*

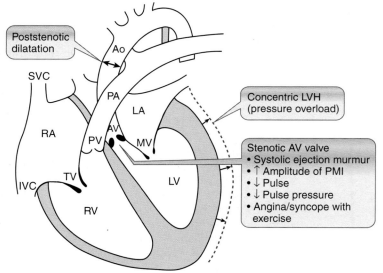

10-18: Aortic stenosis. See text for discussion. Ao, aorta; AV, aortic valve; IVC, inferior vena cava; LA, left atrium; LV, left ventricle; LVH, left ventricular hypertrophy; MV, mitral valve; PA, pulmonary artery; PH, pulmonary hypertension; PMI, point of maximal impulse; PV, pulmonary valve; RA, right atrium; RV, right ventricle; SVC, superior vena cava; TV, tricuspid valve. *(From Goljan EF: Star Series: Pathology. Philadelphia, WB Saunders, 1998.)*

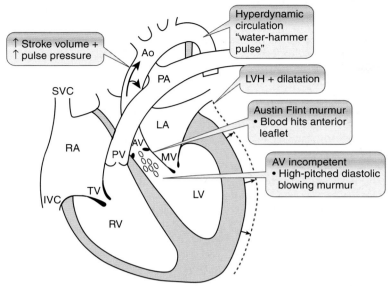

10-19: Aortic regurgitation. See text for discussion. Ao, aorta; AV, aortic valve; IVC, inferior vena cava; LA, left atrium; LV, left ventricle; LVH, left ventricular hypertrophy; MV, mitral valve; PA, pulmonary artery; PV, pulmonary valve; RA, right atrium; RV, right ventricle; SVC, superior vena cava; TV, tricuspid valve. *(From Goljan EF: Star Series: Pathology. Philadelphia, WB Saunders, 1998.)*

2. Pathophysiology (Fig. 10-19)
   a. Retrograde blood flow into the left ventricle
     (1) Due to an incompetent valve or dilated AV ring
     (2) Decreases diastolic pressure
       • Due to drop in arterial volume as blood flows back into the left ventricle
     (3) Volume overload of the left ventricle
       • Increases stroke volume (Frank-Starling mechanism)
   b. Increased pulse pressure (difference between systolic and diastolic pressure)
     • Produces hyperdynamic circulation (e.g., bounding pulses)
3. Clinical findings
   a. Early diastolic murmur; S_3 and S_4 heart sounds (see Box 10-1)
   b. Signs of a hyperdynamic circulation are caused by a widened pulse pressure.
     (1) Left ventricular volume markedly increases due to the incompetent valve.
     (2) Frank-Starling mechanisms increase in stroke volume.
       • Increases systolic pressure
     (3) Blood regurgitating into the left ventricle produces a drop in the diastolic blood pressure.
       • Recall that the diastolic blood pressure represents the amount of blood in the arterial system while the heart is filling up in diastole.
     (4) An increase in systolic pressure plus a decrease in diastolic pressure widens the pulse pressure (difference between systolic pressure and diastolic pressure), which causes the hyperdynamic findings, including:
       (a) Bounding pulses (Corrigan's water hammer pulse)
       (b) Head nodding with systole (de Musset's sign)
       (c) Pulsating nail bed with elevation of the nail (Quincke's pulse)
   c. Austin Flint murmur
     (1) Regurgitant stream from incompetent AV hits the anterior MV leaflet producing a diastolic murmur (functional mitral stenosis).
     (2) Presence of this murmur indicates the need for replacement of the valve.
G. Tricuspid valve (TV) regurgitation
   1. Etiology
   a. Functional TV regurgitation (stretching of TV ring)
     (1) Most common cause in adults
     (2) Examples—RHF, pulmonary hypertension, dilated cardiomyopathy, right ventricular infarction

AV regurgitation: ↑pulse pressure

AV regurgitation: early diastolic murmur; bounding pulses; S_3, S_4; no ↑ intensity with inspiration

AV regurgitation: hyperdynamic circulation

Austin Flint murmur: sign for AV replacement

TV regurgitation: functional most common cause adults

b. Congenital cardiac abnormalities
   - Most common cause in young adults

TV regurgitation: infective endocarditis, carcinoid heart disease

   c. Infective endocarditis in intravenous drug abuse
   d. Carcinoid heart disease
2. Pathophysiology
   a. Retrograde blood flow into the right atrium during systole
      (1) Due to stretching of the valve ring or damage to the valve
      (2) Causes right ventricular overload and RHF
      (3) Causes right atrial dilation and hypertrophy
   b. Produces volume overload in the right atrium and right ventricle
3. Clinical findings
   a. Pulsating liver
      - Blood regurgitates into the venous system with systole.

TV regurgitation: pansystolic murmur; S_3/ S_4; ↑ intensity with deep held inspiration

   b. Giant c-v wave jugular venous pulse (see Box 10-1)
      - Sign of severe TV regurgitation
   c. Pansystolic murmur; S_3 and S_4 heart sounds (see Box 10-1)

H. Pulmonary valve (PV) stenosis
1. Uncommon valvular lesion
2. Associated with carcinoid heart disease
3. Systolic ejection murmur (see Box 10-1)
4. Right ventricular hypertrophy

I. Pulmonary valve regurgitation

PV regurgitation: pulmonary hypertension

1. Most often a functional murmur from stretching of the PV ring
   - Example—pulmonary hypertension (called a Graham Steell murmur)
2. Diastolic murmur; S_3 and S_4 heart sounds (see Box 10-1)

J. Carcinoid heart disease
1. Due to liver metastasis from a carcinoid tumor of small intestine (refer to Chapter 17)
2. Serotonin causes fibrosis of the tricuspid and pulmonary valves.
   - Produces TV regurgitation and PV stenosis

Carcinoid heart disease: PV stenosis, TV regurgitation

K. Infective endocarditis (IE)
1. Epidemiology
   a. Risk factors for IE
      (1) Diabetes mellitus, HIV infection
      (2) Poor dental hygiene, congenital heart disease
      (3) Mitral valve prolapse, aortic stenosis
      (4) Hemodialysis, prosthetic heart valve
      (5) Intravenous catheters, intravenous drug abuse (IVDA)
   b. Microbial pathogens
      (1) *Streptococcus viridans*
         (a) Most common overall cause of IE (30–40% of cases)
         (b) Typically produces subacute IE

Streptococcus viridans: most common cause of IE

      (2) *Staphylococcus aureus*
         (a) Most common cause of IE in IVDA
         (b) High mortality rate

Staphylococcus aureus: most common pathogen producing IE in IV drug abuse

      (3) *Staphylococcus epidermidis*
         (a) Most common cause of IE after insertion of prosthetic valves
            - Usually occurs within 2 months of insertion
         (b) Most common cause of nosocomial endocarditis from intravenous catheters

Staphylococcus epidermidis: most common pathogen producing nosocomial and prosthetic valve IE

      (4) *Streptococcus bovis*
         - Most common cause of IE in ulcerative colitis or colorectal cancer
   c. Valves involved in IE
      (1) Majority of valves involved are left-sided (>90%).
         - Right-sided valves with IE are usually associated with IVDA.

Streptococcus bovis: most common pathogen producing IE in ulcerative colitis/colorectal cancer

      (2) Mitral valve
         - Most common overall valve involved in IE
      (3) Tricuspid valve and aortic valve
         - Most common valves involved in IE due to IVDA

TV regurgitation in IVDA is due to infective endocarditis

2. Pathogenesis
   a. Turbulent blood flow damages the valve → adherence of fibrin and platelets → trapping of circulating bacteria/fungi → proliferation of pathogens + laying down of fibrin to encase the vegetation
   b. *Streptococcus viridans* infects previously damaged valves.

c. *Staphylococcus aureus* infects normal or previously damaged valves.
3. Pathology
   a. Vegetations destroy the valve leaflet and chordae tendineae (Fig. 10-20).
   b. Valve destruction leads to regurgitation murmurs.
4. Clinical findings
   a. Fever is the most consistent sign (98% of cases).
      • Common cause of fever of unknown origin
   b. Immunocomplex vasculitis (if IE is subacute)
      • Examples—glomerulonephritis, Roth's spot (irregular red area with central white dot)
   c. Microembolization findings
      (1) Splinter hemorrhages in nail beds (Fig. 10-21)
      (2) Janeway's lesions (painless lesions on palms and feet)
      (3) Osler's nodes (painful nodules on pads of the fingers or toes)
      (4) Mucosal petechiae
      (5) Infarctions in different tissue sites (e.g., digits, brain)
   d. Splenomegaly (if IE is subacute)
   e. Hematuria with RBC casts (glomerulonephritis)
   f. Hematuria without RBC casts (infarction)
5. Laboratory findings
   a. Positive blood cultures are present in 80% of cases.
      • Reflects the fact that many patients are taking antibiotics
   b. Neutrophilic leukocytosis occurs in acute IE.
   c. Monocytosis occurs in subacute bacterial endocarditis.
   d. Mild anemia
      • Usually anemia of chronic disease
   e. Transesophageal echocardiography
      • Useful in detecting vegetations on the valves
6. Treatment
   a. Initial treatment is directed at the most likely organism.
   b. Antibiotic after identification of the pathogen is guided by susceptibility testing.
L. Libman-Sacks endocarditis
1. Associated with systemic lupus erythematosus (SLE) in 30% to 50% of cases
2. Sterile vegetations are located over the mitral valve surface and chordae.
   • Produces valve deformity and MV regurgitation
M. Nonbacterial thrombotic endocarditis (marantic endocarditis)
1. Paraneoplastic syndrome (refer to Chapter 8)
2. Sterile, nondestructive vegetations on the mitral valve
   • Procoagulant effect of circulating mucin from mucin-producing tumors of the colon/pancreas

Margin notes:

IE: fever most consistent sign

IE signs: microembolization, immunocomplex vasculitis

IE: positive blood culture majority of cases

Libman-Sacks endocarditis: associated with SLE; MV involved

Marantic endocarditis: sterile vegetations; paraneoplastic syndrome

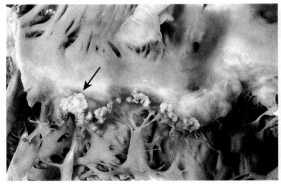

10-20: Acute bacterial endocarditis. Large, friable, and irregular vegetation (*arrow*) is present on the margin of the mitral valve. Smaller vegetations are present along the line of closure of the valve. (*From Damjanov I, Linder J: Pathology: A Color Atlas. St. Louis, Mosby, 2000, p 11, Fig. 1-16.*)

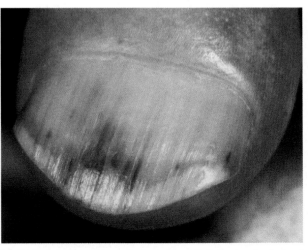

10-21: Splinter hemorrhages in the nail bed. Note the longitudinal red hemorrhages in the nail bed. (*From Swartz MH: Textbook of Physical Diagnosis, 5th ed. Philadelphia, Saunders Elsevier, 2006, p 147, Fig. 8-10.*)

3. Complications
   a. Embolization
   b. May be secondarily infected

VII. Myocardial and Pericardial Disorders

A. Myocarditis

1. Epidemiology
   a. Major cause of sudden death (15–20%) in adults < 40 years of age
   b. Etiology
      (1) Microbial pathogens
         (a) Coxsackievirus (most common cause)
         (b) *Trypanosoma cruzi* (Chagas' disease)
            • Trypanosomes with flagella circulate in blood; amastigotes (no flagella) infect cardiac muscle.
         (c) Lyme disease (*Borrelia burgdorferi*)
      (2) Acute rheumatic fever
      (3) Toxins
         • Examples—diphtheria, carbon monoxide
      (4) Drugs
         • Examples—doxorubicin, daunorubicin, cocaine
      (5) Collagen vascular
         • Examples—SLE, systemic sclerosis
      (6) Sarcoidosis
2. Pathology
   a. Global enlargement of the heart and dilation of all chambers
   b. Lymphocytic infiltrate with focal areas of necrosis (Fig. 10-22)
      • Highly predictive of coxsackievirus
3. Clinical findings
   a. Fever
   b. Chest pain
   c. Pericardial friction rub (see below)
   d. Biventricular heart failure
   e. Heart murmurs
      • MV regurgitation most common
4. Laboratory findings
   a. Increased CK-MB and troponins I and T
   b. Detection of antibodies of pathogens
5. Treatment
   a. Treat the underlying cause.
   b. Approximately 50% of patients will die within 5 years.

B. Pericarditis

1. Etiology
   a. Similar to disorders listed for myocarditis
   b. Coxsackievirus is the most common overall known cause.
      • Most are idiopathic, the cause unknown.

Margin notes:

Coxsackievirus: most common cause of myocarditis and pericarditis

Chagas' disease: most common cause of myocarditis leading to CHF in Central/South America

Drugs: doxorubicin, daunorubicin

Myocarditis: ↑ CK-MB, troponins I and T

Pericarditis: most common cause is coxsackievirus

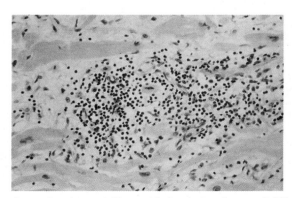

10-22: Myocarditis. The biopsy shows a lymphocytic infiltrate with dissolution of myocardial fibers. *(From Damjanov I, Linder J: Pathology: A Color Atlas. St. Louis, Mosby, 2000, p 15, Fig. 1-28.)*

2. Pathology
   a. Fibrinous type of pericardial exudate
      • Often accompanied by an effusion
   b. Dense scar tissue with dystrophic calcification may cause constrictive pericarditis.
3. Clinical and laboratory findings
   a. Tachycardia
   b. Fever
   c. Precordial chest pain
      (1) Pain is relieved when leaning forward.
      (2) Pain increases when leaning back.

> Pericarditis: precordial rub; pain relieved by leaning forward

   d. Pericardial friction rub
      (1) Scratchy, three-component rub (systole, early, and late diastole)
         (a) Best heard with the patient leaning forward
         (b) All three components are heard in ~50% of cases.
      (2) Does *not* disappear when the patient holds his breath
   e. Serum CK-MB usually normal
   f. Troponins I and T are increased in 35% to 50% of cases.
      • Usually indicates myocarditis present as well
   g. Often accompanied by a pericardial effusion
      (1) Muffled heart sounds
         (a) Fluid surrounds the heart (Fig. 10-23).
         (b) All pressures are equal in all chambers of the heart.

> Young woman with pericarditis and effusion: most likely has SLE

      (2) Hypotension associated with pulsus paradoxus
         (a) Drop in systolic blood pressure > 10 mm Hg during inspiration
         (b) Inspiration increases the flow of venous blood into the right side of the heart (refer to Box 10-1).
            • Increased pressure of blood in the right ventricle displaces the interventricular septum to the left causing a decrease in the left ventricular volume and a corresponding drop in systolic blood pressure.

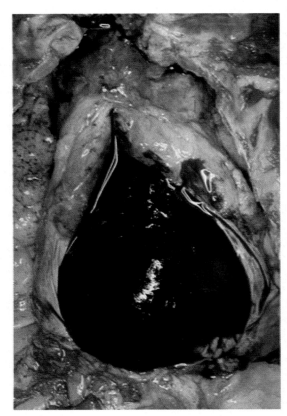

10-23: Hemopericardium. Note the "water bottle" configuration of the blood in the pericardial cavity. *(From Klatt E: Robbins and Cotran's Atlas of Pathology. Philadelphia, WB Saunders, 2006, p 52, Fig. 2-82.)*

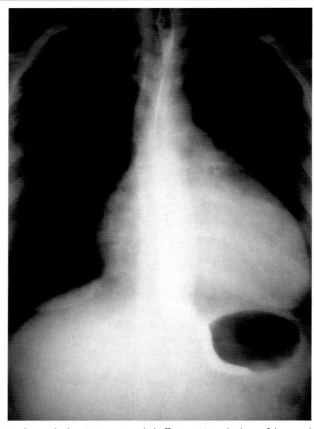

10-24: Posteroanterior chest radiograph showing a pericardial effusion. Note the loss of the usual heart borders and the "water bottle" configuration similar to that seen in the hemopericardium in Fig. 10-23. *(Courtesy of Sven Paulin, MD.)*

Pericardial effusion on inspiration: neck vein distention, ↓ systolic blood pressure > 10 mm Hg

Constrictive pericarditis: incomplete filling of chambers; pericardial knock

Cardiomyopathy: dilated, hypertrophic, restrictive

        (3) Neck vein distention on inspiration
           (a) Blood cannot easily enter the right atrium, due to fluid surrounding the heart.
           (b) Some blood refluxes back into the jugular vein (Kussmaul's sign).
        (4) Chest radiograph shows a "water bottle" configuration (Fig. 10-24).
     h. Constrictive pericarditis
        (1) Etiology
           (a) Tuberculosis is the most common cause worldwide.
           (b) Most cases in the United States are idiopathic or secondary to scarring from previous open heart surgery.
           (c) Pericardial calcification is seen on a chest radiograph in ~25% of cases.
        (2) Pathophysiology
          • Incomplete filling of the cardiac chambers due to thickening of the parietal pericardium
        (3) Pericardial knock
          • Due to the ventricles hitting the thickened parietal pericardium
   4. Treatment of pericarditis
     • Treat the underlying cause if it is known
   5. Treatment of pericardial effusion
     • Pericardiocentesis to remove fluid

VIII. Cardiomyopathy
   A. Definition
     • Group of diseases that primarily involve the myocardium and produce myocardial dysfunction
   B. Types of cardiomyopathy
     1. Dilated (congestive)
     2. Hypertrophic
     3. Restrictive

C. Dilated cardiomyopathy

1. Epidemiology
   a. Most common cardiomyopathy
   b. Etiology
      (1) Idiopathic (most common)
      (2) Genetic causes (25–35%)
      (3) Myocarditis
         • Most common known cause; see Section VII
      (4) Alcohol (15–40%)
         • Direct toxic effect or due to thiamine deficiency (refer to Chapter 7)
      (5) Drugs
         • Examples—doxorubicin, daunorubicin, cocaine
      (6) Postpartum state
         • Last trimester or within 6 months postpartum
      (7) Organic solvents ("glue sniffers heart")
      (8) Acromegaly
      (9) Myxedema heart in severe hypothyroidism
2. Pathophysiology
   a. Decreased contractility
   b. Systolic dysfunction type of LHF
3. Clinical findings
   a. Global enlargement of the heart (Fig. 10-25)
      (1) All chambers are dilated.
      (2) Echocardiography shows poor contractility.
   b. Biventricular CHF
   c. Heart murmurs (MV and TV regurgitation)
   d. Left- and right-sided S_3 and S_4 heart sounds
   e. Narrow pulse pressure
      • Due to decreased stroke volume
   f. Arrhythmias
      (1) Bundle branch blocks
      (2) Atrial and ventricular arrhythmias
   g. Ejection fraction is usually <40% (normal, ≥55%).
4. Treatment
   • If medical therapy is ineffective, cardiac transplantation is the only other option.

D. Hypertrophic cardiomyopathy (HCM)

1. Epidemiology
   a. Most common cause of sudden death in young individuals
   b. Familial form
      (1) Most common form

Dilated cardiomyopathy: most common cardiomyopathy

Dilated cardiomyopathy: myocarditis most common cause

Dilated cardiomyopathy: doxorubicin, daunorubicin

Dilated cardiomyopathy: global enlargement of heart

Hypertrophic cardiomyopathy: most common cause of sudden death in young individuals

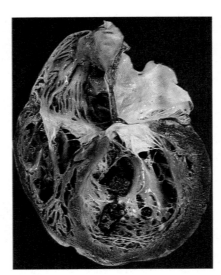

10-25: Dilated cardiomyopathy. Note the global enlargement of the heart and the dilated ventricle on the right and atrium on the left. *(From Damjanov I, Linder J: Pathology: A Color Atlas. St. Louis, Mosby, 2000, p 17, Fig. 1-35.)*

         (2) Autosomal dominant with nearly complete penetrance

         (3) Occurs in young individuals

         (4) Genes mapped to chromosome 14

            (a) Missense mutation in 1 of at least 10 genes that code for proteins of cardiac sarcomeres

            (b) Example—mutation in myosin heavy chain gene

    c. Sporadic form

      • Occurs in elderly people

  2. Pathophysiology

    a. Hypertrophy of the myocardium

        (1) Disproportionately greater hypertrophy of interventricular septum (IVS) than the free left ventricular wall.

        (2) IVS hypertrophy may obstruct blood flow through the outflow tract.

        (3) Most patients do *not* have severe obstruction of the outflow tract.

HCM: obstruction *below* the aortic valve

    b. Obstruction to blood flow, if present, is *below* the aortic valve.

      • As blood exits the left ventricle, the anterior leaflet of the mitral valve is drawn against the asymmetrically hypertrophied IVS (Figs. 10-26 and 10-27).

    c. Aberrant myofibers are present in the conduction system; fatal arrhythmias

    d. Left ventricle is noncompliant.

      • Muscle thickening restricts filling.

  3. Clinical findings

    a. Harsh systolic ejection murmur

      • Best heard along the left sternal border

    b. Palpable double apical impulse

HCM: preload changes on murmur intensity opposite of those for AV stenosis

    c. Murmur intensity increases (obstruction worsens) with decreased preload.

      • Examples—standing up, Valsalva maneuver (increases positive intrathoracic pressure), use of inotropic drugs (e.g., digitalis)

    d. Murmur intensity decreases (obstruction lessens) with increased preload.

        (1) Examples—reclining, drugs decreasing cardiac contractility (e.g., β-blockers), sustained clenching of hands, squatting

        (2) Increasing preload opens the outflow track.

    e. Angina or syncope with exercise

      • Similar to aortic stenosis

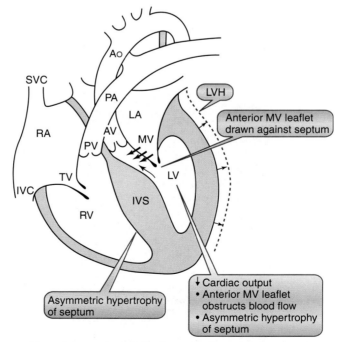

10-26: Schematic of hypertrophic cardiomyopathy. Refer to the text for discussion. Ao, aorta; AV, aortic valve; IVC, inferior vena cava; IVS, interventricular septum; LA, left atrium; LV, left ventricle; LVH, left ventricular hypertrophy; MV, mitral valve; PA, pulmonary artery; PV, pulmonary valve; RA, right atrium; RV, right ventricle; SVC, superior vena cava; TV, tricuspid valve.

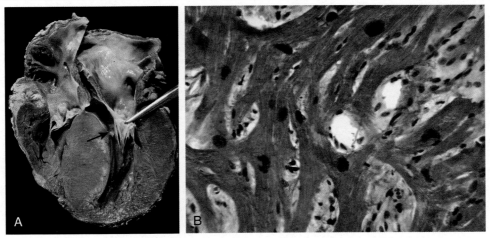

10-27: Hypertrophic cardiomyopathy. The heart (**A**) shows asymmetric hypertrophy of the interventricular septum (*black arrow*) with marked narrowing of the outflow tract. The histologic section of the conduction system in the septum (**B**) shows aberrant myofibers. (*A from Schoen FJ: Interventional and Surgical Cardiovascular Pathology: Clinical Correlations and Basic Principles. Philadelphia, Saunders, 1989; B from Kumar V, Abbas AK, Fausto N, Mitchell RN: Robbins Basic Pathology, 8th ed. Philadelphia, Saunders Elsevier, 2007, p 413, Fig. 11-25.*)

f. Sudden death is due to ventricular tachycardia/fibrillation.
  • Correlates with left ventricular wall thickness
4. Treatment
  a. Avoid strenuous exertion.
  b. Avoid drugs that decrease preload (e.g., diuretics) or increase force of contraction (e.g., digitalis).
  c. β-Blockers are the mainstay of therapy.
    (1) Decreased heart rate prolongs diastole.
      • Increases preload
    (2) Decrease myocardial contractility
  d. Implantable cardioconvertor defibrillator
    • Prevents ventricular tachycardia/fibrillation and sudden cardiac death
5. Screen all first-degree relatives.
  a. Two-dimensional echocardiography is used.
  b. Screening for mutations is likely in the future.
E. Restrictive cardiomyopathy
1. Etiology
  a. Most frequently caused by the following:
    (1) Amyloidosis
    (2) Myocardial fibrosis after open-heart surgery
    (3) Radiation
  b. Infiltrative diseases
    • Examples—Pompe's glycogenosis, hemochromatosis
  c. Endocardial fibroelastosis in a child
    • Thick fibroelastic tissue in the endocardium
  d. Sarcoidosis
  e. Systemic sclerosis
2. Pathophysiology
  a. Decreased ventricular compliance
  b. Diastolic dysfunction type of LHF
3. Clinical findings
  a. Progressive LHF and RHF
  b. ECG is low voltage with ST-T wave changes.
4. Treatment
  a. Treat the underlying cause.
    • Examples—treat hemochromatosis with phlebotomy; treat sarcoidosis with corticosteroids
  b. No effective therapy for most causes

HCM: sudden death due to ventricular tachycardia/fibrillation

HCM: Treat with β-blockers

Restrictive cardiomyopathy: least common cardiomyopathy; low-voltage ECG

Restrictive cardiomyopathy: ↓ ventricular compliance

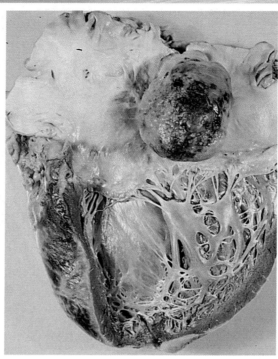

10-28: Cardiac myxoma in the left atrium. Note the large red mass in the left atrium. *(From Damjanov I, Linder J: Pathology: A Color Atlas. St. Louis, Mosby, 2000, p 27, Fig. 1-65A.)*

IX. **Tumors of the Heart**
   A. **Epidemiology**

Heart tumors: metastasis > primary tumors

   1. Metastasis is more common than primary tumors.
      • Example—extension of a primary lung cancer
   2. Pericardium is the most common site for metastasis.
      • Leads to pericarditis and effusions
   3. Primary tumors or tumor-like conditions:
      • Cardiac myxoma, rhabdomyoma
   B. **Cardiac myxoma**
   1. Most common primary adult tumor
   2. Pathology

Cardiac myxoma: most common in left atrium

      a. Benign primary mesenchymal tumor
      b. Approximately 90% arise from the left atrium (Fig. 10-28)
      c. Sessile or pedunculated
      d. "Ball-valve" effect blocks the mitral valve orifice
         • Blocks diastolic filling of the ventricle, simulating mitral valve stenosis
   3. Clinical findings
      a. Nonspecific findings
         • Fever, fatigue, malaise, anemia
      b. Complications
         • Embolization, syncopal episodes (blocks mitral valve orifice)
   4. Diagnosis
      a. Transesophageal ultrasound
      b. Most useful study for viewing the left atrium
         • The left atrium is the most posteriorly located chamber.
   C. **Rhabdomyoma**

Myxomas occur in adults; rhabdomyomas occur in children.

   1. Most common primary tumor of the heart in infants and children
      • Major association with tuberous sclerosis (refer to Chapter 25)
   2. Hamartoma (non-neoplastic) arising from cardiac muscle

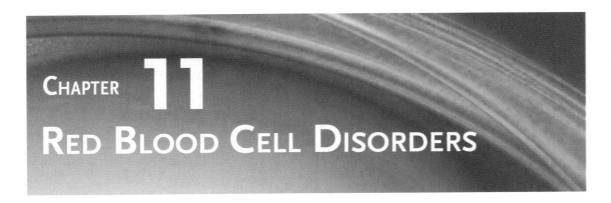

CHAPTER 11

RED BLOOD CELL DISORDERS

I. Erythropoiesis
- Erythropoiesis refers to the production of RBCs in the bone marrow and is dependent on the release of erythropoietin from the kidneys.
  A. Erythropoiesis and erythropoietin (EPO)
    1. Primarily synthesized in the renal cortex by interstitial cells in the peritubular capillary bed
    2. Stimuli for EPO release
        - Hypoxemia, severe anemia, left-shifted O_2-binding curve (OBC), high altitude
    3. Increased O_2 content suppresses EPO release (e.g., polycythemia vera).

> **EPO** increases the O_2-carrying capacity of blood by stimulating erythroid stem cells to divide. Epoetin alfa, a form of EPO produced by recombinant DNA technology, is frequently abused by athletes to increase their energy level. It also is used in the treatment of anemia associated with renal failure, chronic disease, and chemotherapy.

    4. Other sources of EPO
        - Ectopic production by renal cell carcinoma and hepatocellular carcinoma
    5. Peripheral blood markers of erythropoiesis
        a. Reticulocytes are newly released RBCs from the bone marrow.
        b. Identified with supravital stains
            - Detect thread-like RNA filaments in the cytoplasm (Fig. 11-1)
        c. In 24 hours, they become mature RBCs.
  B. Reticulocyte count
    1. Marker of effective erythropoiesis
        - Bone marrow response to anemia
    2. Develop into a mature RBC in 24 hours
        - Maturation occurs with the help of splenic macrophages.
    3. Reticulocyte count is reported as a percentage (normal < 3%).
        a. Percentage count is falsely increased in anemia (Fig. 11-2).
        b. Initial percentage must be corrected for the degree of anemia.
        c. Corrected reticulocyte count = (actual Hct/45) × reticulocyte count, where 45 represents the normal hematocrit (Hct)
        d. Example
            (1) Hct 15%, reticulocyte count 18%
            (2) Corrected reticulocyte count is 6% (15/45 × 18% = 6%)
        e. Additional correction is required if RBC polychromasia is present.
            (1) Polychromatic RBCs are even younger RBCs than reticulocytes (Fig. 11-3).
            (2) Appear when there is a very brisk hemolytic anemia
            (3) Require 2 to 3 days before becoming mature RBCs
            (4) Falsely increase the initial reticulocyte count, because they have RNA filaments and are counted as reticulocytes
            (5) Correction is made by dividing the initial reticulocyte count corrected for the degree of anemia by 2.
                - In the above example, if polychromasia was present, the additional correction would be 6%/2 = 3%, which is still a good response to anemia.

EPO: synthesized by interstitial cells in peritubular capillary bed

Stimuli for EPO: hypoxemia, left-shifted OBC, high altitude

Reticulocyte count: measure of effective erythropoiesis

Reticulocyte count: must correct for degree of anemia.

Correction: Hct/45 × reticulocyte count

Polychromasia: divide original correction by 2

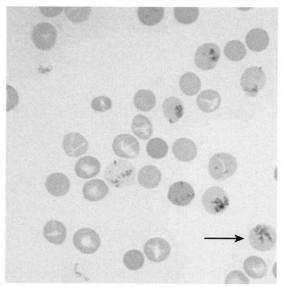

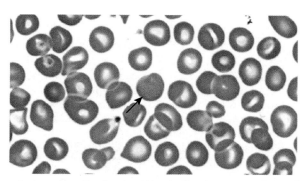

11-2: Correction of the reticulocyte count for degree of anemia. Note that the normal reticulocyte count is 3% when 3 reticulocytes (pale blue RBCs) are expressed as a percentage of 100 RBCs (red blood cells) in the microscopic field. However, the same 3 reticulocytes account for 10% of the RBCs in the patient with anemia, who has only 30 RBCs in the microscopic field. *(From Goljan EF, Sloka KI: Rapid Review Laboratory Testing in Clinical Medicine. St. Louis, Mosby Elsevier, 2008, p 146, Fig. 5-3.)*

11-1: Peripheral blood reticulocytes with supravital stain (new methylene blue). Red blood cells with thread-like material in the cytosol represent residual RNA filaments and protein (*arrow*). *(From Hoffbrand AV: Color Atlas: Clinical Hematology, 3rd ed. St. Louis, Mosby, 2000, Fig. 1-43B.)*

Corrected reticulocyte count: <3% ineffective erythropoiesis; ≥3% effective erythropoiesis

    4. Corrected reticulocyte count ≥ 3%
       a. Good bone marrow response to anemia (i.e., effective erythropoiesis)
       b. Examples—hemolytic anemia; after treatment of iron deficiency with iron
    5. Corrected reticulocyte count < 3%
       a. Poor bone marrow response to anemia (i.e., ineffective erythropoiesis)
       b. Examples—untreated iron deficiency; aplastic anemia
C. Extramedullary hematopoiesis (EMH)
    • RBC, WBC, and platelet production that occurs outside the bone marrow

EMH: most often occurs in the liver and spleen

    1. Common sites of EMH are the liver and spleen.
    2. Pathogenesis
       a. Intrinsic bone marrow disease (e.g., myelofibrosis)
       b. Accelerated erythropoiesis (e.g., severe hemolysis in sickle cell disease)
         (1) Expands the bone marrow cavity
         (2) Radiograph of the skull shows a "hair-on-end" appearance (Fig. 11-4).

EMH: hepatosplenomegaly

    3. EMH produces hepatosplenomegaly.

In the fetus, hematopoiesis (blood cell formation) begins in the yolk sac and subsequently moves to the liver and finally the bone marrow by the fifth to sixth months of gestation.

11-3: Polychromasia. The *arrow* depicts a blue discolored red blood cell without a central area of pallor. *(From Naeim F: Atlas of Bone Marrow and Blood Pathology. Philadelphia, WB Saunders, 2001, Fig. 1-15A.)*

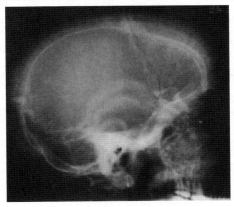

11-4: Skull radiograph showing "hair-on-end" due to expansion of the bone marrow cavity from accelerated erythropoiesis (e.g., severe hemolysis in sickle cell disease). *(From Bouloux P: Self-Assessment Picture Tests: Medicine, Vol. 1. London, Mosby-Wolfe, 1997, p 49, Fig. 97.)*

II. Complete Blood Cell Count (CBC) and Other Studies
A. Components of a CBC
1. Hemoglobin (Hb), Hct, RBC count
2. RBC indices, RBC distribution width (RDW)
3. WBC count with a differential count, platelet count
4. Evaluation of the peripheral blood morphology

B. Hb, Hct, and RBC counts
1. Factors affecting the normal range (reference interval)
   a. Premature newborns
      (1) Variable Hb concentration depending on gestational age
      (2) Anemia in prematurity
         (a) Iron deficiency
            • Due to loss of the daily supply of iron from mother's iron stores
         (b) Blood loss from excessive venipunctures

   Anemia prematurity: loss of iron from mother; blood loss from venipuncture

   b. Newborns
      (1) Newborns have higher normal ranges than do infants and children.
      (2) HbF ($2\alpha/2\gamma$ globin chains) shifts the OBC to the left causing the release of EPO.
         • EPO causes an increase in Hb, Hct, and RBC count.
      (3) After birth, the Hb drops from ~18.5 to 11 g/dL (physiologic anemia).

   Fetal Hb: left-shifts OBC causing an increase in Hb

> Fetal RBCs containing HbF are destroyed by splenic macrophages over the ensuing 6 to 9 months. The unconjugated bilirubin derived from the initial destruction of fetal RBCs is responsible for physiologic jaundice of the newborn, which occurs ~3 days from birth.

      (4) HbF-containing cells are replaced by RBCs containing HbA (>97%), HbA_2 (<2.5%), and HbF (<1%).
   c. Children
      (1) Have a lower Hb concentration than adults
      (2) Due to higher serum phosphorus levels
         (a) Increased serum phosphorus increases synthesis of 2,3-bisphosphoglycerate (BPG).
         (b) Increased 2,3-BPG right-shifts the OBC.
         (c) Greater release of O_2 to tissue overrides the need to have a higher Hb.

   Children: more right-shifted OBCs than adults

   d. Adult men and women
      (1) Men have higher Hb levels than women.
         (a) Due to increased testosterone
            • Stimulates erythropoiesis
         (b) Due to lack of cyclic bleeding
      (2) Anemia in an adult male is an Hb < 13.5 g/dL.
      (3) Anemia in a nonpregnant woman is an Hb < 12.5 g/dL.

   Anemia in adult male: <13.5 g/dL

   Anemia in nonpregnant female: <12.5 g/dL

e. Pregnancy
   (1) Pregnant women have lower normal ranges than nonpregnant women.
      (a) Due to an increase in plasma volume and RBC mass (i.e., more RBCs are produced).
      (b) Plasma volume is twice greater than RBC mass causing a slight decrease in Hb (dilutional effect).
   (2) In a pregnant woman, anemia is a Hb < 11 g/dL.
2. Changes in thalassemia (i.e., a genetic globin chain disorder)
   a. Hb and Hct are decreased.
   b. RBC count is increased.
   c. Mean corpuscular volume (MCV)/RBC count ratio < 13.
3. Anemia
   a. Decrease in Hb, Hct, or RBC concentration
   b. O_2 saturation and Pao_2 are normal; decreased O_2 content (refer to Chapter 1).
   c. Sign of an underlying disease rather than a specific diagnosis
   d. General clinical findings
      (1) Fatigue
      (2) Dyspnea with exertion
      (3) Inability to concentrate
      (4) Dizziness
      (5) Pulmonary flow murmur
        • Decreased blood viscosity in severe anemia
      (6) Pallor of skin, conjunctivae, palmar creases
        • Indications of severe anemia
      (7) High-output cardiac failure
        • Decreased blood viscosity in severe anemia (<5 g/dL)

C. RBC indices
1. MCV
   a. Average volume of RBCs
   b. Used to classify anemia (Fig. 11-5)
      (1) Microcytic (<80 μm³)

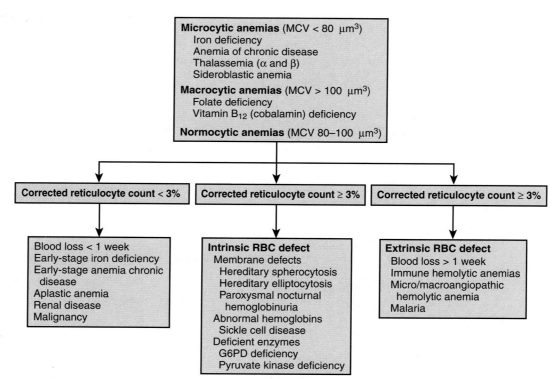

11-5: Classification of anemia using mean corpuscular volume (MCV). An intrinsic RBC defect indicates a structural or biochemical flaw in the RBCs. An extrinsic RBC defect indicates that the RBCs are structurally normal, but that other factors cause the anemia. G6PD, glucose-6-phosphate dehydrogenase.

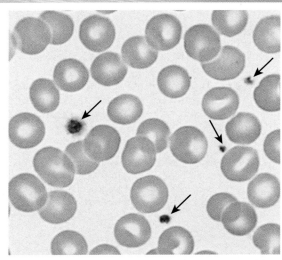

11-6: Normal peripheral blood smear showing RBCs. The RBCs are uniform in size, and the central areas of pallor are slightly less than half the total diameter of an RBC. The four dark objects (*arrows*) outside the RBCs are platelets. *(From Hoffbrand AV: Color Atlas: Clinical Hematology, 3rd ed. St. Louis, Mosby, 2000, p 22, Fig. 1-62.)*

    (2) Normocytic (80–100 μm^3)
    (3) Macrocytic (>100 μm^3)
2. Mean corpuscular hemoglobin concentration (MCHC)
  a. Average Hb concentration in RBCs (Fig. 11-6)
  b. Decreased MCHC
    (1) Correlates with decreased synthesis of Hb
      • Example—all the microcytic anemias
    (2) Central area of pallor is greater than normal.
      • Called hypochromasia (see Fig. 11-11)
  c. Increased MCHC
    (1) Correlates with the presence of spherical RBCs
      • Example—hereditary spherocytosis (see Fig. 11-25)
    (2) RBCs lack the central area of pallor.
3. RDW
  a. Reflects variation in size of peripheral blood RBCs
    (1) Size variation is called anisocytosis.
    (2) RDW is significant only if it is increased.
  b. Increased if RBCs are *not* uniformly the same size
    • Example—mixture of microcytic and normocytic cells
  c. Iron deficiency
    (1) Only microcytic anemia with an increased RDW
    (2) Due to a mixture of normocytic and microcytic RBCs

D. Characteristics of mature RBCs
1. Lack mitochondria; therefore:
  a. No citric acid cycle
  b. No β-oxidation of fatty acids
  c. No ketone body synthesis
2. Anaerobic glycolysis
  a. Main source of adenosine triphosphate (ATP)
  b. Lactic acid is the end-product of RBC metabolism.
    (1) Converted by the liver into glucose via gluconeogenesis
    (2) Glucose is utilized by RBCs for synthesizing ATP.
      • This is called the Cori cycle.
3. Pentose phosphate pathway
  a. Synthesizes glutathione (GSH)
    • Antioxidant that neutralizes hydrogen peroxide (refer to Chapter 2)
  b. Hydrogen peroxide is a product of oxidative metabolism.
4. Methemoglobin reductase pathway (refer to Chapter 1)
  a. Methemoglobin (metHb) refers to heme iron that is oxidized (Fe^{+3}).
    • MetHb *cannot* bind O_2.

Margin notes:

MCHC: ↓ in microcytic anemias; ↑ in spherocytosis

RDW: measure of size variation of RBCs

Iron deficiency: ↑ RDW

Mature RBC: anaerobic glycolysis; lactic acid end-product

Cori cycle: lactic acid converted to glucose in liver→ glucose to RBC

GSH: neutralizes peroxide and other free radicals

MetHb reductase: reduces
Fe^{+3} to Fe^{+2}

2,3-BPG: product of the
glycolytic cycle

Unconjugated bilirubin:
end-product of
heme degradation in
macrophages

Ferritin: synthesized
in bone marrow
macrophages

   b. Reductase system converts iron to ferrous (Fe^{+2}) so that the RBCs can bind O_2.
5. Luebering-Rapaport pathway
   a. Synthesizes 2,3-BPG
   b. Required to right-shift the OBC (i.e., release O_2 to tissue; refer to Chapter 1)
6. Senescent RBCs
   a. Phagocytosed in the cords of Billroth by splenic macrophages
   b. Heme degradation by macrophages produces unconjugated bilirubin.
7. Lack human leukocyte antigens on their membranes (refer to Chapter 3)

E. WBC count and differential

A 100 cell differential count divides leukocytes by percentage (neutrophils, lymphocytes, etc.) and further subdivides neutrophils into segmented and band neutrophils. Multiplication of the percentage times the total white blood cell count gives the absolute number of a particular leukocyte. Example—lymphocytes 30%, total WBC count 10,000/mm³. Absolute lymphocyte count is 0.30 × 10,000 = 3000/mm³.

F. Platelet count
1. Platelets are anucleate cells.
2. They are derived from cytoplasmic budding of megakaryocytes.
3. Platelets and their disorders are discussed in Chapter 14.

G. Iron studies (Fig. 11-7)
1. Serum ferritin
   a. Ferritin is a soluble iron-binding storage protein.
      (1) Primary storage site is in the bone marrow macrophages.
         • See shaded area in the small box in Figure 11-7A.

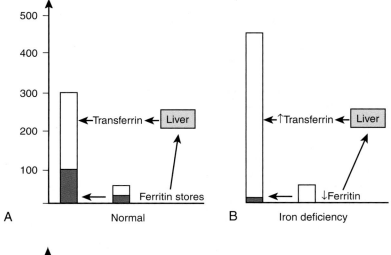

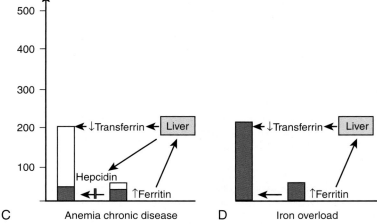

11-7: Iron studies in normal people (**A**) and those with iron deficiency (**B**), anemia of chronic disease (**C**), and iron-overload diseases (**D**). See text for discussion.

(2) Serum levels directly correlate with ferritin stores in the macrophages.
(3) Synthesis of ferritin in macrophages increases in inflammation.
  • Due to release of interleukin 1 and tumor necrosis factor-α
b. Decreased serum ferritin
  • Diagnostic of iron deficiency (see Fig. 11-7B)
c. Increased serum ferritin
  (1) Anemia of chronic disease (ACD) (Fig. 11-7C)
  (2) Iron overload disease (Fig. 11-7D)
d. Hemosiderin
  (1) Insoluble degradation product of ferritin
  (2) Decreased and increased levels correlate with changes in ferritin stores.

> Serum ferritin: ↓ iron deficiency; ↑ ACD, iron overload disease

2. Serum iron
  a. Represents iron bound to transferrin
    (1) Binding protein of iron
    (2) Synthesized in the liver
  b. Serum iron is the shaded area of the column in Figure 11-7A.
    • Note that the normal serum iron level is ~100 μg/dL.
  c. Decreased serum iron
    (1) Iron deficiency (see Fig. 11-7B)
    (2) ACD (see Fig. 11-7C).
  d. Increased serum iron
    (1) Iron overload diseases (see Fig. 11-7D)
    (2) Examples—sideroblastic anemia, hemochromatosis

> Serum iron: ↓ iron deficiency, ACD; ↑ iron overload disease

3. Serum total iron-binding capacity (TIBC)
  a. Serum TIBC correlates with the concentration of transferrin.
    (1) Height of the column in Figure 11-7A correlates with serum transferrin and TIBC.
    (2) Note that the normal TIBC is ~300 μg/dL.

> ↓ TIBC = ↓ transferrin; ↑ TIBC = ↑ transferrin

  b. Relationship of transferrin synthesis with ferritin stores in macrophages
    (1) Decreased ferritin stores cause increased liver synthesis of transferrin (see Fig. 11-7B).
      • Increase in transferrin and TIBC is present in iron deficiency.
    (2) Increased ferritin stores causes decreased liver synthesis of transferrin (see Fig. 11-7C and D).
      • Decrease in transferrin and TIBC occurs in ACD (see Fig. 11-7C) and iron overload disease (see Fig. 11-7D).

> ↓ Ferritin stores = ↑ TIBC; iron deficiency; ↑ ferritin stores = ↓ TIBC; ACD, iron overload

4. Iron saturation (%)
  a. Percentage of binding sites on transferrin occupied by iron
    (1) Iron saturation (%) = serum iron/TIBC × 100
    (2) In Figure 11-7A, the normal % saturation is 100/300 × 100, or 33%.
  b. Decreased iron saturation
    (1) Iron deficiency (see Fig. 11-7B)
    (2) ACD (see Fig. 11-7C)
  c. Increased iron saturation
    • Iron overload disease (see Fig. 11-7D)

> ↓ Iron saturation: iron deficiency, ACD; ↑ iron saturation: iron overload disease

H. Hb electrophoresis
1. Used to detect hemoglobinopathies (Fig. 11-8).
  a. Abnormality in globin chain structure (e.g., sickle cell disease)
  b. Abnormality in globin chain synthesis (e.g., thalassemia)
2. Types of normal Hb detected (Fig. 11-8A)
  a. HbA has 2α/2β globin chains (97% in adults).
  b. HbA₂ has 2α/2δ globin chains (2% in adults).
  c. HbF has 2α/2γ globin chains (1% in adults).

> HbA: 2α/2β
> HbA₂: 2α/2δ
> HbF: 2α/2γ

3. Examples of abnormal Hb detected
  • Sickle Hb, HbH, Hb Bart

III. Microcytic Anemias
A. Types of microcytic anemias
1. Iron deficiency (most common)
2. Anemia of chronic disease (ACD)
3. Thalassemia (α and β)
4. Sideroblastic anemias (least common)

Pattern	Type of Anemia	Interpretation and Discussion
A. A2 (2%), S, F (1%), A (97%)	None	Normal Hb electrophoresis
B. A2 (2%), S, F (1%), A (97%)	Microcytic	α-Thal trait. Note that the proportion of the Hb types remains the same; however, the patient has a microcytic anemia.
C. A2 (5%), S, F (2%), A (93%)	Microcytic	β-Thal minor. Note that HbA is decreased, because β-globin chain synthesis is decreased. There is a corresponding increase in HbA₂ and HbF.
D. A2 (10%), S, F (90%), A	Microcytic	β-Thal major. Note that there is no synthesis of HbA.
E. A2 (2%), S (45%), F (1%), A (52%)	No anemia	Sickle cell trait. Note that there is not enough HbS to cause spontaneous sickling in the peripheral blood.
F. A2 (2%), S (90%), F (8%), A	Normocytic	Sickle cell disease. Note that there is no HbA. There is enough HbS to cause spontaneous sickling.

11-8: Hemoglobin electrophoresis in various hemoglobinopathies. See text for discussion. *(From Goljan EF, Sloka KI: Rapid Review Laboratory Testing in Clinical Medicine. St. Louis, Mosby Elsevier, 2008, p 159, Fig. 5-12.)*

B. **Pathogenesis** (Fig. 11-9)
1. Defects in the synthesis of Hb
   - Hb = heme + globin chains
2. Defects in the synthesis of heme (i.e., iron + protoporphyrin)
   - Iron deficiency, ACD, sideroblastic anemias
3. Defects in the synthesis of globin chains (i.e., α or β)
   - α-Thalassemia, β-thalassemia (thal)

C. **Iron deficiency anemia**
1. Iron reabsorption
   a. Approximately 10% of dietary iron (1–2 mg/day) is reabsorbed in the duodenum.
      (1) Iron from plants is in a nonheme, oxidized form (ferric, Fe^{+3}).
         - Oxidized form *cannot* be reabsorbed in the duodenum.

Microcytic anemias: defects in the synthesis of Hb (heme + globin chains)

Types of iron: reduced Fe^{+2} (heme iron in meat), oxidized Fe^{+3} (nonheme iron in plants)

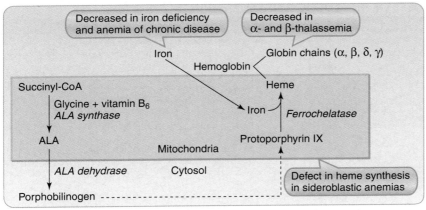

11-9: Pathophysiology of microcytic anemias. See text for discussion. ALA, aminolevulinic acid.

(2) Iron from meat is in a heme, reduced form (ferrous, Fe^{+2})
- Reduced form is directly reabsorbed in the duodenum.

b. Percentage of iron reabsorbed from the diet is increased in the following:
(1) Normal women who have cyclic bleeding
(2) Pregnancy and lactation
(3) Any anemia, regardless of type
- Danger of iron overload, if iron supplements are improperly prescribed

c. Most of the iron is attached to the four heme groups in Hb; the remainder is stored in the following:
(1) Marrow macrophages
- Approximately 1000 mg in men and 400 mg in women
(2) Myoglobin
- Contains one heme group
(3) Enzymes, as a cofactor

d. Gastric acid frees elemental iron from heme and nonheme products.
- Underscores why achlorhydria (absent stomach acid) decreases availability of iron for reabsorption

e. Ascorbic acid is important in iron reabsorption.
- Reduces Fe^{+3} in nonheme foods to the absorbable Fe^{+2}

f. Maintenance of iron homeostasis
(1) Regulation of the amount of iron reabsorbed
(a) HFE (hemochromatosis) gene product facilitates binding of plasma transferrin with its mucosal cell transferrin receptor.
- This allows transferrin to be endocytosed (reabsorbed) by intestinal cells.
(b) Amount of endocytosed transferrin determines how much mucosal cell iron is released into the plasma to bind with transferrin.

2. Epidemiology of iron deficiency
a. It is the most common anemia.
b. Most common nutritional deficiency worldwide
c. Greatest prevalence
(1) Toddlers ages 1 to 2 years old
- Due to inadequate intake
(2) Females ages 12 to 49 years old
- Due to menstrual loss
d. Causes of iron deficiency (Table 11-1)

3. Pathogenesis
- Decreased synthesis of heme (see Fig. 11-9)

4. Clinical and laboratory findings
a. Plummer-Vinson syndrome
(1) Caused by chronic iron deficiency
(2) Esophageal web
- Dysphagia for solids but *not* liquids
(3) Achlorhydria
- Absent acid in the stomach

Margin notes:

Oxidized Fe^{+3} must be reduced to Fe^{+2} for reabsorption in duodenum

Iron: majority stored in marrow macrophages

Ascorbic acid: reduces nonheme iron to Fe^{+2}

Iron deficiency: most common overall anemia

Iron deficiency: most commonly caused by bleeding

Koilonychia: spoon nails; sign of iron deficiency

TABLE 11-1. CAUSES OF IRON DEFICIENCY ANEMIA

CLASSIFICATION	CAUSES	DISCUSSION
Blood loss	Gastrointestinal loss	Meckel's diverticulum (older children)
		PUD (most common cause in adult men)
		Gastritis (e.g., NSAID)
		Hookworm infestation
		Polyps/colorectal cancer (most common cause in adults > 50 years of age); positive stool for blood
	Menorrhagia	Most common cause in women < 50 years of age
Increased utilization	Pregnancy/lactation	Daily iron requirement in pregnancy is 3.4 mg and 2.5–3 mg in lactation
		Net loss of 500 mg of iron if *not* on iron supplements
	Infants/children	Iron required for tissue growth and expansion of blood volume
Decreased intake	Prematurity	Loss of iron each day fetus is not in utero
		Blood loss from phlebotomy
	Infants/children	Most common cause of iron deficiency in young children
	Elderly	Restricted diets with little meat (lack of heme iron)
Decreased absorption	Celiac sprue	Absence of villous surface in the duodenum
	Post-gastric surgery	Rapid transit; absent acid, which helps in iron reabsorption
Intravascular hemolysis	Microangiopathic hemolytic anemia	Chronic loss of Hb in urine leads to iron deficiency
	PNH	

Hb, hemoglobin; PNH, paroxysmal nocturnal hemoglobinuria; PUD, peptic ulcer disease.

(4) Glossitis
- Inflammation of the tongue

(5) Spoon nails (koilonychia; Fig. 11-10)

b. Some patients have a craving (pica) for ice.

c. Laboratory findings

(1) Decreased MCV

(2) Decreased serum iron, iron saturation

(3) Decreased serum ferritin (<30 ng/mL)

(4) Increased TIBC, RDW

Iron deficiency: ↓ iron, % saturation, ferritin; ↑ TIBC, RDW

The **stages of iron deficiency** in sequence are as follows: absent iron stores; decreased serum ferritin; decreased serum iron, increased TIBC, decreased iron saturation; normocytic normochromic anemia; microcytic hypochromic anemia.

Stages of iron deficiency: all lab studies abnormal *before* anemia is present

---

(5) Microcytic and normocytic cells with increased central area of pallor (Fig. 11-11)

(6) Increased serum free erythrocyte protoporphyrin (FEP)
- Less iron combines with protoporphyrin.

(7) Thrombocytosis
(a) Common finding in chronic iron deficiency
(b) Reactive phenomenon to increase blood viscosity

(8) Leukocyte count is usually normal.
- Eosinophilia occurs in hookworm infestations.

5. Treatment

a. Ferrous sulfate, given orally

b. Hct should increase 0.5% to 1%/day after the initial lag period.

c. Lack of response
(1) Noncompliance
(2) Continued blood loss
(3) Iron is not being reabsorbed.

D. Anemia of chronic disease (ACD)

1. Epidemiology

a. Most common anemia in hospitalized patients

b. Common causes
(1) Chronic inflammation
- Examples—rheumatoid arthritis, tuberculosis

Thrombocytosis: common finding in chronic iron deficiency

Rx iron deficiency: ferrous sulfate

ACD: most common anemia in hospitalized patients

ACD: most common anemia in malignancy, alcohol excess

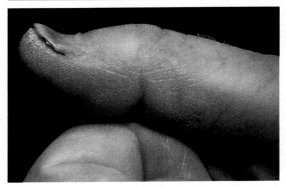

11-10: Koilonychia. Note the spoon shape of the nail bed. *(From Savin JAA, Hunter JAA, Hepburn NC: Diagnosis in Color: Skin Signs in Clinical Medicine. London, Mosby-Wolfe, 1997, p 118, Fig. 4.60.)*

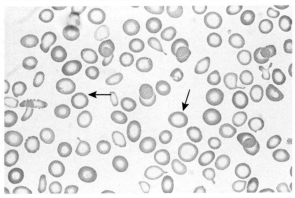

11-11: Peripheral blood smear in iron deficiency anemia. The enlarged central area of pallor in the red blood cell (*arrows*) indicates a decrease in hemoglobin synthesis, which is characteristic of the microcytic anemias. The mean corpuscular hemoglobin concentration is decreased. *(From Wickramasinghe SE, McCullough J: Blood and Bone Marrow Pathology. Philadelphia, Churchill Livingstone, 2003, Fig. 11-6.)*

(2) Alcoholism
- Most common overall anemia

(3) Malignancy
- Most common overall anemia

2. Pathogenesis
   a. Decreased synthesis of heme (see Fig. 11-9)
   b. Decrease renal production of EPO (some cases)
   c. Liver synthesis and release of hepcidin
      (1) Antimicrobial peptide released by the liver in response to inflammation
          - Acute phase reactant (refer to Chapter 2)
      (2) Enters macrophages in the bone marrow
          - Prevents the release of iron to transferrin
      (3) Ferritin synthesis and iron stores increase in bone marrow macrophages.
          - Iron comes into the macrophage but only a little goes out.

3. Laboratory findings
   a. Decreased MCV
   b. Decreased serum iron, TIBC, iron saturation
   c. Increased serum ferritin (>100 ng/mL)
   d. Increased serum FEP
      - Less iron combines with protoporphyrin.
   e. Anemia rarely <9 g/dL.

4. Treatment
   a. Treat the underlying disease causing the inflammation.
   b. In some cases, giving EPO increases the Hb concentration.

E. Thalassemia (thal; α and β)
1. Epidemiology
   a. Autosomal recessive disorders
   b. α-Thal is common in Southeast Asians and in blacks.
   c. β-Thal is common in blacks, Greeks, and Italians.
2. Pathogenesis of α-thal
   a. Decrease in α-globin chain synthesis due to gene deletions (see Fig. 11-9)
      - Four genes control α-globin chain synthesis.
   b. One gene deletion produces a silent carrier.
      - *Not* associated with anemia
   c. The combination of two gene deletions is called α-thal trait (Fig. 11-12).
      (1) Mild anemia with an increased RBC count
      (2) In blacks
          - Associated with a loss of one gene on *each* chromosome (α/– α/–)

Margin notes:

Hepcidin: antimicrobial peptide synthesized/released by liver

Hepcidin: ↑ macrophage iron stores; "reticuloendothelial cell block"

ACD: ↓ iron, TIBC, % saturation; ↑ ferritin

Blacks: can have α- or β-thalassemia

α-Thal: due to gene deletions

α-Thal trait: two gene deletions

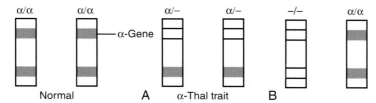

11-12: Gene deletions in α-thalassemia in the black population (**A**) and Asian population (**B**). Four α-genes are involved in α-globin chain synthesis. The black population type is associated with a loss of one gene on each chromosome (*trans* configuration: α/– α/–; schematic A). In the Asian type, there is a loss of both genes on the same chromosome (*cis* configuration: –/– α/α, B). *(From Goljan EF, Sloka KI: Rapid Review Laboratory Testing in Clinical Medicine. St. Louis, Mosby Elsevier, 2008, p 158, Fig. 5-11.)*

      (3) In Asians
         (a) Associated with a loss of both genes on the *same* chromosome (–/– α/α)
         (b) Increased risk for developing more severe types of α-thal
      (4) Decreased MCV, Hb, and Hct
      (5) Increased RBC count
      (6) Normal RDW, serum ferritin, serum FEP, Hb electrophoresis

α-Thal trait: ↓ HbA, HbA₂, HbF (normal electrophoresis); ↑ RBC count

> Hb electrophoresis is normal, because all Hb types require α-globin chains. The Hb concentration is decreased; however, the relative proportions of the normal Hbs remains the same (see Fig. 11-8B).

      (7) Tear drop RBCs in peripheral blood.
        • Damage to RBC membrane from removal of excess globin chains
      (8) There is no treatment.
        • Do *not* treat with iron; danger of iron overload.

HbH: four β-chains

   d. The combination of three gene deletions is called HbH (four β-chains) disease.
      (1) Severe hemolytic anemia
        • Excess β-chain inclusions cause macrophage destruction of the RBCs (hemolytic anemia).
      (2) Hb electrophoresis detects HbH.

Hb Bart: four γ-chains

   e. The combination of four gene deletions is called Hb Bart (four γ-chains) disease.
      (1) Incompatible with life
      (2) Hb electrophoresis shows an increase in Hb Bart.
  3. Pathogenesis of β-thal
   a. Decrease in β-globin chain synthesis (see Fig. 11-9)

β-Thal: mild—DNA splicing defect; severe—stop codon

      (1) Mild anemia is most often due to DNA splicing defects.
      (2) Severe anemia is due to a nonsense mutation with formation of a stop codon.
        • Premature termination of β-globin chain synthesis or absent β-globin chain synthesis.
   b. Normal synthesis of α-, δ-, γ-globin chains

> Normal β-globin chain synthesis is designated β; some β-globin chain synthesis is designated β⁺; absence of β-globin chain synthesis is designated β°.

β-Thal minor: β/β⁺

   c. β-Thal minor (β/β⁺)
      (1) Mild microcytic anemia
      (2) Mild protective effect against falciparum malaria
        • RBC life span is shorter than normal.
      (3) Decreased MCV, Hb, and Hct
      (4) Increased RBC count
      (5) Normal RDW, serum ferritin, FEP
        • Serum FEP is normal because heme synthesis is normal.
      (6) Hb electrophoresis (see Fig. 11-8C)

β-Thal minor: ↓HbA; ↑ RBC count, HbA₂, HbF

        (a) Decreased HbA (2α/2β)
        (b) Increased HbA₂ (2α/2δ) and HbF (2α/2γ)

(7) There is no treatment.
- Do *not* treat with iron; danger of iron overload.

d. β-Thal major (Cooley's anemia; β^0/β^0)

β-Thal major: β^0/β^0

   (1) Severe hemolytic anemia
      (a) RBCs with α-chain inclusions are removed by macrophages in the spleen.
         - Causes an increase in unconjugated bilirubin (jaundice)
      (b) RBCs with α-chain inclusions undergo apoptosis in the bone marrow (ineffective erythropoiesis).
   (2) Extramedullary hematopoiesis
   (3) Increased RDW and reticulocytes
   (4) Hb electrophoresis (see Fig. 11-8D)
      (a) *No* synthesis of HbA

β-Thal major: no HbA;
↑ HbA_2, HbF

      (b) Increase in HbA_2 and HbF
   (5) Long-term transfusion requirement
      - Danger of iron overload (called hemosiderosis)

F. Sideroblastic anemia

1. Epidemiology
   a. Chronic alcoholism (most common cause)
   b. Pyridoxine (vitamin B_6) deficiency
   c. Lead (Pb) poisoning
   d. Hereditary types
      - X-linked recessive inheritance
2. Pathogenesis
   a. Defect in heme synthesis within the mitochondria (see Fig. 11-9)
      (1) Heme is the end-product of porphyrin synthesis.
      (2) Heme has a negative feedback relationship with δ-aminolevulinic acid synthase.
         - δ-Aminolevulinic acid synthase is the rate-limiting enzyme of heme synthesis.

Sideroblastic anemia:
defect in heme synthesis
in the mitochondria;
ringed sideroblasts

   b. Iron accumulates in the mitochondria forming ringed sideroblasts (Fig. 11-13).
   c. Iron-overload type of anemia
      (1) Increase in iron stores in the bone marrow macrophages
      (2) Sideroblasts die in the marrow, and iron is added to the macrophages.
3. Chronic alcoholism
   a. Alcohol is a mitochondrial toxin.
      - Damages heme biosynthetic pathways in the mitochondria

Sideroblastic anemia:
alcohol most common
cause

   b. Sideroblastic anemia occurs in ~30% of hospitalized chronic alcoholics.
4. Pyridoxine deficiency
   a. Vitamin B_6 is a cofactor for δ-aminolevulinic acid synthase.
      - Rate-limiting reaction of heme synthesis (see Fig. 11-9)
   b. Most common cause of deficiency is isoniazid (INH) therapy.
      (1) INH is used in the treatment of tuberculosis.

Pyridoxine deficiency:
INH most common cause

      (2) INH complexes with pyridoxine.
5. Lead (Pb) poisoning
   a. Epidemiology
      (1) Most common in children ages 1 to 5 years old

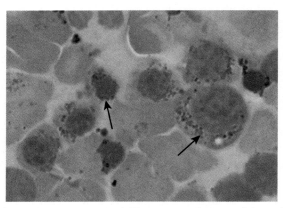

11-13: Ringed sideroblasts in a bone marrow aspirate. Dark blue iron granules around the nucleus of developing normoblasts (*arrows*) represent iron trapped within mitochondria and indicate a defect in mitochondrial heme synthesis. (*From Forbes C, Jackson W: Color Atlas and Text of Clinical Medicine, 2nd ed. St. Louis, Mosby, 2003, p 431, Fig. 10-27.*)

Pb poisoning: paint,
batteries

Pb: denatures
ferrochelatase, ALA
dehydrase, ribonuclease

Pb poisoning: coarse
basophilic stippling

Pb poisoning: Pb deposits
in epiphyses

(2) Causes
   (a) Pica (abnormal craving) for eating lead-based paint
     • Common cause of childhood lead poisoning in inner cities
   (b) Pottery glazes commercial and homemade
(3) Working in a battery or ammunition factory
(4) Radiator repair mechanics
(5) Air contamination from smelter
b. Pb denatures enzymes
  (1) Ferrochelatase (heme synthase)
    (a) Iron cannot bind with protoporphyrin to form heme.
    (b) Increase in serum FEP, which is proximal to the enzyme block
  (2) Aminolevulinic acid (ALA) dehydrase
    • Causes an increase in δ-ALA, which is proximal to the enzyme block
  (3) Ribonuclease
    (a) Ribosomes cannot be degraded and persist in the RBC.
    (b) Produces coarse basophilic stippling (Fig. 11-14)
c. Clinical and laboratory findings
  (1) Abdominal colic with diarrhea
    (a) Pb is visible in the gastrointestinal tract on plain abdominal radiographs (Fig. 11-15).
    (b) Usually occurs in children
  (2) Encephalopathy in children
    (a) δ-ALA damages neurons, increases vessel permeability (cerebral edema), and causes demyelination.
    (b) Learning disabilities in children
  (3) Growth retardation in children
    (a) Pb deposits in the epiphysis of growing bone (Fig. 11-16).
    (b) Radiographs show increased density in the epiphyses.
  (4) Peripheral neuropathy in adults
    • Examples—foot drop (peroneal nerve palsy), wrist drop (radial nerve palsy), claw hand (ulnar nerve palsy)
  (5) Nephrotoxic damage to proximal renal tubules

Tubular damage by lead produces Fanconi syndrome. The syndrome includes proximal renal tubular acidosis (loss of bicarbonate in urine), aminoaciduria, phosphaturia, and glucosuria.

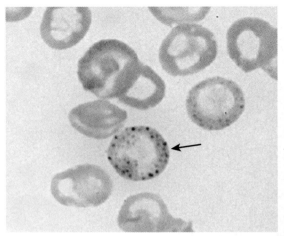

11-14: Peripheral blood with coarse basophilic stippling of red blood cells in lead poisoning. Note the mature red blood cell containing numerous dots representing ribosomes (*arrow*). Lead denatures ribonuclease; hence, the ribosomes persist in the cytoplasm. (*From Naeim F: Atlas of Bone Marrow and Blood Pathology. Philadelphia, WB Saunders, 2001, p 27, Fig. 2-22M.*)

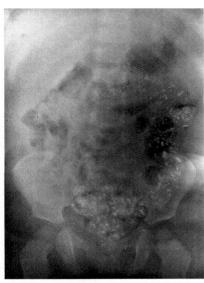

11-15: Abdominal radiograph showing numerous metallic foci representing lead chips. (*From Katz D, Math K, Groskin S: Radiology Secrets. Philadelphia, Hanley & Belfus, 1998, p 310, Fig. 6.*)

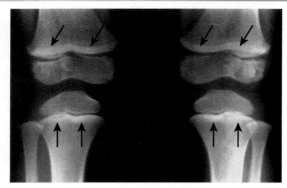

11-16: Bone radiograph showing densities (lead deposits; *arrows*) in the epiphysis of the distal femur and proximal tibia. *(From Katz D, Math K, Groskin S: Radiology Secrets. Philadelphia, Hanley & Belfus, 1998, p 310, Fig. 5.)*

      (6) Pb line in the gums
        • Usually in adults with Pb poisoning and gingivitis
      (7) Increased whole blood and urine Pb levels
        • Best screen and confirmatory test for Pb poisoning
    d. Treatment
      • Chelation therapy—succimer, dimercaprol, EDTA (ethylenediaminetetra-acetic acid)

> Rx Pb poisoning: chelation therapy

  6. Laboratory findings in sideroblastic anemias
    a. Increased serum iron, iron saturation, and ferritin
    b. Decreased MCV and TIBC
    c. Ringed sideroblasts are present in a bone marrow aspirate.
  7. Summary table of microcytic anemias (Table 11-2)

> Sideroblastic anemia: ↑ serum iron, iron saturation, ferritin; ↓ MCV, TIBC

IV. Macrocytic Anemias

• Macrocytic anemias are subdivided into megaloblastic (e.g., folate or vitamin B_{12} deficiency) and nonmegaloblastic anemia (e.g., macrocytosis related to alcohol intoxication).

A. Vitamin B_{12} metabolism

  1. Present in meat, eggs, and dairy products
  2. Parietal cells synthesize intrinsic factor (IF) and hydrochloric acid (HCl).
  3. Gastric acid converts pepsinogen to pepsin.
    • Pepsin frees vitamin B_{12} from ingested proteins.
  4. Free vitamin B_{12} is bound to R-binders synthesized in the salivary glands.
  5. Pancreatic enzymes in the duodenum cleave off the R-binders.
    • Vitamin B_{12} binds to IF to form a complex.
  6. Vitamin B_{12}-IF complex is reabsorbed in the terminal ileum.
  7. Vitamin B_{12} binds to transcobalamin II and is secreted into plasma.
    • Delivered to metabolically active cells or stored in the liver (6–9 years)

> Vitamin B_{12}: only present in animal products
>
> Parietal cells: synthesize IF and HCl
>
> Vitamin B_{12}: reabsorbed in terminal ileum

TABLE 11-2. LABORATORY FINDINGS IN MICROCYTIC ANEMIAS

TEST	IRON DEFICIENCY	ANEMIA OF CHRONIC DISEASE	α-THAL/β-THAL MINOR	LEAD POISONING
MCV	↓	↓	↓	↓
Serum iron	↓	↓	Normal	↑
TIBC	↑	↓	Normal	↓
Percent saturation	↓	↓	Normal	↑
Serum ferritin	↓	↑	Normal	↑
RDW	↑	Normal	Normal	Normal
RBC count	↓	↓	↑	↓
Hb electrophoresis	Normal	Normal	α-Thal trait: normal	—
Ringed sideroblasts	None	None	None	Present
Coarse basophilic stippling	None	None	None	Present

Hb, hemoglobin; MCV, mean corpuscular volume; RDW, red blood cell distribution width; Thal, thalassemia; TIBC, total iron-binding capacity.

TABLE 11-3. **CAUSES OF VITAMIN B$_{12}$ DEFICIENCY**

CLASSIFICATION	CAUSES	DISCUSSION
Decreased intake	Pure vegan diet Malnutrition	Breast-fed infants of pure vegans may develop deficiency May occur in elderly patients
Malabsorption	↓ Intrinsic factor ↓ Gastric acid ↓ Intestinal reabsorption	Autoimmune destruction of parietal cells (i.e., pernicious anemia) Cannot activate pepsinogen to release vitamin B$_{12}$ Crohn's disease or celiac disease involving terminal ileum (destruction of absorptive cells) Bacterial overgrowth (bacterial utilization of available vitamin B$_{12}$) Fish tapeworm Chronic pancreatitis (cannot cleave off R-binder)
Increased utilization	Pregnancy/lactation	Deficiency is more likely in a pure vegan

Vitamin B$_{12}$ deficiency: pernicious anemia most common cause

Intestinal conjugase: inhibited by phenytoin

Monoglutamate reabsorption: inhibited by alcohol and oral contraceptives

Folate deficiency: alcohol most common cause

Vitamin B$_{12}$/folate deficiency: delayed nuclear maturation; megaloblasts

Vitamin B$_{12}$/folate deficiency: pancytopenia; apoptosis, macrophage phagocytosis

B. Causes of vitamin B$_{12}$ deficiency (Table 11-3)

C. Folate metabolism

1. Present in green vegetables and animal proteins
   - In the form of polyglutamates
2. Converted to monoglutamates by intestinal conjugase
   - Intestinal conjugase is inhibited by phenytoin.
3. Monoglutamates are reabsorbed in the jejunum.
   a. Converted to methyltetrahydrofolate, the circulating form of folate
   b. Reabsorption is blocked by alcohol and oral contraceptives.
   c. There is only a 3- to 4-month supply of folate in the liver.

D. Causes of folate deficiency (Table 11-4)

E. Pathogenesis of macrocytic anemia in folate and vitamin B$_{12}$ deficiency

1. Impaired DNA synthesis
   a. Delayed nuclear maturation
      (1) Causes a block in cell division leading to large, nucleated hematopoietic cells
      (2) Enlarged cells are called megaloblasts (Fig. 11-17).
   b. Affects all rapidly dividing cells
      - Examples—RBCs, leukocytes, platelets, intestinal epithelium
   c. Cellular RNA and protein synthesis continue unabated.
      - Cytoplasmic volume continues to expand.
2. Ineffective erythropoiesis
   a. Megaloblastic precursors outside the bone marrow sinusoids are phagocytosed by macrophages.
   b. Megaloblastic precursors undergo apoptosis causing pancytopenia.
      - Anemia, neutropenia, and thrombocytopenia

F. Vitamin B$_{12}$ and folate in DNA synthesis (Fig. 11-18)

1. Vitamin B$_{12}$ removes the methyl group from methyltetrahydrofolate (N^5-methyl-FH$_4$).
   a. Produces tetrahydrofolate (FH$_4$)

TABLE 11-4. **CAUSES OF FOLATE DEFICIENCY**

CLASSIFICATION	CAUSES	DISCUSSION
Decreased intake	Malnutrition Infants/elderly Chronic alcoholics Goat milk	Decreased intake most common cause of folate deficiency
Malabsorption	Celiac disease Bacterial overgrowth	Deficiency usually occurs in association with other vitamin deficiencies (fat and water soluble)
Drug inhibition	5-Fluorouracil Methotrexate, trimethoprim- sulfamethoxazole Phenytoin Oral contraceptives, alcohol	Inhibits thymidylate synthase Inhibit dihydrofolate reductase Inhibits intestinal conjugase Inhibit uptake of monoglutamate in jejunum Alcohol also inhibits the release of folate from the liver.
Increased utilization	Pregnancy/lactation Disseminated malignancy Severe hemolytic anemia	Increased utilization of folate in DNA synthesis

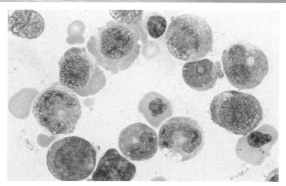

11-17: Megaloblasts in a bone marrow aspirate. Note the open chromatin pattern and enlarged nuclei of red blood cell and white blood cell precursors indicating a lack of nuclear maturation. *(From Goldman L, Ausiello, D: Cecil's Textbook of Medicine, 23rd ed. Philadelphia, Saunders Elsevier, 2008, p 1239, Fig. 170-4.)*

b. Methyl-vitamin B_{12} transfers the methyl group to homocysteine to produce methionine.
  • Deficiency of vitamin B_{12} traps N^5-methyl-FH_4 in its circulating form; may falsely increase the serum folate in 30% of cases.
c. Deficiency of folate or vitamin B_{12} increases plasma homocysteine.

↑ Homocysteine: folate (most common) and vitamin B_{12} deficiency

Folate deficiency is the most common cause of increased serum homocysteine levels in the United States. Homocysteine damages endothelial cells leading to vessel thrombosis.

2. Thymidylate synthase converts deoxyuridine monophosphate (dUMP) to deoxythymidine monophosphate (dTMP).
  • Thymidylate synthase is irreversibly inhibited by 5-fluorouracil.
3. Dihydrofolate reductase converts dihydrofolate (FH_2) to FH_4.
  • Dihydrofolate reductase is inhibited by methotrexate and trimethoprim.

Thymidylate synthase: irreversibly inhibited by 5-fluorouracil

Dihydrofolate reductase: inhibited by methotrexate (reversible), trimethoprim

G. Vitamin B_{12} in odd-chain fatty acid metabolism (Fig. 11-19)
1. Propionyl CoA is converted to methylmalonyl CoA.
2. Methylmalonyl CoA is converted to succinyl CoA.
  • Vitamin B_{12} is a cofactor for methylmalonyl CoA mutase.
3. Vitamin B_{12} deficiency causes an increase in propionyl and methylmalonyl CoA and their corresponding acids.
  • Propionyl CoA replaces acetyl CoA in neuronal membranes resulting in demyelination.

Vitamin B_{12}: odd chain fatty acid metabolism

H. Clinical findings in vitamin B_{12} deficiency
1. Findings in pernicious anemia (PA)
  a. Increased incidence in blood group A individuals

PA: ↑ incidence blood group A

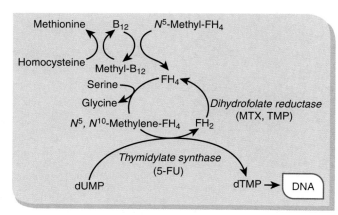

11-18: Vitamin B_{12} and folate in DNA metabolism. See text for discussion. dTMP, deoxythymidine monophosphate; dUMP, deoxyuridine monophosphate; FH_2, dihydrofolate; FH_4, tetrahydrofolate; FU, fluorouracil; MTX, methotrexate; TMP, trimethoprim. *(From Pelley J, Goljan EF: Rapid Review: Biochemistry. St. Louis, Mosby, 2004, Fig. 4-3.)*

Odd-chain
fatty acid
oxidation

ATP + CO$_2$ ADP

Propionyl   *Propionyl CoA*   Methylmalonyl ——— *Methylmalonyl*   Succinyl ——— Citric
CoA   *carboxylase*   CoA   *CoA mutase*   CoA   acid
(3 carbons) *(biotin)*   *(vitamin B$_{12}$)*   cycle

Methionine
Isoleucine
Valine   Gluconeogenesis

11-19: Odd-chain fatty acid metabolism. See text for discussion. *(From Pelley J, Goljan E: Rapid Review Biochemistry, 2nd ed. Philadelphia, Mosby, 2007, p 117, Fig. 7-4.)*

PA: ↑ incidence blood
group A

PA: type II hypersensitivity

PA: ↑ antibodies, gastrin
levels

    b. Achlorhydria (lack of gastric acid) due to destruction of parietal cells
      (1) Maldigestion of food
      (2) Hypergastrinemia
        • Due to loss of acid inhibition of gastrin
    c. Antibodies associated with pernicious anemia (type II hypersensitivity)
      (1) Antibodies directed against the proton pump in parietal cells (85–90% of cases)
      (2) Antibodies that block binding of vitamin B$_{12}$ to IF (60–75% of cases)
        • Most specific test for pernicious anemia
      (3) Antibodies that prevent binding of vitamin B$_{12}$-IF complexes to ileal receptors (30–50% of cases)
    d. Antibody destruction of parietal cells causes chronic atrophic gastritis of the body and fundus.
      • Increased incidence of gastric adenocarcinoma
  2. Smooth, sore tongue with atrophy of papillae
  3. Neurologic disease

Vitamin B$_{12}$ deficiency:
posterior columns, lateral
corticospinal tract, dorsal
spinocerebellar tract

Macrocytic anemia
neurologic disease:
vitamin B$_{12}$ deficiency

↑ Methylmalonic acid:
most sensitive test for
vitamin B$_{12}$ deficiency

    a. Peripheral neuropathy with sensorimotor dysfunction
    b. Subacute combined degeneration (demyelination) of the spinal cord (Fig. 11-20)
      (1) Posterior column dysfunction
        • Decrease in vibratory sensation and proprioception (joint sense)
      (2) Lateral corticospinal tract dysfunction with spasticity
    c. Dorsal spinocerebellar tract demyelination
      • Produces ataxia
    d. Dementia
    e. Possible to have neurologic disease without anemia
I. Laboratory findings in vitamin B$_{12}$ deficiency
  1. Decreased serum vitamin B$_{12}$
  2. Increased serum homocysteine and methylmalonic acid (95% of cases)

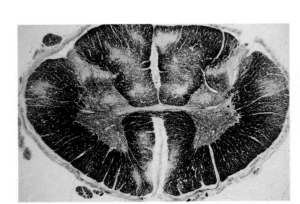

11-20: Subacute combined degeneration of the thoracic cervical cord. Note the pale areas of demyelination in the posterior columns and the lateral corticospinal tracts. *(From Wickramasinghe SN, McCullough J: Blood and Bone Marrow Pathology. London, Churchill Livingstone, 2003, p 237, Fig. 12-10B.)*

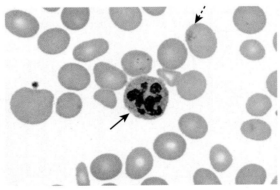

11-21: Peripheral blood in megaloblastic anemia showing a hypersegmented neutrophil *(solid arrow)* with nine lobes. Neutrophils normally have less than five nuclear segments. Hypersegmented neutrophils are excellent markers of folate and vitamin B$_{12}$ deficiency. The enlarged, egg-shaped red blood cells (macro-ovalocytes; *interrupted arrow)* characteristic of macrocytic anemias are associated with problems in DNA maturation. *(From Naeim F: Atlas of Bone Marrow and Blood Pathology. Philadelphia, WB Saunders, 2001, p 180, Fig. 14-10B.)*

3. Peripheral blood findings
   a. Pancytopenia
   b. Oval macrocytes
   c. Hypersegmented neutrophils (Fig. 11-21)
      • More than five nuclear lobes
4. Bone marrow findings
   • Megaloblastic nucleated cells with primitive open (lacy) chromatin pattern
5. Schilling test localizes some of the causes of vitamin B_{12} deficiency.
   • Although it is *not* routinely performed anymore, it is a good review of causes of vitamin B_{12} deficiency.

Hypersegmented neutrophil: marker for folate or vitamin B_{12} deficiency

Schilling test: defines the cause of vitamin B_{12} deficiency

The **Schilling test** has been used in the past to demonstrate impairment of reabsorption of vitamin B_{12}. This is achieved indirectly by combining orally administered radioactive vitamin B_{12} with IF, or with pancreatic extract, or alone after pretreatment with antibiotics followed by a 24-hour urine collection to measure radioactive vitamin B_{12}. Lack of reabsorption of radioactive vitamin B_{12} excludes a potential cause of impaired reabsorption, while the presence of reabsorption confirms the cause of the impaired reabsorption. For example, if the combination of radioactive vitamin B_{12} + IF leads to an increase in radioactive vitamin B_{12} in the urine, the patient has pernicious anemia; if it does not, the diagnosis of pernicious anemia is excluded. Similarly, correction with pancreatic extract implicates chronic pancreatitis as the cause or bacterial overgrowth as the cause, if antibiotics correct the reabsorption.

J. Clinical findings in folate deficiency
   1. Similar to vitamin B_{12} deficiency with the *exception* of neurologic disease
   2. Increased risk for open neural tube defects in the fetus
      • Due to decreased maternal intake of folate *prior* to conception
K. Laboratory findings in folate deficiency
   1. Peripheral blood and bone marrow findings are similar to vitamin B_{12} deficiency.
   2. Decreased serum folate and RBC folate (best screening test)
L. Treatment of vitamin B_{12} and folate deficiency
   1. Treatment of vitamin B_{12} deficiency
      a. Intramuscular injection of vitamin B_{12}
      b. Treatment is indefinite in pernicious anemia.
   2. Treatment of folate deficiency
      • Oral administration of monoglutamic folic acid

↓ Maternal intake of folate: increased risk for open neural tube defect in newborn

RBC folate: best indicator of folate stores

It is important to distinguish folate from vitamin B_{12} deficiency. Pharmacologic doses of folate will correct the hematologic findings in both folate and vitamin B_{12} deficiency; however, neurologic disease is *not* corrected.

M. Comparison table of vitamin B_{12} and folate deficiency (Table 11-5)
N. Nonmegaloblastic macrocytosis
   1. General differences from megaloblastic macrocytic anemias
      a. Macrocytes are round rather than oval

TABLE 11-5. CLINICAL AND LABORATORY FINDINGS IN VITAMIN B_{12} AND FOLATE DEFICIENCIES

LABORATORY/CLINICAL FINDING	PERNICIOUS ANEMIA	OTHER VITAMIN B_{12} DEFICIENCIES	FOLATE DEFICIENCY
Achlorhydria	Present	Absent	Absent
Autoantibodies	Present	Absent	Absent
Chronic atrophic gastritis	Present	Absent	Absent
Gastric carcinoma risk	↑	None	None
Hypersegmented neutrophils	Present	Present	Present
Mean corpuscular volume	↑	↑	↑
Neurologic disease	Present	Present	None
Pancytopenia	Present	Present	Present
Plasma homocysteine	↑	↑	↑
Serum gastrin level	↑	Normal	Normal
Urine methylmalonic acid	↑	↑	Normal

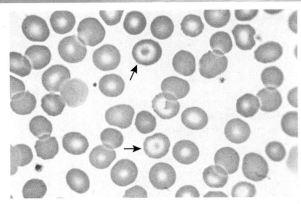

11-22: Round macrocytes and target cells in chronic alcoholism. Note the round macrocytes with target cell formation (*arrows*). (*From Wickramasinghe SN, McCullough J: Blood and Bone Marrow Pathology. London, Churchill Livingstone, 2003, Fig. 6-2F.*)

b. Hypersegmented neutrophils are *not* present.
c. Leukocytes and platelets are quantitatively normal.
d. Absence of glossitis and neuropathy
e. Anemia may *not* be present.
f. Alcohol excess is the most common cause for all types of the macrocytosis.

2. Liver disease associated with alcohol

a. MCV ranges from $105 \pm 10 \ \mu m^3$.

Alcohol liver disease: round macrocytic target cells

b. Thin, round, macrocytic target cells (Fig. 11-22)
• Excess RBC membrane due to increased membrane cholesterol
c. Life span of the RBCs is *not* decreased; there is no anemia.

3. Direct toxic effect of alcohol

a. MCV ranges from 100 to 110 μm^3.
b. Vacuolization of RBC precursors in bone marrow
c. Abstinence from alcohol reverses the macrocytosis and anemia.

V. **Normocytic Anemias: Corrected Reticulocyte Count or Index < 3%**

A. **Acute blood loss**

1. Epidemiology

Acute blood loss: external, internal

a. External blood loss
• Examples—open fractures, knife wound
b. Internal blood loss
• Examples—ruptured abdominal aortic aneurysm; ruptured spleen
c. Most common cause of hypovolemic shock

Signs volume depletion: ↓ blood pressure, ↑ pulse

2. Clinical and laboratory findings (refer to Chapter 4)
3. Requires 5 to 7 days *before* a reticulocyte response is observed

B. **Early iron deficiency or ACD**

1. Anemia is normocytic *before* it becomes microcytic.
• ACD is microcytic in only 10% to 30% of cases.
2. Serum ferritin is most useful in distinguishing the two anemias.

Aplastic anemia: most cases idiopathic; drugs most common known cause

C. **Aplastic anemia**

1. Causes (Table 11-6)

TABLE 11-6. CAUSES OF APLASTIC ANEMIA

CLASSIFICATION	EXAMPLES AND DISCUSSION
Idiopathic	Approximately 50–70% of cases are idiopathic
Drugs	Most common known cause of aplastic anemia Dose-related causes are usually reversible (e.g., alkylating agents) Idiosyncratic reactions are frequently irreversible (e.g., chloramphenicol)
Chemical agents	Toxic chemicals in industry and agriculture (e.g., benzene, insecticides–DDT, parathion)
Infection	May involve all hematopoietic cell lines (pancytopenia) or erythroid cell line alone (pure RBC aplasia) Examples—EBV; CMV; parvovirus; non-A, non-B hepatitis, HCV
Physical agents	Whole-body ionizing radiation (therapeutic or nuclear accident)
Miscellaneous	Thymoma (may be associated with pure RBC aplasia) Paroxysmal nocturnal hemoglobinuria

CMV, cytomegalovirus; EBV, Epstein-Barr virus; HCV, hepatitis C.

2. Pathogenesis
   a. Antigenic alteration of myeloid stem cells
      • Causes T-cell activation and release of cytokines that suppress myeloid stem cells
   b. Defective or deficient myeloid stem cells (acquired or hereditary)
3. Clinical findings
   a. Fever due to infection associated with neutropenia
   b. Bleeding due to thrombocytopenia
   c. Fatigue due to anemia

Aplastic anemia: fever, bleeding, fatigue

4. Laboratory findings
   a. Pancytopenia
   b. Reticulocytopenia
   c. Hypocellular bone marrow (Fig. 11-23)

Aplastic anemia: pancytopenia

5. Complete recovery occurs in < 10% of cases.
6. Treatment
   a. Discontinue drug, if it is responsible
   b. Broad-spectrum antibiotics to prevent infection
   c. Transfusions with irradiated blood (if not a bone marrow transplant candidate)
      • Prevents graft-versus-host reaction (refer to Chapter 3)
   d. Immunosuppressive therapy
      • Examples—antilymphocyte globulin, cyclophosphamide, cyclosporin
   e. Bone marrow transplantation
      • Good prognosis if patient is young and a compatible donor is found

D. Chronic renal failure (CRF)
1. Pathogenesis
   • Decreased synthesis of EPO (most common cause)

Anemia CRF: ↓ EPO most common cause

2. Laboratory findings
   a. Normocytic anemia
   b. Presence of burr cells (i.e., RBCs with an undulating membrane)
   c. Platelet dysfunction
      (1) Thrombocytopenia
      (2) Defect in platelet aggregation that is reversible with dialysis
         • Prolonged bleeding time

CRF: platelet dysfunction

E. Malignancy
1. ACD most common anemia
2. Gastrointestinal bleeding (e.g., colorectal cancer)
   • Could be normocytic or microcytic
3. Metastasis to bone marrow
   a. Malignant cells displace normal marrow hematopoietic cells into peripheral blood
      • Called myelophthisic anemia
   b. Presence of nucleated RBCs and immature myeloid cells into the peripheral blood is called leukoerythroblastic smear (see Fig. 12-1).
4. Immune hemolytic anemia (IHA)
   • Example—cold type IHA in chronic lymphocytic leukemia

Anemia malignancy: ACD, blood loss, metastasis to marrow, immunologic

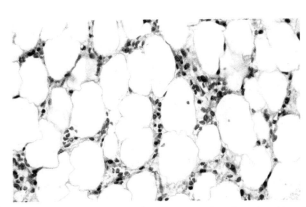

11-23: Bone marrow biopsy in aplastic anemia. The biopsy shows a marrow largely replaced by adipose cells. Scattered lymphocytes are present in between adipose cells. *(From Kumar V, Fausto N, Abbas A: Robbins and Cotran's Pathologic Basis of Disease, 7th ed. Philadelphia, WB Saunders, 2004, Fig. 13-27B.)*

VI. Normocytic Anemias: Corrected Reticulocyte Count ≥ 3%
A. Pathogenesis of hemolytic anemias
1. Intrinsic or extrinsic hemolytic anemias
   a. Intrinsic refers to a defect in the RBC causing the anemia.
      - Examples—membrane defects, abnormal Hb, enzyme deficiency
   b. Extrinsic refers to factors outside the RBC causing hemolysis.
      - Examples—stenotic aortic valve, immune destruction
2. Mechanisms of hemolysis (Fig. 11-24)
   a. Extravascular hemolysis
      (1) RBC phagocytosis by macrophages in the spleen (most common site) and liver
      (2) Reasons for phagocytosis
         (a) RBCs coated by IgG with or without C3b
         (b) Abnormally shaped RBCs (e.g., spherocytes, sickle cells)
      (3) Increase in serum unconjugated bilirubin
         - End-product of macrophage degradation of Hb
      (4) Increased serum lactate dehydrogenase (LDH) from hemolyzed RBCs
   b. Intravascular hemolysis
      (1) Hemolysis occurs within blood vessels.
      (2) Causes of hemolysis
         (a) Enzyme deficiency (e.g., deficiency of glucose-6-phosphate dehydrogenase)
         (b) Complement destruction (e.g., IgM-mediated hemolysis)
         (c) Mechanical damage (e.g., calcific aortic valve stenosis)
      (3) Increased plasma and urine Hb
      (4) Hemosiderinuria
         - Renal tubules convert iron in Hb into hemosiderin.
      (5) Decreased serum haptoglobin

Types hemolytic anemia: intrinsic (defect in RBC), extrinsic (factors outside RBC)

Extravascular hemolysis: macrophage phagocytosis; unconjugated hyperbilirubinemia

Intravascular hemolysis: ↓ serum haptoglobin; hemoglobinuria

> **Haptoglobin** is an acute phase reactant that combines with Hb to form a complex that is phagocytosed and degraded by macrophages causing a decrease in serum haptoglobin. The amount of Hb in the complexes is so small that unconjugated bilirubin is *not* significantly increased enough to produce jaundice in most cases.

   (6) Increased serum LDH from hemolyzed RBCs.

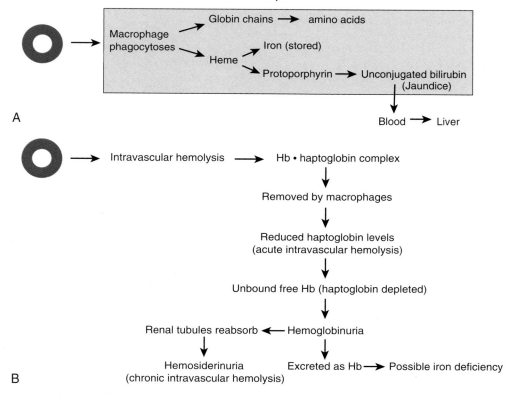

11-24: Extravascular (**A**) and intravascular (**B**) hemolysis of red blood cells. See text for discussion. *(From Goljan EF: Star Series: Pathology. Philadelphia, WB Saunders, 1998, Fig. 12-2.)*

B. Hereditary spherocytosis
1. Pathogenesis
   a. Autosomal dominant disorder
   b. Intrinsic defect with extravascular hemolysis
   c. Membrane protein defect results in the loss of RBC membrane and spherocyte formation.
      (1) Mutation in ankyrin is the most common defect.
      (2) Mutation in band 2, spectrin (α and β), or band 3 account for other defects.
   d. Increased permeability of spherocytes to sodium
      • Due to membrane defect and dysfunctional Na^+/K^+-ATPase pump
2. Clinical findings
   a. Jaundice due to increased unconjugated bilirubin
   b. Increased incidence of calcium bilirubinate gallstones
      • Due to increased concentration of conjugated bilirubin in bile
   c. Splenomegaly
   d. Aplastic crisis
      • May occur in children especially after a viral infection (e.g., parvovirus)
3. Laboratory findings
   a. Normocytic anemia with spherocytosis (Fig. 11-25)
      • Other causes of spherocytosis—warm immune hemolytic anemia, ABO hemolytic disease of newborn
   b. Increased MCHC
   c. Increased RBC osmotic fragility
      (1) Increased permeability of spherocytes to sodium and water
      (2) Spherocytes rupture in mildly hypotonic salt solutions.
4. Treatment is splenectomy.
   • Spherocytes remain in the peripheral blood.

C. Hereditary elliptocytosis
1. Pathogenesis
   a. Autosomal dominant disorder
   b. Defective spectrin and band 4.1
2. Clinical findings
   a. Majority have no anemia or a mild hemolytic anemia.
   b. Splenomegaly
3. Laboratory findings
   a. Elliptocytes > 25% of RBCs in peripheral blood (Fig. 11-26)
   b. Increased osmotic fragility
4. Treatment is splenectomy in symptomatic patients.

D. Paroxysmal nocturnal hemoglobinuria (PNH)
1. Pathogenesis
   a. Acquired membrane defect in myeloid stem cells
      (1) Mutation causes loss of the anchor for decay accelerating factor (DAF).

Margin notes:
Hereditary spherocytosis: intrinsic defect, extravascular hemolysis

Hereditary spherocytosis: mutation in ankyrin in cell membrane

Hereditary spherocytosis: black, calcium bilirubinate gallstones

Aplastic crisis: parvovirus induced

Hereditary spherocytosis: ↑ RBC osmotic fragility

Hereditary elliptocytosis: >25% elliptocytes in peripheral blood

PNH: loss of anchor for DAF

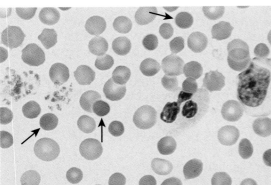

11-25: Peripheral blood with spherocytes in hereditary spherocytosis. Numerous, round, dense red blood cells without central areas of pallor represent spherocytes (*arrows*). The mean corpuscular hemoglobin concentration is increased. *(From Damjanov I, Linder J: Pathology: A Color Atlas. St. Louis, Mosby, 2000, p 75, Fig. 5-7.)*

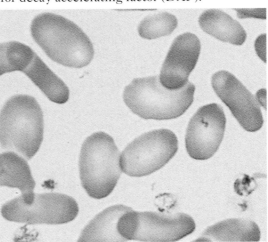

11-26: Peripheral blood with elliptocytes. In hereditary elliptocytosis, elliptocytes constitute more than 25% of the red blood cells, as in this smear. *(From Damjanov I, Linder J: Pathology: A Color Atlas. St. Louis, Mosby, 2000, Fig. 5-8A.)*

(2) Normally DAF destabilizes C3 and C5 convertase adhering to RBCs, platelets, and neutrophils (refer to Chapter 3).
  • Prevents activation of the membrane attack complex and subsequent lysis of RBCs, neutrophils, and platelets
  b. Intravascular complement-mediated lysis of RBCs, neutrophils, and platelets
    • Occurs at night, because respiratory acidosis enhances complement attachment to these cells
    • PNH: intrinsic defect, intravascular hemolysis
2. Clinical findings
  a. Episodic hemoglobinuria
    • May cause iron deficiency
  b. Increased incidence of vessel thrombosis (e.g., hepatic vein)
    • Due to the release of aggregating agents from destroyed platelets
  c. Increased risk for developing acute myelogenous leukemia
3. Peripheral blood findings
  a. Normocytic anemia with pancytopenia
    • Microcytic if iron deficiency develops from hemoglobinuria
  b. Decreased leukocyte alkaline phosphatase
  c. Decreased serum haptoglobin
  d. Increased serum/urine Hb
4. Diagnosis
  a. Identify the defect on hematopoietic cells
    • Most sensitive test
  b. Older tests
    (1) Screening test is the sucrose hemolysis test (sugar water test).
      • Sucrose enhances complement destruction of RBCs.
    (2) Confirmatory test is the acidified serum test (Ham test).
      • Acidified serum activates the alternative pathway causing hemolysis.

E. Sickle cell anemia
1. Epidemiology
  a. Autosomal recessive disorder
  b. Most common hemoglobinopathy in blacks
  c. Heterozygote condition (sickle cell trait, HbAS) has no anemia.
    • Present in ~10% of blacks
  d. Homozygous condition (HbSS) produces anemia.
  e. Pedigree with sickle cell trait persons
    (1) Normal child 25%
    (2) Sickle cell trait 50%
    (3) Sickle cell disease 25%
  f. Protective against *Plasmodium falciparum* malaria
2. Pathogenesis
  a. Predominantly extravascular hemolysis of sickle cells
  b. Missense point mutation
    • Substitution of valine for glutamic acid at sixth position of β-globin chain
  c. Causes of sickling
    (1) HbS molecules aggregate and polymerize into long needle-like fibers.
      • RBCs assume a sickle or boat-like shape (Fig. 11-27).
    (2) Sickle Hb (HbS) concentration greater than 60% is the most important factor for sickling.
      • HbS concentration is too low in HbAS to produce sickling in the peripheral blood.
    (3) Increase in deoxyhemoglobin (correlates with decreased O_2 saturation) increases the risk for sickling.
      (a) Acidosis
        • Right-shifts the OBC causing O_2 release from RBCs
      (b) Volume depletion
        • Intracellular dehydration causes an increase in concentration of deoxyhemoglobin
      (c) Hypoxemia
        • Decrease in arterial Po_2 decreases O_2 saturation of Hb.
  d. Reversible and irreversible sickling
    (1) Initial sickling is reversible with administration of O_2.

PNF: intrinsic defect, intravascular hemolysis

PNH: pancytopenia

PNH: screen—sucrose hemolysis test; confirm—acidified serum test

Trait × trait: 25% normal, 50% trait, 25% disease

Sickle cell anemia: intrinsic defect, extravascular hemolysis

Sickle cell anemia: missense mutation; substitution of valine for glutamic acid

Sickling: ↑ HbS, ↑ deoxyHb

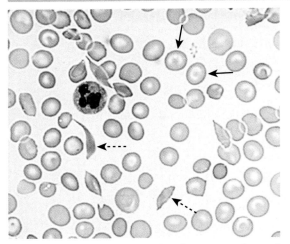

11-27: Peripheral blood with sickle cells (*interrupted arrows*) and target cells, showing the dense, boat-shaped sickle cells. Cells with a bull's-eye appearance are target cells (*solid arrows*), which have excess RBC membrane that bulges in the center of the cell. (*From Hoffbrand AV: Color Atlas: Clinical Hematology, 3rd ed. St. Louis, Mosby, 2000, p 103, Fig. 5-85A.*)

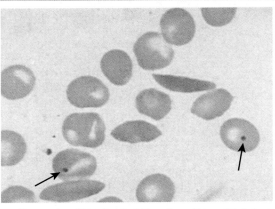

11-28: Peripheral blood with sickle cells and Howell-Jolly bodies. The three dense boat-shaped sickle cells and the two cells containing a single dark, round inclusion (*arrows*) represent nuclear remnants. Howell-Jolly bodies in sickle cell disease indicate splenic dysfunction. (*From Henry JB: Clinical Diagnosis and Management by Laboratory Methods, 20th ed. Philadelphia, WB Saunders, 2001, Fig. 26-2A.*)

    (2) Recurrent sickling causes irreversible sickling due to membrane damage.
    (3) Irreversibly sickled cells have increased adherence to endothelial cells in the microcirculation.
       • Microvascular occlusions (vaso-occlusive crises) produce ischemic damage.
  e. HbF prevents sickling.
    (1) Increased HbF at birth prevents sickling in HbSS for 5 to 6 months.
    (2) Hydroxyurea increases the synthesis of HbF.
  f. Key pathologic processes in HbSS
    (1) Severe hemolytic anemia
    (2) Painful vaso-occlusive crises
 3. Clinical findings in HbSS
  a. Dactylitis (hand-foot syndrome)
    (1) Painful swelling of hands and feet
       • Pain due to bone infarctions
    (2) Occurs in infants (usually 6–9 months old)
  b. Acute chest syndrome
    (1) Most common cause of death in adults
    (2) Precipitated by
      (a) Pneumonia
        • *Streptococcus pneumoniae*, *Mycoplasma*, viruses
      (b) Infarction
      (c) Fat embolism
    (3) Clinical findings
      (a) Chest pain
      (b) Wheezing
      (c) Dyspnea
    (4) Laboratory
      • Hypoxemia
    (5) Chest x-ray reveals lung infiltrates.
  c. Aseptic necrosis of the femoral head (see Fig. 23-6)
  d. Autosplenectomy
    (1) Spleen is enlarged but dysfunctional by 2 years of age.
      • Nuclear remnants (Howell-Jolly bodies) appear in RBCs indicating loss of macrophage function (Fig. 11-28).
    (2) Spleen is fibrosed and diminished in size in young adults.

Irreversible sickle cell: increased adherence to endothelial cells

Sickling: HbF prevents sickling
Hydroxyurea: ↑ HbF

Sickle cell anemia: severe hemolytic anemia; vaso-occlusive crises

Dactylitis: most common presentation in infants

Acute chest syndrome: most common cause of death in adults

Howell-Jolly bodies: sign of splenic dysfunction

e. Increased susceptibility to infections
   (1) Due to dysfunctional spleen
      • Impaired opsonization of encapsulated bacteria
   (2) Children are at risk for *Streptococcus pneumoniae* sepsis.
      (a) Most common cause of death in children
      (b) Prophylactic penicillin recommended
   (3) Increased incidence of osteomyelitis
      • Most often due to *Salmonella paratyphi*; less frequently to *Staphylococcus aureus*

f. Aplastic crisis
   (1) Reticulocytopenia
   (2) Association with parvovirus
g. Sequestration crisis
   (1) Rapid splenic enlargement
      • Entrapment of RBCs causing hypovolemia
   (2) Reticulocytosis

h. Increased risk for calcium bilirubinate gallstones
   • Due to increased conjugated bilirubin in bile from chronic hemolysis
i. Strokes
4. Renal findings in HbAS (also in HbSS)
   a. Sickling may occur in peritubular capillaries in the medulla.
      • Due to the low O_2 tension in the medulla
   b. Presents with microhematuria due to infarctions
      • Always order a sickle cell screen in black patients with unexplained hematuria.
   c. Renal papillary necrosis may occur.
      • Loss of concentration and dilution

5. Laboratory findings
   a. Sickle cell screen
      • Sodium metabisulfite reduces O_2 tension, which induces sickling.
   b. Hb electrophoresis (see Fig. 11-8E and F)
      (1) HbAS profile—HbA 55% to 60%, HbS 40% to 45%
      (2) HbSS profile—HbS 90% to 95%, HbF 5% to 10%, no HbA
   c. Peripheral blood findings
      (1) Normal peripheral blood in HbAS
      (2) In HbSS, there are sickle cells and target cells.
   d. Prenatal screening
      • Analysis of fetal DNA to detect the point mutation

6. Treatment
   a. Treat infections
   b. Pain relief (e.g., morphine)
   c. Transfusion
      • Acute chest syndrome, aplastic crisis
7. Preventive measures
   a. Hydroxyurea
   b. Routine immunizations all current
   c. Pneumococcal vaccine
   d. Folic acid supplementation

F. Glucose-6-phosphate dehydrogenase (G6PD) deficiency
1. Epidemiology
   a. X-linked recessive disorder
   b. Subtypes of G6PD deficiency
      (1) Mediterranean variant in Greeks and Italians
      (2) Black variant
   c. Protective against *Plasmodium falciparum* malaria

2. Pathogenesis
   a. Intrinsic defect with predominantly intravascular hemolysis
      • Mild component of extravascular hemolysis
   b. Decreased synthesis of reduced form of nicotinamide adenine dinucleotide phosphate (NADPH) and glutathione (GSH) in the pentose phosphate pathway (Fig. 11-29)
      (1) GSH normally neutralizes hydrogen peroxide, an oxidant product in RBC metabolism.
      (2) In G6PD deficiency, peroxide oxidizes Hb, which precipitates in the form of Heinz bodies.

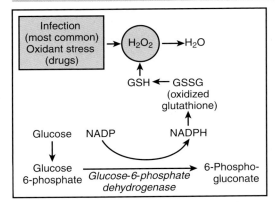

11-29: Pentose phosphate pathway. The enzyme glucose-6-phosphate dehydrogenase catalyzes the irreversible reaction that converts glucose-6-phosphate to 6-phosphogluconate. NADPH (reduced form of nicotinamide adenine dinucleotide phosphate [NADP]) is produced in this reaction and reduces oxidized glutathione (GSSG) to glutathione (GSH), which neutralizes peroxide and converts it to water. *(From Goljan EF: Pathology: Saunders Text and Review Series. Philadelphia, WB Saunders, 1998, Fig. 12-10.)*

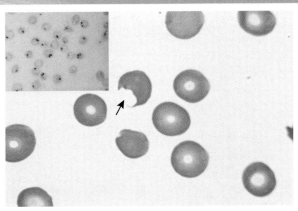

11-30: Peripheral blood smear with a bite cell and inset showing Heinz bodies in glucose-6-phosphate dehydrogenase deficiency. The *arrow* shows a bite cell with part of the red blood cell membrane removed. The *inset* shows a peripheral blood smear with a supravital stain visualizing punctate inclusions representing denatured hemoglobin (Heinz bodies). *(From Kumar V, Fausto N, Abbas A: Robbins and Cotran's Pathologic Basis of Disease, 7th ed. Philadelphia, WB Saunders, 2004, Fig. 13-8; inset from Wickramasinghe SN, McCullough J: Blood and Bone Marrow Pathology. London, Churchill Livingstone, 2003, Fig. 8-8.)*

    (a) Heinz bodies damage the RBC membranes causing intravascular hemolysis.
    (b) Heinz bodies removed from RBC membranes by splenic macrophages produce bite cells.
  c. Half-life of G6PD in the Mediterranean variant is markedly reduced.
    • Produces a severe, chronic hemolytic anemia
  d. Half-life of G6PD in the black variant is moderately reduced.
    • Episodic type of hemolytic anemia *after* exposure to oxidant stresses
  e. Oxidant stresses inducing hemolysis
    (1) Infection (most common)

> G6PD deficiency: oxidant damage with Heinz bodies and bite cells

Decrease in NADPH impairs neutrophils and monocyte killing of bacteria by the O_2-dependent myeloperoxidase (MPO) system (refer to Chapter 2), which requires NADPH as a cofactor for NADPH oxidase.

> G6PD deficiency: O_2-dependent MPO system dysfunctional; lack of NADPH cofactor

    (2) Drugs
      • Examples—primaquine, chloroquine, dapsone, sulfonamides, nitrofurantoin
    (3) Fava beans (mainly in Mediterranean variant)
  3. Clinical findings
    • Sudden onset of back pain with hemoglobinuria 2 to 3 days after an oxidant stress
  4. Laboratory findings
    a. Normocytic anemia
    b. Heinz bodies (Fig. 11-30)
      (1) Identified with a supravital stain
      (2) Best screen during active hemolysis
    c. RBC enzyme analysis
      • Confirmatory test *after* hemolysis has subsided
    d. Peripheral blood findings
      • Bite cells (macrophage removal of membrane; see Fig. 11-30)
G. Pyruvate kinase (PK) deficiency
  1. Epidemiology
    a. Autosomal recessive disease
    b. Most common enzyme deficiency in the Embden-Meyerhof pathway (Fig. 11-31)
      • PK normally converts phosphoenolpyruvate to pyruvate leading to a net gain of 2 ATP.

> Drugs: primaquine, dapsone, sulfonamides

> G6PD deficiency: active hemolysis screen with Heinz body prep

> Confirmatory test: enzyme analysis

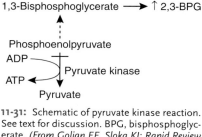

1,3-Bisphosphoglycerate ⟶ ↑ 2,3-BPG

Phosphoenolpyruvate

ADP ⟶ Pyruvate kinase

ATP ⟵

Pyruvate

11-31: Schematic of pyruvate kinase reaction. See text for discussion. BPG, bisphosphoglycerate. *(From Goljan EF, Sloka KI: Rapid Review Laboratory Testing in Clinical Medicine. St. Louis, Mosby Elsevier, 2008, p 183, Fig. 5-26.)*

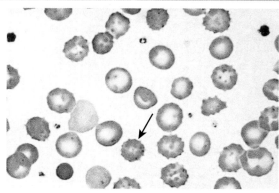

11-32: Peripheral blood smear in pyruvate kinase deficiency. The *arrow* shows one of many red blood cells with thorny projections (echinocytes) extending from the red blood cell membrane. *(From Wickramasinghe SN, McCullough J: Blood and Bone Marrow Pathology. London, Churchill Livingstone, 2003, Fig. 8-10.)*

PK deficiency: intrinsic defect, extravascular hemolysis

2. Pathogenesis
   a. Intrinsic defect with extravascular hemolysis
   b. Chronic lack of ATP causes membrane damage.
      • Results in dehydration of the RBC (echinocytes; Fig. 11-32)
3. Clinical findings
   a. Hemolytic anemia with jaundice beginning at birth
   b. Increase in 2,3-BPG synthesis proximal to enzyme block

PK deficiency: ↑ 2,3-BPG right-shifts OBC; offsets clinical effects of anemia

      • Right shift of OBC causes increased release of O_2, which somewhat offsets the clinical effects of the anemia.
4. Laboratory findings
   a. Normocytic anemia
   b. RBCs with thorny projections (echinocytes)
   c. RBC enzyme assay is the confirmatory test.
H. Immune hemolytic anemias
   • Group of extrinsic hemolytic anemias with extravascular or intravascular hemolysis
   1. Classification (Table 11-7)
      a. Autoimmune

Immune hemolytic anemia: autoimmune warm type (IgG) most common cause

         (1) Most common type of immune hemolytic anemia
         (2) More common in women than men
            • Systemic lupus erythematosus (SLE) is the most common cause of autoimmune hemolytic anemia (AIHA).
         (3) 70% are warm type (IgG antibodies) of AIHA
         (4) 30% are cold type (IgM antibodies) of AIHA

Drug-induced: drug adsorption (penicillin), immunocomplex (quinidine), autoantibody (methyldopa)

      b. Drug-induced (see Table 11-7)
      c. Alloimmune (refer to Chapter 15)

TABLE 11-7. CLASSIFICATION OF IMMUNE HEMOLYTIC ANEMIAS

TYPE OF IMMUNE HEMOLYTIC ANEMIA	EXAMPLES
Autoimmune	
Warm antibodies (IgG)	Primary or idiopathic (no underlying cause)
	Secondary (e.g., SLE)
Cold antibodies (IgM)	Primary or idiopathic
	Secondary
	Mycoplasma pneumoniae (anti-I antibodies)
	Infectious mononucleosis (anti-i antibodies)
Chronic lymphocytic leukemia	Warm and cold immune hemolytic anemia
Drug-induced	Drug adsorption (e.g., penicillin): IgG antibody directed against the drug attached to the RBC membrane
	Immunocomplex (e.g., quinidine): drug-IgM immunocomplex deposits on the RBC causing intravascular hemolysis
	Autoantibody induction (e.g., α-methyldopa): drug alters Rh antigens on RBCs causing synthesis of autoantibodies against Rh antigens
Alloimmune	Hemolytic transfusion reaction (refer to Chapter 15)
	ABO hemolytic disease of newborn (refer to Chapter 15)
	Rh hemolytic disease of newborn (refer to Chapter 15)

SLE, systemic lupus erythematosus.

2. Pathogenesis
   a. IgG-mediated hemolysis
      (1) RBCs coated by IgG are phagocytosed by splenic macrophages.
         • Extravascular hemolysis
      (2) Spherocytes are produced if a small portion of the membrane is removed.
   b. Complement-mediated hemolysis
      (1) RBCs coated by C3b alone are phagocytosed by liver macrophages.
         • Extravascular hemolysis
      (2) RBCs coated by C5-C9 (membrane attack complex)
         • Intravascular hemolysis
      (3) RBCs coated by IgG and C3b are phagocytosed by liver and splenic macrophages (e.g., SLE).
         • Extravascular hemolysis
   c. IgM-mediated hemolysis
      (1) Extravascular or intravascular depending on the degree of complement activation
      (2) Most often intravascular hemolysis
3. Clinical findings
   a. Jaundice due to unconjugated hyperbilirubinemia
      • Occurs in extravascular types of hemolysis
   b. Hepatosplenomegaly
      • Due to work hyperplasia of splenic and liver macrophages
   c. Raynaud's phenomenon (refer to Chapter 9)
      • May occur in cold types of AIHA
4. Laboratory findings
   a. Positive direct antihuman globulin test (DAT; Coombs' test)
      • DAT detects RBCs sensitized with IgG and/or C3b (Fig. 11-33A).
   b. Positive indirect antihuman globulin test (indirect Coombs' test; Fig. 11-33B)
      • Detects antibodies in the serum (e.g., anti-D antibodies)
   c. Unconjugated hyperbilirubinemia if extravascular hemolysis is present.
   d. Hemoglobinuria, decreased serum haptoglobin in intravascular hemolysis
   e. Peripheral blood findings
      (1) Normocytic anemia
      (2) Spherocytosis due to macrophage removal of RBC membrane (IgG type)
      (3) RBC agglutination (IgM type; Fig. 11-34)

IgG-mediated: extravascular hemolysis; spherocytosis

Complement-mediated: intravascular or extravascular hemolysis

IgM-mediated: intravascular (most common) or extravascular hemolysis

DAT: most important marker of immune hemolytic anemia

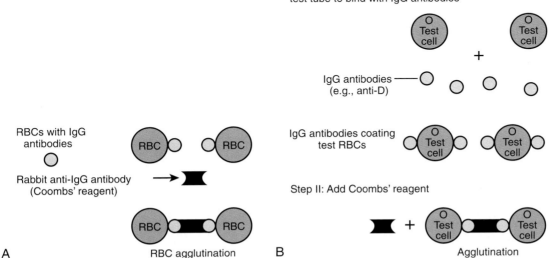

Step I: Add test blood group O RBCs to the test tube to bind with IgG antibodies

IgG antibodies (e.g., anti-D)

RBCs with IgG antibodies

Rabbit anti-IgG antibody (Coombs' reagent)

IgG antibodies coating test RBCs

Step II: Add Coombs' reagent

A   RBC agglutination

B   Agglutination

11-33: Schematic of the direct Coombs' test (**A**) and indirect Coombs' test (**B**). **A,** In the direct Coombs' test, red blood cells (RBCs) sensitized with IgG antibodies (or C3b) are agglutinated when Coombs' reagent (rabbit anti-IgG antibody) is added to the test tube. **B,** In the indirect Coombs' test, IgG antibodies (e.g., anti-D) in the serum must first bind to blood group type O test RBCs added to the test tube. Addition of Coombs' reagent causes the sensitized type O test RBCs to agglutinate, indicating that IgG antibodies are present in the serum. The specificity of the antibodies (e.g., anti-D IgG antibodies) is determined by other tests performed in the blood bank. *(From Goljan EF: Pathology: Saunders Text and Review Series. Philadelphia, WB Saunders, 1998, p 289, Fig. 12-11.)*

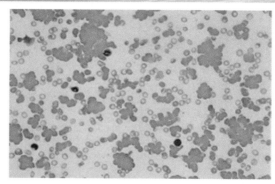

11-34: Red blood cell agglutination in a patient with a cold (IgM) immune hemolytic anemia. *(Courtesy of Jean Schafer.)*

5. Treatment
   a. Discontinue any offensive drug
   b. Corticosteroids
   c. Immunosuppressive agents if corticosteroids are not effective
   d. Splenectomy in selected cases
   e. Intravenous immunoglobulin
      (1) IgG coats all the macrophage receptors so they cannot phagocytose RBCs.
      (2) Only used when most of the above treatments are not working

I. **Micro- and macroangiopathic hemolytic anemias (MHA)**

1. Causes (Table 11-8)
2. Pathogenesis
   a. Extrinsic defect with intravascular hemolysis
   b. Microangiopathic
      • Microcirculatory lesions cause RBC fragmentation (schistocytes; Fig. 11-35)
   c. Macroangiopathic
      • Hemolytic process caused by valvular defects (e.g., aortic stenosis)

MHA: aortic stenosis most common cause

MHA: extrinsic, intravascular hemolysis

Schistocytes: sign of MHA

TABLE 11-8 CAUSES OF MICRO- AND MACROANGIOPATHIC HEMOLYTIC ANEMIA

TYPES	EXAMPLES
Microangiopathic	
Platelet thrombi	Hemolytic uremic syndrome (refer Chapter 14) Thrombotic thrombocytopenic purpura (refer Chapter 14)
Fibrin thrombi	Disseminated intravascular coagulation (refer Chapter 14) HELLP syndrome: H, hemolytic anemia; EL, elevated transaminases; LP, low platelets; associated with preeclampsia
Macroangiopathic	Aortic stenosis (most common cause) Prosthetic heart valves

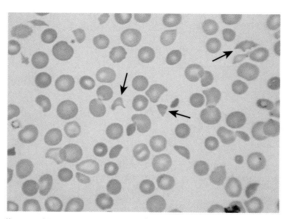

11-35: Fragmented red blood cells, or schistocytes (*arrows*), in the peripheral blood. Note their helmet shapes. *(From Goldman L, Ausiello D: Cecil's Textbook of Medicine, 23rd ed. Philadelphia, Saunders Elsevier, 2008, p 1174, Fig. 161-10.)*

3. Laboratory findings
   a. Normocytic anemia
      - Long-standing hemoglobinuria causes iron deficiency anemia.
   b. Decreased serum haptoglobin, hemoglobinuria
   c. Schistocytes in the peripheral blood

J. Malaria
1. Epidemiology
   - Female *Anopheles* mosquito transmits *Plasmodia* to humans.
2. Pathogenesis
   a. Intraerythrocytic parasite causes intravascular hemolysis.
      - Correlates with fever spikes
   b. Extrinsic defect with predominantly intravascular hemolysis
      - Minor component of extravascular hemolysis
3. Clinical findings
   a. Fever and splenomegaly
   b. *Plasmodium vivax*
      (1) Most common type
      (2) Duffy (Fy) antigen on RBCs is the binding site.
         - Fy antigen often absent in blacks; protective
      (3) Tertian fever pattern (every 48 hours)
   c. *Plasmodium falciparum*
      (1) Most lethal type
      (2) Quotidian fever pattern (daily spikes with no pattern)
   d. *Plasmodium malariae*
      (1) Association with nephrotic syndrome
      (2) Quartan fever pattern (every 72 hours)
4. Laboratory findings
   a. Thick smears identify organisms in RBCs (Fig. 11-36).
   b. Immunologic tests have excellent sensitivity (98%) and specificity (99%).
5. Medications
   a. Prophylaxis (prevention)
      (1) Chloroquine
         (a) Safe during pregnancy
         (b) Kills blood schizonts
         (c) Gametocidal to all malaria species *except P. falciparum*
      (2) Resistant strains *P. falciparum*
         (a) Use atovaquone-proguanil
         (b) Mefloquine alternative
   b. Treatment *P. vivax/ovale*
      - Chloroquine + primaquine
   c. Treatment *P. falciparum*
      (1) If chloroquine sensitive—chloroquine without primaquine
      (2) If chloroquine resistant—quinine sulfate + doxycycline

K. Summary table of normocytic anemias (Table 11-9)

Malaria: *Anopheles* mosquito

Malaria: intravascular hemolysis correlates with fever spikes

Malaria: extrinsic, intravascular hemolysis

Malaria: *P. vivax* most common type; fever every 48 hours

Malaria: *P. falciparum* most lethal type; fever quotidian

Malaria: *P. malariae* fever every 72 hours

Malaria: chloroquine prevention

Malaria Rx *P. vivax/ovale*: chloroquine + primaquine

Malaria Rx *P. falciparum*: chloroquine sensitive—chloroquine alone; resistant—quinine sulfate + doxycycline

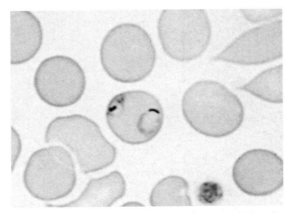

11-36: *Plasmodium falciparum* ring forms in RBCs. This RBC has two ring forms. Multiple infestation of an RBC is characteristic of *P. falciparum* malaria. *(From Hoffbrand AV: Color Atlas: Clinical Hematology, 3rd ed. St. Louis, Mosby, 2000, p 315, Fig. 18-4C.)*

TABLE 11-9. **SUMMARY OF NORMOCYTIC ANEMIAS**

ANEMIA	PATHOGENESIS	DISCUSSION
Reticulocytosis < 3%		
Acute blood loss	Loss of whole blood	Initial Hb and Hct normal Infusion of normal saline uncovers anemia Signs of volume depletion (e.g., absolute neutrophilic leukocytosis) commonly present; positive tilt test (refer to Chapter 4)
Early iron deficiency	Decreased iron stores	Normocytic *before* microcytic Iron studies abnormal ($\downarrow$ serum ferritin)
Early ACD	Iron trapped in macrophages by hepcidin	Normocytic *before* microcytic Iron studies abnormal ($\uparrow$ serum ferritin)
Aplastic anemia	Suppression or deficiency of myeloid stem cells	Pancytopenia Hypocellular marrow
Chronic renal failure	Deficiency of EPO	Presence of burr cells
Reticulocytosis $\geq$ 3%		
Hereditary spherocytosis	AD disorder Defect in ankyrin Extravascular hemolysis	Increased osmotic fragility Treat with splenectomy
Hereditary elliptocytosis	AD disorder Defect in spectrin and band 4.1 Extravascular hemolysis	Elliptocytes > 25%
Paroxysmal nocturnal hemoglobinuria	Loss of anchor for DAF in myeloid stem cell Complement destruction of hematopoietic cells Intravascular hemolysis Detect defect on hematopoietic cells	Pancytopenia Positive sugar water test (screen) and acidified serum test (confirmatory test)
Sickle cell anemia	AR disorder Valine substitution for glutamic acid β-globin chain Extravascular hemolysis	HbAS: HbA 55–60%; HbS 40–45% HbSS: HbS 90–95%; HbF 5–10%; no HbA
G6PD deficiency	XR disorder Deficiency GSH causes oxidant damage to Hb and RBC membrane Intravascular hemolysis	Heinz body preparation: screen during active hemolysis Enzyme assay: confirmatory test when hemolysis subsides
Pyruvate kinase deficiency	AR disease $\downarrow$ ATP synthesis Extravascular hemolysis	$\uparrow$ 2,3-BPG right shifts OBC Dehydrated RBCs with thorny projections (echinocytes)
Acute blood loss	Loss of whole blood Reticulocytosis 5–7 days	$\downarrow$ Hb, Hct, RBC count
Warm AIHA	IgG with or without C3b Extravascular hemolysis	Positive direct Coombs' test SLE most common cause
Cold AIHA	IgM with C3b Extravascular or intravascular hemolysis	Association with *Mycoplasma pneumoniae*; EBV Positive direct Coombs' test
Drug-induced immune hemolytic anemia	Drug hapten: penicillin Extravascular hemolysis Immunocomplex: quinidine Intravascular hemolysis Autoantibody: methyldopa Extravascular hemolysis	Positive direct Coombs' test
Alloimmune hemolytic anemia	Antibodies against foreign RBC antigens Extravascular hemolysis	Hemolytic transfusion reaction ABO and Rh HDN Positive direct Coombs' test
Micro- and macroangiopathic hemolytic anemia	Mechanical destruction of RBCs with formation of schistocytes Intravascular hemolysis	Calcific aortic stenosis most common cause Chronic hemoglobinuria causes iron deficiency
Malaria	Transmitted by female *Anopheles* mosquito Intravascular hemolysis	Rupture of RBCs corresponds with fever

ACD, anemia of chronic disease; AD, autosomal dominant; AIHA, autoimmune hemolytic anemia; AR, autosomal recessive; ATP, adenosine triphosphate; BPG, bisphosphoglycerate; DAF, decay accelerating factor; EBV, Epstein-Barr virus; EPO, erythropoietin; G6PD, glucose-6-phosphate dehydrogenase; GSH, glutathione; Hb, hemoglobin; HbAS, sickle cell trait; HbSS, homozygous for sickle cell disease; Hct, hematocrit; OBC, oxygen-binding curve; Rh HDN, Rhesus hemolytic disease of the newborn; SLE, systemic lupus erythematosus; XR, X-linked recessive.

CHAPTER 12
WHITE BLOOD CELL DISORDERS

I. Benign Qualitative White Blood Cell Disorders
A. Pathogenesis
1. Defects in leukocyte structure
   - Example—membrane fusion defect in Chédiak-Higashi syndrome (refer to Chapters 1 and 2)
2. Defects in leukocyte function
   a. Leukocyte adhesion defect
      - Example—deficient selectin or CD11a/CD18 (refer to Chapter 2)
   b. Phagocytosis defect
      - Example—decreased opsonins in Bruton's agammaglobulinemia (refer to Chapters 2 and 3)
   c. Microbicidal defect
      - Example—deficiency of myeloperoxidase (refer to Chapter 2)

B. Clinical findings
1. Unusual pathogens (e.g., coagulase-negative *Staphylococcus*)
2. Frequent infections and growth failure in children
3. Lack of an inflammatory response (e.g., production of "cold" abscesses)
4. Severe gingivitis

Job's syndrome is an autosomal recessive disorder of neutrophils, characterized by abnormal chemotaxis leading to "cold" soft tissue abscesses due to *Staphylococcus aureus*. Patients have red hair, a leonine face, chronic eczema, and increased IgE (hyperimmune E syndrome).

C. Unusual benign leukocyte reactions
1. Leukemoid reaction
   a. Absolute leukocyte count usually >50,000 cells/mm^3
      - May involve neutrophils, lymphocytes, or eosinophils
   b. Etiology
      (1) Perforated appendicitis (neutrophils)
      (2) Whooping cough (lymphocytes)
      (3) Cutaneous larva migrans (eosinophils)
   c. Pathogenesis
      - Exaggerated response to infection
2. Leukoerythroblastic reaction (Fig. 12-1)
   a. Immature bone marrow cells enter the peripheral blood.
   b. Pathogenesis
      (1) Bone marrow infiltrative disease
      (2) Examples—fibrosis, metastatic breast cancer
   c. Peripheral blood findings
      (1) Myeloblasts, progranulocytes
      (2) Nucleated RBCs, tear drop RBCs (if fibrosis is present)

II. Benign Quantitative WBC Disorders
A. Disorders involving neutrophils
1. Neutrophilic leukocytosis
   a. Absolute neutrophil count > 7000 cells/mm^3 (see Fig. 2-12)

Margin notes:

Qualitative WBC defects: defects in structure and function

Qualitative WBC defects: unusual pathogens, "cold" abscesses, frequent infections

Job's syndrome: defect in chemotaxis; ↑ IgE

Absolute count = % leukocytes × total WBC count

Leukemoid reaction: benign, exaggerated leukocyte response

Leukoerythroblastic reaction in woman > 50 years of age: usually due to metastatic breast cancer

Neutrophilic leukocytosis: neutrophil count > 7000 cells/mm^3

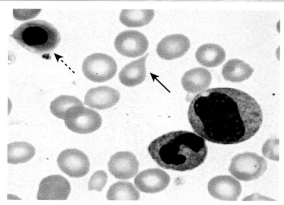

12-1: Leukoerythroblastic reaction. The *solid arrow* shows a tear drop RBC. Immature myeloid cells are also present in a nucleated RBC (*interrupted arrow*). *(From Naeim F: Atlas of Bone Marrow and Blood Pathology. Philadelphia, WB Saunders, 2001, Fig. 4-10B.)*

b. Etiology
    (1) Infection (e.g., acute appendicitis)
    (2) Sterile inflammation with necrosis (e.g., acute myocardial infarction)
    (3) Drugs (e.g., corticosteroids)
c. Pathogenesis
    (1) Increased bone marrow production or release of neutrophils
    (2) Decreased activation of neutrophil adhesion molecules
        (a) Fewer neutrophils adhere to endothelial cells
        (b) Examples—corticosteroids, catecholamines, lithium

2. Neutropenia

> Neutropenia: neutrophil count < 1500 cells/mm³

a. Absolute neutrophil count < 1500 cells/mm³
b. Etiology
    (1) Aplastic anemia
    (2) Immune destruction
        • Example—systemic lupus erythematosus (SLE)
    (3) Septic shock
c. Pathogenesis
    (1) Decreased production
    (2) Increased destruction
        • Destruction by complement, macrophages
    (3) Activation of neutrophil adhesion molecules
        (a) Increase the number of neutrophils adhering to endothelium
        (b) Example—endotoxins

B. Disorders involving eosinophils
1. Eosinophilia (Fig. 12-2A)

> Eosinophilia: eosinophil count > 700 cells/mm³

a. Absolute eosinophil count > 700 cells/mm³
b. Etiology
    (1) Type I hypersensitivity reaction
        • Examples—bronchial asthma, reaction to penicillin, hay fever
    (2) Invasive helminthic infection
        (a) Examples—strongyloidiasis, hookworm infection
        (b) Pinworms and adult ascariasis do *not* have eosinophilia (noninvasive).
    (3) Polyarteritis nodosa
    (4) Addison's disease (cortisol deficiency)

> Eosinophilia: type I hypersensitivity, invasive helminths, hypocortisolism

c. Pathogenesis
    (1) Release of eosinophil chemotactic factor from mast cells
        • Type I hypersensitivity reaction
    (2) No sequestering of eosinophils in lymph nodes
        • Example—hypocortisolism

2. Eosinopenia; etiology:

> Eosinopenia: hypercortisolism

a. Hypercortisolism
    • Examples—Cushing syndrome, corticosteroids
b. Corticosteroids sequester eosinophils in lymph nodes.

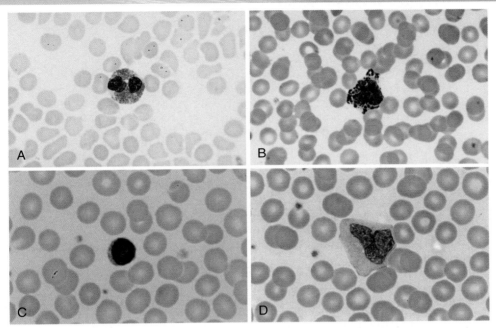

12-2: Normal morphology of eosinophil (**A**), basophil (**B**), lymphocyte (**C**), and monocyte (**D**). The cytoplasm of an eosinophil (**A**) is packed with reddish-orange granules that do *not* cover the nucleus. The cytoplasm of a basophil (**B**) is packed with large purplish black granules that cover the usually bilobed nucleus. The cytoplasm of a small lymphocyte (**C**) is scant and surrounds a nucleus that is usually round (sometimes indented) and contains condensed nuclear chromatin. The cytoplasm of a monocyte (**D**) is grayish blue and contains many fine azurophilic granules and one or more clear vacuoles. The nucleus is large, eccentrically located, and either round, kidney- or horseshoe-shaped (monocyte in the picture), or lobulated. *(From Wickramasinghe SE, McCullough J: Blood and Bone Marrow Pathology. London, Churchill Livingstone, 2003, Fig. 1-1.)*

C. **Disorders involving basophils; basophilia**
  1. Absolute basophil count > 110 cells/mm^3 (Fig. 12-2B)
  2. Etiology
     • Chronic myeloproliferative disorders (e.g., polycythemia vera)
D. **Disorders involving lymphocytes**
  1. Lymphocytosis
     a. Absolute lymphocyte count > 4000 cells/mm^3 in adults or >8000 cells/mm^3 in children (Fig. 12-2C)
     b. Etiology
        (1) Viral
           • Examples—mononucleosis, cytomegalovirus (CMV)
        (2) Bacterial
           • Example—whooping cough
        (3) Drugs
           • Example—phenytoin
        (4) Graves' disease
     c. Pathogenesis
        (1) Increased production
        (2) Decreased entry into lymph nodes
           • Example—due to lymphocytosis-promoting factor produced by *Bordetella pertussis*
  2. Atypical lymphocytosis
     a. Etiology
        (1) Infection
           • Examples—mononucleosis, viral hepatitis, CMV infection, toxoplasmosis
        (2) Drugs (e.g., phenytoin)
     b. Pathogenesis
        (1) Antigenically stimulated lymphocytes
        (2) Prominent nucleoli and abundant blue cytoplasm

Basophilia: consider myeloproliferative disease

Lymphocytosis: lymphocyte count > 4000 cells/mm^3 (adult); >8000 cells/mm^3 (child)

Atypical lymphocytes: antigenically stimulated

3. Infectious mononucleosis
   a. Caused by Epstein-Barr virus (EBV)
   b. Pathogenesis
      (1) Primarily transmitted by kissing
          • EBV initially replicates epithelial cells in oropharynx.
      (2) Infection spreads to B cells in lymph nodes
          (a) Attaches to CD21 receptors on B cells.
          (b) Causes B-cell proliferation and increased synthesis of IgM antibodies
          (c) Virus remains dormant in B cells.
              • Recurrences may occur.
   c. Clinical findings
      (1) Severe fatigue
      (2) Exudative tonsillitis
      (3) Hepatosplenomegaly
          • Danger of splenic rupture in contact sports
      (4) Generalized painful lymphadenopathy
      (5) Rash develops if treated with ampicillin.
   d. Laboratory findings
      (1) Atypical lymphocytosis
          (a) Usually more than 20% of the total WBC count
          (b) Atypical lymphocytes are antigenically stimulated T cells (Fig. 12-3).
      (2) Positive heterophil antibody test
          (a) Initial screening test
          (b) Detects IgM antibodies against horse (most common), sheep, and bovine RBCs
          (c) Sensitivity 87%, specificity 91%
      (3) Antiviral capsid antigen (VCA) antibodies
          (a) High sensitivity and specificity
          (b) Develops early in the infection
          (c) Persists for life
      (4) Anti-early antigen (EA) antibodies
          • Increased with chronic infections
      (5) Anti-Epstein Barr nuclear antigen (EBNA) antibodies
          (a) High sensitivity and specificity
          (b) Develops late in the infection
          (c) Persists for life
      (6) Increased serum transaminases from hepatitis
          • Jaundice is rare.

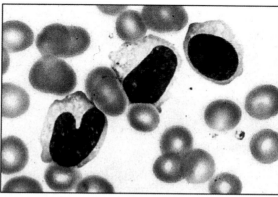

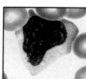
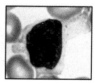

12-3: Peripheral blood with atypical lymphocytes. The lymphocytes are large and have abundant blue-gray cytoplasm. Nuclei are irregular and have dark chromatin with inconspicuous nucleoli. *(From Naeim F: Atlas of Bone Marrow and Blood Pathology. Philadelphia, WB Saunders, 2001, Fig. 13-1.)*

4. Lymphopenia
   a. Absolute lymphocyte count < 1500 cells/mm^3 in adults or <3000 cells/mm^3 in children
   b. Etiology
     (1) HIV
     (2) Immunodeficiency
       (a) DiGeorge syndrome (T-cell deficiency)
       (b) Severe combined immunodeficiency (B- and T-cell deficiency)
     (3) Immune destruction (e.g., SLE)
     (4) Corticosteroids (apoptosis)
     (5) Radiation
       • Lymphocytes most sensitive cells to destruction by radiation (refer to Chapter 6)
   c. Pathogenesis
     (1) Increased destruction
       • Examples—lysis CD4 helper T cells by HIV; apoptosis by corticosteroids; immune destruction (SLE)
     (2) Decreased production
       • Example—Bruton's agammaglobulinemia

E. Disorders involving monocytes; monocytosis
   1. Absolute monocyte count > 800 cells/mm^3 (see Fig. 12-2D)
   2. Etiology
     a. Chronic infection
       • Examples—tuberculosis, subacute infective endocarditis
     b. Autoimmune disease
       • Examples—rheumatoid arthritis, cirrhosis
     c. Malignancy
       • Examples—carcinoma, malignant lymphoma
   3. Pathogenesis
     • Response to chronic inflammation or malignancy

III. Leukemias (Acute and Chronic)
  A. Epidemiology
   1. Malignant diseases of bone marrow stem cells
     • May involve all cell lines
   2. More common in males than females
   3. Risk factors
     a. Chromosomal abnormalities
       • Examples—Down syndrome, chromosome instability syndromes
     b. Ionizing radiation
       • Example—nuclear plant explosion
     c. Chemicals
       • Example—benzene for myeloid leukemia
     d. Alkylating agents
       • Particularly busulfan
     e. Chronic myeloproliferative diseases
       • Example—polycythemia vera
     f. Paroxysmal nocturnal hemoglobinuria
     g. Cigarette smoking
     h. Immunodeficiency diseases
       • Example—Wiskott-Aldrich syndrome
   4. Age ranges for common leukemias
     a. More common in adults than children
     b. Newborn to 14 years old
      (1) Acute lymphoblastic leukemia (ALL)
      (2) Most common leukemia in children
      (3) Most common cancer in children
     c. Persons 15 to 39 years old
      • Acute myeloblastic leukemia (AML)
     d. Persons 40 to 60 years old
      (1) AML (>60% of cases)
      (2) Chronic myelogenous leukemia (CML; ~40% of cases)
       • May occur in patients > 60 years old
     e. Persons > 60 years of age
      • Chronic lymphocytic leukemia (CLL)

Margin notes:

Lymphopenia: lymphocyte count < 1500 cells/mm^3 (adult); <3000 cells/mm^3 (child)

Lymphopenia in HIV: lysis of CD4 helper T cells by the virus

Corticosteroids produce neutrophilic leukocytosis, eosinopenia, and lymphopenia.

Monocytosis: chronic infection, autoimmune disease, malignancy

Leukemia: malignant transformation of marrow stem cells

ALL: most common leukemia and cancer in children

AML: 15–60 years old

CML: 40–60+ years old

Most common overall type of leukemia: CLL

B. **Pathogenesis**
1. Block in stem cell differentiation
   a. Monoclonal proliferation of neoplastic leukocytes behind the block
   b. Acute leukemia
      • Block occurs at an early stage
   c. Chronic leukemia
      (1) Block occurs at a later stage
      (2) Some evidence of maturation

Leukemia: arises in the marrow and disseminates

2. Leukemic cells
   a. Replace most of the bone marrow
      • Replace normal hematopoietic cells
   b. Enter the peripheral blood
   c. Metastasize throughout the body

C. **Clinical findings in acute leukemia**
1. Abrupt onset of signs and symptoms
2. Clinical findings
   a. Fever usually from infection
   b. Bleeding from thrombocytopenia

Acute leukemia: abrupt onset

   c. Fatigue from anemia
3. Metastatic disease
   a. Hepatosplenomegaly
   b. Generalized painless lymphadenopathy

Skin involvement: T cell leukemias

CNS, testicle involvement: ALL

   c. Central nervous system (CNS) involvement
      • Especially in ALL
   d. Skin involvement
      • Especially T-cell leukemias
   e. Testicles
      • Especially in ALL
4. Bone pain and tenderness
   • Due to bone marrow expansion by leukemic cells

D. **Laboratory findings in acute leukemia**
1. Peripheral WBC count

Most important test for diagnosing leukemia: bone marrow examination

   a. Below 10,000 cells/mm^3 (normal) to >100,000 cells/mm^3
   b. Blast cells usually present
      • Examples—myeloblasts, lymphoblasts, monoblasts
2. Normocytic to macrocytic anemia
   • Macrocytic if folate is depleted in production of leukemic cells
3. Thrombocytopenia
   • Usually <100,000 cells/mm^3
4. Bone marrow findings

Acute leukemia: key finding of blasts >20% in bone marrow

Chronic leukemia: insidious onset

   a. Hypercellular with >20% blasts
   b. Often completely replaced by blasts

E. **Clinical findings in chronic leukemia**
   a. Insidious onset
   b. Slightly more common than acute leukemia
   c. Hepatosplenomegaly
   d. Generalized painless lymphadenopathy

F. **Laboratory findings in chronic leukemia**
   a. Peripheral WBC count
      (1) Similar to that of acute leukemia

Chronic leukemia: key finding of blasts <10% in bone marrow

      (2) Blast cells usually <10%
      (3) Evidence of maturation of cells
   b. Normocytic to macrocytic anemia
      • Macrocytic if folate is depleted in production of leukemic cells
   c. Thrombocytopenia (usually <100,000 cells/mm^3)
      • *Exception* in CML, in which thrombocytosis occurs in 40% of cases
   d. Bone marrow findings
      • Hypercellular with <10% blasts

Acute versus chronic leukemia: bone marrow aspirate with blast count

G. **Survival rates**
1. Acute lymphoblastic leukemia: 87% 5-year survival rate
2. Acute myelogenous leukemia: 21% 5-year survival rate
3. Chronic lymphocytic leukemia: 75% 5-year survival rate

4. Chronic myelogenous leukemia: 89% 5-year survival rate
IV. Neoplastic Myeloid Disorders
A. Overview
1. Myeloid disorders are neoplastic stem cell disorders.
   - May involve one or more stem cell lines
2. Classification
   a. Chronic myeloproliferative disorders
   b. Myelodysplastic syndrome
   c. Acute myeloblastic leukemia
B. Chronic myeloproliferative disorders
1. Classification
   a. Polycythemia vera
   b. Chronic myelogenous leukemia
   c. Myeloid metaplasia with myelofibrosis
   d. Essential thrombocythemia
2. General characteristics
   a. Splenomegaly
   b. Propensity for reactive bone marrow fibrosis ("spent phase")
   c. Propensity for transformation to acute leukemia
3. Polycythemia (Fig. 12-4)
   a. Increased hemoglobin (Hb), hematocrit (Hct), and RBC count
   b. Plasma volume (PV) varies with the type of polycythemia.
   c. RBC count versus RBC mass
      (1) RBC count is the number of RBCs per microliter (μL) of blood.
      (2) RBC mass is the total number of RBCs in the body in mL/kg.
      (3) RBC count is the ratio of RBC mass to PV.
         - Figure 12-4A shows the normal relationship between RBC count, RBC mass, PV, erythropoietin (EPO), and O_2 saturation (Sao_2).
   d. Relative polycythemia (Fig. 12-4B)
      (1) Overall most common polycythemia
      (2) Increased RBC count due to a decrease in PV
         - Example—volume depletion from sweating
      (3) RBC mass is normal.
         - *No* increase in bone marrow production of RBCs
      (4) EPO and Sao_2 are normal.
      (5) Fluid replacement corrects the polycythemia.
   e. Absolute polycythemia
      (1) Increase in bone marrow production of RBCs
         - Increased RBC count and RBC mass
      (2) Appropriate absolute polycythemia (Fig. 12-4C)
         (a) There is a hypoxic stimulus for EPO release.
         (b) Examples—primary lung disease, cyanotic congenital heart disease, high altitude
         (c) Decreased O_2 saturation (Sao_2)
         (d) Increased RBC count, RBC mass, EPO
         (e) Normal PV
      (3) Inappropriate absolute polycythemia: ectopic EPO production (Fig. 12-4D)
         (a) No hypoxic stimulus for EPO release
            - Ectopic release of EPO from renal cell carcinoma
         (b) Increased RBC count, RBC mass, EPO
         (c) Normal PV and Sao_2
4. Polycythemia vera (Fig. 12-4E)
   a. Inappropriate absolute polycythemia
   b. Pathogenesis
      (1) Clonal expansion of the myeloid stem cell
      (2) Most due to mutation of *JAK2* gene on short arm of chromosome 9
         - Same mutation may manifest as myelofibrosis and myeloid metaplasia or essential thrombocythemia
      (3) Increased production of RBCs, granulocytes (neutrophils, eosinophils, basophils), mast cells, and platelets
   c. Clinical findings
      (1) Hepatosplenomegaly

Myeloid disorders: neoplastic stem cell disorders

Polycythemia vera: most common chronic myeloproliferative disorder

RBC count = RBC mass/PV

Relative polycythemia: ↑ RBC count; ↓ PV; normal RBC mass, Sao_2, EPO

Appropriate absolute polycythemia: ↑ RBC mass, EPO; normal PV; ↓ Sao_2

Inappropriate absolute polycythemia (ectopic secretion EPO): ↑ RBC mass, EPO; normal PV, normal Sao_2

Inappropriate absolute polycythemia (PRV): ↑ RBC mass, ↓ EPO; ↑ PV, normal Sao_2

PRV: mutation of *JAK2* gene

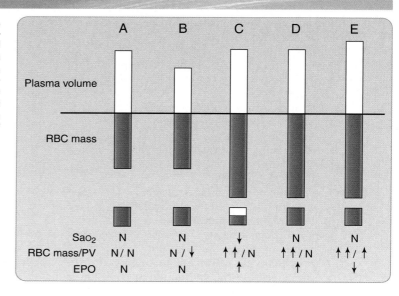

12-4: Schematic showing RBC count, RBC mass, plasma volume (PV), erythropoietin (EPO) concentration, and O_2 saturation (Sao_2) in polycythemia and the normal (N) state: normal (**A**), relative polycythemia (**B**), appropriate absolute polycythemia (**C**), inappropriate absolute polycythemia due to ectopic production of EPO (**D**), polycythemia vera (**E**). See text for discussion.

(2) Ruddy (plethoric) face
 • Due to vessel congestion
(3) Thrombotic events
  (a) Due to hyperviscosity related to increased RBC count
  (b) Examples—hepatic vein thrombosis, dural sinus thrombosis, retinal vein thrombosis
(4) Impaired CNS circulation
  (a) Headache
  (b) Blurred vision
  (c) Retinal vein engorgement
  (d) Vertigo
  (e) Transient ischemic attack
  (f) Stroke

(5) Signs of increased histamine released from mast cells
  (a) Pruritus after bathing
   • Very common initial complaint; mast cells degranulate with change in skin temperature
  (b) Peptic ulcer disease
   • Histamine stimulates production of gastric acid.
(6) Gout
  (a) Increased breakdown of nucleated cells with release of purines
  (b) Purines are converted to uric acid.
 d. Laboratory findings in polycythemia vera
  (1) Increased RBC count, RBC mass, PV

  (2) Decreased EPO
   • Best initial test for polycythemia vera
  (3) Normal Sao_2
 e. Major and minor criteria for diagnosing polycythemia vera
  • Three major criteria or first two major criteria plus two minor criteria
  (1) Major criteria
   (a) Increased RBC mass: >36 mL/kg, >32 mL/kg in women
   (b) Normal Sao_2 (>92%)
   (c) Splenomegaly
  (2) Minor criteria
   (a) Absolute leukocytosis: >12,000 cells/mm³
   (b) Thrombocytosis: >400,000 cells/mm³
   (c) Increased serum leukocyte alkaline phosphatase: >100 score
   (d) Increased serum vitamin B_{12}: >900 pg/mL or vitamin B_{12} binding protein > 2200 pg/mL
  (3) Hypercellular bone marrow with fibrosis in later stages

TABLE 12-1. LABORATORY FINDINGS IN POLYCYTHEMIAS

POLYCYTHEMIA	RBC MASS	PLASMA VOLUME	Sao₂	EPO
Polycythemia vera	↑	↑	Normal	↓
Appropriate polycythemia (e.g., COPD, cyanotic congenital heart disease)	↑	Normal	↓	↑
Inappropriate polycythemia: ectopic EPO (e.g., renal cell carcinoma)	↑	Normal	Normal	↑
Relative polycythemia (e.g., volume depletion)	Normal	↓	Normal	Normal

COPD, chronic obstructive pulmonary disease; EPO, erythropoietin; Sao₂, oxygen saturation.

    f. Treatment
       (1) Nonpharmacologic
           • Phlebotomy to reduce hyperviscosity
       (2) Pharmacologic
          (a) Hydroxyurea + phlebotomy
          (b) Interferon-α
    g. Prognosis
        • Median survival 6 to 18 months
    h. Summary table of the polycythemias (Table 12-1)
  5. CML
    a. Epidemiology
       (1) Usually occurs 40 to 60+ years of age
       (2) Accounts for 15% of adult leukemias
       (3) Risk factors
           • Exposure to ionizing radiation and benzene
    b. Pathogenesis
       (1) Neoplastic clonal expansion of the pluripotential stem cell
           • This stem cell has the capacity to differentiate into a lymphoid or myeloid stem cell.
       (2) t9;22 translocation of *ABL* proto-oncogene
          (a) Proto-oncogene fuses with the break cluster region (BCR) on chromosome 22 (*BCR-ABL* fusion gene).
          (b) Chromosome 22 with translocation is called Philadelphia chromosome.
    c. Clinical findings
       (1) Hepatosplenomegaly and generalized painless lymphadenopathy
           • Due to metastasis
       (2) Blast crisis
          (a) Usually occurs in ~5 years
          (b) Increase in numbers of myeloblasts or lymphoblasts
          (c) Myeloblasts do *not* contain Auer rods (see below).
    d. Laboratory findings
       (1) Peripheral WBC count 50,000 to 200,000 cells/mm³ (Fig. 12-5)
          (a) Myeloid series in all stages of development
          (b) Basophilia

Margin notes:

Polycythemia vera: phlebotomy reduces viscosity-induced thrombosis

CML: 40–60+ years of age

Philadelphia chromosome = chromosome 22 with translocation

CML blast crisis: myeloblasts or lymphoblasts; no Auer rods

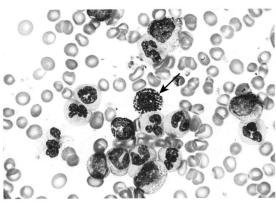

12-5: Peripheral blood in chronic myelogenous leukemia. Marked leukocytosis shows neutrophils at different stages of development (segmented and band neutrophils, metamyelocytes, and myelocytes). The cell in the center (*arrow*) depicts a basophil with dark granules in the cytosol and overlying the nucleus. Basophilia is prominent in chronic myeloproliferative diseases. (*From Damjanov I, Linder J: Pathology: A Color Atlas. St. Louis, Mosby, 2000, p 80, Fig. 5-26.*)

(2) Normocytic to macrocytic anemia
  • Macrocytic if folate is depleted in the production of leukemic cells
(3) Platelet count
  (a) Thrombocytosis in 40% to 50% of cases (uncommon in leukemia)
  (b) Thrombocytopenia in the remainder of cases
(4) Bone marrow findings
  (a) Myeloblasts < 10%
  (b) Hypercellular
(5) Positive Philadelphia chromosome (95% of cases)
  (a) It is *not* specific for CML and is present in other leukemias (e.g., ALL).
  (b) It is *not* lost during therapy unless α-interferon is used.
(6) *BCR-ABL* fusion gene (100% of cases)
  • Fusion gene is the most sensitive and specific test for CML.
(7) Decreased leukocyte alkaline phosphatase (LAP) score
  • LAP is absent in neoplastic granulocytes and present in benign granulocytes.
e. Treatment
  (1) Imatinib mesylate
    (a) Oral tyrosine kinase inhibitor
    (b) <35% Philadelphia chromosome positive cells after treatment
  (2) Allogenic stem cell transplantation
f. Prognosis
  • ~90% 5-year survival rate
6. Myelofibrosis and myeloid metaplasia (MMM)
  a. Epidemiology
    (1) Occurs in patients > 50 years old
    (2) Most common cause of splenomegaly in this group
  b. Pathogenesis
    (1) Clonal myeloproliferative disease
    (2) Most due to mutation of *JAK2* gene on short arm of chromosome 9
      • Same mutation may manifest as polycythemia vera or thrombocythemia.
    (3) Ineffective erythropoiesis, dysplastic megakaryocytes, immature granulocytes, reactive myelofibrosis
      • Marrow fibrosis occurs earlier than in the other chronic myeloproliferative diseases.
    (4) Hematopoiesis moves to the spleen, liver, and other sites (extramedullary hematopoiesis, EMH).
  c. Clinical findings
    (1) Massive splenomegaly with portal hypertension
    (2) Splenic infarcts with left-sided pleural effusions
  d. Laboratory findings
    (1) Bone marrow fibrosis (Fig. 12-6)
    (2) Peripheral WBC count 10,000 to 50,000 cells/mm^3
    (3) Normocytic anemia
      (a) Tear drop cells (damaged RBCs)
      (b) Leukoerythroblastic reaction (see Fig. 12-1)
    (4) Platelet count is variable.
      • Platelets have abnormal morphology.
    (5) Serum leukocyte alkaline phosphatase score is normal to increased.
      (a) Decreased in chronic myelogenous leukemia
      (b) Increased in polycythemia vera
  e. Treatment
    (1) Hydroxyurea
    (2) Interferon-α
7. Essential thrombocythemia (ET)
  a. Pathogenesis
    (1) Clonal myeloproliferative disease with excess formation of dysplastic and defective platelets
    (2) Most due to mutation of *JAK2* gene on short arm of chromosome 9
      • Same mutation may manifest as polycythemia vera or myelofibrosis and myeloid metaplasia.

Margin notes:

CML: only leukemia with thrombocytosis

BCR-ABL fusion gene: most sensitive and specific test for CML

MMM: mutation of *JAK2* gene

MMM: EMH; marrow fibrosis; massive splenomegaly

MMM: tear drop RBCs; leukoerythroblastic smear

ET: dysplastic/nonfunctional platelets; ↑ platelets

ET: mutation of *JAK2* gene

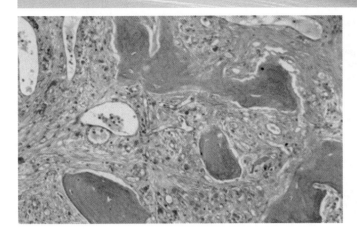

12-6: Bone marrow with myelofibrosis: The bone marrow is replaced by fibrous tissue and the spicules are sclerotic. *(From Goldman L, Ausiello D: Cecil's Textbook of Medicine, 23rd ed. Philadelphia, Saunders Elsevier, 2008, p 1125, Fig. 177-6.)*

    b. Clinical findings
        (1) Bleeding
            (a) Usually gastrointestinal with concomitant iron deficiency
            (b) Platelets nonfunctional
        (2) Splenomegaly
    c. Laboratory findings
        (1) Thrombocytosis
            (a) Platelets > 600,000 cells/mm³; often >1 million cells/mm³
            (b) Platelet morphology is abnormal.
        (2) Mild neutrophilic leukocytosis
        (3) Basophilia
        (4) Hypercellular bone marrow with abnormal megakaryocytes
    d. Treatment
      • Hydroxyurea

C. Myelodysplastic syndromes (MDS)
    1. Epidemiology
      • Usually occurs in men between 50 and 80 years old
    2. Pathogenesis
      a. Group of acquired clonal disorders affecting stem cells
      b. Cytopenias and hypercellular marrow
      c. Classification
        (1) Refractory anemia
        (2) Refractory anemia with ringed sideroblasts
        (3) Chronic myelomonocytic leukemia
        (4) Refractory anemia with excess blasts in transformation
      d. Frequently progresses to acute myeloblastic leukemia (AML; 30% of cases)
    3. Laboratory findings
      a. Severe pancytopenia
        (1) Normocytic to macrocytic anemia
          • Dimorphic RBC population (microcytic and macrocytic)
        (2) Leukoerythroblastic reaction
      b. Bone marrow findings
        (1) Ringed sideroblasts (nucleated RBCs with excess iron)
        (2) Myeloblasts < 20%
          • If >20%, disease is progressing to AML.

D. Acute myeloblastic leukemia
    1. Epidemiology
      a. Usually occurs between 15 and 59 years of age
      b. French-American-British (FAB) classification is used (Table 12-2).
    2. Cytogenetic abnormalities are common.
      • Example—t(15;17) in acute promyelocytic leukemia (M3)
    3. Clinical findings
      a. Disseminated intravascular coagulation (DIC) is common.
        • Invariable in acute promyelocytic leukemia
      b. Gum infiltration is common in acute monocytic leukemia (M5).

MDS: cytopenias; hypercellular marrow

MDS: >30% progress to acute leukemia

Acute promyelocytic leukemia: t(15;17)

Acute monocyte leukemia: gum infiltration

TABLE 12-2. **FRENCH-AMERICAN-BRITISH CLASSIFICATION OF ACUTE MYELOBLASTIC LEUKEMIA (AML)**

CLASS	COMMENTS
M0: Minimally differentiated AML	No Auer rods
M1: AML without differentiation: 20%	Rare Auer rods
M2: AML with maturation	Most common type (30–40% of cases). Auer rods present 15–59-year-old age bracket
M3: Acute promyelocytic	Numerous Auer rods DIC is invariably present t(15;17) translocation Abnormal retinoic acid metabolism: high doses of all-trans-retinoic acid may induce remission by maturing cells
M4: Acute myelomonocytic	Auer rods uncommon
M5: Acute monocytic	No Auer rods Gum infiltration
M6: Acute erythroleukemia	Bizarre, multinucleated erythroblasts Myeloblasts present
M7: Acute megakaryocytic	Myelofibrosis in bone marrow Increased incidence in Down syndrome in children < 3 years old

DIC, disseminated intravascular coagulation.

AML: Auer rods in the cytoplasm of myeloblasts

Auer rods: only in AML; not in CML

4. Auer rods
    a. Splinter-shaped to rod-shaped structures in the cytosol of myeloblasts
        • Auer rods are fused azurophilic granules (Fig. 12-7).
    b. Only present in AML (M2 and M3)
        • They are *not* present in myeloblasts in CML.
5. Treatment
    a. Induction therapy: cytarabine + daunorubicin
    b. Consolidation therapy: aggressive chemotherapy with or without radiation
    c. Maintenance therapy: cytarabine

V. **Lymphoid Leukemias**
  A. **Acute lymphoblastic leukemia**
    1. Epidemiology

ALL: most common cancer and leukemia in children

    a. Most common leukemia and cancer in children (newborn to 14 years of age)
    b. Subtypes
        (1) Early pre–B-cell ALL (80%)
        (2) Pre–B-, B-, and T-cell ALL
    2. Pathogenesis
        • Clonal lymphoid stem cell disease
    3. Early pre–B-cell ALL

ALL: CD10 and TdT positive; most common type

ALL: t(12;21) offers favorable prognosis

    a. Positive marker studies for common ALL antigen (CALLA, CD10)
    b. Positive marker studies for terminal deoxynucleotidyl transferase (TdT)
    c. t(12;21) translocation offers a favorable prognosis.

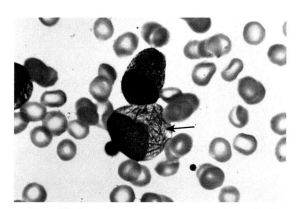

12-7: Peripheral blood with promyelocyte filled with Auer rods in acute promyelocytic leukemia. The neoplastic promyelocyte has numerous splinter-shaped inclusions in the cytoplasm (*arrow*) representing Auer rods. (*From Damjanov I, Linder J: Pathology: A Color Atlas. St. Louis, Mosby, 2000, p 79, Fig. 5-21.*)

d. Greater than 90% achieve complete remission.
  • At least two thirds of patients can be considered cured.

ALL: around two thirds cured

4. T-cell ALL
  • CD10 negative and TdT positive
5. Clinical findings
  a. Metastatic sites similar to those of AML
  b. B-cell types
    • Commonly metastasize to the CNS and testicles
  c. T-cell type
    • Presents as anterior mediastinal mass or acute leukemia
6. Laboratory findings
  a. Peripheral WBC count 10,000 to 100,000 cells/mm^3 (Fig. 12-8)
    • Over 20% lymphoblasts in peripheral blood
  b. Normocytic anemia with thrombocytopenia
  c. Bone marrow findings
    • Bone marrow often totally replaced by lymphoblasts
7. Treatment
  a. Induction therapy: vincristine, prednisone, L-asparaginase
  b. Consolidation therapy: aggressive chemotherapy with or without radiation
  c. Maintenance therapy: methotrexate + 6-mercaptopurine
  d. Bone marrow transplantation is an option.

B. Adult T-cell leukemia
  1. Epidemiology
    a. Malignant leukemia associated with human T-cell leukemia virus (HTLV-1)
    b. May present as a malignant lymphoma

Adult T-cell leukemia: association with HTLV-1

  2. Pathogenesis
    a. Activation of *TAX* gene, which inhibits the *TP53* suppressor gene
    b. Leads to monoclonal proliferation of neoplastic CD4 helper T cells

TAX gene: inhibits *TP53* suppressor gene

  3. Clinical findings
    a. Hepatosplenomegaly and generalized lymphadenopathy
    b. Skin infiltration
      • Common finding in all T-cell malignancies
    c. Lytic bone lesions

Adult T-cell leukemia: skin lesions; lytic bone lesions with hypercalcemia

      (1) Due to lymphoblast release of osteoclast-activating factor
      (2) Associated with hypercalcemia
  4. Laboratory findings
    a. Peripheral WBC count 10,000 to 50,000 cells/mm^3
      (1) Over 20% lymphoblasts

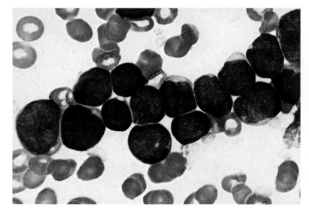

12-8: Peripheral blood in acute lymphoblastic leukemia. Lymphoblasts show condensed nuclear chromatin, small nucleoli, and scant cytoplasm. *(From Kumar V, Fausto N, Abbas A: Robbins and Cotran's Pathologic Basis of Disease, 7th ed. Philadelphia, WB Saunders, 2004, Fig. 14-5A.)*

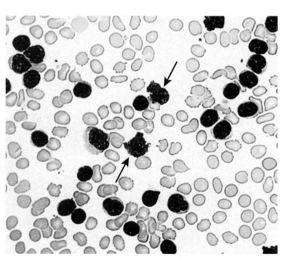

12-9: Peripheral blood in chronic lymphocytic leukemia. Note the increased number of lymphocytes with dense nuclear chromatin and scant cytoplasmic borders. The lymphocytes are extremely fragile and produce characteristic "smudge" cells *(arrows)* during preparation of a slide. *(From Hoffbrand AV: Color Atlas: Clinical Hematology, 3rd ed. St. Louis, Mosby, 2000, p 179, Fig. 10-11.)*

(2) Positive CD4 marker study

(3) Negative for TdT

b. Normocytic anemia and thrombocytopenia

c. Bone marrow findings

- Replaced by CD4 lymphoblasts

C. Chronic lymphocytic leukemia

1. Epidemiology

a. Occurs in individuals > 60 years old

b. Most common overall leukemia

c. Most common cause of generalized lymphadenopathy in the same age bracket

2. Pathogenesis

- Neoplastic disorder of virgin B cells (B cells that cannot differentiate into plasma cells)

3. Clinical findings

a. Generalized lymphadenopathy

b. Metastatic sites similar to those of AML

c. Increased incidence of immune hemolytic anemia

- Both warm (IgG) and cold (IgM) types

4. Laboratory findings

a. Peripheral WBC count 15,000 to 200,000 cells/mm^3 (Fig. 12-9)

b. Lymphoblasts < 10%

c. Neutropenia

d. Numerous "smudge" cells (fragile leukemic cells)

e. Normocytic anemia (50% of cases) and thrombocytopenia (40% of cases)

f. Bone marrow findings

(1) Usually completely replaced by neoplastic B cells

(2) Lymphoblasts < 10%

g. Hypogammaglobulinemia is common.

- Neoplastic B cells do not form plasma cells

5. Treatment

- Chlorambucil

D. Hairy cell leukemia (HCL)

1. Type of B-cell leukemia

- Most common in middle-aged men

2. Clinical findings

a. Splenomegaly (90% of cases)

- Primary site for proliferation of neoplastic cells

b. Absence of lymphadenopathy

- Only leukemia *without* lymphadenopathy

c. Hepatomegaly (20% of cases)

d. Autoimmune vasculitis and arthritis

3. Laboratory findings

a. Pancytopenia

b. Leukemic cells have hair-like projections (Fig. 12-10)

Margin notes:

CLL: most common leukemia

CLL: most common cause of generalized lymphadenopathy in those >60 years old

CLL: hypogammaglobulinemia; smudge cells

HCL: spleen primary site for neoplastic cells

HCL: absence of lymphadenopathy

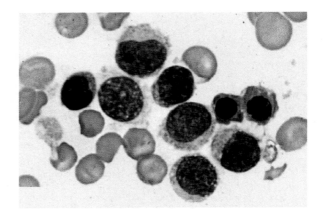

12-10 Peripheral blood in hairy cell leukemia. Clusters of neoplastic cells show dense chromatin and cytoplasmic projections. *(From Naeim F: Atlas of Bone Marrow and Blood Pathology. Philadelphia, WB Saunders, 2001, Fig. 8-20A.)*

  c. Bone marrow
    (1) Packed with neoplastic cells
    (2) Increased reticulin fibers
  d. Positive tartrate-resistant acid phosphatase (TRAP) stain
4. Treatment
  • Drugs of choice are purine analogs; e.g., 2-chloro-2 deoxyadenosine
E. **Summary table of the lymphoid leukemias** (Table 12-3)

HCL: positive TRAP stain

HCL: dramatic response to purine nucleosides

TABLE 12-3. **SUMMARY OF ACUTE AND CHRONIC LYMPHOID LEUKEMIAS**

LEUKEMIA	DESCRIPTION
Acute lymphoblastic (early pre-B type)	Most common leukemia in children Newborn to 14 years old CALLA (CD10) and TdT positive t(12;21) offers a good prognosis
Chronic lymphocytic	Virgin B-cell leukemia Patients > 60 years old Most common cause generalized lymphadenopathy in same age bracket Hypogammaglobulinemia
Adult T cell	HTLV-1 association Leukemic cells CD4 positive and TdT negative Skin infiltration Lytic bone lesions with hypercalcemia
Hairy cell	B cell leukemia Cytoplasmic projections TRAP stain positive Splenomegaly (site of proliferation neoplastic cells) Absence of lymphadenopathy Pancytopenia Dramatic response to purine nucleosides

CALLA, common acute lymphoblastic leukemia antigen; HTLV, human T-cell leukemia; TdT, terminal deoxynucleotidyl transferase; TRAP, tartrate-resistant acid phosphatase.

CHAPTER 13
LYMPHOID TISSUE DISORDERS

I. Lymphadenopathy

    A. Locations of lymphoid tissue

        1. Locations

           a. Regional lymph nodes

           b. Tonsils and adenoids (Waldeyer's ring)

           c. Peyer's patches and appendix

           d. White pulp of the spleen

        2. B cells (Fig. 13-1)

           a. Germinal follicles in lymph nodes

           b. Peripheral areas of spleen white pulp

        3. T cells (see Fig. 13-1)

           a. Paracortex (parafollicular) in lymph nodes

           b. Periarteriolar sheath in spleen

           c. Thymus

        4. Histiocytes

           a. Sinuses in lymph nodes (see Fig. 13-1)

           b. Skin (Langerhans cells)

        5. Locations of lymphoid disorders (Fig. 13-2)

    B. Lymphadenopathy (Fig. 13-3)

        1. Epidemiology

           a. Age

               (1) Patients < 30 years old

                  • Nodal enlargement is usually benign disease (~80% of cases).

               (2) Patients > 30 years old

                  • Nodal enlargement is usually malignant disease (~60% of cases).

           b. Causes

               (1) Reactive lymphadenitis

                  • Hyperplasia of B cells, T cells, or histiocytes

               (2) Infiltrative disease

                  • Examples—metastasis (most common), malignant lymphoma

        2. Clinical findings

           a. Painful nodes imply inflammation (e.g., infection)

               (1) Localized

                  (a) Drain sites of infection (e.g., tonsillitis)

                  (b) Most common sites

                      • Anterior cervical nodes, inguinal nodes

               (2) Generalized

                  (a) Systemic disease

                  (b) Examples—infectious mononucleosis, systemic lupus erythematosus (SLE)

           b. Painless nodes imply a malignancy.

               (1) Lymph nodes are indurated and often fixed to surrounding tissue.

               (2) Localized

                  (a) Nodes draining a primary cancer site

                      • Example—axillary nodes in breast cancer

                  (b) Hodgkin's lymphoma (HL)

Margin notes:

B cells: germinal follicles

T cells: paracortex, thymus

Histiocytes: sinuses, skin (Langerhans cell)

Nodule enlargement: <30 usually benign; >30 usually malignant

Painful lymphadenopathy: inflammation

Painless lymphadenopathy: metastasis or primary malignant lymphoma

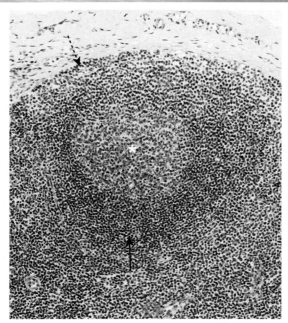

13-1: Lymph node cortex, light micrograph (×132). The *white asterisk* shows a germinal follicle containing B cells; the *solid arrow* shows the paracortex containing T cells; and the *interrupted arrow* shows the subcapsular sinus where histiocytes are located. *(From Gartner L, Hiatt J: Color Textbook of Histology, 3rd ed. Philadelphia, WB Saunders, 2001, p 292, Fig. 12-8.)*

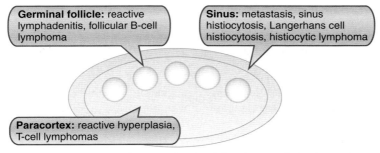

Germinal follicle: reactive lymphadenitis, follicular B-cell lymphoma

Sinus: metastasis, sinus histiocytosis, Langerhans cell histiocytosis, histiocytic lymphoma

Paracortex: reactive hyperplasia, T-cell lymphomas

13-2: Sites of pathologic processes in lymph nodes. Some lymphoid disorders initially localize in the germinal follicles, where B cells are located; others localize in the paracortex, where T cells are located. Mixed B- and T-cell reactions also may occur. Histiocytic disorders involve the sinuses.

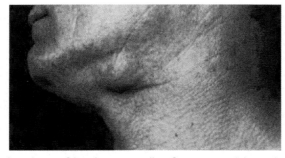

13-3: Patient with cervical lymph node. Painful nodes are usually inflammatory, while painless nodes are usually malignant. *(From Bouloux P: Self-Assessment Picture Tests: Medicine, Vol. 1. London, Mosby-Wolfe, 1997, p 41, Fig. 81.)*

(3) Generalized
  (a) Metastasis in leukemia
  (b) Follicular B-cell lymphoma
c. Key nodal groups involved in primary or metastatic cancer
  (1) Submental
    • Metastatic squamous cell carcinoma in the floor of the mouth
  (2) Cervical
    (a) Metastatic head and neck tumors (e.g., larynx; thyroid, nasopharynx)
    (b) HL

  (3) Left-sided supraclavicular (Virchow's nodes)
    • Metastatic abdominal cancers (e.g., stomach; pancreas)
  (4) Right-sided supraclavicular
    (a) Metastatic lung and esophageal cancers
    (b) HL
  (5) Axillary
    • Metastatic breast cancer
  (6) Epitrochlear
    (a) Unilateral—hand infection, non-Hodgkin's lymphoma (NHL)
    (b) Bilateral—sarcoidosis

  (7) Hilar
    • Metastatic lung cancer
  (8) Mediastinal
    (a) Metastatic lung cancer
    (b) HL (particularly nodular sclerosing type)
    (c) T-cell lymphoblastic lymphoma
  (9) Tonsillar (superior jugular node)
    • Metastatic squamous cancers in oral cavity
  (10) Para-aortic

    (a) Metastatic testicular cancer
      • Testicles migrate to the scrotum from an abdominal location.
    (b) Burkitt's lymphoma
  (11) Inguinal
    • Metastatic vulvar and penis cancers

C. Types of reactive lymphadenitis
  1. Follicular hyperplasia
    a. B-cell antigenic response (see Fig. 13-1)
      (1) Germinal follicles are sharply demarcated from the paracortex.
      (2) Cells are in different stages of development.
    b. Examples
      (1) Early stages of HIV infection
      (2) Examples—rheumatoid arthritis, SLE

  2. Paracortical hyperplasia
    a. T-cell antigenic response
    b. Dermatopathic lymphadenitis
      (1) Nodes draining chronic dermatitis (e.g., psoriasis)
      (2) Nodes contain macrophages with phagocytosis of melanin pigment.
        • Simulates metastatic malignant melanoma

    c. Examples—phenytoin, viral infections
  3. Mixed B- and T-cell hyperplasia
    a. Cat-scratch disease
      (1) Granulomatous microabscesses in regional lymph nodes (e.g., axillary, cervical)
      (2) Due to *Bartonella henselae*
      (3) Treatment is azithromycin.

    b. Toxoplasmosis
      (1) Approximately 50% of the population has been infected with *Toxoplasma gondii*.
      (2) Produces a mononucleosis-like syndrome with painful cervical lymphadenopathy

    c. Tularemia
      (1) Epidemiology
        (a) *Francisella tularensis*
        (b) Gram-negative intracellular coccobacillus

(c) Zoonosis often seen in hunters, trappers
(d) Reservoirs
  • Rodents, deer, rabbits (90%)
(e) Transmission
  • Bites by *Dermacentor* ticks; skin contact with animal hide; aerosol
(2) Ulceroglandular type
  • Most common presentation in the United States
  (a) Localized papular lesion at the point of inoculation (bite) →
  (b) Ulceration of the papule →
  (c) Regional lymphadenitis (noncaseating granulomatous inflammation) →
    • Draining of lymph nodes
  (d) Sepsis leading to dissemination throughout the body (e.g., spleen, liver)
(3) Treatment is gentamicin.
4. Sinus histiocytosis
  a. Benign histiocytic response in lymph nodes draining a tumor
  b. Favorable sign in the axillary nodes in breast cancer

II. **Non-Hodgkin's Lymphomas**
  A. **Epidemiology**
    1. Account for ~60% of adult lymphomas
      • More than 80% are of B-cell origin and derive from the germinal follicle.
    2. Second most common cancer in HIV
    3. Approximately one third arise from extranodal sites.
      • Examples—stomach (most common), Peyer's patches, central nervous system (CNS) (in HIV infections)
    4. Childhood lymphomas
      a. NHL accounts for 60% of cases.
        • Usually T-cell lymphoblastic lymphoma or Burkitt's lymphoma
      b. Generally more aggressive than adult lymphomas
    5. Risk factors for NHL
      a. Viruses
        (1) Epstein-Barr virus (EBV)
          (a) Burkitt's lymphoma
          (b) Diffuse large B-cell lymphoma
          (c) Primary CNS lymphoma
            • Associated with AIDS
        (2) Human T-cell leukemia virus type I
          • Adult T-cell lymphoma or leukemia
        (3) Hepatitis C virus
          • B-cell lymphoma
      b. *Helicobacter pylori*
        (1) Malignant lymphoma derives from mucosa-associated lymphoid tissue in the stomach.
        (2) Treatment of peptic ulcer disease caused by *H. pylori* reduces the risk for developing this lymphoma.
      c. Autoimmune disease
        (1) Sjögren's syndrome
          • Predisposes to salivary gland and gastrointestinal lymphomas
        (2) Hashimoto's thyroiditis
          • Predisposes to thyroid malignant lymphoma
      d. Immunodeficiency syndromes
        (1) Chromosome instability syndromes (e.g., Bloom syndrome)
        (2) AIDS
      e. Immunosuppressive therapy
        • Recipients of organ or bone marrow transplants
      f. High-dose radiation
        • Treatment of HL
  B. **Pathogenesis**
    1. Mutation produces a block at a specific stage in development of B or T cells.
    2. Example—accumulation of small cleaved B cells in follicular lymphoma
  C. **B-cell lymphomas** (Table 13-1 and Figs. 13-4 and 13-5)

Tularemia: zoonosis (rabbits); ulceroglandular type most common

Sinus histiocytosis axillary nodes: favorable sign in breast cancer

NHL: majority β-cell origin

Extranodal sites: stomach, CNS, Peyer's patch

NHL: most common malignant lymphoma adults/children

Epstein-Barr virus: Burkitt's lymphoma, CNS lymphoma

H. pylori: malignant lymphoma of stomach

Lymphoma in autoimmune disease: Sjögren's syndrome, Hoshimoto's thyroiditis

TABLE 13-1. **COMMON TYPES OF B-CELL NON-HODGKIN'S LYMPHOMA**

TYPE	EPIDEMIOLOGY	DESCRIPTION/IMMUNOPHENOTYPE	CLINICAL FINDINGS
Burkitt's lymphoma (see Fig. 13-4)	30% of children with NHL	EBV relationship with t(8;14) "Starry sky" appearance with neoplastic B cells (dark of night) and reactive histiocytes with phagocytic debris (stars)	*American type:* GI tract, para-aortic nodes *African type:* jaw Bone marrow involvement Leukemic phase common
Diffuse large B-cell lymphoma	50% of adults with NHL; elderly and childhood populations	Derives from germinal center	Localized disease with extranodal involvement: GI tract, brain (EBV association with AIDS)
Extranodal marginal zone lymphoma	Association with *Helicobacter pylori* gastritis	Derives from MALT	Low-grade malignant lymphoma of the stomach
Follicular lymphoma (see Fig. 13-5)	40% of adults with NHL; elderly patients	Derives from germinal center t(14;18) causing overexpression of *BCL2* antiapoptosis gene	Generalized lymphadenopathy Bone marrow involvement
Small lymphocytic lymphoma (SLL)	Patients usually >60 years of age	Neoplasm of small, mature B lymphocytes SLL if confined to lymph nodes CLL if leukemic phase is present	Generalized lymphadenopathy

CLL, chronic lymphocytic leukemia; EBV, Epstein-Barr virus; GI, gastrointestinal; MALT, mucosa-associated lymphoid tissue; NHL, non-Hodgkin's lymphoma.

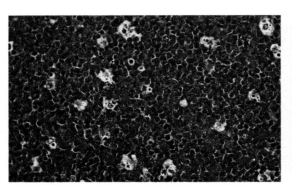

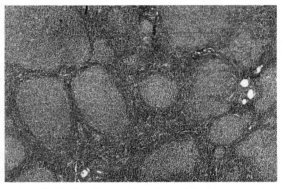

13-4: Burkitt's lymphoma. The node is completely effaced with a monomorphic infiltrate of lymphocytes. Interspersed are clear spaces with reactive histiocytes containing phagocytic debris. At low power the node has a "starry sky" appearance, with the stars represented by the reactive histiocytes. This type of lymphoma is associated with a t(8;14) translocation. *(From Rosai J, Ackerman LV: Surgical Pathology, 9th ed. St. Louis, Mosby, 2004, p 1955, Fig. 21-103.)*

13-5: Follicular lymphoma. Note the nodular aggregates that are present throughout the lymph node. Unlike germinal centers, these nodules are composed of a monomorphic infiltrate of lymphoma cells. This type of lymphoma is associated with the t(14;18) translocation leading to overexpression of the BCL-2 protein product (antiapoptosis gene). *(Courtesy of Dr. Robert W. McKenna, Department of Pathology, University of Texas Southwestern Medical School, Dallas, Texas.)*

D. T-cell lymphomas
   1. Precursor T-cell lymphoblastic leukemia/lymphoma
      a. Precursor T-cell lymphoma accounts for 40% of childhood lymphomas.
         (1) Primarily involves the anterior mediastinum and cervical nodes
         (2) Bone marrow and central nervous system involvement is common.
      b. Precursor T-cell lymphoblastic leukemia
         • Leukemic variant of this lymphoma
   2. Mycosis fungoides and Sézary syndrome
      a. Epidemiology
         (1) Both conditions involve neoplastic peripheral CD4 T helper (T_H) cells.
         (2) Usually involves adults 40 to 60 years of age
      b. Mycosis fungoides
         (1) Begins in skin (rash to plaque to nodular masses)
            • Progresses to lymph nodes, lung, liver, and spleen
         (2) Groups of neoplastic cells in the epidermis are called Pautrier's microabscesses.

Mycosis fungoides: neoplasm of CD4 T_H cells; skin involvement

      c. Sézary syndrome
         (1) Mycosis fungoides with a leukemic phase
         (2) Circulating cells are called Sézary cells (prominent nuclear cleft).

E. NHL survival statistics
- Five-year survival rate is 63%; 10-year survival rate is 51%.

III. Hodgkin's Lymphoma

A. Epidemiology
1. Accounts for ~40% of adult lymphomas
2. Age and sex
   a. Slightly more common in men
     - *Exception*—nodular sclerosing type is more common in women.
   b. More common in adults than children
   c. More common in whites than blacks
3. Bimodal age distribution
   a. First large peak: 15 to 34 years old
   b. Second smaller peak: >50 years old
   c. Involves younger age bracket than NHL
4. Most common site of initial involvement is the neck region.
5. EBV association
   - EBV is identified in more than 50% of cases of mixed cellularity HL.
6. Defects in cellular immunity
   - Defects in cutaneous anergy to common antigens (anergy)
7. Classification (Table 13-2)
   a. Lymphocyte predominant
   b. Nodular sclerosing (most common type)
   c. Mixed cellularity
   d. Lymphocyte depletion (not discussed)

B. Pathogenesis
1. Possible genetic predisposition
2. Unknown factors (EBV, retrovirus) cause B and T cells to become neoplastic Reed-Sternberg cells.

C. Pathologic findings
1. Involves localized groups of nodes and has contiguous spread
   a. Often involves cervical or supraclavicular nodes
   b. Cut section has a bulging "fish-flesh" appearance
2. Reed-Sternberg (RS) cells
   a. Neoplastic cell of HL
     (1) Transformed germinal center B cell (some cases)
     (2) CD15 and CD30 positive
   b. Classic RS cell
     - Two mirror image nuclei, each with an eosinophilic nucleolus surrounded by a clear halo (Fig. 13-6)

Margin notes:

Sézary syndrome: mycosis fungoides in leukemic phase

Nodular sclerosing HL: female dominant

EBV: association with mixed cellularity HL

Nodular sclerosing HL: most common type of HL

RS cell: neoplastic cell of HL; CD15+, CD30+

TABLE 13-2. SOME TYPES OF HODGKIN'S LYMPHOMA (HL)

TYPE	EPIDEMIOLOGY	CLINICAL FINDINGS
Lymphocyte predominant	5% of cases Occurs mainly in males	Asymptomatic young male with cervical or supraclavicular nodal enlargement Difficult to find classic RS cells L and H variants present Best survival statistics
Nodular sclerosing (see Fig. 13-7)	60% of cases Occurs mainly in females	Usually involves anterior mediastinal nodes (seen on chest x-ray) and either cervical or supraclavicular nodes RS cells infrequent Lacunar cells present Collagen separates nodular areas
Mixed cellularity	30% of cases Men > 50 years of age Strong Epstein-Barr virus association	RS cells numerous; mononuclear variants ↑ Eosinophils, plasma cells, histiocytes
Lymphocyte depletion	5% of cases Men > 50 years of age	Most aggressive HL RS cells frequent Poorest survival statistics

RS, Reed-Sternberg.

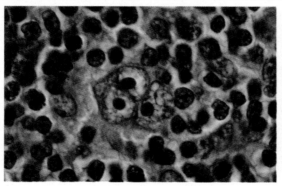

13-6: Classic Reed-Sternberg (RS) cell. The large, multilobed cell with prominent nucleoli is surrounded by a halo of clear nucleoplasm. Classic RS cells are more easily found in mixed-cellularity Hodgkin's lymphoma than in lymphocyte-predominant and nodular-sclerosing Hodgkin's lymphoma. *(From Damjanov I, Linder J: Anderson's Pathology, 10th ed. St. Louis, Mosby, 1996, p 1145, Fig. 42-47A.)*

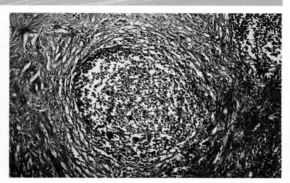

13-7: Nodular-sclerosing Hodgkin's lymphoma. The lymphoid nodule is encased by fibrous tissue. Note the spaces in the nodule within which are Reed-Sternberg variants called lacunar cells. *(From Rosai J, Ackerman LV: Surgical Pathology, 9th ed. St. Louis, Mosby, 2004, p 1924, Fig. 21-56.)*

     c. RS variants
       (1) L and H variant
         (a) Large, pale staining, multilobed cell ("popcorn cell")
         (b) Present in lymphocyte predominant type
       (2) Lacunar cells (Fig. 13-7)
         (a) Pale cell with multilobed nucleus containing many small nucleoli
         (b) Cell lies within a clear space in formalin-fixed tissue.
         (c) Present in nodular sclerosing type
       (3) Mononuclear variants
         (a) Single nucleus with a prominent nucleolus
         (b) Seen in mixed cellularity type

RS cell: required to make the diagnosis of HL

   3. Diagnosis of HL
     a. Presence of a classic RS cell is required
     b. Presence of RS variant cells in a background of reactive cells
       • Reactive cells include eosinophils, plasma cells, histiocytes.
   4. Differences from NHL
     • Less commonly involves Waldeyer's ring, mesenteric nodes, and extranodal sites

D. Clinical findings and prognosis
   1. Constitutional signs
     a. Fever, unexplained weight loss, night sweats
     b. Pruritus

HL: Pel-Ebstein fever

     c. Pel-Ebstein fever (uncommon variant of fever)
       • Alternating bouts of fever followed by remissions
   2. Hematologic findings
     a. Normocytic anemia
     b. Painless enlargement of single groups of lymph nodes
       • Usually cervical, supraclavicular, or anterior mediastinal nodes

Prognosis: stage more important than type of HL

   3. Main factors determining prognosis
     a. Clinical stage is more important than the type of HL.

Nodular sclerosing HL: anterior mediastinal mass + single group of nodes above diaphragm

     b. Majority have lymphadenopathy above the diaphragm (stages I and II).
       • Usually involves supraclavicular nodes and anterior mediastinal nodes

Rx for HL: ↑ risk for second malignancies

   4. Increased risk for second malignancies
     a. Acute myelogenous leukemia or NHL
     b. Complication of treatment with radiation and alkylating agents

E. Treatment
   • Radiotherapy and chemotherapy depending on the stage

F. HL survival statistics
   • Five-year survival rate is 85%; 10-year survival rate is 80%.

IV. **Langerhans Cell Histiocytoses (Histiocytosis X)**
  A. **Epidemiology**
    1. Langerhans histiocytes
      a. CD1 positive
      b. Contain Birbeck granules (tennis racket appearance; Fig. 13-8)
        • Visible only with electron microscopy
    2. Primarily occurs in children and young adults
    3. Classification
      a. Letterer-Siwe disease
      b. Hand-Schüller-Christian disease
      c. Eosinophilic granuloma
  B. **Letterer-Siwe disease**
    1. Malignant histiocytosis
    2. Epidemiology
      • Occurs in infants and children < 2 years old
    3. Clinical findings
      a. Diffuse eczematous rash (Fig. 13-9)
      b. Multiple organ involvement
      c. Lytic lesions in the skull, pelvis, and long bones
      d. Rapidly fatal
  C. **Hand-Schüller-Christian (HSC) disease**
    1. Malignant histiocytosis
    2. Epidemiology
      • Mainly affects children
    3. Clinical findings
      a. General
        (1) Fever
        (2) Localized rash on scalp and in ear canals
      b. Classic triad due to infiltrative disease
        (1) Lytic lesion in the skull
        (2) Diabetes insipidus due to invasion of posterior pituitary
        (3) Exophthalmos from infiltration of the orbit
      c. Intermediate prognosis

Histiocytes: CD1+ contain Birbeck granules

Malignant histiocytoses: skin involvement is common; lytic bone lesions

HSC: lytic skull lesion, diabetes insipidus, exophthalmos

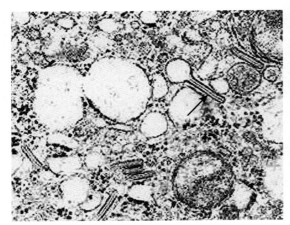

13-8: Electron micrograph showing racket shaped Birbeck granules in a histiocyte. (Courtesy of William Meek, Professor and Vice Chairman of Anatomy and Cell Biology, Oklahoma State University, Center for Health Sciences, Tulsa, Oklahoma.)

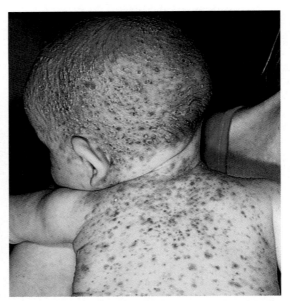

13-9: Child with Letterer-Siwe disease (Langerhans histiocytosis). Note the eczematous type rash over the body surface due to malignant histiocytes infiltrating the skin and dermis. *(From Kumar V, Fausto N, Abbas A: Robbins and Cotran's Pathologic Basis of Disease, 7th ed. Philadelphia, WB Saunders, 2004, p 1249, Fig. 25-18A.)*

D. **Eosinophilic granulomas**
1. Benign histiocytosis
2. Epidemiology
   • Occurs in adolescents and young adults
3. Clinical findings
   a. Unifocal lytic lesions in bone (skull, ribs, and femur)
   b. Bone pain and pathologic fractures are common.

V. **Mast Cell Disorders**
A. **Overview**
1. Presentation
   a. Localized—urticaria pigmentosum, solitary mastocytoma
   b. Systemic—systemic mastocytosis
2. Signs and symptoms relate to mast cell release of histamine.
   • Pruritus and swelling of tissue
B. **Urticaria pigmentosum (UP)**
1. Skin lesions
   a. Multiple oval, red-brown, nonscaling macules (flat lesions) or papules (Fig. 13-10)
   b. Scratching results in erythematous swelling of the lesions and pruritus.
      • Called Darier's sign
   c. Dermatographism
      • Dermal edema occurs when apparently normal skin is stroked with a pointed object.
   d. Lesions remain hyperpigmented when they regress.
   e. Skin biopsy
      (1) Mast cells have metachromatic granules.
      (2) Granules stain positive with toluidine blue and Giemsa stain.
2. Pruritus and flushing may be triggered by foods, alcohol, drugs (e.g., codeine).
VI. **Plasma Cell Dyscrasias**
A. **Overview**
1. Monoclonal B-cell disorders
   a. Increase in a single immunoglobulin
   b. Increase in the corresponding light chain
2. Immunoglobulin is detected as a monoclonal spike (M component) on serum protein electrophoresis (Fig. 13-11).
3. Clinical significance of M components
   a. Most commonly due to an increase in IgG
      • Other plasma cell clones are suppressed.
   b. Bence Jones (BJ) protein
      (1) Refers to κ or λ light chains excreted in urine
      (2) Associated with a plasma cell malignancy and Waldenström's macroglobulinemia

Sidebar notes (left margin):

Eosinophilic granuloma: benign histiocytosis; unifocal lytic lesions in bone

Mast cell disease: pruritus, swelling, hyperpigmentation

UP: dermatographism; lesions remain hyperpigmented

Mast cells: metachromatic granules

Plasma cell dyscrasia: monoclonal spike; usually IgG

BJ protein: light chains in the urine

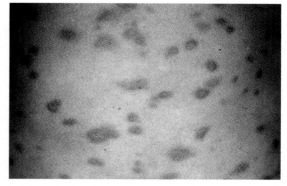

13-10: Urticaria pigmentosum. Note the numerous red-brown, round to oval macules and papules that are distributed over the trunk. These lesions are pruritic as a result of the release of histamine from the dermal mast cells. The lesions gradually darken over time because of increased melanin pigmentation. *(Courtesy of R.A. Marsden, MD, St. George's Hospital, London.)*

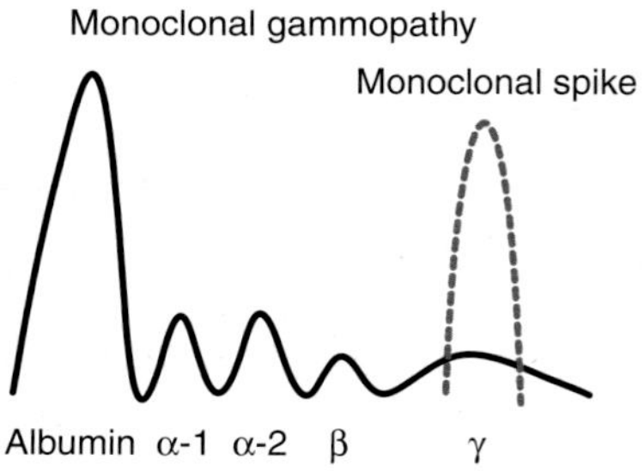

Monoclonal gammopathy

Monoclonal spike

Albumin α-1 α-2 β γ

13-11: Serum protein electrophoresis (SPE) showing a schematic of a monoclonal gammopathy. *(From Goljan EF, Sloka KI: Rapid Review Laboratory Testing in Clinical Medicine. St. Louis, Mosby Elsevier, 2008, p 284, Fig. 9-1C.)*

c. Immunoelectrophoresis or immunofixation
  • These techniques identify the immunoglobulin and light chain in serum and light chains in urine.

B. Multiple myeloma
  1. Epidemiology
    a. More common in blacks than in whites
    b. Rare under 40 years of age
    c. Peak incidence in 50 to 60 year olds
    d. Accounts for 10% of all hematologic malignancies
    e. Increased risk with radiation or benzene exposure
    f. M-spike occurs in 80% to 90% of cases.
      (1) Usually IgG κ light chain followed by IgA and pure light chain myeloma
      (2) BJ represents excess light chains in urine.
      (3) Urine BJ protein is positive in 60% to 80% of cases.
  2. Pathophysiology
    a. Chromosome abnormalities (deletions, translocations)
    b. Possible evolution from normal plasma cells → monoclonal gammopathy of undetermined significance (MGUS) → multiple myeloma
  3. Pathologic findings
    a. Sheets of malignant plasma cells in a bone marrow aspirate/biopsy (Fig. 13-12)
    b. Plasma cells account for >10% of cells in the aspirate.
  4. Skeletal system findings
    a. Bone pain
      (1) Due to "punched out" lytic lesions (Fig. 13-13)
        (a) Myeloma cells produce an inhibitor of osteoblast differentiation
        (b) Myeloma cells release interleukin 1 (osteoclast activating factor)
      (2) Vertebra is the most common site.
      (3) Other sites include ribs, skull, pelvis.
      (4) Commonly presents with pathologic fractures
        • Particularly rib lesions
    b. Hypercalcemia (25% of cases)
  5. Renal findings
    a. Renal failure (30–50% of cases)
    b. Myeloma kidney has different presentations.
      (1) Proteinaceous tubular casts
        (a) Composed of BJ protein
        (b) BJ protein damages tubular epithelium
        (c) Intratubular multinucleated giant cell reaction
      (2) Nephrocalcinosis
        (a) Metastatic calcification of tubular basement membranes in the collecting ducts (refer to Chapter 1)
        (b) Common cause of acute renal failure in multiple myeloma

Myeloma: rare <40 years of age

Myeloma: normal plasma cell → MGUS → myeloma

Bone findings in myeloma: lytic lesions, pathologic fractures, hypercalcemia

BJ renal disease in myeloma: proteinaceous casts with multinucleated giant cell reaction

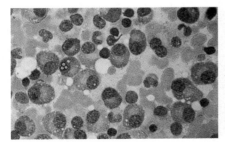

13-12: Malignant plasma cells in multiple myeloma. The majority of malignant plasma cells show a dark blue cytoplasm, peripherally located nuclei, and perinuclear clearing. Occasional cells have vacuoles containing immunoglobulin. *(From Goldman L, Ausiello D: Cecil's Textbook of Medicine, 23rd ed. Philadelphia, Saunders Elsevier, 2008, p 1430, Fig. 198-4.)*

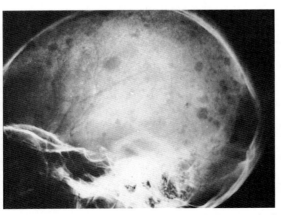

13-13: Radiograph of a skull showing multiple "punched out" lytic lesions in multiple myeloma. When these lesions are located in other areas, such as the ribs, pathologic fractures frequently occur. *(From Damjanov I, Linder J: Anderson's Pathology, 10th ed. St. Louis, Mosby, 1996, p 1105, Fig. 41-61.)*

(3) Metastatic disease to interstitial tissue

(4) Primary amyloidosis (10% of cases)

    (a) Light chains are converted into amyloid (refer to Chapter 3).

    (b) Produces a nephrotic syndrome

6. Hematologic findings

  a. Normocytic anemia with rouleaux (see Fig. 2-17)

  b. Increased erythrocyte sedimentation rate

  c. Prolonged bleeding time

    • Due to a defect in platelet aggregation

7. Radiculopathy from bone compression and vertebral fractures

8. Recurrent infection is a common cause of death.

  • Sepsis due to *Haemophilus influenzae*, *Streptococcus pneumoniae*

9. Treatment

  a. High-dose chemotherapy

  b. Autologous stem cell transplantation

10. Prognosis

  • Median survival after diagnosis is 3 years.

C. Other plasma cell dyscrasias (Table 13-3)

VII. Spleen Disorders

A. Clinical anatomy and physiology

1. Red pulp

  • Contains the cords of Billroth with fixed macrophages and sinusoids

2. White pulp

  • Contains B and T cells

3. Important functions of the spleen

  a. Blood filtration; macrophages remove:

    (1) Hematopoietic elements (e.g., old red blood cells)

    (2) Intraerythrocytic parasites (e.g., malaria)

Marginalia:

Myeloma: sepsis and renal failure common causes of death

MGUS: most common monoclonal gammopathy

Red pulp: fixed macrophages

White pulp: B and T cells

TABLE 13-3. ADDITIONAL PLASMA CELL DYSCRASIAS

TYPE	DISCUSSION
MGUS	Most common monoclonal gammopathy Small IgG M spike in elderly patients Plasma cells < 3% in bone marrow No BJ protein Increased risk for developing multiple myeloma, Waldenstrom's macroglobulinemia
Solitary skeletal plasmacytoma	Bone sites: vertebra, ribs, pelvis Slight increase in monoclonal protein No plasmablasts in bone marrow No BJ protein 75% develop multiple myeloma
Extramedullary plasmacytoma	Sites: upper respiratory tract (nasopharynx, sinuses, larynx) Slight increase in monoclonal protein Absence of malignant plasma cells in the bone marrow Absence of BJ protein Small percentage may develop multiple myeloma
Lymphoplasmacytic lymphoma (Waldenström's macroglobulinemia)	Neoplastic lymphoplasmacytoid B cells Elderly male-dominant disease Main risk factor is MGUS M spike with IgM BJ protein is present Generalized lymphadenopathy (not present in myeloma) Anemia and bone marrow (no lytic lesions like myeloma), liver, and spleen involvement Hyperviscosity syndrome due to increased IgM: retinal hemorrhages, strokes, platelet aggregation defects; plasmapheresis important to remove IgM Median survival, 5 years
Heavy-chain diseases	M protein heavy chain *without* light chains Absence of BJ protein α-Heavy-chain disease: neoplastic infiltration of the jejunum, leading to malabsorption or localized upper respiratory tract disease γ-Heavy-chain disease: presents as a lymphoma μ-Heavy-chain disease: often associated with chronic lymphocytic leukemia or lymphoma

BJ, Bence Jones; MGUS, monoclonal gammopathy of undetermined significance.

(3) Encapsulated bacteria
- Examples—*Streptococcus pneumoniae*
b. Antigen trapping and processing in macrophages
c. Reservoir for one third of the peripheral blood platelet pool
d. Site for extramedullary hematopoiesis (refer to Chapter 11)

B. Splenomegaly
1. Causes of splenomegaly
a. Autoimmune disorders
- Examples—SLE, immune thrombocytopenia, and anemia
b. Infectious mononucleosis
- Due to antigenic stimulation of T cells
c. Parasitic infections
- Malaria is the most common cause of splenomegaly in developing countries.
d. Primary and reactive (secondary) amyloidosis
e. Lysosomal storage diseases
(1) Gaucher's disease
(a) Deficiency of glucocerebrosidase
- Lysosomal accumulation of glucocerebrosides
(b) Macrophages have a fibrillary appearance (Fig. 13-14).
(2) Niemann-Pick disease
(a) Deficiency of sphingomyelinase
- Lysosomal accumulation of sphingomyelin
(b) Macrophages have soap bubble appearance (Fig. 13-15).
f. Acute and chronic leukemias
g. Hereditary spherocytosis
h. Portal hypertension in cirrhosis
i. Chronic myeloproliferative diseases
- Polycythemia vera, myelofibrosis and myeloid metaplasia, essential thrombocythemia
2. Clinical findings
a. Left upper quadrant pain
- May be associated with splenic infarctions causing friction rubs and a left-sided pleural effusion
b. Hypersplenism (see later)

C. Portal hypertension in cirrhosis
1. Gross findings
- Spleen is often surfaced by a thickened ("sugar-coated") capsule from perisplenitis.
2. Microscopic findings
- Calcium and iron concretions called Gamna-Gandy bodies are present in collagen.

D. Hypersplenism
1. Definition
a. Exaggeration of normal splenic function
b. RBCs, WBCs, and platelets, either singly or in combination, are sequestered and destroyed.

Malaria: most common cause splenomegaly in developing countries

Gaucher's disease: ↓ glucocerebrosidase, ↑ glucocerebroside

Niemann-Pick: ↓ sphingomyelinase, ↑ sphingomyelin

Massive splenomegaly: infarctions common with pain, friction rub, and left-sided pleural effusion

Splenomegaly in cirrhosis: "sugar-coated" spleen

Hypersplenism: destruction of hematopoietic cells producing cytopenias

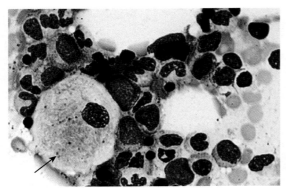

13-14: Gaucher's disease. Note the fibrillary appearance of the cytoplasm in the macrophages (*arrow*). (*From Naeim F: Atlas of Bone Marrow and Blood Pathology. Philadelphia, WB Saunders, 2001, p 157, Fig. 11-14B.*)

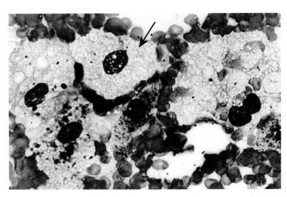

13-15: Niemann-Pick disease. Note the soap bubble appearance of the cytoplasm in the macrophages (*arrow*). (*From Naeim F: Atlas of Bone Marrow and Blood Pathology. Philadelphia, WB Saunders, 2001, p 159, Fig. 11-17B.*)

2. Portal hypertension associated with cirrhosis is the most common cause.
3. Clinical findings
    a. Splenomegaly
    b. Peripheral blood cytopenias
        • Anemia, thrombocytopenia, neutropenia alone or in combination
    c. Compensatory reactive bone marrow hyperplasia
        • Attempt by the marrow to replace lost cells
    d. Correction of cytopenias with splenectomy
E. **Splenic dysfunction and splenectomy**
1. Splenic dysfunction
    a. Presence of Howell-Jolly bodies (nuclear remnants) in peripheral blood RBCs
    b. Predisposition to infections by encapsulated pathogens
        (1) Infections include septicemia, peritonitis, osteomyelitis.
        (2) Pathogens include:
            • *Streptococcus pneumoniae, Haemophilus influenzae, Salmonella, Neisseria meningitidis*
        (3) Mechanisms
            (a) Concentration of IgM drops leading to a decrease in complement system activation
                • The spleen is a site for IgM synthesis.
            (b) Macrophages are *not* present to phagocytose the opsonized encapsulated pathogens.
            (c) Loss of tuftsin, which is normally synthesized in the spleen
                • Tuftsin activates receptors on macrophages to increase their phagocytic activity.
        (4) Pathogens commonly involved
            (a) *Streptococcus pneumoniae*
            (b) Other pathogens include *Haemophilus influenzae* and *Salmonella paratyphi* (osteomyelitis in sickle cell disease).
                • Immunization helps prevent infectious complications.
2. Splenectomy
    a. Increases the risk for infections (see earlier)
    b. Hematologic findings
        (1) Nucleated RBCs
        (2) Howell-Jolly bodies
        (3) Target cells (excess membrane cannot be removed)
        (4) Thrombocytosis
            • Platelets normally sequestered in the spleen are now circulating.

Splenic dysfunction: ↑ risk for *Streptococcus pneumoniae* sepsis

Mechanisms: ↓ IgM, ↓ tuftsin, ↓ splenic macrophages

CHAPTER 14
HEMOSTASIS DISORDERS

I. Normal Hemostasis and Hemostasis Testing
- Prevention of blood loss while maintaining maximal perfusion requires the interaction of the blood vessels, platelets, coagulation factors, and fibrinolytic agents.

A. Factors preventing thrombus formation in small blood vessels
- Small blood vessels include capillaries, venules, arterioles.
  1. Heparin-like molecules
     a. Enhance antithrombin III (ATIII) activity
     b. Neutralize activated serine protease coagulation factors
        - Factors XII, XI, IX, and X; thrombin (activated prothrombin)
  2. Prostaglandin (PG) I_2 (prostacyclin)
     a. Synthesized by intact endothelial cells
     b. PGH_2 is converted by prostacyclin synthase to PGI_2.
     c. Vasodilator; inhibits platelet aggregation
     d. Aspirin does *not* inhibit synthesis of PGI_2 by endothelial cells.
  3. Proteins C and S
     a. Vitamin K–dependent factors
     b. Inactivate factors V and VIII
     c. Enhance fibrinolysis
  4. Tissue plasminogen activator (tPA)
     a. Synthesized by endothelial cells
     b. Activates plasminogen to release plasmin
     c. Plasmin degrades coagulation factors and lyses fibrin clots (thrombi).

B. Factors enhancing thrombus formation in small vessel injury
  1. Thromboxane A_2 (TXA_2)
     a. Synthesized by platelets
        (1) PGH_2 is converted into TXA_2 by thromboxane synthase.
        (2) Aspirin *irreversibly* inhibits platelet cyclooxygenase.
           - Prevents formation of PGH_2, the precursor for TXA_2
        (3) Other NSAIDs *reversibly* inhibit platelet cyclooxygenase.
        (4) Prostacyclin synthase in endothelial cells is minimally affected by NSAIDs.
     b. Functions of TXA_2 in hemostasis
        - Vasoconstrictor, enhances platelet aggregation
  2. Von Willebrand factor (vWF)
     a. Synthesized by endothelial cells and megakaryocytes
        (1) Synthesized in Weibel-Palade bodies in endothelial cells
        (2) Platelets carry vWF in their α-granules.
     b. Functions of vWF
        (1) Platelet adhesion molecule
           (a) Binds platelets to exposed collagen
           (b) Platelets have glycoprotein (Gp) Ib receptors for vWF.
        (2) Complexes with factor VIII coagulant activity (factor VIII:c) in the circulation
           (a) Factor VIII:c is synthesized by the liver and other sites.
           (b) VIII:vWF complexes with VIII:c in the circulation.
              - Prevents degradation of factor VIII:c
           (c) Decrease in vWF secondarily decreases VIII:c activity.

Heparin-like molecules: enhance ATIII activity

ATIII: neutralizes activated serine protease coagulation factors

PGI_2: vasodilator, inhibits platelet aggregation

Proteins C and S: inactivate factors V and VIII, enhance fibrinolysis

tPA: activates plasminogen to release plasmin

TXA_2: vasoconstrictor; enhances platelet aggregation

vWF: platelet adhesion molecule; synthesized in Weibel-Palade bodies in endothelial cells

Factor VIII:c: synthesized in the liver

vWF: ↓ vWF causes ↓ VIII:c

vWF: platelet adhesion; prevents degradation of VIII:c in plasma

Factor VIII:c is synthesized by the liver and reticuloendothelial tissues. When VIII:c is activated by thrombin, it dissociates from the VIII:vWF complex and performs its procoagulant function in the intrinsic coagulation cascade system.

3. Tissue thromboplastin (factor III)
   a. Noncirculating ubiquitous substance
      • Released from injured tissue
   b. Activates factor VII in the extrinsic coagulation system
4. Extrinsic and intrinsic coagulation systems (see later)

C. Platelet structure and function
1. Derivation
   a. Cytoplasmic fragmentation of megakaryocytes
   b. Approximately 1000 to 3000 platelets are produced per megakaryocyte.
2. Locations
   a. Peripheral blood (live for ~9–10 days)
   b. Approximately one third of the total platelet pool is stored in the spleen.
3. Platelet receptors
   a. Glycoprotein (Gp) receptors for vWF are designated GpIb.
   b. Glycoprotein receptors for fibrinogen are designated GpIIb-IIIa.
      (1) Ticlopidine and clopidogrel
         (a) Inhibit adenosine diphosphate (ADP)-induced expression of platelet GpIIb-IIIa receptors
         (b) Prevents fibrinogen binding and platelet aggregation
      (2) Abciximab
         • Monoclonal antibody that is directed against the GpIIb-IIIa receptor
4. Platelet factor 3 (PF3)
   a. Located on the platelet membrane
   b. Phospholipid substrate required for the clotting sequence
5. Platelet structure
   a. Contractile element
      (1) Called thrombosthenin
      (2) Helps in clot retraction
   b. Dense bodies contain:
      (1) ADP, an aggregating agent
      (2) Calcium, a binding agent for vitamin K–dependent factors
   c. α-Granules contain:
      (1) vWF, fibrinogen
      (2) Platelet factor 4 (PF4)
         • Heparin neutralizing factor
6. Platelet function
   a. Fill gaps between endothelial cells in small vessels
      (1) Prevents leakage of RBCs into the interstitium
      (2) Platelet dysfunction causes leakage of RBCs, producing petechiae.
   b. Formation of the hemostatic plug in small vessel injury
   c. Platelet-derived growth factor stimulates smooth muscle hyperplasia.
      • Important in the pathogenesis of atherosclerosis

D. Coagulation system (Fig. 14-1)
1. Coagulation cascade
   a. Extrinsic system (factor VII)
   b. Intrinsic system (factors XII, XI, IX, VIII)
2. Extrinsic system
   a. Factor VII is activated (factor VIIa) by tissue thromboplastin.
   b. Factor VIIa activates factor X in the final common pathway.
3. Intrinsic system
   a. Factor XII (Hageman factor) is activated by:
      (1) Exposed subendothelial collagen
      (2) High-molecular-weight kininogen (HMWK)
   b. Functions of factor XIIa
      (1) Activates factor XI
      (2) Activates plasminogen (produces plasmin)
      (3) Activates the kininogen system (produces kallikrein and bradykinin)

Marginal notes:

Tissue thromboplastin: activates factor VII in extrinsic coagulation system

Platelet receptors: GpIb (binds to vWF); GpIIb-IIIa (binds to fibrinogen)

Ticlopidine, clopidogrel, abciximab: interfere with GpIIb-IIIa receptor function

Important platelet storage proteins: ADP, vWF, fibrinogen

Platelet function: stabilizes intercellular adherens junctions in venular endothelial cells

Extrinsic system: factor VII

Intrinsic system: factors XII, XI, IX, VIII

Factor XIIa: activates the kininogen system

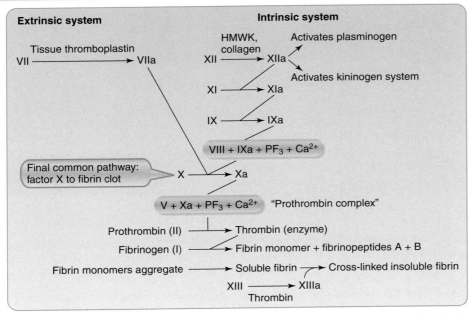

14-1: Coagulation cascade. Both the extrinsic and intrinsic coagulation systems use the final common pathway for the formation of a fibrin clot. a, activated; HMWK, high-molecular-weight kininogen; PF3, platelet factor 3.

    c. Factor XIa activates factor IX to form factor IXa.
        (1) Four-component complex is formed (IXa, VIII, PF3, calcium).
        (2) Complex activates factor X in the final common pathway.
        (3) Calcium binds factor IXa, a vitamin K–dependent coagulation factor.
  4. Final common pathway
    a. Includes factors X, V, prothrombin (II), and fibrinogen (I)
    b. Prothrombin complex
        (1) Four-component system consisting of factor Xa, factor V, PF3, and calcium
        (2) Calcium binds factor Xa, a vitamin K–dependent coagulation factor.
        (3) Complex cleaves prothrombin into thrombin (enzyme).
    c. Functions of thrombin
        (1) Acts on fibrinogen to produce fibrin monomers plus fibrinopeptides A and B
        (2) Activates fibrin stabilizing factor XIII
           (a) Factor XIIIa converts soluble fibrin monomers to insoluble fibrin.
           (b) Enhances protein-protein cross-linking to strengthen the fibrin clot
             • Cross-links are detected in D-dimer assay.
        (3) Activates VIII:c in the intrinsic system
  5. Vitamin K–dependent factors
    a. Factors II, VII, IX, X, protein C, and protein S
    b. Synthesized in the liver as nonfunctional precursor proteins
    c. Function of vitamin K
        (1) Vitamin K is activated in the liver by epoxide reductase.
           • Majority of vitamin K is synthesized by colonic bacteria.
        (2) Activated vitamin K γ-carboxylates each factor.
           • Carboxylated factors can bind to calcium and PF3 in the cascade sequence.
  6. Certain coagulation factors are consumed in the formation of a fibrin clot.
    • Consumed factors are fibrinogen (I), factor V, factor VIII, and prothrombin (II)

> When blood is drawn into a clot tube (no anticoagulant is added), a fibrin clot is formed. When the tube is spun down in a centrifuge, the supranate is called serum, which, unlike plasma, is missing fibrinogen, prothrombin (II), factor V, and factor VIII.

E. Fibrinolytic system
  1. Activation
    a. tPA activates plasminogen to release the enzyme plasmin.
        • Alteplase and reteplase are recombinant forms of tPA used in thrombolytic therapy.

Margin notes:

Final common pathway: factors X, V, II, I

Factor XIII: cross-links insoluble fibrin monomers

Vitamin K–dependent factors: procoagulants II, VII, IX, X; anticoagulants protein C and S

Vitamin K: liver activated by epoxide reductase

Calcium: binds γ-carboxylated vitamin K–dependent factors

Factors consumed in a clot: I, II, V, VIII; serum

Plasminogen activators: tPA, streptokinase, urokinase

Aminocaproic acid: inhibits plasminogen

D-Dimers: cross-linked fibrin monomers

  b. Other activators of plasminogen
    (1) Factor XIIa
    (2) Streptokinase
      • Derived from streptococci
    (3) Anistreplase
      • Complex of streptokinase and plasminogen
    (4) Urokinase (derived from human urine)
  c. Aminocaproic acid
    • Competitively blocks plasminogen activation, thereby inhibiting fibrinolysis
  2. Functions of plasmin
    a. Cleaves insoluble fibrin monomers and fibrinogen into fibrin(ogen) degradation products (FDPs)
      • Fragments of cross-linked insoluble fibrin monomers are called D-dimers.
    b. Degrades factors V, VIII, and fibrinogen
    c. α_2-Antiplasmin inactivates plasmin.
      • Synthesized in the liver
F. **Small vessel hemostasis response to injury** (Fig. 14-2)
  1. Sequence involves vascular, platelet, coagulation, and fibrinolytic phases.
  2. Vascular phase
    a. Transient vasoconstriction occurs directly after injury.
    b. Factor VII (extrinsic system) is locally activated by tissue thromboplastin.
    c. Exposed collagen activates factor XII (intrinsic system).
    d. Thrombin produced changes fibrinogen holding platelets together into fibrin at the end of the platelet phase.
  3. Platelet phase
    a. Platelet adhesion
      • Platelet GpIb receptors adhere to exposed vWF in damaged endothelial cells.
    b. Platelet release reaction
      (1) Release of ADP
      (2) Produces conformational changes in GpIIb-IIIa receptor
    c. Platelet synthesis and release of TXA$_2$
      (1) TXA$_2$ is a vasoconstrictor, which reduces blood flow.
      (2) TXA$_2$ is a platelet aggregator.
        • Enhances fibrinogen attachment to GpIIb-IIIa receptors
    d. Temporary platelet plug stops bleeding.
      (1) Unstable plug that can easily be dislodged
      (2) Only held together by fibrinogen (no cross-links)
      (3) Correlates with the end of the bleeding time (BT)
  4. Coagulation phase
    a. Fibrinogen attached to GpIIb-IIIa receptors is converted by thrombin (see above) to insoluble fibrin monomers (cross-linked).
    b. Stable platelet plug is formed.
      • Held together by fibrin, *not* fibrinogen

Platelet sequence in hemostasis: adhesion, release reaction, synthesis TXA$_2$, temporary plug

TXA$_2$: enhances fibrinogen attachment to GpIIb-IIIa receptors

Temporary platelet plug: held together by fibrinogen

Stable platelet plug: held together by fibrin

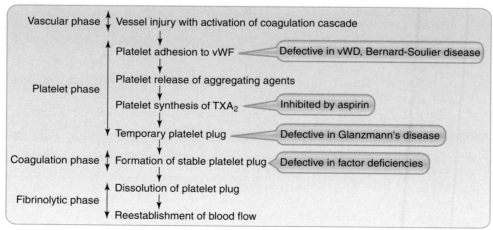

14-2: Small vessel hemostasis response to injury. See the text for discussion. TXA$_2$, thromboxane A$_2$; vWD, von Willebrand disease; vWF, von Willebrand factor.

TABLE 14-1. **CAUSES OF PROLONGED BLEEDING TIME**

CAUSE	NATURE OF DEFECT	DISCUSSION
Aspirin or NSAIDs	Platelet aggregation defect Inhibition of platelet COX, which ultimately inhibits synthesis of TXA_2	Normal platelet count
Bernard-Soulier syndrome	Platelet adhesion defect Autosomal recessive disease Absent GpIb platelet receptors for vWF	Thrombocytopenia, giant platelets Lifelong bleeding problem
Glanzmann's disease	Platelet aggregation defect Autosomal recessive disease Absent GpIIb-IIIa fibrinogen receptors Absent thrombosthenin	Lifelong bleeding problem
Renal failure	Platelet aggregation defect Inhibition of platelet phospholipid by toxic products	Reversed with dialysis and desmopressin acetate
Scurvy	Vascular defect Caused by vitamin C deficiency Defective collagen resulting from poor cross-linking	May cause ecchymoses and hemarthroses
Thrombocytopenia	Decreased platelet number	Increased bleeding time when platelet count < 90,000 cells/mm³
Von Willebrand disease	Platelet adhesion defect Autosomal dominant disorder Absent or defective vWF Decreased VIII:c	Combined platelet and coagulation factor disorder

COX, cyclooxygenase; TXA_2, thromboxane A_2; vWF, von Willebrand factor.

5. Fibrinolytic phase
   a. Plasmin cleaves the insoluble fibrin monomers holding the platelet plug together.
   b. Blood flow is eventually re-established.

G. Platelet tests
   1. Platelet count
      a. Normal count is 150,000 to 400,000 cells/mm³.
      b. A normal count does *not* guarantee normal platelet function.
   2. Bleeding time
      a. Evaluates platelet function up to the formation of the temporary platelet plug
         (1) Normal reference interval is 2 to 7 minutes.
         (2) Many laboratories have discontinued the BT.
      b. Disorders causing a prolonged BT are listed in Table 14-1.
   3. Platelet aggregation test
      a. Evaluates platelet aggregation in response to aggregating reagents
      b. Aggregating agents include ADP, epinephrine, collagen, and ristocetin.
   4. Tests for vWF
      a. Ristocetin cofactor assay
         (1) Evaluates vWF function
         (2) Abnormal assay
            (a) Classic von Willebrand disease (deficiency of vWF)
            (b) Bernard-Soulier disease (absent GpIb receptor)
      b. vWF antigen assay
         (1) Measures the quantity of vWF regardless of function
         (2) Decreased in classic von Willebrand disease

H. Coagulation tests (Fig. 14-3)
   1. Prothrombin time (PT)
      a. Evaluates the extrinsic system down to formation of the fibrin clot
         • Factors evaluated include VII, X, V, II, and I.
      b. Normal reference interval for PT is 11 to 15 seconds.
         • Only prolonged when a factor level is 30% to 40% of normal
      c. International normalized ratio (INR)
         (1) Standardizes the PT for use in warfarin therapy
         (2) Results are the same regardless of the reagents used to perform the test.
         (3) Usual range for INR is 2 to 3.
      d. Uses of PT
         (1) Follow patients who are taking warfarin for anticoagulation
         (2) Evaluate liver synthetic function
            • Increased PT indicates severe liver dysfunction.
         (3) Detect factor VII deficiency

BT: test of platelet function to formation of temporary plug

Ristocetin cofactor assay: test of vWF function

PT: evaluates factors VII, X, V, II, and I

INR: standardizes PT for warfarin therapy

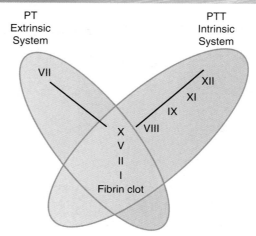

PT
Extrinsic
System

PTT
Intrinsic
System

14-3: Prothrombin time (PT) and partial thromboplastin time (PTT). See the text for discussion.

2. Partial thromboplastin time (PTT)
   a. Evaluates the intrinsic system down to formation of a fibrin clot
      • Factors evaluated include XII, XI, IX, VIII, X, V, II, and I.
   b. Normal reference interval for PTT is 25 to 40 seconds.
      • Only prolonged when a factor level is 30% to 40% of normal
   c. Uses of PTT
      (1) Follow heparin therapy
          (a) Heparin enhances ATIII activity.
          (b) PTT is *not* required to follow low-molecular-weight heparin therapy.
      (2) Detect factor deficiencies in the intrinsic system

PTT: evaluates factors XII, XI, IX, VIII, X, V, II, I

Whether the patient is anticoagulated with heparin or warfarin, both the PT and PTT are prolonged, because both inhibit factors in the final common pathway. Experience has shown that the PT performs better in monitoring warfarin, while the PTT performs better in monitoring heparin.

I. **Fibrinolytic system tests**
    1. Fibrin(ogen) degradation products (FDPs)
       • Detects fragments associated with plasmin degradation of fibrinogen or insoluble fibrin in fibrin clots
    2. D-Dimer assay
       a. Detects cross-linked insoluble fibrin monomers in a fibrin clot
       b. Does *not* detect fibrinogen degradation products (not cross-linked)
       c. Most specific test for evidence of degradation of a fibrin clot (thrombus); examples:
          (1) Thrombolytic therapy for coronary artery thrombosis
              • Thrombus is composed of platelets held together by fibrin (refer to Chapter 4).
          (2) Screening test for pulmonary thromboembolism
              • Thrombus is composed of RBCs, platelets, WBCs held together by fibrin (refer to Chapter 4).
          (3) Screening test for disseminated intravascular coagulation (DIC)
              • Thrombus is composed of RBCs, platelets, and WBCs held together by fibrin (see Section III).

FDPs: increased with lysis of fibrinogen and fibrin in fibrin thrombi

D-Dimer assay: specific for lysis of fibrin thrombi (clots); detects cross-links

II. **Platelet Disorders**
    A. **Classification of platelet disorders**
       1. Quantitative platelet disorders
          a. Thrombocytopenia
          b. Thrombocytosis
       2. Qualitative (functional) platelet disorders
    B. **Pathogenesis**
       1. Thrombocytopenia (Table 14-2)
          • Decreased number of platelets
          a. Decreased production
             • Examples—aplastic anemia, leukemia

TTP/HUS: platelet consumption + hemolytic anemia with schistocytes

TABLE 14-2. **DISORDERS PRODUCING THROMBOCYTOPENIA**

DISEASE	COMMENTS
Acute idiopathic thrombocytopenic purpura (ITP)	Most common cause thrombocytopenia in children 2–6 years of age IgG antibodies directed against GpIIb-IIIa receptors (type II reaction) Abrupt onset 1–3 weeks after a viral infection. Present with epistaxis, easy bruising, petechiae Absence of lymphadenopathy and splenomegaly *Treatment* varies with the platelet count Responds well to corticosteroids
Chronic ITP	Most common cause of thrombocytopenia in adults Most common in women 20–40 years of age IgG antibodies directed against GpIIb-IIIa receptors (type II reaction) Insidious onset Often resistant to steroids and requires splenectomy; IV γ-globulin temporarily stops serious bleeding (IgG blocks macrophage Fc receptors) Newborn infants of mothers with ITP may have transient thrombocytopenia due to transplacental passage of IgG antibodies Secondary causes: SLE, HIV, lymphoproliferative diseases
Neonatal alloimmune thrombocytopenia (NAIT)	Accounts for 20% of cases of thrombocytopenia in neonates Feto-maternal incompatibility for platelet specific antigens (e.g., Pl^{A1}); Pl^{A1} is absent from the 2% of population Pl^{A1}-negative mother develops IgG antibodies during pregnancy or from a previous pregnancy or transfusion Transplacental passage of IgG antibodies targets fetal Pl^{A1} positive platelets leading to macrophage destruction of platelets (type II hypersensitivity) May produce petechial hemorrhages in first few days of life or CNS hemorrhages in severe cases
Post-transfusion purpura	Primarily occurs in multiparous women Patient receiving blood has antibodies against Pl^{A1} or other platelet antigens that are present on donor platelets Severe thrombocytopenia with destruction of donor and patient platelets occurs 7–10 days after a blood transfusion
Heparin-induced thrombocytopenia	Most common cause of thrombocytopenia in hospitalized patients Macrophage removal of platelets surfaced by IgG antibody directed against heparin attached to PF4 (type II hypersensitivity) Occurs 5–14 days after Rx; must stop heparin; release of PF4 (anti-heparin factor) after platelet destruction may result in vessel thrombosis
Thrombotic thrombocytopenic purpura (TTP)	Occurs in adult females Acquired or genetic deficiency in vWF-cleaving metalloprotease in endothelial cells Increase in circulating multimers of vWF increases platelet adhesion to areas of endothelial injury at arteriole-capillary junctions Platelets are consumed owing to production of platelet thrombi in areas of injury (*not* DIC) Enhanced by other factors that damage endothelial cells (e.g., ticlopidine, clopidogrel, cyclosporine, oral contraceptives; hypertension, postpartum) Clinical pentad: fever, thrombocytopenia, renal failure, microangiopathic hemolytic anemia with schistocytes (damage by platelet thrombi), CNS deficits *Treatment*: plasma exchange; corticosteroids; vincristine Mortality rate, 10–20%
Hemolytic uremic syndrome (HUS)	Primarily occurs in children < 10 years old Most often caused by endothelial damage at arteriole-capillary junction due to Shiga-like toxin of O157:H7 serotype of *E. coli* Organisms proliferate in undercooked beef May also be caused by drugs and other infections (e.g., *Shigella*, *Salmonella*) Clinical findings similar to TTP; however, CNS findings are less frequent Bloody diarrhea in 75% of cases Triad: thrombocytopenia, acute renal failure, microangiopathic hemolytic anemia *Treatment*: plasma exchange transfusions; corticosteroids Mortality rate, 3–5%

DIC, disseminated intravascular coagulation; PF4, platelet factor 4; Rx, treatment; SLE, systemic lupus erythematosus; vWF, von Willebrand factor

    b. Increased destruction
        (1) Immune
            • Examples—idiopathic thrombocytopenic purpura, drugs
        (2) Nonimmune
            • Examples—thrombotic thrombocytopenic purpura, DIC
    c. Sequestration in the spleen
        • Hypersplenism in portal hypertension

Thrombocytosis:
chronic iron deficiency,
malignancy, splenectomy

Aspirin: most common
cause of a qualitative
platelet defect

Petechiae: only with
thrombocytopenia

2. Thrombocytosis
- Increased platelet count
  a. Primary thrombocytosis
     - Examples—essential thrombocythemia, polycythemia vera (refer to Chapter 12)
  b. Secondary (reactive) thrombocytosis
     - Examples—chronic iron deficiency, infections, splenectomy, malignancy
3. Qualitative platelet disorders
   - Acquired (e.g., aspirin) or hereditary (e.g., Glanzmann's disease)

C. Clinical findings associated with platelet dysfunction
1. Epistaxis (nosebleeds) is the most common symptom.
2. Petechiae and multiple small ecchymoses (purpura); only with thrombocytopenia
   a. Petechiae are pinpoint areas of hemorrhage in subcutaneous tissue (Fig. 14-4).
      - RBCs leak through postcapillary venular gaps in the endothelium.
   b. Ecchymoses are the size of a quarter.

Senile purpura: vessel
instability

> **Ecchymoses (purpura)** can be caused by a variety of disorders unrelated to thrombocytopenia. Palpable purpura (purpura that can be felt) is a sign of a small vessel vasculitis (refer to Chapter 9). Because vasculitis is a type of acute inflammation, the lesions are palpable due to increased vessel permeability and *not* a platelet disorder. Ecchymoses are also present in scurvy (vitamin C deficiency), and are due to vessel weakness related to lack of cross-bridging between tropocollagen molecules (refer to Chapter 7). Senile purpura is a normal finding in elderly patients and is due to vessel instability normally associated with aging (Fig. 14-5). Ecchymoses develop in areas of trauma (e.g., back of the hands, shins).

Platelet dysfunction
(e.g., aspirin): bleeding
from superficial scratches,
easy bruising

Thrombocytopenia:
petechia and above
findings

3. Bleeding from superficial scratches
   - No temporary platelet plug is present to stop bleeding from injury to small vessels.
4. Other findings
   a. Menorrhagia, hematuria
   b. Bleeding from tooth extraction sites
   c. Easy bruiseability
   d. Gastrointestinal and intracranial bleeding

III. Coagulation Disorders
  A. Classification of coagulation disorders
1. Acquired
   - Single or multiple coagulation factor deficiencies
2. Hereditary
   - Usually a single coagulation factor deficiency

  B. Pathogenesis
1. Decreased production
   - Examples—hemophilia A, cirrhosis
2. Pathologic inhibition
   - Example—acquired circulating antibodies (inhibitors) against coagulation factors

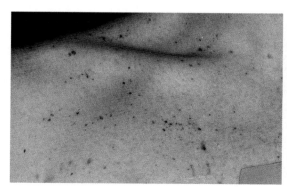

14-4: Petechiae in idiopathic thrombocytopenic purpura showing pinpoint hemorrhages, a sign of platelet dysfunction, in the skin over the thorax and shoulders. When touched, petechiae do not blanch with pressure. (*From Forbes C, Jackson W: Color Atlas and Text of Clinical Medicine, 2nd ed. St. Louis, Mosby, 2003, Fig. 10-10.*)

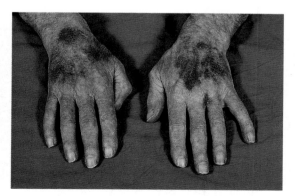

14-5: Senile purpura showing the large, irregular areas of hemorrhage on the backs of both hands. This benign condition primarily occurs in body areas that are frequently traumatized. It is due to the normal vessel instability that is associated with aging. (*From Forbes C, Jackson W: Color Atlas and Text of Clinical Medicine, 2nd ed. St. Louis, Mosby, 2003, Fig. 10-112.*)

3. Excessive consumption
   - Example—disseminated intravascular coagulation

C. Clinical findings in coagulation disorders
   1. Late rebleeding after surgery or wisdom tooth extraction
      a. Temporary platelet plug is the only mechanical block preventing bleeding.
      b. Lack of thrombin prevents formation of a stable platelet plug held together by fibrin.
   2. Findings in severe factor deficiencies
      a. Hemarthroses
      b. Retroperitoneal and deep muscular bleeding
   3. Findings similar to platelet disorders
      a. Ecchymoses, epistaxis
      b. Menorrhagia, hematuria
      c. Bleeding from tooth extraction sites
      d. Easy bruiseability
      e. Gastrointestinal and intracranial bleeding

D. Hemophilia A
   1. Epidemiology
      a. X-linked recessive
         (1) Females are asymptomatic carriers.
         (2) Females transmit the abnormal X chromosome to 50% of their sons.
      b. Absent family history of hemophilia
         - Most likely due to a new mutation (30% of cases)
      c. Female carriers with symptomatic disease
         (1) Due to inactivation of more maternal than paternal X chromosomes
         (2) Females become "homozygous" for the abnormal X chromosome.
   2. Pathogenesis
      - Decreased synthesis of factor VIII:c, a coagulation factor in the intrinsic system
   3. Clinical findings in hemophilia A
      a. Signs and symptoms correlate with the level of factor VIII:c activity
         (1) Mild disease is 5% to 25% of normal.
         (2) Moderate disease is 1% to 4% of normal.
         (3) Severe disease is <1% of normal.
      b. Bleeding problems may occur in newborns (10–15% of cases).
         - Excessive bleeding may occur after circumcision or umbilical cord separation.

> **Hemophilia B** (Christmas disease) is an X-linked recessive disorder involving a deficiency of factor IX. It is clinically indistinguishable from hemophilia A.

      c. Laboratory findings in hemophilia A
         (1) Increased PTT and a normal PT
         (2) Decreased factor VIII:c activity
         (3) Detection of female carriers
            - DNA techniques are most sensitive.
   4. Treatment of hemophilia A
      a. Mild cases respond to desmopressin acetate
         - Increases release of VIII:c from storage sites
      b. Severe cases require infusion of recombinant factor VIII
         - *No* risk for HIV

E. Classic von Willebrand disease
   1. Epidemiology
      a. Autosomal dominant disorder
      b. Most common hereditary coagulation disorder
      c. Several subtypes
         - Type I (80%; only one discussed), type IIA, type IIB, type III
         (1) Some differ in inheritance pattern.
         (2) Some differ in ristocetin cofactor assay results.
         (3) Some have abnormal multimer patterns on agar electrophoresis.
         (4) Some differ in ristocetin-induced platelet aggregation.
         (5) Some differ in VIII:c activity.
      d. Associations
         (1) Mitral valve prolapse (MVP)

Coagulation disorders: ↓ production, inhibition, consumption

Coagulation disorders: late rebleeding; hemarthroses (severe deficiency)

Hemophilia A: X-linked recessive

Hemophilia A: % VIII:c never changes; correlates with severity of disease

Hemophilia B: X-linked recessive; factor IX deficiency

Hemophilia A: ↓ VIII:c; ↑ PTT

vWD: AD inheritance

vWD associations: MVP, Marfan syndrome, angiodysplasia

vWD: most common hereditary coagulation disorder

vWD: combined platelet and coagulation factor disorder

(2) Marfan syndrome
(3) Angiodysplasia
2. Pathogenesis
   • Decreased vWF and factor VIII:c activity
3. Clinical findings in vWD
   a. Menorrhagia
   b. Epistaxis
   c. Easy bruiseability

vWD: ↑ PTT, bleeding time; ↓ VIII:c, vWF

4. Laboratory findings in vWD
   a. Increased PTT and a normal PT
   b. Increased bleeding time
      • Due to a platelet adhesion defect
   c. Abnormal ristocetin cofactor assay
   d. Decreased vWF antigen
   e. Decreased VIII:c activity
5. Treatment of vWD

Rx vWD: desmopressin acetate, OCP

   a. Desmopressin acetate or estrogen in oral contraceptive pills (OCPs) (women)
      • Increases release of vWF and VIII:c from storage sites
   b. Severe cases require infusion of recombinant factor VIII

F. **Circulating anticoagulants (inhibitors)**
   1. Pathogenesis
      a. Coagulation factor is destroyed by antibodies.
      b. Most common type is antibodies against factor VIII:c (e.g., postpartum).
   2. Clinical findings
      • Similar to those with coagulation factor deficiencies due to decreased production
   3. Laboratory findings
      a. Prolonged PT or PTT, depending on the factor deficiency
         • Does *not* differentiate immune destruction versus decreased production
      b. Mixing studies

Circulating anticoagulant: PT and PTT *not* corrected with mixing study

         (1) Normal plasma is mixed with patient plasma in a test tube.
         (2) *No* correction of PT or PTT indicates immune destruction.
         (3) Correction of PT and PTT indicates decreased production.

G. **Vitamin K deficiency**
   1. Function of vitamin K
      • γ-Carboxylates vitamin K–dependent factors II, VII, IX, X and proteins C and S

Vitamin K–dependent factors: II, VII, IX, X, protein C and S; γ-carboxylation activates them

   2. Causes of vitamin K deficiency
      a. Decreased synthesis of vitamin K by colonic bacteria
         (1) Newborns lack bacterial colonization of the bowel.
            (a) Vitamin K levels normally decrease between days 2 and 5.
            (b) Danger of severe bleeding (e.g., intracerebral hemorrhage)
            (c) Newborns require an intramuscular injection of vitamin K at birth.
               • Breast milk contains very little vitamin K.

Newborns: lack bacterial colonization in bowel; no synthesis vitamin K

         (2) Prolonged treatment with antibiotics
            (a) Antibiotics sterilize the bowel causing decreased production of vitamin K.
            (b) Most common cause of vitamin K deficiency in a hospitalized patient

Vitamin K deficiency in hospitalized patient: due to antibiotic therapy

      b. Decreased small bowel reabsorption of vitamin K
         (1) Malabsorption of fat causes malabsorption of fat-soluble vitamins.
         (2) Example—celiac disease
      c. Decreased activation of vitamin K by epoxide reductase in the liver
         (1) Warfarin inhibits epoxide reductase.
            (a) Vitamin K–dependent factors are nonfunctional.

Rat poison: contains warfarin

            (b) Rat poison contains warfarin.
            (c) Children may have exposure to warfarin from elders living in the household.

Warfarin: inhibits epoxide reductase; vitamin K is nonfunctional

Warfarin is an anticoagulant that inhibits epoxide reductase, which prevents any further γ-carboxylation of the vitamin K–dependent coagulation factors. However, full anticoagulation does *not* immediately occur, because previously γ-carboxylated factors are still present. Prothrombin has the longest half-life; therefore, full anticoagulation requires at least 3–4 days before all functional prothrombin has disappeared. This explains why patients are initially placed on both heparin and warfarin, because heparin immediately anticoagulates the patient by enhancing ATIII activity.

(2) Cirrhosis
    (a) Decreased activation of vitamin K and synthesis of vitamin K–dependent coagulation factors
    (b) Prolonged PT is *not* corrected with intramuscular injection of vitamin K.

3. Clinical findings of vitamin K deficiency
  a. Gastrointestinal bleeding
  b. Bleeding into subcutaneous tissue
  c. Bleeding at the time of circumcision
  d. Intracranial hemorrhage

4. Treatment of vitamin K deficiency
  a. If bleeding is *not* severe, treatment is an intramuscular injection of vitamin K.
    • Corrects bleeding in a few hours
  b. If bleeding is severe, treatment is with fresh frozen plasma.
    (1) Immediate correction
    (2) Vitamin K–dependent factors are γ-carboxylated.

> Cirrhosis: ↓ synthesis of vitamin K–dependent factors, ↓ activation of vitamin K

H. Hemostasis disorders in liver disease

1. Pathogenesis
  a. Decreased synthesis of coagulation factors
    (1) Multiple coagulation factor deficiencies
    (2) Decreased γ-carboxylation of vitamin K–dependent factors
  b. Decreased synthesis of anticoagulants
    • Examples—ATIII, proteins C and S
  c. Decreased synthesis of fibrinolytic agents (e.g., plasminogen)
  d. Decreased clearance of FDPs and D-dimers
    • Interfere with platelet aggregation and polymerization of fibrin
  e. Decreased clearance of tPA and decreased synthesis of α_2-antiplasmin
    • May produce primary fibrinolysis (see section IV)

2. Laboratory findings in liver disease
  a. Increased PT and PTT
  b. Increased FDPs and D-dimers
  c. Increased bleeding time

> Cirrhosis: multiple hemostasis abnormalities

I. Disseminated intravascular coagulation

1. Causes of DIC
  a. Sepsis (>50% of cases)
    (1) Common pathogens are *E. coli* (most common) and *Neisseria meningitidis*.
    (2) Others include Rocky Mountain spotted fever and malaria.
  b. Disseminated malignancy
    (1) Acute promyelocytic leukemia
    (2) Pancreatic cancer with release of procoagulants in mucin
  c. Other causes
    (1) Crush injuries
    (2) Rattlesnake envenomation
    (3) Amniotic fluid embolism
    (4) Disseminated malignancy
    (5) Abruptio placentae

> Sepsis: most common cause of DIC

2. Pathogenesis
  a. Activation of the coagulation cascade
    • Due to release of tissue thromboplastin or endothelial cell injury
  b. Fibrin thrombi develop in the microcirculation.
    (1) Thrombi obstruct blood flow.
    (2) Thrombi consume coagulation factors (I, II, V, VIII) and trap platelets.
  c. Activation of the fibrinolytic system
    • Secondary fibrinolysis due to activation of plasminogen by factor XII

> DIC: consumption of coagulation factors

3. Clinical findings in DIC
  a. Thrombohemorrhagic disorder
    (1) Ischemia from occlusive fibrin thrombi
    (2) Bleeding from anticoagulation
     • Factors I, II, V, and VIII are consumed in production of the fibrin thrombi.
    (3) Bleeding from interference with platelet aggregation by fibrinogen degradation products
  b. Hypovolemic shock due to blood loss

> DIC: thrombohemorrhagic disorder

c. Diffuse oozing of blood from all breaks in the skin and mucous membranes

d. Petechiae and ecchymoses from thrombocytopenia

4. Laboratory findings in DIC

a. Coagulation abnormalities

(1) Increased PT and PTT

(2) Decreased fibrinogen

b. Platelet abnormalities

(1) Thrombocytopenia

(2) Increased bleeding time

c. Fibrinolysis abnormalities

• Presence of FDPs and D-dimers

d. Normocytic anemia

(1) Bleeding from different sites

(2) Microangiopathic hemolytic anemia with schistocytes

• RBCs are damaged by fibrin thrombi.

5. Treatment

a. Treating the underlying disease is most important!

b. Transfuse blood components

(1) Fresh frozen plasma for multiple coagulation factor deficiencies

(2) Packed RBCs for anemia

(3) Platelet concentrates for thrombocytopenia

(4) Cryoprecipitate for fibrinogen deficiency (if warranted)

c. Low-dose heparin in selected cases (controversial)

IV. **Fibrinolytic Disorders**

A. **Primary fibrinolysis**

1. Causes

a. Open heart surgery

• Cardiopulmonary bypass causes a decrease in α_2-antiplasmin and increase in tPA.

b. Radical prostatectomy

• Causes increased release of urokinase

c. Diffuse liver disease

• Causes a decrease in the synthesis of α_2-antiplasmin

2. Pathogenesis

a. FDPs interfere with platelet aggregation.

b. Plasmin degrades coagulation factors causing multiple factor deficiencies.

3. Clinical findings

• Severe bleeding

4. Laboratory findings

a. Increased PT and PTT

• Due to multiple factor deficiencies

b. Increased bleeding time

• Due to interference with platelet aggregation

c. Positive test for FDPs

d. Negative D-dimer assay

• *No* fibrin thrombi are present.

e. Normal platelet count

5. Treatment

• Aminocaproic acid

B. **Secondary fibrinolysis**

1. Compensatory reaction in the presence of DIC

2. Increase in both FDPs and D-dimers

V. **Summary of Laboratory Test Results in Hemostasis Disorders** (Table 14-3)

VI. **Thrombosis Syndromes**

A. **Acquired thrombosis syndromes**

1. Antiphospholipid syndrome (APLS)

a. Epidemiology

(1) Highest association with SLE

(2) Other diseases: rheumatoid arthritis, Sjögren's syndrome, HIV infection

b. Pathogenesis

(1) Presence of antiphospholipid antibodies (APAs)

• Directed against phospholipids bound to plasma proteins

Margin notes:

Lab findings: ↑ PT, PTT, D-dimers, BT; ↓ platelets

D-Dimers: most sensitive screen for DIC

DIC Rx: treat underlying disease most important; component replacement

Primary fibrinolysis: open heart surgery, prostatectomy, diffuse liver disease

Primary fibrinolysis: − test for FDPs, D-dimers; normal platelet count; ↑ PT and PTT

Secondary fibrinolysis: D-dimer and FDPs; ↓ platelet count; ↑ PT and PTT

APAs: anticardiolipin antibody, lupus anticoagulant

TABLE 14-3. LABORATORY FINDINGS IN COMMON HEMOSTASIS DISORDERS

DISORDER	PLATELET COUNT	BLEEDING TIME	PT	PTT
Thrombocytopenia ITP, TTP, HUS	↓	↑	Normal	Normal
Von Willebrand disease	Normal	↑	Normal	↑
Hemophilia A	Normal	Normal	Normal	↑
DIC	↓	↑	↑	↑
Primary fibrinolysis	Normal	↑	↑	↑
Aspirin or NSAIDs	Normal	↑	Normal	Normal
Warfarin or heparin	Normal	Normal	↑	↑

DIC, disseminated intravascular coagulation; HUS; hemolytic uremic syndrome; ITP, idiopathic thrombocytopenic purpura; PT, prothrombin time; PTT, partial thromboplastin time; TTP, thrombotic thrombocytopenic purpura.

(2) APAs include:
    (a) Anticardiolipin antibody and lupus anticoagulant
       • Anticardiolipin antibody reacts with the cardiolipin reagent in the rapid plasma reagin test for syphilis.
    (b) Lupus anticoagulant
    (c) Anti-β_2 glycoprotein-1 antibodies
  (3) Produce arterial and venous thrombosis syndromes
    • Venous thrombi more common than arterial

c. Clinical findings in APLS
  (1) Repeated spontaneous abortions
    • Due to thrombosis of placental bed vessels
  (2) Strokes
  (3) Deep vein thrombosis
  (4) Hepatic vein thrombosis

d. Laboratory findings
  (1) False positive syphilis serologic test
    • If anticardiolipin antibodies are present
  (2) Lupus anticoagulant
    • Prolonged PTT that does *not* correct with mixing studies
  (3) Anticardiolipin antibodies
    • Most sensitive and specific test (>80%)
  (4) Anti-β_2 glycoprotein-1 antibodies

e. Treatment
  (1) Depends on the clinical presentation
  (2) In general, initiate anticoagulation with heparin and keep on lifelong warfarin treatment

2. Other acquired causes of thrombosis
  a. Postoperative state with stasis of blood flow
  b. Malignancy
    (1) Increase in coagulation factors
    (2) Thrombocytosis
    (3) Release of procoagulants from tumors, particularly pancreatic cancers
  c. Folate or vitamin B_{12} deficiency
    • Due to increased plasma homocysteine levels
  d. OCPs
    • Estrogen increases the synthesis of coagulation factors and decreases ATIII
  e. Hyperviscosity
    (1) Polycythemia syndromes
    (2) Waldenström's macroglobulinemia

B. Hereditary thrombosis syndromes
1. Epidemiology
  a. Autosomal dominant syndromes
  b. Deep venous thrombosis and pulmonary emboli occur at an early age.
  c. Venous thromboses often occur in unusual places.
    • Examples—hepatic vein, dural sinus
2. Factor V Leiden
  a. Most common hereditary thrombosis syndrome
  b. Mutant form of factor V *cannot* be degraded by protein C and protein S.

APLS: thrombosis syndrome

Anticardiolipin antibody: false positive syphilis serologic test

APLS: spontaneous abortions, strokes, deep vein thrombosis, hepatic vein thrombosis

Other thrombosis syndromes: post-op state, malignancy, OCPs, ↓ folate/B_{12}, hypersensitivity

Factor V Leiden: most common hereditary thrombosis syndrome

3. Antithrombin III (ATIII) deficiency
    a. Functions of ATIII
        (1) Activity is enhanced by heparin.
        (2) Neutralizes activated serine proteases
            • Example—factors XII, XI, IX, X, thrombin
    b. *No* prolongation of PTT after injecting a standard dose of heparin
    c. Treatment
        (1) Infuse a greater dose of heparin than normal
            • PTT eventually increases due to enhancement of whatever ATIII is present.
        (2) Send the patient home on warfarin.
4. Proteins C and S deficiency
    a. Pathogenesis
        • Cannot inactivate factors V and VIII
    b. Treatment
        (1) Begin with heparin and a very low dose of warfarin to reduce the risk for developing hemorrhagic skin necrosis.
        (2) Send the patient home on warfarin.

ATIII deficiency: normal PTT after standard dose heparin

Hemorrhagic skin necrosis: associated with warfarin therapy in protein C deficiency

There is a potential for heterozygote carriers of protein C deficiency to develop hemorrhagic skin necrosis when placed on warfarin. Heterozygote carriers have ~50% protein C activity. Protein C has a short half-life (~6 hours). When these patients are placed on warfarin, protein C activity falls to zero activity in 6 hours, causing a hypercoagulable state due to increased activity of factors V and VIII. This causes cutaneous vessel thrombosis and concomitant skin necrosis. This complication is not likely to occur in normal people.

I. ABO Blood Group Antigens
   A. Definition of ABO blood group antigens
      • They are glycoproteins attached to the RBC surface.
   B. Blood group O characteristics
      1. Most common blood group
         • *No* blood group antigens are present on the RBC membrane.
      2. Natural antibodies (isohemagglutinins) in serum
         a. Anti-A-IgM, anti-B-IgM
         b. Most people have anti-A and B-IgG antibodies.

Blood group antibodies are natural antibodies that are synthesized in Peyer's patches. A and B antigens that are normally present in food are trapped by specialized epithelial cells called M cells that overlie Peyer's patches. M cells have close proximity to B lymphocytes lying within the epithelium. M cells transport the A and B antigens to these lymphocytes, resulting in the development of natural antibodies against the antigens. Natural antibodies develop against antigens that are *not* present on the RBC, which explains why blood group O patients have antibodies against both A and B antigens.

      3. Increased incidence of duodenal ulcers
   C. Blood group A characteristics
      1. Anti-B-IgM antibodies
      2. Increased incidence of gastric carcinoma
   D. Blood group B characteristics
      • Anti-A-IgM antibodies
   E. Blood group AB characteristics
      1. Least common blood group
      2. *No* natural antibodies
   F. Newborns
      1. Do *not* have natural antibodies at birth
      2. IgG antibodies are of maternal origin.
         • IgG antibodies cross the placenta.
   G. Elderly people
      • Frequently lose their natural antibodies

Elderly patients may *not* have a hemolytic transfusion reaction if they are transfused with the wrong blood group because they frequently lose their natural antibodies.

   H. Paternity issues in newborns
      1. Blood group AB parents *cannot* have an O child.
      2. Blood group O parents *cannot* have an AB, A, or B child.
      3. Blood group A and B parents can have O children if both have AO and BO phenotypes (Fig. 15-1).
   I. Determining the ABO group (Fig. 15-2)
      1. Forward type

Sidebar notes:
Blood group O: most common blood group

Group O: anti-A-IgM, anti-B-IgM, anti-A and B-IgG

M cells: transport A and B antigens in Peyer's patches to B lymphocytes

Group A: anti-B-IgM

Group B: anti-A-IgM

Group AB: no natural antibodies

Newborns: lack natural antibodies

Elderly people: frequently lose natural antibodies

Blood group AB parents: cannot have O child

Blood group O parents: cannot have AB, A, or B child

	B	O	Father
Mother	A	AB	AO
	O	BO	**OO**

15-1: Possible children phenotypes if father is BO and mother is AO. See text for discussion. *(Adapted from Goljan EF: Star Series: Pathology. Philadelphia, WB Saunders, 1998.)*

Blood group	Forward Type		Back Type	
	Anti-A	Anti-B	A RBCs	B RBCs
O	−	−	+	+
A	+	−	−	+
B	−	+	+	−
AB	+	+	−	−

15-2: Forward and back type to identify ABO blood groups. Forward type identifies the blood group antigen by reacting anti-A and anti-B against patient RBCs. Back type identifies the natural antibodies in the patient serum by reacting A RBCs and B RBCs against the patient serum. Refer to the text for discussion of the blood groups and their natural antibodies.

Forward typing: identifies blood group antigen

  a. Identifies the blood group antigen
    • Patient RBCs are added to test tubes that contain either anti-A or anti-B test serum.
  b. Example—blood group A RBCs
    • Agglutination reaction with anti-A test serum but *not* with anti-B test serum
 2. Back type

Back typing: identifies natural antibodies

  a. Identifies the natural antibodies
    • Patient serum is added to test tubes containing either A or B test RBCs.
  b. Example—blood group A serum
    • Patient anti-B-IgM antibodies agglutinate B test RBCs but *not* A test RBCs.

II. Rh and Non-Rh Antigen Systems
A. Rh antigen system

 1. It has three adjoining gene loci.

Five Rh antigens: D, C, c, E, e

  a. Locus coding for D antigen (no d antigen)
  b. Locus coding for C and c antigen
  c. Locus coding for E and e antigen
 2. Autosomal codominant inheritance
  a. One of the sets of three Rh antigens from each parent is transmitted to each child.
    (1) Example—child with cDe from the mother and cde from the father (Fig. 15-3)
      • Note that the child lacks E antigen.
    (2) Absence of D antigen on a chromosome is designated d even though the antigen does *not* exist.
  b. Possible Rh antigen profiles
    (1) DD, Dd, or dd
    (2) CC, Cc, or cc
    (3) EE, Ee, or ee

Rh positive: D antigen positive

 3. An individual who is Rh positive is D antigen positive.
 4. Approximately 85% of the population has D antigen.
    • Individuals lacking D antigen are considered Rh negative.
 5. Rh phenotype of an individual
  a. RBCs are reacted with test antisera against each of the Rh antigens.
  b. Example—Rh phenotype that is positive for C, c, D, and E antigens but negative for e antigen (phenotype is CcDE)

Alloimmunization: antibodies develop against foreign antigens

B. Alloimmunization

 1. Production of an antibody against a foreign antigen *not* present on an individual's RBCs
  a. Patient exposure to Rh antigen he is lacking (e.g., D antigen)
  b. Patient exposure to non-Rh antigen she is lacking (e.g., Kell antigen)
  c. These antibodies are called atypical antibodies.
    • The individual is considered sensitized if atypical antibodies are present.

Atypical antibodies: may produce an HTR

 2. Significance of atypical antibodies
  a. May produce a hemolytic transfusion reaction (HTR)

	cde	CDE	Father
Mother	cDe	cDe/cde	cDe/CDE
	CDE	CDE/cde	CDE/CDE

15-3: Possible Rh phenotypes in children if the father is cde/CDE and the mother is cDE/CDE. See text for discussion. *(Adapted from Goljan EF: Star Series: Pathology. Philadelphia, WB Saunders, 1998.)*

(1) Occurs when blood containing the foreign antigen is infused into an individual
(2) Example—individual with anti-Kell antibodies is exposed to Kell antigen positive RBCs.
(3) IgG antibodies are more likely to produce an HTR than IgM antibodies.
   • IgG antibodies react best in warm temperatures, but IgM antibodies react best in cold temperatures.
b. Transfusion requirements in an individual with atypical antibodies
   (1) Individual must receive blood that is negative for the foreign antigen.
   (2) Example—individual with anti-Kell antibodies must receive Kell antigen negative blood.

Individual with an atypical antibody must receive blood lacking the antigen.

C. Clinically important non-Rh antigens
1. Duffy (Fy) antigens
   a. Fy antigens are the binding site for infestation of RBCs by *Plasmodium vivax*.
   b. Majority of blacks lack the Fy antigen.
      • Offers protection against contracting *P. vivax* malaria
2. I and i antigen systems
   a. IgM antibodies (cold agglutinins) may develop against I or i antigen.
   b. Increased risk for developing a cold autoimmune hemolytic anemia (refer to Chapter 11)
      (1) Anti-i hemolytic anemia may occur in infectious mononucleosis.
      (2) Anti-I hemolytic anemia may occur in *Mycoplasma pneumoniae* infections.

Fy antigen negative RBCs: protection against P. vivax malaria

III. Blood Transfusion Therapy
A. Blood donors
1. Autologous transfusion
   a. Process of collection, storage, and reinfusion of the individual's own blood
   b. Safest form of transfusion
2. Tests performed on donor blood
   a. Group (ABO) and type (Rh)
   b. Antibody screen (indirect Coombs' test)
      • Detects atypical antibodies (e.g., anti-D, anti-Kell)
   c. Screening tests for infectious disease
      • Examples—syphilis, hepatitis B and C, human immunodeficiency virus (HIV-1 and 2), human T-lymphotrophic virus (HTLV-1)

Autologous transfusion: safest transfusion

CMV: most common pathogen transmitted by transfusion

There is a risk for **transmitting infection when transfusing blood**, because there is an incubation period *before* specific antibodies are developed against the pathogen. The risk for developing an infection per unit of blood in the post-nucleic acid testing era has markedly reduced the risk for transmission of HBV, HCV, and HIV. The most common infectious agent transmitted by blood transfusion is cytomegalovirus (CMV), which is present in donor lymphocytes. When newborns receive transfusions, the blood must be irradiated to destroy lymphocytes that may be carrying CMV. Because a newborn's cellular immunity is *not* fully developed, a CMV infection would likely be disseminated.

Newborn transfusion: must irradiate blood to destroy lymphocytes

B. Patient crossmatch
1. Components of a standard crossmatch
   a. ABO group and Rh type
   b. Antibody screen for atypical antibodies
   c. Direct Coombs' test to identify atypical IgG antibodies on patient RBCs
   d. Major crossmatch
2. Major crossmatch
   a. Purpose of a major crossmatch
      • Detect atypical antibodies that are directed against foreign antigens on donor RBCs
   b. Patient serum is mixed with a sample of RBCs from a donor unit.
      (1) Each unit of donor blood must have a separate crossmatch.
      (2) Lack of RBC agglutination or hemolysis indicates a compatible crossmatch.

Major crossmatch: patient serum + donor RBCs

Patients with a negative antibody screen should have a compatible crossmatch. However, a compatible crossmatch does *not* guarantee that the recipient will not develop atypical antibodies, a transfusion reaction, or an infection.

A negative antibody screen ensures that a major crossmatch will be compatible.

3. Use of blood group O–packed RBCs for transfusion
   a. Can be transfused into any patient, regardless of the blood group
      (1) Blood group O RBCs lack A and B antigens.

Blood group O
individuals: universal
donors

(2) Blood group O individuals are considered universal donors.
  • Anti-A-IgM and anti-B-IgM cannot hemolyze O RBCs.
4. Blood group AB individuals can be transfused with blood from any blood group.
  a. They lack natural antibodies.
  b. They are considered universal recipients.

Blood group AB
individuals: universal
recipients

Before blood is transfused into newborns or patients with T-cell deficiencies, it must be irradiated to kill donor lymphocytes. This prevents the patient from developing a graft-versus-host reaction (refer to Chapter 3) or a disseminated CMV infection.

C. Blood component therapy (Table 15-1)
D. Transfusion reactions
  1. Allergic reaction
    a. Most common transfusion reaction
    b. Type I IgE-mediated hypersensitivity reaction against proteins in the donor blood
    c. Clinical findings
      (1) Urticaria with pruritus
      (2) Fever, tachycardia, wheezing
      (3) Potential for anaphylactic shock
      (4) Mild cases are treated with antihistamines.

Allergic transfusion
reaction: IgE-mediated

IgA deficient patients:
must receive IgA
deficient blood products

Individuals who are **deficient in IgA** and who have antibodies directed against IgA from previous exposure to a blood product may develop a severe anaphylactic reaction. IgA-deficient individuals must receive blood or blood products that lack IgA.

  2. Febrile reaction
    a. Pathogenesis
      (1) Recipient has anti–human leukocyte antigen (HLA) antibodies directed against foreign HLA antigens on donor leukocytes (refer to Chapter 3).
        • There are *no* HLA antigens on RBCs.
      (2) Type II hypersensitivity reaction
    b. Clinical findings
      (1) Fever, chills, headache, and flushing
      (2) Treated with antipyretics

Febrile transfusion
reaction: anti-HLA
antibodies against donor
leukocytes

Anti-HLA antibodies: come
from previous exposure
to HLA antigens (blood
transfusion, transplant)

Anti-HLA antibodies develop when individuals are exposed to foreign HLA antigens (e.g., previous blood transfusion or organ transplant). Women commonly have these reactions owing to pregnancy, when there is an increased risk for exposure to fetal blood during delivery or after a spontaneous abortion.

TABLE 15-1. BLOOD COMPONENTS

COMPONENT	DISCUSSION
Packed RBCs	Purpose: increase O_2 transport to tissues Packed RBCs have less volume and a higher Hct than whole blood Each unit of packed RBCs should raise the Hb by 1 g/dL and the Hct by 3%; lack of an increment implies a hemolytic transfusion reaction or continued blood loss in the patient *Yersinia enterocolitica*, a pathogen that thrives on iron, is the most common contaminant of stored blood
Platelets	Purpose: stop medically significant bleeding related to thrombocytopenia or qualitative platelet defects (e.g., aspirin) Platelets have HLA antigens and ABO antigens on their surface; however, they lack Rh antigens Each unit of platelets should raise the platelet count by 5000–10,000 cells/mm³
Fresh frozen plasma	Purpose: treatment of multiple coagulation deficiencies (e.g., DIC, cirrhosis) or treatment of warfarin over-anticoagulation if bleeding is life-threatening
Cryoprecipitate	Purpose: treatment of coagulation factor deficiencies involving fibrinogen and factor VIII (e.g., DIC) Cryoprecipitate contains fibrinogen, factor VIII, and factor XIII Desmopressin acetate is used instead of cryoprecipitate in treating mild hemophilia A and von Willebrand disease

DIC, disseminated intravascular coagulation; Hb, hemoglobin; Hct, hematocrit.

3. Acute hemolytic transfusion reaction (HTR)
  a. May be intravascular or extravascular hemolytic reactions (refer to Chapter 11)
  b. Intravascular hemolysis
    (1) ABO blood group incompatibility
    (2) Example—group B patient receives group A donor blood.
      • Anti-A-IgM attaches to A positive donor RBCs producing intravascular hemolysis; type II hypersensitivity reaction
  c. Extravascular hemolysis
    (1) An atypical antibody reacts with a foreign antigen on donor RBCs.
      (a) Recipient's splenic macrophages will phagocytose and destroy donor RBCs coated by the atypical antibody
      (b) Type II hypersensitivity reaction
    (2) Jaundice commonly occurs.
      • Unconjugated bilirubin is the end-product of macrophage degradation of hemoglobin (Hb).

Acute HTRs are due to blood group incompatibility or presence of an atypical antibody.

Acute HTRs: intravascular or extravascular hemolysis

Individuals who have been infused with blood in the past may have been exposed to a foreign blood group antigen and developed atypical antibodies that are no longer circulating; therefore, the pretransfusion antibody screen is negative. However, memory B cells are present and reexposure to the foreign antigen causes them to produce antibodies, resulting in an extravascular hemolytic anemia. This reaction may occur within hours to 3 to 10 days after the transfusion.

  d. Clinical findings
    (1) Fever
    (2) Back pain
    (3) Hypotension
  e. Potential complications
    (1) Disseminated intravascular coagulation
    (2) Acute renal failure
  f. Laboratory findings
    (1) Positive direct Coombs' test
      • IgG antibody or C3b is coating donor RBCs.
    (2) Positive indirect Coombs' test
      • Atypical antibody is present in serum.
    (3) *No* significant increase in Hb over pretransfusion levels
    (4) Hemoglobinuria
      • Sign of intravascular hemolysis (refer to Chapter 11)
    (5) Jaundice
      • Sign of extravascular hemolysis
4. Suspected transfusion reactions
  a. Immediately stop the blood transfusion
  b. Keep the intravenous line in place
    • Keep the line open with normal saline
  c. Send the unit of blood to the blood bank
  d. Blood bank will do a transfusion reaction workup

Suspected HTRs: keep IV open with normal saline; discontinue transfusion

IV. **Hemolytic disease of the newborn (HDN)**
  • HDN results from the transplacental passage of maternal IgG antibodies (e.g., anti-D antibodies, anti-A and B antibodies in group O mothers) resulting in an extravascular hemolytic anemia in the fetus.
  A. **ABO HDN** (Fig. 15-4A)
    1. Epidemiology
      a. Most common HDN
        • Present in 20% to 25% of all pregnancies
      b. Mothers are blood group O and the fetus is either blood group A or B.
    2. Pathogenesis
      a. Blood group O individuals have anti-A and B-IgG antibodies.
        (1) IgG antibodies cross the placenta and attach to fetal A or B RBCs.
        (2) Fetal splenic macrophages phagocytose RBCs, causing a mild anemia.
        (3) Unconjugated bilirubin from extravascular hemolysis is disposed of in the mother's liver.
      b. May affect the firstborn or any future pregnancy if ABO incompatibility exists

ABO HDN: most common HDN

ABO HDN: mother group O, fetus blood group A or B

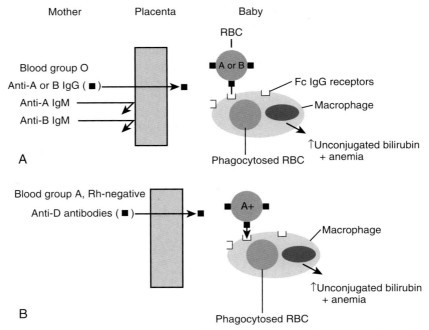

15-4: ABO and Rh hemolytic disease of the newborn. See text for discussion. *(From Goljan EF: Star Series: Pathology. Philadelphia, WB Saunders, 1998, Fig. 14-1.)*

3. Clinical and laboratory findings
   a. Jaundice develops within the first 24 hours after birth.
      (1) ABO HDN is the most common cause of jaundice in this period.
         • Newborn liver cannot handle the excess bilirubin load.
      (2) Risk for kernicterus is very small (see later).
   b. Anemia
      (1) Mild normocytic anemia or no anemia at all
      (2) Exchange transfusions are rarely indicated.
   c. Positive direct Coombs' test on fetal cord blood RBCs
      • Due to anti-A or B-IgG antibodies coating fetal A or B RBCs
   d. Spherocytes are present in the cord blood peripheral smear.
      • Due to macrophage removal of a portion of the RBC membrane

B. Rh HDN (Fig. 15-4B)
1. Pathogenesis
   a. Mother is Rh (D antigen) negative and the fetus is Rh positive.
   b. Mother is exposed to fetal Rh positive blood (fetomaternal bleed).
      (1) Occurs during the last trimester or during childbirth itself
      (2) Cytotrophoblast is absent during the last trimester.
         • Increases the risk for a fetomaternal bleed
   c. Mother develops anti-D-IgG antibodies when exposed to fetal Rh positive cells.
      • First Rh incompatible pregnancy does *not* affect the firstborn.
   d. Subsequent Rh incompatible pregnancies result in extravascular hemolytic anemia in the fetus.
      (1) Anti-D-IgG antibodies cross the placenta and attach to fetal Rh positive RBCs.
      (2) Fetal splenic macrophages phagocytose RBCs, causing severe anemia.
         (a) Fetus may develop high-output cardiac failure leading to hydrops fetalis and death.
         (b) Hydrops fetalis is a combined left- and right-sided heart failure with ascites and edema.
         (c) Extramedullary hematopoiesis is present in the liver and spleen.
         (d) Unconjugated bilirubin is conjugated in the mother's liver.
2. Clinical and laboratory findings
   a. Degree of anemia is more severe than with ABO HDN.
   b. Jaundice develops shortly after birth.
      (1) Level of unconjugated bilirubin is much higher than with ABO HDN.
         • Most of the unconjugated bilirubin is *not* bound by albumin and circulates free in the blood.

Jaundice in first 24 hours: most common cause is ABO HDN

ABO HDN: positive direct Coombs' test on fetal cord RBCs

Rh HDN: mother Rh negative, fetus Rh positive

Rh HDN: anemia and amount of unconjugated bilirubin > ABO HDN

Rh HDN: unconjugated bilirubin is free (not bound)

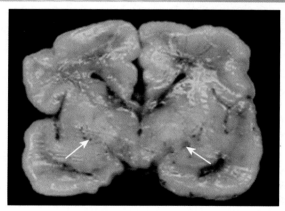

15-5: Cross section of the brain of a newborn with kernicterus. *Arrows* depict yellow bilirubin pigment deposited in the basal ganglia. Bilirubin is toxic to neurons and produces long-term neurologic sequelae. *(From Kumar V, Fausto N, Abbas A: Robbins and Cotran's Pathologic Basis of Disease, 7th ed. Philadelphia, WB Saunders, 2004, p 487, Fig. 10-16.)*

(2) Increased risk for kernicterus
    • The free, unbound lipid-soluble unconjugated bilirubin poses the greatest risk for bilirubin entry into the brain (Fig. 15-5).

Kernicterus: free unconjugated bilirubin deposits in basal ganglia

Kernicterus refers to deposition of free (not bound to albumin) lipid-soluble unconjugated bilirubin in the basal ganglia owing to an incompletely formed blood-brain barrier. Bilirubin damages neurons in the brain, causing severe dysfunction.

   c. Positive direct and indirect Coombs' tests on fetal cord blood
   d. Spherocytes are *not* present in cord blood.
     • Macrophages phagocytose the entire RBC.
   e. Exchange transfusions are required.
     (1) Newborn's blood is removed and replaced with fresh blood.
     (2) Transfusion corrects anemia and removes antibodies and unconjugated bilirubin.

Rh HDN: positive direct Coombs' test on fetal RBCs

ABO incompatibility protects the mother from developing Rh sensitization. For example, in a mother who is O negative and carrying a fetus who is A positive, any A positive fetal RBCs entering her circulation will be destroyed by maternal anti-A-IgM antibodies, thereby preventing sensitization.

ABO incompatibility: protects mother from Rh sensitization

3. Prevention of Rh HDN in Rh negative mothers without anti-D
   a. Receive anti-D globulin (Rh immune globulin) during the 28th week of pregnancy
   b. Anti-D globulin does *not* cross the placenta.
   c. Anti-D globulin protects the mother from sensitization to fetal Rh positive cells that may enter her circulation during the last trimester.
   d. Anti-D globulin lasts ~3 months in the mother's blood.
   e. Additional anti-D globulin is given to the mother after delivery if the baby is Rh positive.

Prevention of Rh HDN: Rh immune globulin (anti-D globulin)

Special tests are performed on the mother's blood that detect fetal RBCs in her blood. The amount of fetal blood is quantified so that the appropriate amount of anti-D globulin is given to the mother. Anti-D globulin masks the antigenic sites on the fetal RBCs or destroys the fetal RBCs so that the mother does *not* host an antibody response against the D antigen. If the patient develops anti-D antibodies, there is no indication for giving the globulin either during or after delivery, because its main purpose is to prevent sensitization.

4. Tests performed on sensitized (anti-D positive) women
   a. Women are followed with sequential antibody titers and periodic amniocentesis.
   b. Amniotic fluid is submitted to spectrophotometric analysis to identify bilirubin pigment.
     (1) Bilirubin has absorbance at a wavelength of 450 nm.

Bilirubin absorbance: 450 nm

ΔOD 450: bilirubin
wavelength in amniotic
fluid; degree of increase
correlates with severity of
hemolysis

(2) A Δ OD 450 value is obtained on the fluid.
- Height of the bilirubin spike on the spectrophotometer reading from the baseline.
(3) Δ OD 450 is sequentially plotted on a Liley chart.
- Correlates Δ OD 450 with gestational age of the fetus
(4) Graph provides an indication of the degree of severity of the RBC hemolysis.
(5) Very severe cases at an early gestational age may require an in-utero exchange transfusion.

C. Use of blue fluorescent light

Blue fluorescent light:
converts bilirubin in skin
to water-soluble dipyrrole

1. Used as a treatment of jaundice in the newborn
2. Unconjugated bilirubin in the skin absorbs light energy from blue fluorescent light.
3. Photoisomerization converts unconjugated bilirubin to a nontoxic water-soluble dipyrrole (called lumirubin).
- Lumirubin is excreted in bile or urine.

CHAPTER 16

UPPER AND LOWER RESPIRATORY DISORDERS

I. **Symptoms and Signs of Respiratory Disease** (Tables 16-1 and 16-2)
II. **Pulmonary Function Tests**
   A. **Calculation of the alveolar-arterial (A-a) gradient**
   1. A-a gradient is the difference in the partial pressure of oxygen (Po_2) between the alveolar Po_2 (Pao_2) and arterial Po_2 (Pao_2).
      a. A-a gradient is normally due to a mismatch between ventilation and perfusion in the lungs.
         • Example—An A-a gradient exists when perfusion is greater than ventilation in the lower lobes.
      b. It is useful in differentiating causes of hypoxemia (decreased Pao_2; refer to Chapter 1).
         (1) Hypoxemia due to pulmonary causes increases A-a gradient.
         (2) Hypoxemia due to extrapulmonary causes has a normal A-a gradient.
   2. Calculation of the A-a gradient
      a. $Pao_2 = \% \ O_2 \ (713) -$ arterial $Pco_2/0.8$
         • % O_2 is the percentage of O_2 the patient is breathing; 713 is the atmospheric pressure (760 mm Hg) minus the water vapor pressure (47 mm Hg); and 0.8 is the respiratory quotient.
      b. Example using normal values
         (1) Normal $Pao_2 = 0.21 \ (713) - 40/0.8 = 100$ mm Hg
         (2) Normal $Pao_2 = 95$ mm Hg
         (3) Normal A-a gradient = 100 mm Hg − 95 mm Hg = 5 mm Hg
         (4) Medically significant A-a gradient ≥ 30 mm Hg
            (a) A-a gradient normally increases with age.
            (b) A-a ≥ 30 mm Hg is set for highest specificity.
   3. Causes of hypoxemia with an increased A-a gradient (refer to Chapter 1)
      a. Ventilation defect
         (1) Impaired O_2 delivery to the alveoli for gas exchange
         (2) Example—airway collapse due to the respiratory distress syndrome
      b. Perfusion defect
         (1) Decreased or absent blood flow to the alveoli
         (2) Example—pulmonary embolus
      c. Diffusion defect
         (1) O_2 cannot diffuse through the alveolar-capillary interface.
         (2) Examples—interstitial fibrosis, pulmonary edema
      d. Right-to-left cardiac shunt
         • Example—tetralogy of Fallot

↑ A-a gradient: hypoxemia of pulmonary origin

Normal A-a gradient: hypoxemia of extrapulmonary origin

$Pao_2 = \% \ O_2 \ (713) -$ arterial $Pco_2/0.8$

A-a ≥ 30 mm Hg

Hypoxemia + ↑ A-a: ventilation, perfusion, diffusion defects; right-to-left cardiac shunts

Calculation of the A-a gradient in a patient breathing 0.30 O_2 who has a Pco_2 of 80 mm Hg and Pao_2 of 40 mm Hg: $Pao_2 = 0.30 \ (713) - 80/0.8 = 114$ mm Hg. A-a gradient = 114 − 40 = 74 mm Hg, which is medically significant and indicates one or more of the above-mentioned lung disorders or a right-to-left shunt in the heart.

TABLE 16-1. **COMMON SYMPTOMS OF RESPIRATORY DISEASE**

SYMPTOM	CAUSES/DISCUSSION
Dyspnea	Difficulty with breathing Due to stimulation of J receptors causing decrease in full inspiration Causes: 　Decreased compliance (e.g., interstitial fibrosis) 　Increased airway resistance (e.g., chronic bronchitis) 　Chest bellows disease (e.g., obesity, kyphoscoliosis) 　Interstitial inflammation/fluid accumulation (e.g., left-sided heart failure)
Cough	Cough receptors: located at bifurcations in airways, larynx, distal esophagus Cough with a normal chest x-ray 　Postnasal discharge is the most common cause Nocturnal cough with: 　GERD: due to acid reflux in tracheobronchial tree at night 　Bronchial asthma: due to bronchoconstriction Productive cough with: 　Chronic bronchitis: due to smoking cigarettes 　Typical bacterial pneumonia 　Bronchiectasis Drugs causing cough: 　ACE inhibitors: inhibit degradation of bradykinin; causes mucosal swelling and 　　irritation in tracheobronchial tree 　Aspirin: causes an increase in LT C-D-E$_4$ (bronchoconstrictors)
Hemoptysis	Coughing up blood-tinged sputum Mechanisms: 　Parenchymal necrosis 　Bronchial and/or pulmonary vessel damage Causes: 　Chronic bronchitis (most common cause) 　Pneumonia, bronchogenic carcinoma 　TB, bronchiectasis, aspergilloma (fungus living in a cavitary lesion)

ACE, angiotensin-converting enzyme; GERD, gastroesophageal reflux disease; LT, leukotriene; TB, tuberculosis.

TABLE 16-2. **SIGNS OF RESPIRATORY DISEASE**

SIGN	DISCUSSION
Tachypnea	Normal respiratory rate: 14–20 breaths per minute (bpm) in adults; up to 44 bpm in 　children Tachypnea: rapid shallow breathing (>20 bpm) Causes: restrictive lung disease; pleuritic chest pain; pulmonary embolus with 　infarction (key finding)
Chest Palpation	
Tracheal shift	Due to large changes in pleural fluid volume Causes: 　Pressure in contralateral lung: large tension pneumothorax, large pleural effusion 　Decreased volume in ipsilateral lung: large spontaneous pneumothorax, 　　resorption atelectasis
Vocal tactile fremitus	Palpable thrill (vibration) transmitted through chest when patient says "E" or "1, 2, 　3" or "99" *Decreased* vocal tactile fremitus with emphysema or asthma, with increased AP 　diameter from an increase in total lung capacity *Absent* vocal tactile fremitus with atelectasis (collapse of airways); fluid (effusion); air 　(pneumothorax) in pleural space *Increased* tactile fremitus (sound travels well through consolidations) with alveolar 　consolidation (e.g., lobar pneumonia)
Percussion	*Dull* percussion with pleural effusion; lung consolidation; atelectasis (no air in the alveoli) *Hyperresonant* percussion with pneumothorax; asthma; emphysema
Lung Sounds	
General breath sounds	Origin for normal breath sounds: trachea Mechanism: air velocity and turbulence induce vibrations in airway walls Sites modifying breath sound: terminal airway and alveolar disease modify breath 　sounds; sounds heard with the stethoscope are produced in more central 　(hilar) regions and are altered in intensity and tonal quality as they pass through 　pulmonary tissue to the periphery Site for normal airway resistance: segmental bronchi (turbulent air flow) Site for laminar air flow: begins at the terminal bronchioles—"small airway" 　Parallel branching: increases cross-sectional area of airways; converts turbulent 　　into laminar air flow Effects of inflammation of small airways (e.g., asthma, chronic bronchitis): air 　trapping, wheezing, increased airway resistance

TABLE 16-2. **SIGNS OF RESPIRATORY DISEASE—cont'd**

SIGN	DISCUSSION
Lung Sounds—cont'd	

Tubular breath sounds	Sound like blowing air through a tube
	Tracheal breath sound: normal sound over lateral neck or suprasternal notch
	Bronchial breath sounds: always an abnormal sound
	   Loud, high-pitched sound with a peculiar hollow or tubular quality
	   Expiratory sounds longer than inspiratory
	   Significance: consolidation (e.g., lobar/bronchopneumonia)
	   Mechanism: bronchi must be patent and partially collapsed
	
	Alveolar consolidation (exudate, transudate) Partially collapsed bronchus
	
	Associated with an "air bronchogram": air-filled bronchi silhouetted against airless consolidated parenchyma

Vesicular breath sounds	Normal breath sounds: tracheal sounds that are modified (filtered) in alveoli
	   Sites: most lung fields *except* trachea and central bronchi
	      Inspiratory-to-expiratory ratio is 3:1
	Present in: normal lungs; chronic bronchitis; emphysema
	Diminished in: emphysema and asthma due to increased AP diameter
	Absent in: pneumothorax; atelectasis; effusion

Bronchovesicular breath sounds	Normal breath sounds heard over main bronchi Abnormal if heard in lung periphery Inspiratory and expiratory breath sounds are equal in length
Adventitial sounds	Extra sounds that are normally absent in respiratory cycle
Crackles	Crackles: usually inspiratory Early and midinspiratory crackles: due to secretions in proximal large to medium-sized airways (e.g., chronic bronchitis); clear with coughing Late inspiratory crackles: due to reopening of distal airways partially occluded by increased interstitial pressure (e.g., interstitial fluid—pus, transudate in CHF); do *not* clear with coughing; vary from fine to coarse Causes: pulmonary edema; lobar pneumonia; interstitial fibrosis (e.g., sarcoidosis)
Wheezing	Wheezing: high-pitched musical sound usually heard in expiration; sometimes inspiration and expiration; expiration longer than inspiration Causes: inflammation segmental bronchi, small airways (e.g., asthma, chronic bronchitis); pulmonary edema constricting airway (called cardiac asthma); pulmonary infarction (release of TXA_2 from platelets in embolus causes bronchoconstriction)
Rhonchi	Rhonchi: low-pitched snoring sound heard during inspiration or expiration; due to secretions in large airways (bronchus, trachea); usually clear with coughing; common in chronic bronchitis
Inspiratory stridor	Inspiratory stridor: high-pitched inspiratory sound; sign of upper airway obstruction Causes: epiglottitis (*Haemophilus influenzae*); croup (parainfluenza virus) Inspiratory and expiratory stridor: sign of fixed upper airway obstruction (e.g., from cancer)
Pleural friction rub	Pleural friction rub: two inflamed surfaces (pleural and parietal) rubbing against each other Timing: end of inspiration and early part of expiration Disappears: large effusion is present (separates inflamed surfaces); holding breath (continues with pericardial friction rub) Causes: pleuritis due to cancer, infarction, pneumonia, serositis (SLE)
Grunting in newborns	Grunting in newborns: always abnormal after 24 hours; common finding in RDS
Transmitted voice sounds	Bronchophony (sound of bronchi) Normal lung: spoken syllables or numbers (e.g., 99) are *indistinctly heard* Alveolar consolidation: syllables/numbers heard louder and more distinctly Whispered pectoriloquy (Latin for "voice of chest"): clear and intelligible words (e.g., patient whispering "1, 2, 3") Egophony (Greek for "voice of goat"): patient saying "E" sounds like "A"

AP, anteroposterior; bpm, breaths per minute; CHF, congestive heart failure; RDS, respiratory distress syndrome; SLE, systemic lupus erythematosus; TXA_2, thromboxane A_2.

Hypoxemia + normal
A-a: depress respiratory
center, upper airway
obstruction, chest bellows
disease

4. Causes of hypoxemia with a normal A-a gradient
   a. Depression of the respiratory center in the medulla
     • Examples—barbiturates, brain injury
   b. Upper airway obstruction
     (1) Epiglottitis due to *Haemophilus influenzae*
     (2) Croup due to parainfluenza virus
       • Mucosal edema narrows the trachea.
   c. Chest bellows (muscles of respiration) dysfunction
     (1) Paralyzed diaphragm
     (2) Amyotrophic lateral sclerosis with degeneration of anterior horn cells

> **Calculation of the A-a gradient** in a patient breathing room air who has a Pco_2 of 80 mm Hg and Pao_2 of 40 mm Hg: $Pao_2 = 0.21\ (713) - 80/0.8 = 50$ mm Hg. A-a gradient $= 50 - 40 = 10$ mm Hg, which excludes the lung as the cause of the hypoxemia and indicates an extrapulmonary cause of hypoxemia.

B. Spirometry (Fig. 16-1)
   • Useful in distinguishing restrictive from obstructive lung disease
   1. Volumes and capacities that are *not* directly measured by spirometry
     a. Functional residual capacity (FRC)
       • Total amount of air in the lungs at the end of a normal expiration
     b. Total lung capacity (TLC)
       • Total amount of air in a fully expanded lung
     c. Residual volume (RV)
       • Volume of air left over in the lung after maximal expiration
   2. Tidal volume (TV)
     • Volume of air that enters or leaves the lungs during normal quiet respiration
   3. Forced vital capacity (FVC), forced expiratory volume in 1 second (FEV$_{1\,sec}$), and FEV$_{1\,sec}$/FVC
     a. FVC is the total amount of air expelled after a maximal inspiration.
       • Normal FVC is 5 L (see Fig. 16-1A).
     b. Forced expiratory volume in 1 second (FEV$_{1\,sec}$)
       (1) Amount of air expelled from the lungs in 1 second after a maximal inspiration
       (2) Normal FEV$_{1\,sec}$ is 4 L (see Fig. 16-1A).
     c. Ratio of FEV$_{1\,sec}$/FVC is normally 4/5, or 80%.
   4. Expiratory reserve volume (ERV)
     a. ERV refers to the amount of air forcibly expelled at the end of a normal expiration.
     b. ERV is commonly used to calculate residual volume (FRC − ERV = RV).
   5. Comparison of pulmonary function tests in restrictive and obstructive lung disease (Table 16-3)

Volumes *not* directly
measured by spirometry:
TLC, FRC, RV

Normal FEV$_{1\,sec}$/FVC:
4–5 L

FRC − ERV = RV

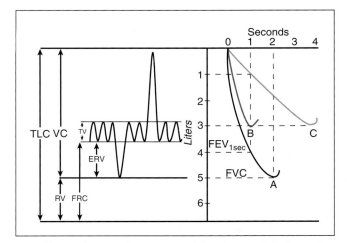

16-1: Spirometry showing normal lung volumes and capacities and forced expiratory volume at 1 second (FEV$_{1\,sec}$) and forced vital capacity (FVC) findings in a normal person (A), a person with restrictive lung disease (B), and a person with obstructive lung disease (C). ERV, expiratory reserve volume; FRC, functional residual capacity; RV, residual volume; TLC, total lung capacity; TV, tidal volume; VC, vital capacity. *(From Goljan EF: Star Series: Pathology. Philadelphia, WB Saunders, 1998, p 229, Fig. 11-1.)*

TABLE 16-3. **COMPARISON OF PULMONARY FUNCTION TESTS IN RESTRICTIVE AND OBSTRUCTIVE LUNG DISEASE**

PARAMETER	RESTRICTIVE	OBSTRUCTIVE
Total lung capacity	Decreased	Increased
Residual volume	Decreased	Increased
$FEV_{1\,sec}$	Decreased	Decreased
FVC	Decreased	Decreased
$FEV_{1\,sec}$/FVC	Normal to increased	Decreased
Pao_2	Decreased	Decreased
A-a gradient	Increased	Increased

A-a, alveolar-arterial; FEV, forced expiratory volume; FVC, forced vital capacity.

C. Flow-volume loop

1. Plot of inspiratory and expiratory flow rate (liters/second) versus lung volume (liters)
   - Patient takes a maximal inspiration followed by a maximal expiration.
2. Loop consists of an inspiration curve and an expiration curve (Fig. 16-2).
   a. Maximal inspiration
      - Begins at point A (RV) and extends to point B (TLC)
   b. Maximal expiration
      (1) Extends from point B to point C (peak expiratory flow, PEF) and then trails off back to point A
      (2) PEF occurs early in expiratory phase of the loop (point B to C).
         - Due to elastic recoil of the lungs into airways with low resistance and large caliber
      (3) Flow rate becomes linear from point C to A.
         - Encounters increased resistance in the small airways
      (4) Volume of air in liters between points A and B is the vital capacity (VC).
3. Flow-volume loop in obstructive lung disease (Fig. 16-3A)
   a. TLC is increased (e.g., ~8.5 L) and RV is increased (e.g., 4 L).
      - Expiratory curve is shifted to the left of the normal curve.
   b. Decreased PEF
   c. Nonuniform emptying of the airways
      - Concave configuration of the curve (arrow) is due to mucus plugs or collapsed small airways.
4. Flow-volume loop findings in restrictive parenchymal disease (Fig. 16-3B)
   a. TLC is decreased (e.g., ~4 L).
   b. RV is decreased (e.g., ~0.3 L).
   c. Expiratory curve is shifted to the right of the normal curve.
      - Expiratory curve is narrow because of decreased lung volumes.

TLC and RV: TLC end of maximal inspiration; RV end of maximal expiration

Obstructive pattern: nonuniform emptying; expiratory curve shift to left of normal curve

Restrictive parenchymal: expiratory curve shifted to right of normal curve

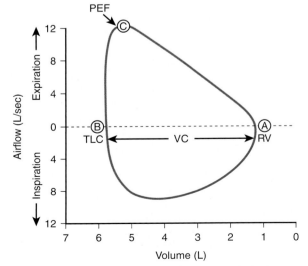

16-2: Flow-volume loop. See text for discussion. PEF, peak expiratory flow; RV, residual volume; TLC, total lung capacity; VC, vital capacity. *(From Goljan EF, Sloka KI: Rapid Review Laboratory Testing in Clinical Medicine. St. Louis, Mosby Elsevier, 2008, p 71, Fig. 3-3.)*

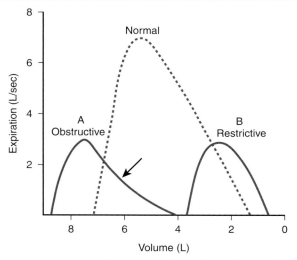

16-3: Flow-volume loops in normal person, obstructive disorder (A), restrictive disorder (B). See text for discussion. *(From Goljan EF, Sloka KI: Rapid Review Laboratory Testing in Clinical Medicine. St. Louis, Mosby Elsevier, 2008, p 72, Fig. 3-4.)*

III. Upper Airway Disorders

Choanal atresia: newborn cannot breathe through the nose; cyanosis when breast-feeding

A. **Choanal atresia**
1. Unilateral or bilateral bony septum between the nose and the pharynx
2. Newborn turns cyanotic when breast-feeding.
   • Crying causes the child to "pink up" again.

B. **Nasal polyps**

Allergic polyp: most common polyp; adults

1. Nasal polyps are non-neoplastic tumefactions (Fig. 16-4).
   • Develop as a response to chronic inflammation
2. Allergic polyps
   a. Most common polyp
   b. Most often seen in adults with a history of IgE-mediated allergies
3. Nasal polyps are associated with aspirin and other nonsteroidal drugs.

Triad asthma: aspirin, nasal polyp, asthma

   a. Epidemiology
      • Most often occur in women with chronic pain syndromes
   b. Pathogenesis
      (1) Drugs block cyclooxygenase leaving the lipoxygenase pathway open.
      (2) Leukotrienes (LT) C-D-E_4 are increased, causing bronchoconstriction.

Nasal polyps in child: order a sweat test to rule out cystic fibrosis

   c. Clinical triad—nonsteroidal drugs, asthma, and nasal polyps
4. Nasal polyps are often associated with cystic fibrosis.

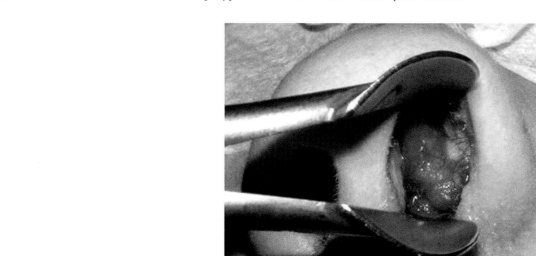

16-4: Nasal polyp. Note the gray-white mass in the left nasal cavity. *(From Swartz MH: Textbook of Physical Diagnosis, 5th ed. Philadelphia, Saunders Elsevier, 2006, p 312, Fig. 11-24.)*

C. Obstructive sleep apnea (OSA)

1. Epidemiology
   a. Excessive snoring with intervals of breath cessation (apnea)
   b. Causes
      (1) Obesity (very common)
         • Pharyngeal muscles collapse due to the weight of tissue in the neck.
      (2) Tonsillar hypertrophy, nasal septum deviation
2. Pathogenesis
   • Airway obstruction causes CO_2 retention, leading to hypoxemia.
3. Clinical findings
   a. Excessive snoring with episodes of apnea
   b. Daytime somnolence often simulating narcolepsy
4. Laboratory findings
   a. Decreased Po_2 and O_2 saturation during apneic episodes
   b. Increase in arterial Pco_2 (respiratory acidosis)
5. Complications
   a. Pulmonary hypertension (PH) leading to right ventricular hypertrophy
      • Called cor pulmonale (see section VII)
   b. Secondary polycythemia
      • Due to a hypoxemic stimulus for erythropoietin release
6. Polysomnography
   • Confirmatory test that documents periods of apnea during sleep
7. Treatment
   a. Nasal continuous positive airway pressure (CPAP)
   b. Surgical correction of any obstructive lesions, weight loss

D. Sinusitis

1. Epidemiology
   a. Maxillary sinus is most often involved in adults.
   b. Ethmoid sinus is most often involved in children.
   c. Causes
      (1) Upper respiratory infections (URIs); e.g., viral, bacterial
         • Block drainage of sinuses into nasal cavity
      (2) Deviated nasal septum
      (3) Allergic rhinitis
      (4) Barotrauma
      (5) Smoking cigarettes
   d. Pathogens causing sinusitis
      (1) Rhinoviruses
      (2) *Streptococcus pneumoniae* (most common)
      (3) Anaerobes (chronic sinusitis)
      (4) Systemic fungi (e.g., *Mucor* or *Aspergillus* species)
         • Diabetics commonly have sinusitis due to *Mucor* species.
2. Pathogenesis
   • Blockage of sinus drainage into the nasal cavity
3. Clinical findings
   a. Fever
   b. Nasal congestion
   c. Pain over sinuses
   d. Postnasal drip
4. Diagnosis
   a. Gold standard for bacterial culture is sinus aspiration
   b. Sinus radiographs
   c. CT scan is the most sensitive test.
      • Recommended if surgery is an option
5. Treatment
   a. Decongestants
   b. Antimicrobial therapy
      (1) Recommendation is *not* to use antibiotics.
         • Most cases are viral and resolve within 2 weeks
      (2) If resolution does *not* occur, antibiotics often used include the following:
         • Amoxicillin (most common drug), erythromycin, trimethoprim-sulfamethoxazole (TMP/SMX)

Margin notes:

OSA: excessive with periods of apnea

OSA: apnea causes respiratory acidosis and hypoxemia

OSA: risk for developing cor pulmonale

Polysomnography: confirmatory test for OSA

Sinus infections: maxillary in adults, ethmoid in children

Viral URI: most common cause of sinusitis

Streptococcus pneumoniae: most common bacterial pathogen causing sinusitis

Sinusitis: blockage of sinus drainage in nasal cavity

Sinusitis: CT scan most sensitive

E. **Nasopharyngeal carcinoma**
1. Epidemiology
   a. Most common malignant tumor of the nasopharynx
   b. Male dominant
   c. Increased incidence in the Chinese and African populations

Nasopharyngeal carcinoma: association with EBV

2. Pathogenesis
   • Causal relationship with Epstein-Barr virus (EBV)
3. Pathologic findings
   a. Squamous cell carcinoma or undifferentiated cancer
   b. Metastasizes to cervical lymph nodes

F. **Laryngeal carcinoma**
1. Epidemiology and pathogenesis
   a. More common in men than in women
   b. Risk factors

Laryngeal carcinoma: cigarette smoking is the most common cause

      (1) Cigarette smoking (most common cause)
      (2) Alcohol (synergistic effect with smoking)
      (3) Squamous papillomas and papillomatosis
         • Human papillomavirus type 6 and 11 association
   c. Majority are located on the true vocal cords (Fig. 16-5).

Laryngeal carcinoma: most on true vocal cords; squamous cancer

2. Majority are keratinizing squamous cell carcinomas.
3. Clinical findings
   • Persistent hoarseness is often associated with cervical lymphadenopathy.
4. Treatment is surgery.

IV. **Atelectasis**
   • Loss of lung volume due to inadequate expansion of the airspaces (collapse)
A. **Resorption atelectasis**
1. Pathogenesis
   a. Airway obstruction by thick secretions prevents air from reaching the alveoli.
      • Obstruction occurs in bronchi, segmental bronchi, or terminal bronchioles.

Resorption atelectasis: most common cause of fever 24 to 36 hours after surgery

   b. Causes of obstruction
      (1) Mucus or mucopurulent plug after surgery
      (2) Aspiration of foreign material
      (3) Centrally located bronchogenic carcinoma
   c. Cause of alveolar collapse
      • Lack of air and distal resorption of preexisting air through the pores of Kohn in the alveolar walls
   d. Collapse may involve all or part of a lung.
2. Clinical findings
   a. Fever and dyspnea
      • Both usually occur within 24 to 36 hours of collapse.
   b. Absent breath sounds

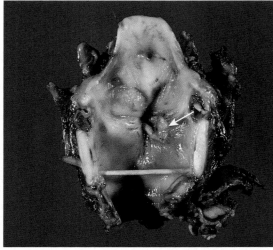

16-5: Laryngeal squamous cell carcinoma involving the right vocal cord (*arrow*). *(From Damjanov I, Linder J: Pathology: A Color Atlas. St. Louis, Mosby, 2000, p 47, Fig. 3-16.)*

c. Absent vocal vibratory sensation (tactile fremitus)
  - Alveoli are collapsed.
d. Ipsilateral elevation of the diaphragm and tracheal deviation
  - Only occurs if large areas of the lung are atelectatic
e. Collapsed lung does *not* expand on inspiration (inspiratory lag).

3. Treatment
  a. Incentive spirometry after surgery
  b. Positive-pressure breathing (CPAP) by face mask
  c. Positive end-expiratory pressure (PEEP) on mechanical ventilation

B. Compression atelectasis
  1. Air or fluid in the pleural cavity under increased pressure collapses small airways beneath the pleura.
  2. Examples
    a. Tension pneumothorax where air compresses the lung
    b. Pleural effusion where fluid compresses the lung

C. Atelectasis due to loss of surfactant
  1. Surfactant
    a. Synthesized by type II pneumocytes
      (1) Stored in lamellar bodies (Fig. 16-6)
      (2) Synthesis begins in 28th week of gestation.
    b. Phosphatidylcholine (lecithin) is the major component.
    c. Synthesis is increased by cortisol and thyroxine.
    d. Synthesis is decreased by insulin.
    e. Surfactant reduces surface tension in the small airways.
      - Prevents collapse on expiration, when collapsing pressure is greatest
  2. Respiratory distress syndrome (RDS) in newborns
    a. Pathogenesis
      (1) Decreased surfactant in the fetal lungs; causes:
        (a) Prematurity
        (b) Maternal diabetes
          - Fetal hyperglycemia increases insulin release.
        (c) Cesarean section
          - Lack of stress-induced increase in cortisol from a vaginal delivery

Women who have to deliver their babies prematurely receive glucocorticoids in order to increase fetal surfactant synthesis, thereby reducing the potential for developing RDS. Good maternal glycemic control decreases the risk for RDS.

      (2) Widespread atelectasis results in massive intrapulmonary shunting.
        - Perfusion without ventilation

Resorption atelectasis: absent vibratory sensation, dullness to percussion, absent breath sounds

Compression atelectasis: air under pressure or fluid in pleural cavity

Surfactant: synthesized in type II pneumocytes

Surfactant: cortisol increases synthesis, insulin inhibits synthesis

Surfactant: ↓ surface tension

RDS: due to a decrease in surfactant

RDS: prematurity, diabetes, C-section

Fetal surfactant: ↑ with maternal intake of glucocorticoids

RDS: intrapulmonary shunting

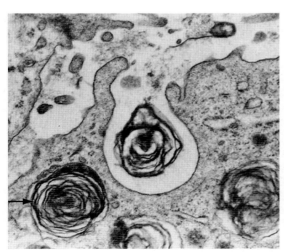

16-6: Electron micrograph of a type II pneumocyte showing a lamellar body *(arrow)* containing surfactant. *(From Corrin B: Pathology of the Lungs. London, Churchill Livingstone, 1999, p 15, Fig. 1-26.)*

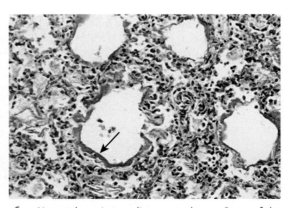

16-7: Neonatal respiratory distress syndrome. Some of the dilated respiratory bronchioles and alveolar ducts are lined with a fibrin-rich membrane (hyaline membrane) *(arrow)*. The subjacent alveoli are collapsed. *(From Damjanov I: Pathology for the Health-Related Professions, 2nd ed. Philadelphia, WB Saunders, 2000, p 128, Fig. 5-25.)*

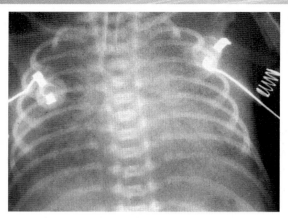

16-8: Chest radiograph in respiratory distress syndrome. Note the fine, uniform granularity distributed throughout both lungs ("ground glass" appearance). *(From Katz D, Math K, Groskin S: Radiology Secrets. Philadelphia, Hanley & Belfus, 1998, p 380, Fig. 2.)*

    b. Collapsed alveoli are lined by hyaline membranes (Fig. 16-7).
        • Derived from proteins leaking out of damaged pulmonary vessels
    c. Clinical findings
        (1) Respiratory difficulty begins within a few hours after birth.
        (2) Grunting (see Table 16-2)
        (3) Tachypnea
        (4) Intercostal retractions
        (5) Infants develop hypoxemia and respiratory acidosis.
    d. Diagnosis
        • Chest radiograph shows a "ground glass" appearance (Fig. 16-8).
    e. Complications
        (1) Superoxide free radical damage from O_2 therapy
            • May result in blindness and permanent damage to small airways (bronchopulmonary dysplasia)
        (2) Intraventricular hemorrhage
        (3) Patent ductus arteriosus
            • Due to persistent hypoxemia
        (4) Necrotizing enterocolitis
            • Intestinal ischemia allows entry of gut bacteria into the intestinal wall.
        (5) Hypoglycemia in newborn
            (a) Excess insulin decreases serum glucose, producing seizures and damage to neurons.
            (b) Must give newborns glucose to prevent hypoglycemia
    f. Treatment
        • CPAP therapy with endotracheal tube with O_2 and surfactant
V. **Acute Lung Injury**
    A. **Pulmonary edema** (refer to Chapters 4 and 10)
        1. Edema due to alterations in Starling pressure (transudate)
            a. Increased hydrostatic pressure in pulmonary capillaries
                • Left-sided heart failure, volume overload, mitral stenosis
            b. Decreased oncotic pressure
                • Nephrotic syndrome, cirrhosis
        2. Edema due to microvascular or alveolar injury (exudate)
            a. Infections
                • Examples—sepsis, pneumonia
            b. Aspiration
                • Examples—drowning (refer to Chapter 6), gastric contents
            c. Drugs
                • Example—heroin (refer to Chapter 6)
            d. High altitude (refer to Chapter 6)
            e. Acute respiratory distress syndrome (ARDS; see later)
    B. **Acute respiratory distress syndrome (ARDS)**
        • Noncardiogenic pulmonary edema resulting from acute alveolar-capillary damage
        1. Epidemiology
            a. Due to direct injury to the lungs or systemic diseases

RDS: grunting, tachypnea, intercostal retractions

RDS O_2 complications: blindness, bronchopulmonary dysplasia

Hypoglycemia in newborn: due to excess insulin in response to fetal hyperglycemia

Left-sided heart failure: most common cause of pulmonary edema

ARDS: noncardiogenic pulmonary edema

    b. Risk factors for ARDS
      (1) Gram-negative sepsis (>40% of cases)
      (2) Gastric aspiration (>30% of cases)
      (3) Severe trauma with shock (>20% of cases)
      (4) Diffuse pulmonary infections
         • Severe acute respiratory syndrome (SARS), hantavirus
      (5) Heroin
      (6) Smoke inhalation
      (7) Acute pancreatitis
      (8) Cardiopulmonary bypass
      (9) Disseminated intravascular coagulation
     (10) Amniotic fluid embolism, fat embolism

> RDS risk: sepsis, gastric aspiration, severe trauma

  2. Pathogenesis
    a. Acute damage to alveolar capillary walls and epithelial cells
    b. Alveolar macrophages and other cells release cytokines.
      (1) Cytokines are chemotactic to neutrophils.
      (2) Neutrophils transmigrate into the alveoli through pulmonary capillaries.
      (3) Capillary damage causes leakage of a protein-rich exudate producing hyaline membranes.
      (4) Neutrophils damage type I and II pneumocytes.
         • Decrease in surfactant causes atelectasis with intrapulmonary shunting.
    c. Late findings
      (1) Repair by type II pneumocytes
      (2) Progressive interstitial fibrosis (restrictive lung disease)

> ARDS: acute alveolar-capillary damage; sepsis most common cause
>
> Alveolar macrophages: cytokines chemotactic to neutrophils
>
> ARDS: neutrophil damage to type I and II pneumocytes

  3. Clinical findings
    a. Dyspnea/tachypnea
    b. Late inspiratory crackles
  4. Laboratory findings
    a. Severe hypoxemia *not* responsive to O_2 therapy
      • $Pao_2 < 50$ mm Hg
    b. Pulmonary artery wedge pressure < 18 mm Hg
      • Important in distinguishing ARDS from cardiogenic pulmonary edema
    c. Respiratory alkalosis or normal $Paco_2$
    d. Increased A-a gradient, due to:
      (1) Intrapulmonary shunting
         • Related to atelectasis
      (2) Diffusion abnormalities
         • Related to hyaline membranes, alveolar infiltrate
    e. Chest x-ray
      (1) Bilateral interstitial infiltrates initially
      (2) Progresses to widespread alveolar consolidation with air bronchograms (80%)

> ARDS: severe hypoxemia, PA wedge pressure < 18 mm Hg, ↑ A-a gradient

  5. Treatment
    a. Treat underlying disease
    b. Hemodynamic monitoring
    c. Mechanical ventilation
    d. Nitric oxide inhalation
    e. Corticosteroids
  6. Poor prognosis (40–50% mortality rate)

VI. Pulmonary Infections
A. Pneumonia
  1. Epidemiology
    a. Classified as community-acquired or nosocomial (hospital-acquired)
    b. Community-acquired pneumonia is further subdivided into typical and atypical.
  2. Typical community-acquired pneumonia
    a. Epidemiology
      (1) Majority are caused by bacterial pathogens.
      (2) Most often due to *Streptococcus pneumoniae* (50–75%; Fig. 16-9A)
    b. Pathogenesis
      (1) Inhalation of aerosol from an infected patient
      (2) Aspiration of nasopharyngeal flora while sleeping
    c. Bronchopneumonia
      (1) Begins as an acute bronchitis and spreads locally into the lungs
      (2) Usually involves the lower lobes or right middle lobe

> *Streptococcus pneumoniae*: most common cause of typical community-acquired pneumonia

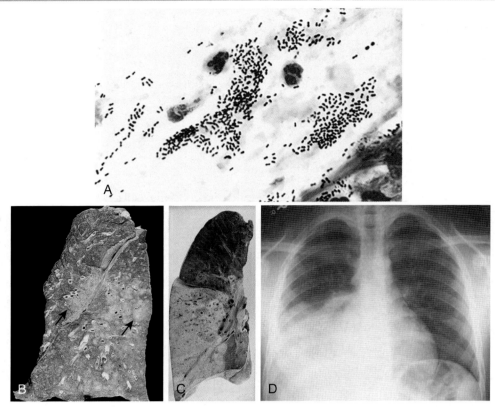

16-9: A, Gram stain of *Streptococcus pneumoniae*. The sputum stain shows numerous lancet-shaped diplococci with the tapered ends pointing to each other. A few neutrophils contain phagocytosed bacteria. **B,** Bronchopneumonia showing patchy areas of consolidation (*arrows*) representing collections of neutrophils in the alveoli and bronchi. **C,** Lobar pneumonia. The lower lobe is uniformally consolidated. **D,** Posteroanterior radiograph of a right lower lobe pneumococcal pneumonia. Note the alveolar consolidation and the visible border of the right ventricle indicating that the middle lobe is *not* involved. (***A*** *from Henry JB: Clinical Diagnosis and Management by Laboratory Methods, 20th ed. Philadelphia, WB Saunders, 2001, Plate 50-1;* ***B*** *from Kumar V, Fausto N, Abbas A: Robbins and Cotran's Pathologic Basis of Disease, 7th ed. Philadelphia, WB Saunders, 2004, p 749, Fig. 15-33;* ***C*** *from Corrin B: Pathology of the Lungs. London, Churchill Livingstone, 2000, p 162, Fig. 5.2.5;* ***D*** *from Kliegman RM, Jenson HB, Behrman RE, Stanton BF: Nelson Textbook of Pediatrics, 18th ed. Philadelphia, Saunders Elsevier, 2007, p 1798, Fig. 397-2A.)*

Bronchopneumonia: acute bronchitis lung parenchyma

(3) Lung has patchy areas of consolidation (Fig. 16-9B).
    • Microabscesses are present in the areas of consolidation.
  d. Lobar pneumonia
    • Complete or almost complete consolidation of a lobe of lung (Fig. 16-9C)
  e. Complications
    (1) Lung abscesses, empyema (pus in the pleural cavity)
    (2) Sepsis
  f. Clinical findings
    (1) Sudden onset of high fever with productive cough
    (2) Chest pain
    (3) Tachycardia

Typical pneumonia: signs of consolidation (alveolar exudate)

    (4) Signs of consolidation (alveolar exudate)
      (a) Dullness to percussion
      (b) Increased vocal tactile fremitus
        • Sound is transmitted well through alveolar consolidations.
      (c) Late inspiratory crackles
      (d) Bronchial breath sounds
      (e) Bronchophony and egophony

Chest radiograph: gold standard for diagnosing pneumonia

    (5) Chest radiograph (gold standard screen)
      (a) Patchy infiltrates (bronchopneumonia) or lobar consolidation (Fig. 16-9D)
      (b) Sensitivity 50% to 85%

Positive Gram stain: more useful than culture

    (6) Laboratory findings
      (a) Positive Gram stain
        1. More useful than culture
          • Cultures are still obtained.

TABLE 16-4. **SUMMARY OF RESPIRATORY MICROBIAL PATHOGENS**

PATHOGEN	DISCUSSION
Viruses	
Rhinovirus	Most common cause of the common cold Transmitted by hand to eye-nose contact Other causes of colds—coronaviruses, adenoviruses, influenza C virus, coxsackievirus
Coxsackievirus	Acute chest syndrome: fever with pleuritis
RSV	Most common viral cause of atypical pneumonia and bronchiolitis (wheezing) in children; otitis media in older children Occurs in late fall and winter Rapid diagnosis with antigen detection in nasopharyngeal wash Passive immunization: palivizumab (monoclonal antibody) reduces hospitalization rates

Parainfluenza (see Fig. 16-10A)	Most common cause of croup (laryngotracheobronchitis) in infants
	    Inspiratory stridor (upper airway obstruction) due to submucosal edema in trachea; brassy cough; signs of respiratory distress
	    Anterior x-ray of neck shows "steeple sign," representing mucosal edema in the trachea (site of obstruction)
	Bronchiolitis in infants
	Treatment: cold water humidifiers and aerosolized racemic epinephrine

CMV (see Fig. 16-10B)	Common pneumonia in immunocompromised hosts (e.g., bone marrow transplants, AIDS) Enlarged alveolar macrophages/pneumocytes, contain basophilic intranuclear inclusions surrounded by a halo
Influenzavirus	Type A viruses are most often involved Hemagglutinins bind virus to cell receptors in the nasal passages Neuraminidase dissolves mucus and facilitates release of viral particles Influenza A: worldwide epidemics; pneumonia may be complicated by a superimposed bacterial pneumonia (usually *Staphylococcus aureus*) Influenza B: causes major outbreaks Antigen drift: minor mutation; does *not* require new vaccine Antigen shift: major mutation in hemagglutinin or neuraminidase; new vaccine required Clinical: fever, headache, cough, myalgias, chest pain Vaccination: mandatory for people > 65 years old, people with chronic illnesses *Treatment*: neuraminidase inhibitors zanamivir, oseltamivir Associations: Reye syndrome with salicylate ingestion; Guillain-Barré syndrome
Rubeola	Fever, cough, conjunctivitis, and excessive nasal mucus production Koplik spots in the mouth *precede* onset of the rash Warthin-Finkeldey multinucleated giant cells are a characteristic finding
SARS	Infects lower respiratory tract and then spreads systemically First transmitted to humans through contact with masked palm civets (China) and then from human-to-human contact through respiratory secretions (e.g., hospitals, families) Develop severe respiratory infection Diagnose with viral detection by PCR assay or detection of antibodies
Hantavirus pulmonary syndrome	Transmission: inhalation of urine/feces from deer mice in Southwestern United States Pulmonary syndrome: ARDS, hemorrhage, renal failure Diagnosis: detect viral RNA in lung tissue No effective treatment High mortality rate
Bacteria	
Chlamydia *Chlamydophilia pneumoniae*	Second most common cause of atypical pneumonia Seroepidemiologic association with coronary artery disease *Treatment*: doxycycline
Chlamydia trachomatis	Newborn pneumonia (passage through birth canal) Afebrile, staccato cough (choppy cough), conjunctivitis, wheezing *Treatment*: erythromycin
Mycoplasma *M. pneumoniae*	Most common cause of atypical pneumonia Common in adolescents and military recruits (closed spaces) Insidious onset with low-grade fever Complications: bullous myringitis, cold autoimmune hemolytic anemia due to anti-I-IgM antibodies. *Treatment*: erythromycin; azithromycin; clarithromycin Cold agglutinins in blood
Coxiella burnetii	Usually transmitted without a vector Contracted by dairy farmers, veterinarians Associated with the birthing process of infected sheep, cattle, and goats, and handling of milk or excrement Atypical pneumonia, myocarditis, granulomatous hepatitis *Treatment*: doxycycline

Continued

TABLE 16-4. **SUMMARY OF RESPIRATORY MICROBIAL PATHOGENS—cont'd**

PATHOGEN	DISCUSSION
Bacteria—cont'd	
Streptococcus pneumoniae (see Fig. 16-9A)	Gram-positive lancet-shaped diplococcus Most common cause of typical community-acquired pneumonia Rapid onset, productive cough, signs of consolidation Urine antigen test excellent screen *Treatment:* penicillin G; amoxicillin
Staphylococcus aureus	Gram-positive cocci in clumps Yellow sputum Commonly superimposed on influenza pneumonia and measles pneumonia Major lung pathogen in cystic fibrosis and IV drug abusers Hemorrhagic pulmonary edema, abscess formation, and tension pneumatocysts (intrapleural blebs), which may rupture and produce a tension pneumothorax. *Treatment:* TMP-SMX
Corynebacterium diphtheriae (see Fig. 16-10C)	Gram-positive rod Toxin inhibits protein synthesis by ADP-ribosylation of elongation factor 2 involved in protein synthesis Toxin also impairs β-oxidation of fatty acids in the heart Toxin-induced pseudomembranous inflammation produces shaggy gray membranes in the oropharynx and trachea; toxic myocarditis (death) *Treatment:* erythromycin
Bacillus anthracis	Gram-positive rod Habitat: soil Capsule inhibits phagocytosis Exotoxins: edema factor (activates adenylate cyclase); lethal factor (inhibits a signal transduction protein involved in cell division); protective antigen (assists entry of above toxins into cells) Transmission: direct contact with animal skins or products (most commonly sheep and cattle) and entry of the organisms through abrasions or cuts; inhalation (use in germ warfare) Cutaneous anthrax (90–95% of cases): occurs through direct contact with infected or contaminated animal products; resembles insect bite but eventually swells to form a black scab, or eschar, with a central area of necrosis ("malignant pustule"); if untreated, death occurs in 20% of patients Pulmonary anthrax: "first sign of the disease is death"; inhalation of spores present in contaminated hides or germ warfare; necrotizing pneumonia, meningitis, pronounced splenomegaly, and dissemination throughout the rest of the body Prevention: vaccine available for high-risk patients; e.g., veterinarians, soldiers entering developing countries *Treatment:* ciprofloxacin
Actinomyces israeli	Gram-positive filamentous bacteria; strict anaerobe; normal flora in tonsils and adenoids Produces draining sinuses in the jaw, chest cavity, and abdomen; pus contains sulfur granules (yellow specks) that contain the bacteria *Treatment:* ampicillin or penicillin G
Nocardia asteroides	Gram-positive filamentous bacteria; strict aerobe; partially acid-fast Produces granulomatous microabscesses in the lungs Frequently disseminates to the CNS and kidneys *Treatment:* TMP-SMX

Bordetella pertussis	Gram-negative rod
	Pili attach to cilia in upper respiratory tract; toxin stimulates adenylate cyclase, which catalyzes the addition of ADP-ribose to the inhibitory subunit of the G protein complex; toxin also produces absolute lymphocytosis (normal-appearing lymphocytes) often in leukemoid reaction range
	Produces whooping cough, transmitted by droplet infection
	  Catarrhal phase: lasts 1–2 weeks; mild coughing, rhinorrhea, conjunctivitis
	  Paroxysmal coughing phase: lasts 2–5 weeks; characteristic 4–5 coughs in succession on expiration followed by an inspiratory whoop; absolute lymphocytosis (20,000–50,000 cells/mm³)
	  Convalescence phase: lasts 1–2 weeks; slow decline in coughing and lymphocytosis
	  Complications: hemorrhage into skin, conjunctiva, bronchus, brain from coughing; otitis media; meningoencephalitis (10%); rectal prolapse from coughing; pneumonia (most common cause of death in children < 3 years old; children < 1 year old have no protection from mother's immunoglobulins)
	Diagnosis: nasopharyngeal swabs using special cough plate; direct immunofluorescence of swab material
	Treatment: erythromycin

Haemophilus influenzae	Gram-negative rod Common cause of sinusitis, otitis media, conjunctivitis ("pinkeye") Inspiratory stridor may be due to acute epiglottitis Swelling of epiglottis produces "thumbprint sign" on lateral x-ray of the neck Most common bacterial cause of acute exacerbation of COPD *Treatment:* cefotaxime; ceftriaxone

TABLE 16-4. SUMMARY OF RESPIRATORY MICROBIAL PATHOGENS—cont'd

PATHOGEN	DISCUSSION
Bacteria—cont'd	
Moraxella catarrhalis	Gram-negative diplococcus Common cause of typical pneumonia, especially in the elderly Second most common pathogen causing acute exacerbation of COPD Common cause of chronic bronchitis, sinusitis, otitis media *Treatment:* amoxicillin-clavulanate
Pseudomonas aeruginosa	Green sputum (pyocyanin) Water-loving bacteria most often transmitted by respirators Most common cause of nosocomial pneumonia and death due to pneumonia in cystic fibrosis Pneumonia often associated with infarction due to vessel invasion *Treatment:* antipseudomonal beta-lactam + aminoglycoside + antipseudomonal quinolone or macrolide
Klebsiella pneumoniae	Gram-negative fat rod surrounded by a mucoid capsule Most common gram-negative organism causing lobar pneumonia and typical pneumonia in elderly patients in nursing homes Common cause of pneumonia in alcoholics; however, *S. pneumoniae* is still the most common pneumonia Atypical pneumonia associated with blood-tinged, thick, mucoid sputum Lobar consolidation and abscess formation are common *Treatment:* ceftriaxone
Legionella pneumophila	Gram-negative rod (requires IF stain or Dieterle silver stain to identify in tissue) Antigens can also be detected in urine Water-loving bacterium (water coolers; mists in produce section of grocery stores; outdoor restaurants in summer; rain forests in zoos) Risk factors: alcoholic, smoker, immunosuppression Pneumonia associated with high fever, dry cough, flu-like symptoms May produce tubulointerstitial disease with destruction of the JG apparatus leading to hyporeninemic hypoaldosteronism (type IV renal tubular acidosis—hyponatremia, hyperkalemia, metabolic acidosis) Urine antigen test excellent screen *Treatment:* fluoroquinolone; azithromycin
Yersinia pestis	Gram-negative rod Cause of plague Transmitted by bite of rat flea; primary reservoir for bacteria are ground squirrels in the Southwest Also transmitted person-to-person by droplet infection Macrophages cannot kill bacteria due to protection by V and W antigens Three types of disease: bubonic (most common), pneumonic (transmitted by aerosol), septicemic Bubonic type: bite by rat flea that has recently bitten an infected ground squirrel; infected lymph nodes enlarge (usually in the groin), mat together, and drain to the surface (buboes) *Treatment:* Pneumonic type: gentamicin + doxycycline Bubonic type: gentamicin or streptomycin
Systemic Fungi	
Cryptococcus neoformans (see Fig. 16-10D)	Budding yeast with narrow-based buds; surrounded by a thick capsule. Found in pigeon excreta (around buildings, outside office windows, under bridges) Primary lung disease (40%): granulomatous inflammation with caseation *Treatment:* fluconazole
Aspergillus fumigatus (see Fig. 16-10E)	Fruiting body and narrow-angled (<45 degrees), branching septate hyphae Aspergilloma: fungus ball (visible on x-ray) that develops in a preexisting cavity in the lung (e.g., old TB site); cause of massive hemoptysis Allergic bronchopulmonary aspergillosis: type I and type III hypersensitivity reactions; IgE levels increased; eosinophilia. Intense inflammation of airways and mucus plugs in terminal bronchioles. Repeated attacks may lead to bronchiectasis and interstitial lung disease; treatment with corticosteroids Vessel invader with hemorrhagic infarctions and a necrotizing bronchopneumonia *Treatment:* voriconazole
Mucor species	Wide-angled hyphae (>45 degrees) without septa Clinical settings: diabetes, immunosuppressed patients Vessel invader and produces hemorrhagic infarcts in the lung Invades the frontal lobes in patients with diabetic ketoacidosis (rhinocerebral mucormycosis) *Treatment:* amphotericin B

Continued

TABLE 16-4. SUMMARY OF RESPIRATORY MICROBIAL PATHOGENS—cont'd

PATHOGEN	DISCUSSION
Systemic Fungi—cont'd	
Coccidioides immitis (see Fig. 16-10F)	Spherules with endospores in tissues Contracted by inhaling arthrospores in dust while living or passing through arid desert areas in the Southwest (valley fever); increased after earthquakes (increased dust) Flu-like symptoms and erythema nodosum (painful nodules on lower legs; inflammation of subcutaneous fat) Granulomatous inflammation with caseous necrosis *Treatment*: usually self-limited; if severe: itraconazole or fluconazole
Histoplasma capsulatum (see Fig. 16-10G, H)	Most common systemic fungal infection Endemic in Ohio and central Mississippi river valleys Inhalation of microconidia in dust contaminated with excreta from bats (increased incidence in cave explorers, spelunkers), starlings, or chickens (common in chicken farmers) Granulomatous inflammation with caseous necrosis Yeast forms are present in macrophages Simulates TB lung disease; produces coin lesions, consolidations, miliary spread, and cavitation Marked dystrophic calcification of granulomas; most common cause of multiple calcifications in the spleen *Treatment*: usually self-limited; if severe, itraconazole or amphotericin B
Blastomyces dermatitidis (see Fig. 16-10I)	Yeasts have broad-based buds and nuclei Occurs in Great Lakes region, central, and southeastern United States Male dominant disease Produces skin and lung disease; skin lesions simulate squamous cell carcinoma Granulomatous inflammation with caseous necrosis *Treatment*: itraconazole or amphotericin B
Pneumocystis jiroveci (see Fig. 3-3)	Cysts and trophozoites present; cysts attach to type I pneumocytes Primarily an opportunistic infection; occurs when CD4 count < 200 cells/mm³. Most common initial AIDS-defining infection Patients develop fever, dyspnea, and severe hypoxemia Diffuse intra-alveolar foamy exudates with cup-shaped cysts best visualized with silver or Giemsa stains Chest x-ray shows diffuse alveolar and interstitial infiltrates *Treatment*: TMP-SMX given prophylactically when CD4 counts < 200 cells/mm³

ARDS, acute respiratory distress syndrome; CMV, cytomegalovirus; COPD, chronic obstructive pulmonary disease; IF, immunofluorescent; JG, juxtaglomerular; PCR, polymerase chain reaction; RSV, respiratory syncytial virus; SARS, severe acute respiratory syndrome; TB, tuberculosis; TMP-SMX, trimethoprim-sulfamethoxazole.

2. Sensitivity 80%
   (b) Neutrophilic leukocytosis
   (c) Blood cultures positive in 20% of cases.
3. Table 16-4 (Fig.16-10A to I) summarizes important respiratory microbial pathogens.
4. Atypical community-acquired pneumonia
   a. Epidemiology
      (1) Usually caused by *Mycoplasma pneumoniae*
      (2) Other pathogens
         (a) *Chlamydophilia pneumoniae*
         (b) Viruses
            • Respiratory syncytial virus, influenzavirus, adenovirus
         (c) *Chlamydia trachomatis* in newborns
   b. Pathogenesis
      • Contracted by inhalation (droplet infection)
   c. Patchy interstitial pneumonia
      (1) Mononuclear infiltrate
      (2) Alveolar spaces usually free of exudate
   d. Clinical findings
      (1) Insidious onset, low-grade fever
      (2) Nonproductive cough
      (3) Chest pain
      (4) Flu-like symptoms
         • Pharyngitis, laryngitis, myalgias, headache
      (5) *No* signs of consolidation
5. Nosocomial pneumonia
   a. Epidemiology; risk factors:
      (1) Severe underlying disease
      (2) Antibiotic therapy

Mycoplasma pneumoniae: most common cause of atypical pneumonia

Atypical pneumonia: interstitial pneumonia; no signs of consolidation

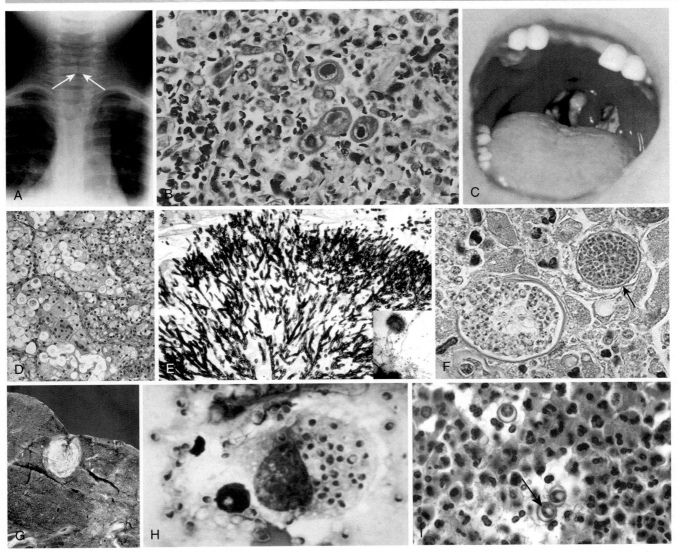

16-10: **A,** Parainfluenza virus producing laryngotracheobronchitis. Frontal radiograph showing narrowing of the trachea (*arrows*) producing the classic steeple sign. **B,** Cytomegalovirus. The enlarged nuclei of many of the type I pneumocytes contain large inclusions (basophilic staining with hematoxylin and eosin stain) surrounded by a clear halo. **C,** Tonsillitis due to *Corynebacterium diphtheriae*. Note the gray, pseudomembrane covering the tonsils. **D,** *Cryptococcus neoformans*. The yeast form produces a clear capsule around a central faint nucleus. **E,** *Aspergillus fumigatus*. Lung biopsy stained with Gomori methenamine-silver shows septated hyphae and fruiting body (*inset*). **F,** *Coccidioides immitis*. Note the spherules containing endospores (*arrow*). **G,** *Histoplasma capsulatum*. Laminated granuloma at the lung periphery produces puckering of the pleural surface. **H,** *Histoplasma capsulatum*. Alveolar macrophage contains intracellular yeast forms. **I,** *Blastomyces dermatidis*. Note the yeast forms with broad-based buds (*arrow*). (**A** *from Pretorius ES, Solomon JA: Radiology Secrets, 2nd ed. St. Louis, Mosby, 2006, p 464, Fig. 57-4;* **B** *from Damjanov I, Linder J: Pathology: A Color Atlas. St. Louis, Mosby, 2000, p 56, Fig. 4-24;* **C** *courtesy of Franklin H. Top, Department of Hygiene and Preventive Medicine, State University of Iowa College of Medicine, Iowa City, Iowa, and Parke, Davis & Company's Therapeutic Notes;* **D** *and* **F** *from Klatt E: Robbins and Cotran's Atlas of Pathology. Philadelphia, WB Saunders, 2006, pp 127, 126, Figs. 5-92, 5-91 on right, respectively;* **E, G, I** *from Kumar V, Fausto N, Abbas A: Robbins and Cotran's Pathologic Basis of Disease, 7th ed. Philadelphia, WB Saunders, 2004, pp 400, 754, 755, Figs. 8-49B, 15-37, 15-39A, respectively;* **H** *from Murray PR, Shea YR: Medical Microbiology, 2nd ed. St. Louis, Mosby, 2002, p 773, Fig. 74-10.)*

(3) Immunosuppression
(4) Respirators
  • Most common source of infection
b. Pathogens
  (1) Gram-negative bacteria
    • *Pseudomonas aeruginosa* (respirators), *Escherichia coli*
  (2) Gram-positive bacteria (e.g., *Staphylococcus aureus*)
6. Pneumonia in immunocompromised hosts
  a. Complication of AIDS and bone marrow transplantation

Pseudomonas aeruginosa: nosocomial pneumonia; contracted from respirators

b. Common opportunistic infections:
   (1) Cytomegalovirus (Fig. 16-10B)
   (2) *Pneumocystis jiroveci* (see Fig. 3-8)
     • Trimethoprim-sulfamethoxazole is used for prophylaxis and treatment.
   (3) *Aspergillus fumigatus* (Fig. 16-10E)
7. Tuberculosis (TB)
  a. Epidemiology and pathogenesis
   (1) Contracted by inhalation of *Mycobacterium tuberculosis*
   (2) Organism resides in phagosomes of alveolar macrophages
     • Produces a protein that prevents fusion of lysosomes with phagosome
   (3) Characteristics
    (a) Strict aerobe, acid-fast (due to mycolic acid in cell wall)
    (b) Cord factor is virulence factor
   (4) Screening
    (a) Purified protein derivative (PPD) intradermal skin test
    (b) Does *not* distinguish active from inactive disease
   (5) Protein in cell wall
     • Responsible for positive PPD
   (6) Drug resistance
    (a) Chromosome mutations involving mycolic acid
    (b) Chromosome mutations involving catalase peroxidase
     • Enzyme is required to activate isoniazid
  b. Primary TB
   (1) Subpleural location (Fig. 16-11)
    (a) Upper part of the lower lobes or lower part of the upper lobes
    (b) Ghon focus (caseous necrosis) in periphery
    (c) Ghon complex (caseous necrosis) in hilar lymph nodes
   (2) Usually resolves
    (a) Produces a calcified granuloma or area of scar tissue
    (b) May be a nidus for secondary TB
  c. Secondary (reactivation) TB
   (1) Due to reactivation of a previous primary TB site
   (2) Involves one or both apices in upper lobes (Fig. 16-12)
     • Ventilation (oxygenation) is greatest in the upper lobes.
   (3) Cavitary lesion due to release of cytokines from memory T cells
  d. Clinical findings
    • Fever, drenching night sweats, weight loss
  e. Complications
   (1) Miliary spread in lungs due to invasion into the bronchus or lymphatics
   (2) Miliary spread to extrapulmonary sites
    (a) Due to invasion of pulmonary vein tributaries
    (b) Kidney is the most common extrapulmonary site.
    (c) Adrenal involvement may result in Addison's disease.

Pneumocystis jiroveci: most common pathogen causing pneumonia in AIDS

TB: acid-fastness due to mycolic acid

TB: cord factor is virulence factor

PPD: does *not* distinguish active from inactive TB

Primary TB: upper part lower lobes; lower part upper lobes; Ghon complex

Reactivation TB: upper lobe cavitary lesion(s)

TB: drenching night sweats, fever, weight loss

Kidneys: most common extrapulmonary site in TB

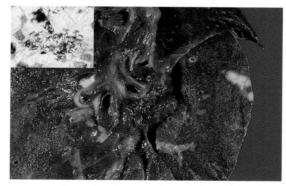

16-11: Primary tuberculosis. Note the tan-yellow subpleural granuloma with caseation necrosis and the tan-yellow area of caseation necrosis in the hilar lymph node in the mid-lung field. The two of these together is called a Ghon complex. The inset shows an acid-fast stain with numerous *Mycobacterium tuberculosis* organisms. *(The gross picture of primary tuberculosis is from Klatt, E: Robbins and Cotran's Atlas of Pathology. Philadelphia, WB Saunders, 2006, p 197, Fig. 8-4; inset from Hoffbrand AV: Color Atlas: Clinical Hematology, 3rd ed. St. Louis, Mosby, 2000, p 136, Fig. 7-85B.)*

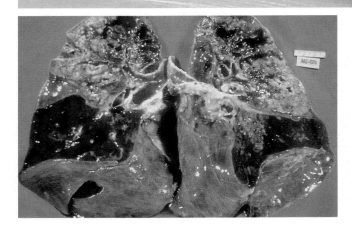

16-12: Reactivation tuberculosis. The apices of both lungs show gray-white areas of caseation necrosis and multiple areas of cavitation. *(From Kumar V, Fausto N, Abbas A: Robbins and Cotran's Pathologic Basis of Disease, 7th ed. Philadelphia, WB Saunders, 2004, p 386, Fig. 8-32.)*

(3) Massive hemoptysis, bronchiectasis, scar carcinoma
(4) Granulomatous hepatitis, spread to vertebra (Pott's disease)
   f. Diagnosis
     (1) Bronchoalveolar lavage best for staining and culture
     (2) Sputum cultures
   g. Treatment
     (1) Isoniazid + rifampin + pyrazinamide
     (2) Noninfectious in 2 to 3 weeks
     (3) Treat for additional 9 to 12 months
       • Kills metabolically inactive persisters in lesions
8. *Mycobacterium avium-intracellulare* complex (MAC)
   a. Atypical mycobacterium
   b. Most common TB in AIDS (often disseminates)
     • Occurs when CD4 T_H count falls below 50 cells/mm³
   c. Treatment
     • Clarithromycin + rifabutin + ethambutol
9. Systemic fungal infections (see Fig. 16-10D to I)
   a. Contracted from inhalation of the pathogen
   b. Produce a granulomatous inflammatory reaction with or without caseation
B. Lung abscess
1. Causes of lung abscesses
   a. Most often due to aspiration of oropharyngeal material (e.g., tonsillar material)
     (1) Risk factors
       (a) Alcoholism
       (b) Loss of consciousness
       (c) Recent dental work
     (2) Microbial pathogens
       (a) Aerobic and anaerobic streptococci
       (b) *Staphylococcus species*
       (c) *Prevotella*
       (d) *Fusobacterium*
   b. Complication of bacterial pneumonia
     • Examples—*Staphylococcus aureus, Klebsiella pneumoniae*
   c. Septic embolism
     • Example—infective endocarditis
   d. Obstructive lung neoplasia
     • From 10% to 15% of abscesses are behind a bronchus obstructed by cancer.
2. Gross findings
   a. Vary in size and location (Fig. 16-13)
   b. Those due to aspiration are primarily located on the right side (Box 16-1).
3. Clinical findings
   a. Spiking fever with productive cough (foul-smelling sputum)
   b. Chest imaging shows cavitation with an air-fluid level (Fig. 16-14).
4. Treatment
   a. Clindamycin
   b. Bronchoscopy if does not resolve

Margin notes:

TB in vertebra: Pott's disease

MAC: most common TB in AIDS

Lung abscesses: most often due to aspiration of oropharyngeal material

Lung abscesses: mixed aerobic/anaerobic infection

Lung abscesses: chest x-ray shows cavitation and fluid level

Superior segment, right lower lobe: most common site for aspiration

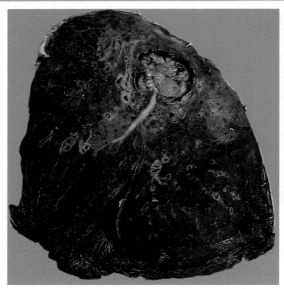

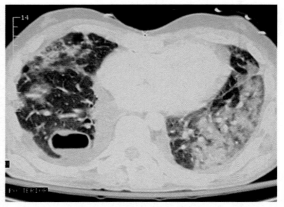

16-14: Lung abscess. The chest computed tomographic scan shows an abscess in the right lower lobe with an air-fluid level. *(From Klatt E: Robbins and Cotran's Atlas of Pathology. Philadelphia, WB Saunders, 2006, p 121, Fig. 5-74.)*

16-13: Lung abscess. Note the large abscess spanning the right upper and lower lobes. It is filled with necrotic material. *(From Corrin B: Pathology of the Lungs. London, Churchill Livingstone, 2000, p 172, Fig. 5.5.16.)*

BOX 16-1 ASPIRATION SITES IN THE LUNGS

Foreign material localizes to different portions of the lung, depending on the position of the patient. In the standing or sitting position, material localizes in the posterobasal segment of the right lower lobe; in the supine position, the superior segment of the right lower lobe; and in the right-sided position, the right middle lobe or the posterior segment of the right upper lobe. The most common aspiration site is the superior segment of the right lower lobe.

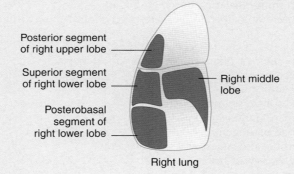

VII. Vascular Lung Lesions

A. Pulmonary thromboembolism

1. Epidemiology and pathogenesis

    a. Source

    - Majority (95%) originate in the femoral vein

    b. Risk factors for thromboembolism (refer to Chapter 4)

    - Stasis of blood flow (e.g., prolonged bed rest), hypercoagulable states

    c. Size of the embolus determines pulmonary vessel that is occluded.

    (1) Large emboli occlude the major vessels (saddle embolus) (Fig. 16-15).

    (2) Small emboli occlude medium-sized and small pulmonary arteries.

    d. Potential consequences of pulmonary artery occlusion

    (1) Increase in pulmonary artery pressure

    (2) Decrease blood flow to pulmonary parenchyma

    - May cause hemorrhagic infarction

Source of pulmonary thromboemboli: femoral veins

Bronchial arteries: protect lungs from infarction

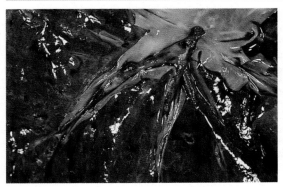

16-15: Saddle embolus occluding the main branches of the pulmonary artery. *(From Damjanov I, Linder J: Pathology: A Color Atlas. St. Louis, Mosby, 2000, p 57, Fig. 4-26.)*

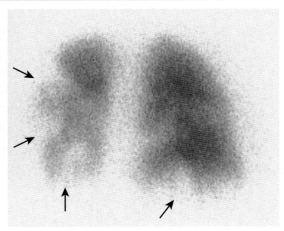

16-16: Radionuclide perfusion scan in the lung. The radionuclide scan shows multiple perfusion defects in both lungs *(arrows)* due to multiple pulmonary emboli. *(From Forbes C, Jackson W: Color Atlas and Text of Clinical Medicine, 2nd ed. Philadelphia, Mosby, 2003, Fig. 4-49.)*

In a patient with normal bronchial artery blood flow (originates from thoracic aorta and intercostal arteries) and ventilation, a pulmonary embolus produces a hemorrhagic infarction in ~10% of cases. However, if the patient has decreased bronchial artery blood flow (e.g., decreased cardiac output), or previously underventilated lung (e.g., obstructive lung disease), then occlusion of the pulmonary vessel will likely result in a hemorrhagic infarction, which significantly increases risk of morbidity and death.

Bronchial arteries: arise from aorta and intercostal arteries

2. Red-blue, raised, wedge-shaped area that extends to the pleural surface (see Fig. 1-11C)
   a. Pleural surface has a fibrinous exudate (produces a pleural friction rub).
      • Hemorrhagic pleural effusion may also occur.
   b. Majority are located in the lower lobes.
      • Perfusion is greater than ventilation in the lower lobes.
3. Clinical findings
   a. Saddle embolus
      (1) Sudden increase in pulmonary artery pressure
      (2) Produces acute right ventricular strain and sudden death
   b. Pulmonary infarction
      (1) Sudden onset of dyspnea and tachypnea
      (2) Fever
      (3) Pleuritic chest pain (pain on inspiration)
      (4) Pleural friction rub
      (5) Pleural effusion
      (6) Expiratory wheezing
         • Due to release of thromboxane A_2 from platelets

Saddle embolus: sudden death

4. Laboratory findings with a pulmonary infarction
   a. Respiratory alkalosis (arterial PCO_2 < 33 mm Hg)
   b. PaO_2 < 80 mm Hg (90% of cases)
   c. Increase in A-a gradient (100% of cases)
   d. Increase in D-dimers
5. Diagnosis
   a. Chest x-ray
      (1) Pleural effusion
      (2) "Cut-off" sign of one or more pulmonary arteries
         • Hypovascularity behind the blocked vessel
      (3) Hampton's hump
         • Wedge-shaped area of consolidation
   b. Abnormal perfusion radionuclide scan
      (1) Ventilation scan is normal, but the perfusion scan is abnormal (Fig. 16-16).

Pulmonary infarction: dyspnea and tachypnea most common symptom and sign; respiratory alkalosis; hypoxemia

(2) Pulmonary angiogram is gold standard confirmatory test.
   • Expensive and not clinically available in smaller hospitals
(3) Spiral (helical) CT is excellent if preexisting lung disease is present.

Diagnosis: V/Q scan +
D-dimers: spira CT

   c. Positive D-dimers (refer to Chapter 14)
   • Usually performed in conjunction with ventilation/perfusion (V/Q) scan or spiral CT
6. Treatment
   • Refer to Chapter 4
7. Prognosis
   a. ~80% overall survival
   b. ~60% resolve without treatment

Pulmonary infarction:
normal ventilation scan,
abnormal perfusion scan;
↑ D-dimers

   c. ~90% resolve with treatment

B. Pulmonary hypertension (PH)
1. Definition
   a. Mean pulmonary artery pressure > 25 mm Hg at rest
   b. Mean pulmonary artery pressure > 30 mm Hg with exercise
2. Epidemiology and pathogenesis
   a. Primary PH
      (1) Primary type is more common in women.
      (2) Genetic predisposition
         • Mutations in genes associated with transforming growth factor-β
      (3) Vascular hyperreactivity with proliferation of smooth muscle
   b. Secondary PH
      (1) Endothelial cell dysfunction
         (a) Loss of vasodilators (e.g., nitric oxide)
         (b) Increase in vasoconstrictors (e.g., endothelin)
      (2) Hypoxemia and respiratory acidosis stimulate vasoconstriction of pulmonary arteries.

Main cause of secondary
PH: respiratory acidosis
and hypoxemia

         • Causes smooth muscle hyperplasia and hypertrophy
      (3) Causes
         (a) Chronic hypoxemia
            • Examples—chronic lung disease; living at high altitude
         (b) Chronic respiratory acidosis
            • Chronic bronchitis (CB); obstructive sleep apnea
         (c) Loss of pulmonary vasculature
            • Increases workload for remaining vessels; emphysema, recurrent pulmonary emboli
         (d) Left-to-right cardiac shunts (refer to Chapter 10)
            • Volume overloading pulmonary vasculature
         (e) Mitral stenosis
            • Backup of blood into pulmonary veins; pulmonary venous hypertension
3. Pathologic findings

PH: atherosclerosis of
main PAs

   a. Atherosclerosis of main elastic pulmonary arteries (PAs)
      • Due to increased pressure on the endothelium leading to injury
   b. Proliferation of myointimal cells and smooth muscle cells
4. Clinical findings

PH: exertional dyspnea
most common symptom

   a. Exertional dyspnea most common presenting sign
   b. Chest pain

PH: tapering of
pulmonary arteries on
chest x-ray

   c. Chest radiograph shows tapering of the pulmonary arteries
   d. Accentuated P_2 (sign of PH)
   e. Left parasternal heave (sign of right ventricular hypertrophy [RVH])
      • PH imposes an increased afterload on the right ventricle.
   f. Right-sided heart failure due to cor pulmonale
5. Diagnosis
   a. Catheterization to measure pressures
      • Can also use transthoracic Doppler echocardiogram
   b. Chest x-ray
      (1) Enlargement of main pulmonary arteries
         • Rapid tapering of distal vessels
      (2) Right ventricular enlargement
6. Treatment
   a. Diuretics
   b. Oxygen

  c. Vasodilators
   • Calcium channel blockers, prostanoids, endothelin receptor antagonists
  d. Lung transplant
 7. Cor pulmonale (Fig. 16-17)
  • Combination of PH and right RVH leading to right-sided heart failure
C. Goodpasture syndrome (refer to Chapter 19)
 • Pulmonary hemorrhage with hemoptysis often precedes renal failure.

VIII. Restrictive Lung Diseases
 • These disorders are characterized by reduced total lung capacity in the presence of a normal or reduced expiratory flow rate.
A. Causes of restrictive disease
 1. Chest wall disorders in the presence of normal lungs
  • Examples—kyphoscoliosis, pleural disease (e.g., mesothelioma), obesity
 2. Acute or chronic interstitial lung diseases
  a. Acute interstitial disease (e.g., ARDS, see section V)
  b. Chronic interstitial disease
   (1) Fibrosing disorders (e.g., pneumoconiosis)
   (2) Granulomatous disease (e.g., sarcoidosis)
B. Pathogenesis of interstitial fibrosis
 1. Earliest manifestation is an alveolitis.
  • Leukocytes release cytokines, which stimulate fibrosis.
 2. Effects of interstitial fibrosis
  a. Decreases lung compliance
   (1) Decreased expansion of the lung parenchyma during inspiration
   (2) Damage to type I/II alveolar cells and endothelial cells
    • Functional loss of alveolar and capillary units
  b. Increases lung elasticity
   • Recoil of the lung on expiration is increased.
 3. Clinical and laboratory findings in all restrictive lung diseases
  a. Dry cough and exertional dyspnea
  b. Late inspiratory crackles in lower lung fields
  c. Potential for cor pulmonale
  d. Pulmonary function test findings and arterial blood gases
   (1) All volumes and capacities are equally decreased.

Cor pulmonale: PH + RVH

Goodpasture syndrome: hemoptysis followed by renal failure

Alveolitis → interstitial fibrosis

Restrictive lung disease: ↓ compliance, ↑ elasticity

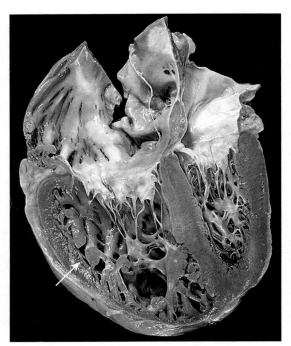

16-17: Cor pulmonale. Note the increased ventricular volume and hypertrophied muscle of the right ventricle (*arrow*). The patient had pulmonary hypertension.

Restrictive lung disease: ↓ volumes/capacities, normal to ↑ FEV$_{1\,sec}$/FVC ratio

(2) Decreased FEV$_{1\,sec}$ (see Fig. 16-1B)
  • Example—3 L (normal 4 L)
(3) Decreased FVC (see Fig. 16-1B)
  • Often the same value as FEV$_{1\,sec}$ (3 L) due to increased lung elasticity
(4) Increased ratio of FEV$_{1\,sec}$/FVC
  • Example—3/3 = 100% (normal is 80%)
(5) Respiratory alkalosis (arterial P$_{CO_2}$ < 33 mm Hg)
(6) Decreased P$_{ao_2}$
  e. Chest radiograph findings
    • Diffuse bilateral reticulonodular infiltrates

C. Pneumoconioses
  1. Epidemiology
    a. Inhalation of mineral dust into the lungs leading to interstitial fibrosis
      (1) Mineral dust includes coal dust, silica, asbestos, and beryllium.
      (2) Accounts for ~25% of cases of chronic interstitial lung disease
    b. Particle size determines site of lung deposition
      (1) 1- to 5-μm particles
        • Reach the bifurcation of the respiratory bronchioles and alveolar ducts
      (2) Smaller than 0.5-μm particles
        • Reach the alveoli and are phagocytosed by alveolar macrophages
    c. Coal dust is the *least* fibrogenic particle.
    d. Silica, asbestos, and beryllium are very fibrogenic.
  2. Coal worker's pneumoconiosis (CWP)
    a. Sources of coal dust (anthracotic pigment)
      • Coal mines, large urban centers, tobacco smoke
    b. Pulmonary anthracosis
      (1) Usually asymptomatic
      (2) Anthracotic pigment in interstitial tissue and hilar nodes
        • Alveolar macrophages with anthracotic pigment are called "dust cells."
    c. Simple CWP
      (1) Fibrotic opacities are smaller than 1 cm in upper lobes and upper portions of lower lobes.
      (2) Coal deposits adjacent to respiratory bronchioles produce centriacinar (centrilobular) emphysema (see section IX).
    d. Complicated CWP (progressive massive fibrosis)
      (1) Fibrotic opacities larger than 1 to 2 cm with or without necrotic centers (Fig. 16-18)
      (2) Crippling lung disease ("black lung" disease)
      (3) *No* increased incidence of TB or primary lung cancer
      (4) Cor pulmonale may occur.
      (5) Caplan syndrome may occur.
        • CWP plus large cavitating rheumatoid nodules in the lungs

Pneumoconiosis: inhalation of mineral dust

Particle size 1–5 μm: bifurcation respiratory bronchioles and alveolar ducts

<0.5 μm: alveoli

CWP: anthracotic pigment; also element of obstructive lung disease

Dust cells: alveolar macrophages with anthracotic pigment

Complicated CWP: black lung disease

CWP: no risk for lung cancer or TB

Caplan syndrome: pneumo-coniosis and cavitating rheumatoid nodules

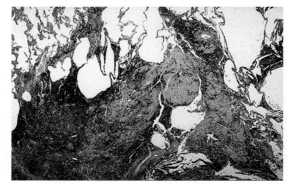

16-18: Coal worker's pneumoconiosis. Note the heavy anthracotic pigment deposition in the fibrotic tissue. Subjacent alveoli are dilated. *(From Klatt E: Robbins and Cotran's Atlas of Pathology. Philadelphia, WB Saunders, 2006, p 113, Fig. 5-48.)*

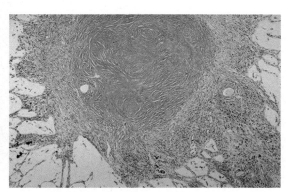

16-19: Silicosis. Note the nodular fibrotic mass in the lung. *(From Klatt E: Robbins and Cotran's Atlas of Pathology. Philadelphia, WB Saunders, 2006, p 113, Fig. 5-49.)*

3. Silicosis
   a. Epidemiology
      (1) Most common occupational disease in the world
      (2) Quartz (crystalline silicone dioxide) is most often implicated.
         • Sources: foundries (casting metal), sandblasting, working in mines
   b. Pathogenesis
      (1) Quartz is highly fibrogenic and deposits in the upper lungs.
      (2) Quartz activates and is cytolytic to alveolar macrophages.
         • Macrophages release cytokines that stimulate fibrogenesis.
   c. Acute exposure; chest x-ray findings:
      • Ground glass appearance in all lung fields
   d. Chronic exposure; chest x-ray findings:
      (1) Nodular opacities in the lungs
         • Concentric layers of collagen with or without central cavitation (Fig. 16-19)
      (2) "Egg-shell" calcification in hilar nodes
         • Rim of dystrophic calcification in the nodes
   e. Complications
      (1) Cor pulmonale, Caplan syndrome
      (2) Increased risk for developing lung cancer and TB
4. Asbestos-related disease
   a. Geometric forms of asbestos
      (1) Serpentine
         (a) Curly and flexible fibers (e.g., chrysotile)
         (b) Produces interstitial fibrosis and lung cancer
      (2) Amphibole
         (a) Straight and rigid (e.g., crocidolite)
         (b) Produces interstitial fibrosis, lung cancer, mesothelioma
      (3) Deposition sites
         • Respiratory bronchioles, alveolar ducts, alveoli
   b. Sources
      (1) Insulation around pipes in old naval ships
      (2) Roofing material, ceiling tiles, floor tiles used >20 years ago
      (3) Demolition of old buildings
   c. Appearance in tissue
      (1) Fibers are coated by iron and protein (called ferruginous bodies)
         • Macrophages phagocytose and coat the fibers with ferritin (synthesized by macrophages)
      (2) Golden, beaded appearance in sputum or in distal, small airways (Fig. 16-20)
   d. Asbestos-related disease
      (1) Benign pleural plaques
         (a) Calcified plaques on the pleura and dome of the diaphragm
         (b) They are *not* a precursor lesion for a mesothelioma.
      (2) Diffuse interstitial fibrosis with or without pleural effusions
      (3) Primary bronchogenic carcinoma
         (a) Risk further increases if the patient smokes cigarettes.
         (b) Occurs ~20 years after first exposure.
      (4) Malignant mesothelioma of pleura
         (a) *No* etiologic relationship with smoking
         (b) Arises from the serosal cells lining the pleura
         (c) Encases and locally invades the subpleural lung tissue (Fig. 16-21)
         (d) Occurs ~25 to 40 years after first exposure
      (5) *No* increased risk for TB
   e. Complications
      • Cor pulmonale, Caplan syndrome
5. Berylliosis
   a. Exposure in the nuclear and aerospace industry
   b. Diffuse interstitial fibrosis with noncaseating granulomas
   c. Increased risk for cor pulmonale and primary lung cancer

Silicosis: most common occupational disease

Silicosis: opacities contain collagen and quartz

Silicosis: "egg-shell" calcification in hilar nodes

Silicosis: ↑ risk lung cancer and TB

Asbestos fibers deposit in the respiratory unit.

Ferruginous bodies: iron-coated asbestos fibers

Benign pleural plaques: most common lesions

Bronchogenic carcinoma: most common asbestos-related cancer

Malignant mesothelioma: arises from serosa of pleura; encases the lung

Asbestos: no risk for TB

Berylliosis: risk for lung cancer

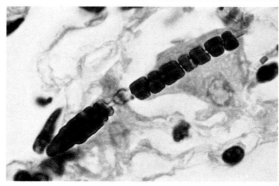

16-20: Asbestos body. The straight, golden-brown, beaded asbestos body represents an asbestos fiber coated by iron and protein. *(From Damjanov I, Linder J: Pathology: A Color Atlas. St. Louis, Mosby, 2000, p 65, Fig. 4-51B.)*

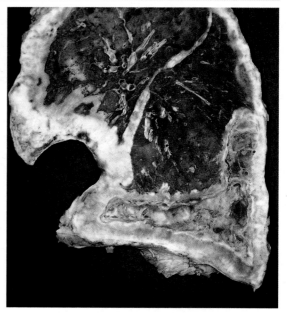

16-21: Malignant mesothelioma encases the lung and invades locally into the lung parenchyma. *(From Corrin B: Pathology of the Lungs. London, Churchill Livingstone, 2000, p 619, Fig. 14.8.)*

Sarcoidosis: most common noninfectious granulomatous disease of the lungs

Sarcoidosis: CD4 T$_H$ cells interact with unknown antigen

Sarcoidosis: noncaseating granulomas

D. Sarcoidosis
- Multisystem granulomatous disease of unknown etiology
1. Epidemiology
   a. Accounts for ~25% of cases of chronic interstitial lung disease
   b. Common in blacks and nonsmokers
   c. More common in women than men
2. Pathogenesis
   a. Disorder in immune regulation
   b. CD4 T$_H$ cells interact with an unknown antigen.
      - Releases cytokines causing formation of noncaseating granulomas
   c. Diagnosis of exclusion
      - Must rule out other granulomatous diseases
3. Lung disease
   a. Primary target organ
      (1) Granulomas located in the interstitium and mediastinal and hilar nodes
      (2) Granulomas contain multinucleated giant cells (Fig. 16-22).
         - Contain laminated calcium concretions (Schaumann bodies) and stellate inclusions (called asteroid bodies)
   b. Dyspnea is the most common symptom.

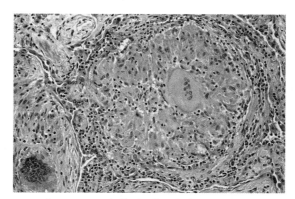

16-22: Sarcoid granuloma showing pink-staining epithelioid cells and foreign body type of multinucleated giant cells. *(From Kumar V, Fausto N, Abbas A: Robbins and Cotran's Pathologic Basis of Disease, 7th ed. Philadelphia, WB Saunders, 2004, p 738, Fig. 15-23.)*

4. Skin lesions
   a. Nodular lesions containing granulomas
   b. Violaceous rash occurs on the nose and cheeks (called lupus pernio).
   c. Erythema nodosum
      (1) Painful nodules on lower extremities
      (2) Inflammation of subcutaneous fat
5. Eye lesions; produces uveitis:
   - Blurry vision, glaucoma, and corneal opacities
6. Liver lesions
   - Granulomatous hepatitis
7. Other multisystem findings
   a. Enlarged salivary and lacrimal glands
   b. Diabetes insipidus (hypothalamic and posterior pituitary disease)
   c. Granulomas in the bone marrow and spleen
8. Laboratory findings
   a. Increased angiotensin-converting enzyme (ACE; 60%)
      - Nonspecific finding
   b. Hypercalcemia (5% of cases)
      - Increased synthesis of 1-α-hydroxylase in granulomas (hypervitaminosis D)
   c. Other findings
      (1) Polyclonal gammopathy
      (2) Cutaneous anergy to common skin antigens (e.g., *Candida*)
         - Due to consumption of CD4 T_H cells in granulomas and loss of cells in alveolar secretions
9. Chest radiograph
   a. Enlarged hilar and mediastinal lymph nodes (called "potato nodes")
   b. Reticulonodular densities throughout the lung parenchyma
10. Treatment
    a. Majority (75–90%) have spontaneous remission in 2 years and do *not* require treatment.
    b. Corticosteroids if treatment is required
    c. Tumor necrosis factor inhibitors
    d. Hydroxychloroquine useful if skin involvement is present
11. Prognosis
    - Approximately 10% to 15% develop severe interstitial fibrosis, leading to cor pulmonale and death.

E. Idiopathic pulmonary fibrosis
1. Epidemiology
   a. Accounts for ~15% of cases of chronic interstitial lung disease
   b. More common in males than in females
   c. Usually occurs in individuals 40 to 70 years old
2. Pathogenesis
   a. Repeated cycles of alveolitis are triggered by an unknown agent.
   b. Release of cytokines produces interstitial fibrosis.
   c. Alveolar fibrosis leads to proximal dilation of the small airways.
      - Lung has a honeycomb appearance.
3. Clinical findings
   a. Fever
   b. Dyspnea with exertion
   c. Chronic, nonproductive cough
   d. Late inspiratory crackles
4. Treatment
   - None very useful
5. Poor prognosis

F. Collagen vascular diseases
1. Account for ~10% of cases of chronic interstitial lung disease
2. Systemic sclerosis (refer to Chapter 3)
   - Most common cause of death is lung disease.
3. Systemic lupus erythematosus (SLE)
   a. Interstitial lung disease occurs in 50% of patients.
   b. Pleuritis with pleural effusions

Margin notes:

Sarcoidosis: skin nodules have granulomas on biopsy

Sarcoidosis: most common noninfectious granulomatous disease of the liver

Sarcoidosis: ↑ ACE

Sarcoidosis: hypercalcemia due to hypervitaminosis D

Sarcoidosis: diagnosis of exclusion; rule out other granulomatous diseases

Idiopathic pulmonary fibrosis: alveolitis leading to interstitial fibrosis; honeycomb lung

Collagen vascular diseases with interstitial fibrosis: systemic sclerosis, SLE, RA

Pleural effusion in young woman: consider SLE

Any unexplained pleural effusion in a young woman is SLE until proved otherwise. Pleural fluid contains an inflammatory infiltrate (exudate), and lupus erythematosus cells (neutrophils with phagocytosed DNA) are sometimes present. One of the key criteria for diagnosing SLE is the presence of serositis, pleuritis with a pleural effusion being an example of this type of inflammation.

    4. Rheumatoid arthritis (RA)
      a. Rheumatoid nodules in lungs plus a pneumoconiosis is called Caplan syndrome.
      b. Pulmonary findings in RA
        (1) Interstitial fibrosis with or without intrapulmonary rheumatoid nodules
          • Nodules often cavitating
        (2) Pleuritis with pleural effusions

G. Hypersensitivity pneumonitis
    1. Extrinsic allergic alveolitis associated with exposure to a *known* inhaled antigen
      • Does *not* involve IgE antibodies (type I hypersensitivity) or have eosinophilia
    2. Farmer's lung

Farmer's lung: antigen is thermophilic actinomyces in moldy hay

      a. Exposure to *Saccharopolyspora rectivirgula* (thermophilic actinomycetes) in moldy hay
      b. First exposure
        • Patient develops precipitating IgG antibodies (present in serum)
      c. Second exposure

Farmer's lung: type III and IV hypersensitivity

        (1) Antibodies combine with inhaled allergens to form immune complexes.
          • Type III hypersensitivity reaction
        (2) Immunocomplexes produce an inflammatory reaction in lung tissue.
      d. Chronic exposure
        • Additional component of granulomatous inflammation (type IV hypersensitivity)
      e. Treatment
        (1) Avoidance of antigen with facial mask
        (2) Corticosteroids
    3. Silo filler's disease

Silo filler's disease: inhalation of gases (oxides of nitrogen)

      a. Inhalation of gases (oxides of nitrogen) from plant material
      b. Causes an immediate hypersensitivity reaction associated with dyspnea
      c. Treatment
        • Corticosteroids
    4. Byssinosis
      a. Epidemiology
        (1) Occurs in workers in textile factories
        (2) Contact with cotton, linen, hemp products
          • Exposure to bacterial endotoxin from gram-negative bacteria growing on the cotton

Byssinosis: contact with cotton, linen, hemp products; "Monday morning blues"

      b. Clinical findings
        (1) Develop dyspnea on exposure to cotton, linen, or hemp products
        (2) Workers feel better over the weekend (no exposure to antigens)
          • Depression occurs when returning to work on Monday ("Monday morning blues")
      c. Treatment
        • Improve dust removal

H. Drugs associated with interstitial fibrosis
    1. Amiodarone
    2. Bleomycin and busulfan
    3. Cyclophosphamide
    4. Methotrexate and methysergide
    5. Nitrosourea and nitrofurantoin

Drugs: amiodarone, bleomycin, cyclophosphamide, methotrexate

I. Radiation-induced lung disease
    1. Acute pneumonitis may occur 1 to 6 months after therapy.
    2. Clinical findings
      a. Fever
      b. Dyspnea
      c. Pleural effusions
      d. Chest x-ray shows infiltrates

Radiation: cause of interstitial lung disease

    3. Some patients develop chronic radiation pneumonitis.

IX. **Obstructive Lung Disease**
  • Obstruction to airflow out of the lungs
  A. **Emphysema**
    1. Permanent enlargement of all or part of the respiratory unit
      • Respiratory bronchioles, alveolar ducts, alveoli
    2. Epidemiology
      a. Causes
        (1) Cigarette smoking is the most common cause.
        (2) α_1-Antitrypsin (AAT) deficiency
      b. Types of emphysema associated with smoking or loss of AAT
        (1) Centriacinar (centrilobular) emphysema
        (2) Panacinar emphysema
    3. Pathogenesis
      a. Increased compliance and decreased elasticity
        (1) Imbalance between elastase and anti-elastases (e.g., AAT)
        (2) Imbalance between oxidants (free radicals) and antioxidants (e.g., glutathione)
        (3) Elastase and oxidants derive from neutrophils and macrophages.
        (4) Net effect of the preceding is destruction of elastic tissue.
      b. Cigarette smoke is chemotactic to neutrophils and macrophages.
        • They accumulate in the respiratory unit and release free radicals and elastases.
      c. Free radicals in cigarette smoke inactivate AAT and antioxidants.
        • Produces a functional AAT deficiency
      d. Normal function of elastic tissue
        (1) Fibers attach to the outside wall of the small airways (Fig. 16-23A).
        (2) Fibers apply radial traction to keep the airway lumens open.
      e. Destruction of elastic tissue causes loss of radial traction.
        • Small airways collapse, particularly on expiration.
      f. Sites of elastic tissue destruction in emphysema
        (1) Distal terminal bronchiole at its junction with the respiratory bronchiole (RB)
        (2) All or part of the respiratory unit
      g. Site of obstruction and air trapping in emphysema
        (1) During expiration, the distal terminal bronchioles collapse preventing egress of air out of the respiratory unit.
        (2) Trapped air distends parts of the respiratory unit that have lost their elastic tissue support.

Margin notes:

Emphysema: targets the respiratory unit

Cigarette smoking: most common cause of emphysema

Emphysema: ↑ compliance, ↓ elasticity

Cigarette smoke: chemotactic to neutrophils; inactivates AAT and glutathione

Destruction of elastic tissue: loss of radial traction

Air trapping behind collapsed distal terminal bronchioles

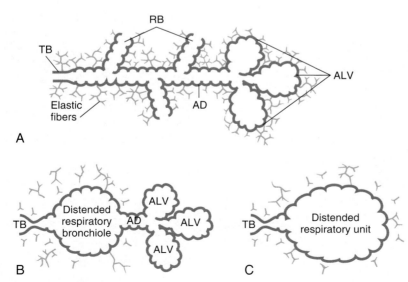

16-23: Types of emphysema. **A,** The schematic shows a normal distal airway, including a terminal bronchiole (TB) leading into the respiratory unit consisting of a respiratory bronchiole (RB), alveolar duct (AD), and alveoli (ALV). Elastic fibers apply radial traction to keep these airways open. **B,** Centriacinar (centrilobular) emphysema is characterized by trapping of air in the respiratory bronchioles. Note how the elastic fibers of the distal TB are destroyed, causing obstruction to airflow. This causes the trapped air to distend the RBs, whose elastic tissue support is destroyed. **C,** Panacinar emphysema is characterized by trapping of air in the entire respiratory unit behind the collapsed TB.

4. Centriacinar (centrilobular) emphysema (Fig. 16-23B)
   a. Epidemiology
      • Most common type of emphysema in smokers
   b. Pathogenesis
      (1) Primarily involves the apical segments of the upper lobes
      (2) Distal terminal bronchioles and the RBs (Fig. 16-24) are the sites of elastic tissue destruction.
      (3) Air trapped behind the collapsed distal terminal bronchioles distends the RBs.
         • The trapped air increases RV and TLC.
5. Panacinar emphysema (see Fig. 16-22C)
   a. Epidemiology
      (1) Associated with AAT deficiency
         • Genetic or acquired causes (cigarette smoke inactivates AAT)
      (2) Genetic type of AAT deficiency
         (a) Autosomal dominant
         (b) MM phenotype is normal.
            • Normal amounts of AAT are synthesized in the liver.
         (c) Homozygous ZZ type has decreased synthesis of AAT by the liver.
      (3) Emphysema develops at an early age in the genetic type.
   b. Pathogenesis
      (1) Primarily affects the lower lobes
      (2) Distal terminal bronchioles and all parts of the respiratory units are the sites of elastic tissue destruction (Fig. 16-25).
      (3) Air trapped behind the collapsed terminal bronchioles distends the entire respiratory unit.
   c. Laboratory finding
      • Absent α_1-globulin peak in a serum protein electrophoresis (SPE)
6. Clinical findings in centriacinar and panacinar emphysema
   a. Progressive dyspnea and hyperventilation
      (1) Dyspnea is severe and occurs early in the disease.
      (2) Sometimes patients are called "pink puffers."
   b. Centriacinar type frequently coexists with chronic bronchitis.
   c. Breath sounds are diminished due to hyperinflation.
   d. Cor pulmonale is uncommon.
7. Chest radiograph (Fig. 16-26)
   a. Hyperlucent lung fields
   b. Increased anteroposterior diameter

Centriacinar emphysema: destruction of the distal terminal bronchioles and RBs; upper lobe

Panacinar emphysema: targets distal terminal bronchioles and the entire respiratory unit; lower lobe

Panacinar emphysema: loss α_1-globulin peak on SPE

Emphysema: pink puffers; blow off CO_2

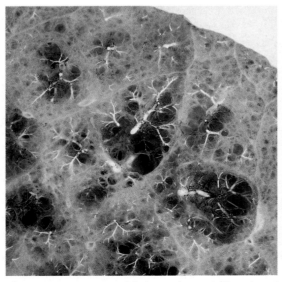

16-24: Centriacinar (centrilobular emphysema). The enlarged spaces in the lung parenchyma are air-filled respiratory bronchioles that have lost their elastic tissue support. *(Reproduced by permission of the late Professor B.E. Heard, Brompton, UK.)*

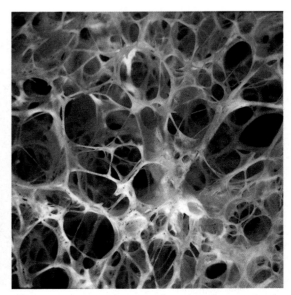

16-25: Panacinar emphysema. The enlarged spaces in the lung parenchyma are air-filled respiratory bronchioles, alveolar ducts, and alveoli that have lost their elastic tissue support. *(Reproduced by permission of the late Professor B.E. Heard, Brompton, UK.)*

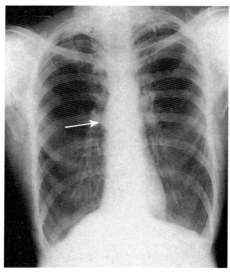

16-26: Chest radiograph in emphysema showing a vertically oriented heart *(arrow)* and depressed diaphragm. *(From Forbes C, Jackson W: Color Atlas and Text of Clinical Medicine, 2nd ed. St. Louis, Mosby, 2003, p 186, Fig. 4-94.)*

  c. Vertically oriented heart
  d. Depressed diaphragms due to hyperinflated lungs
 8. Pulmonary function tests and arterial blood gases
  a. Increased TLC due to an increase in RV
  b. Decreased $FEV_{1\,sec}$ (e.g., 1 L versus 4 L; see Fig. 16-1C)
  c. Decreased FVC (e.g., 3 L versus 5 L; see Fig. 16-1C)
   • Decreased $FEV_{1\,sec}$/FVC ratio (e.g., 1/3 = 33%)
  d. Decreased PaO_2 develops late in the disease.
   • Destruction of the capillary bed matches destruction of the respiratory unit.
  e. Normal to decreased arterial PCO_2 (respiratory alkalosis)
 9. Treatment
  a. Cessation of smoking most important
  b. Pulmonary rehabilitation program
  c. Oxygen, using 1 to 2 L/minute, through nasal prongs
   • Maintain O_2 saturation of 90%
  d. Bronchodilators
   (1) Catecholamine inhalers/nebulizers
   (2) Steroid inhalers controversial
  e. Anticholinergics
 10. Other types of emphysema unrelated to smoking or AAT deficiency
  a. Paraseptal emphysema
   (1) Localized disease in a subpleural location
    • Primarily targets the alveolar ducts and alveoli
   (2) Does *not* produce obstructive airway disease
   (3) Increased incidence of spontaneous pneumothorax
    • Due to rupture of subpleural blebs
  b. Irregular emphysema
   (1) Localized disease is associated with scar tissue.
   (2) Does *not* produce obstructive airway disease
B. Chronic bronchitis
 1. Epidemiology
  a. Productive cough for at least 3 months for 2 consecutive years
  b. Causes
   (1) Smoking cigarettes
   (2) Cystic fibrosis
 2. Pathogenesis
  a. Hypersecretion of mucus in bronchi
  b. Obstruction to airflow in the terminal bronchioles
   • Airflow obstruction is proximal to the obstruction in emphysema.
  c. Irreversible fibrosis of terminal bronchioles

Chest x-ray: hyperlucency, ↑ AP diameter, vertically oriented heart, depressed diaphragms

Emphysema: ↑TLC, RV; ↓$FEV_{1\,sec}$/FVC

Emphysema: normal to ↓ arterial PCO_2 (respiratory alkalosis)

Paraseptal emphysema: risk for spontaneous pneumothorax

Irregular emphysema: scar emphysema

CB: productive cough at least 3 months for 2 consecutive years

Smoking cigarettes: most common cause of CB

Turbulent airflow in the bronchi is converted to laminar airflow in the terminal (nonrespiratory) bronchioles. The terminal bronchioles undergo parallel branching, which reduces airflow resistance and spreads air out over a large cross-sectional area. Small airway disease associated with expiratory wheezing is due to narrowing of the terminal bronchioles by mucus plugs, inflammation, and fibrosis. Mucus plugs located in a proximal terminal bronchiole prevent the exodus of a large amount of CO_2 arising from the distally located airways producing respiratory acidosis.

d. Changes in the bronchi

> CB: hypersecretion of mucous glands

(1) Hypersecretion of submucosal mucus-secreting glands in trachea and bronchi
  • Primarily responsible for sputum overproduction
(2) Acute inflammation (neutrophils) often superimposed on chronic inflammation
(3) Loss of ciliated epithelium and presence of squamous metaplasia
e. Changes in the terminal bronchioles
(1) Mucus plugs in lumens (block the exodus of CO_2)
(2) Goblet cell metaplasia
(3) Hypertrophy of mucus-secreting glands
(4) Chronic inflammation and fibrosis narrowing the lumen
3. Clinical findings
a. Productive cough
b. Dyspnea occurs late in the disease.
c. Cyanosis of skin and mucous membranes

> CB: blue bloaters; retain CO_2 and develop cyanosis

(1) Decreased O_2 saturation from hypoxemia (refer to Chapter 1)
(2) Patients are called "blue bloaters."

> CB: stocky and obese; horizontally oriented heart

d. Tend to be stocky or obese
e. Expiratory wheezing and sibilant rhonchi
f. Cor pulmonale is commonly present.
4. Chest radiograph
a. Large, horizontally oriented heart
b. Increased bronchial markings
5. Pulmonary function tests and arterial blood gases
a. Less increase in TLC and RV than emphysema
b. Chronic respiratory acidosis

> CB: chronic respiratory acidosis and hypoxemia

(1) Arterial P_{CO_2} > 45 mm Hg
(2) Bicarbonate > 30 mEq/L

> CB: hypoxemia early in CB

c. Moderate to severe hypoxemia early in the disease
6. Treatment (see Emphysema)
7. Summary of findings in disease and emphysema (Table 16-5)
C. **Asthma**
1. Epidemiology
a. Episodic and reversible airway disease (most cases)
b. Primarily targets the bronchi and terminal bronchioles
c. Most common chronic respiratory disease in children

> Asthma: episodic and reversible airway disease

(1) More common in children than adults
(2) Majority (50–80%) develop symptoms *before* 5 years of age
d. Extrinsic and intrinsic types
2. Extrinsic asthma

> Extrinsic asthma: type I hypersensitivity reaction

a. Pathogenesis
(1) Type I hypersensitivity reaction with exposure to extrinsic allergens
  • Typically develops in children with an atopic family history to allergies

TABLE 16-5. **COMPARISON OF EMPHYSEMA AND CHRONIC BRONCHITIS**

PARAMETER	EMPHYSEMA	CHRONIC BRONCHITIS
Pa_{O_2}	Decreased	Decreased
Pa_{CO_2}	Normal to decreased	Increased
pH	Normal to increased	Decreased
Cyanosis	Absent	Present
Habitus	Thin	Stocky
Cor pulmonale	Rare	Common
Onset of hypoxemia	Late	Early
Onset of dyspnea	Early	Late

(2) Initial sensitization to an inhaled allergen
 (a) Stimulate induction of subset 2 helper T cells (CD4 T_H2) that release interleukin (IL) 4 and IL-5
 (b) IL-4 stimulates isotype switching to IgE production.
 (c) IL-5 stimulates production and activation of eosinophils.
(3) Inhaled antigens cross-link IgE antibodies on mast cells on mucosal surfaces.
 (a) Release of histamine and other preformed mediators
 (b) Functions of mediators
  • Stimulate bronchoconstriction, mucus production, influx of leukocytes
(4) Late phase reaction (4–8 hours later)
 (a) Eotaxin is produced.
  • Chemotactic for eosinophils and activates eosinophils
 (b) Eosinophils release major basic protein and cationic protein.
  • Damage epithelial cells and produce airway constriction

b. Other mediators involved
 (1) LTC-D-E_4 causes prolonged bronchoconstriction.
 (2) Acetylcholine causes airway muscle contraction.
c. Histologic changes in bronchi
 (1) Thickening of the basement membrane
 (2) Edema and a mixed inflammatory infiltrate
 (3) Hypertrophy of submucosal glands
 (4) Hypertrophy/hyperplasia of smooth muscle cells
d. Histologic changes in the terminal bronchioles
 (1) Formation of spiral-shaped mucus plugs
  (a) Contain shed epithelial cells called Curschmann spirals
  (b) Pathologic effect of major basic protein and cationic protein
 (2) Crystalline granules in eosinophils coalesce to form Charcot-Leyden crystals.
 (3) Patchy loss of epithelial cells, goblet cell metaplasia
 (4) Thick basement membrane
 (5) Smooth muscle cell hypertrophy and hyperplasia
e. Clinical findings
 (1) Episodic expiratory wheezing (inspiratory as well when severe)
 (2) Nocturnal cough
 (3) Increased anteroposterior diameter
  • Due to air trapping and increase in residual volume
f. Laboratory findings
 (1) Initially develop respiratory alkalosis
  (a) Patients work hard at expelling air through inflamed airways.
  (b) May progress into respiratory acidosis if bronchospasm is *not* relieved
   • Normal pH or respiratory acidosis is an indication for intubation and mechanical ventilation.
 (2) Eosinophilia, positive skin tests for allergens
g. Treatment of mild disease
 • Metered-dose inhaler with a β_2-agonist (e.g., albuterol)
h. Treatment of more advanced disease
 (1) Metered low-dose inhaler with corticosteroids
 (2) Use of leukotriene inhibitors
3. Intrinsic asthma
 a. Nonimmune
 b. Causes
  (1) Virus-induced respiratory infection
   • Examples—rhinovirus, parainfluenza virus, respiratory syncytial virus
  (2) Air pollutants

Ozone (O_3) is an air pollutant that derives from interactions of O_2 with oxides of nitrogen and sulfur, and hydrocarbons. It forms highly reactive free radicals in the airways that cause inflammation and irritation, often precipitating asthma.

  (3) Aspirin or nonsteroidal drug sensitivity (see section III)
  (4) Stress, exercise, cigarette smoke

Margin notes:

IL-4: isotype switching to IgE production

IL-5: production and activation of eosinophils

Eosinophils: major basic protein and cationic protein damage epithelial cells

LTC-D-E_4: potent bronchoconstrictors

Curschmann spirals: shed epithelial cells

Eosinophils: granules produce Charcot-Leyden crystals

Asthma: wheezing; ↑ anteroposterior diameter

Bronchial asthma: initially present with respiratory alkalosis

Bronchial asthma: normal pH or respiratory acidosis indicates need for intubation

Intrinsic asthma: nonimmune

O_3: free radical; O_2 combining with oxides of nitrogen and sulfur

D. Bronchiectasis

1. Epidemiology and pathogenesis

   a. Permanent dilation of the bronchi and bronchioles
      • Due to destruction of cartilage and elastic tissue by chronic necrotizing infections
   b. Causes
      (1) Cystic fibrosis (CF)
         • Most common cause in the United States
      (2) Infections
         (a) TB is the most common cause worldwide.
         (b) Adenovirus, *Staphylococcus aureus*, *Haemophilus influenzae*
      (3) Bronchial obstruction
         • Example—proximally located bronchogenic carcinoma occludes the lumen.
      (4) Primary ciliary dyskinesia
         (a) Absent dynein arm in cilia
         (b) Dynein arm contains ATPase (adenosine triphosphatase) for movement of the cilia.
      (5) Allergic bronchopulmonary aspergillosis
2. Gross findings
   a. Most commonly occurs in the lower lobes
   b. Dilated bronchi and bronchioles are filled with pus (Figs. 16-27 and 16-28).
      (1) Dilated airways extend to the lung periphery.
      (2) Dilations are tubelike and/or saccular.
3. Clinical findings
   a. Cough productive of copious sputum (often cupfuls)
   b. Hemoptysis that is sometimes massive
   c. Digital clubbing
   d. Cor pulmonale
4. Chest radiograph findings
   • Crowded bronchial markings extend to the lung periphery.
5. CF
   a. Epidemiology
      (1) Autosomal recessive disease
      (2) Primarily affects whites (>98%)
         • Uncommon in Asians and blacks
      (3) Most common fatal hereditary disorder of whites in United States
      (4) Median age of diagnosis ~5 months
      (5) Median survival age: 30 years
   b. Pathogenesis
      (1) Three nucleotide deletion on chromosome 7
         • Nucleotides normally code for phenylalanine.

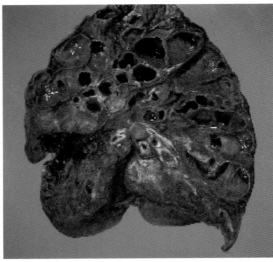

16-27: Bronchiectasis showing dilated airways filled with pus. *(From Corrin B: Pathology of the Lungs. London, Churchill Livingstone, 1999, p 85, Fig. 3-5.)*

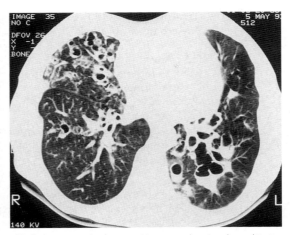

16-28: Computed tomographic scan showing bronchiectasis in both lungs. Note the dilated cystic to saccular appearing airways. *(From Goldman L, Ausiello D: Cecil's Textbook of Medicine, 23rd ed. Philadelphia, Saunders Elsevier, 2008, p 633, Fig. 90-2.)*

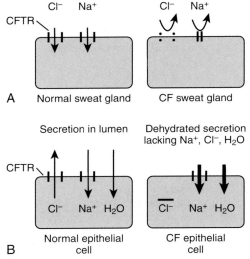

16-29: Schematic showing defect in cystic fibrosis transmembrane regulator (CFTR) in cystic fibrosis (CF) in sweat glands (**A**) and epithelial cells (**B**). See text for discussion.

  (2) Production of a defective CF transmembrane conductance regulator (CFTR) for chloride ions
  (3) CFTR Cl⁻ is degraded in the Golgi apparatus.
    • Due to defective protein folding
  (4) Loss of CFTR Cl⁻ causes decreased Na⁺ and Cl⁻ reabsorption in sweat glands. (Fig. 16-29A)
    • Basis of the sweat test
  (5) Effect of loss of CFTR Cl⁻ in other secretions (Fig. 16-29B)
    (a) Increased Na⁺ and water reabsorption from luminal secretions
    (b) Decreased Cl⁻ secretion out of epithelial cells into luminal secretions
    (c) Net effect is dehydration of body secretions due to lack of NaCl
      • Secretions are dehydrated in bronchioles, pancreatic ducts, bile ducts, meconium, and seminal fluid.
  c. Clinical findings
    (1) Nasal polyps (25% of cases)
    (2) Heat exhaustion
      • Loss of sodium-containing fluid from skin
    (3) Respiratory infections/failure
      (a) *Pseudomonas aeruginosa* is the most common respiratory pathogen.
        • Other common pathogens—*S. aureus, H. influenzae*
      (b) Cor pulmonale commonly occurs.
    (4) Pneumothorax (20%)
      • Rupture of blebs that develop from infection
    (5) Malabsorption (80%)
      (a) Pancreatic exocrine deficiency
      (b) Atrophy of glands from dehydrated secretions blocking the lumens
      (c) Chronic pancreatitis
    (6) Type 1 diabetes mellitus (20%)
      • Due to chronic pancreatitis
    (7) Infertility in males (95%)
      • Atresia of vas deferens
    (8) Infertility in females (20%)
    (9) Meconium ileus (20%)
      • Small bowel obstruction in newborn
    (10) Rectal prolapse
      • Straining at stool
    (11) Gallstones (>50%)
      (a) Usually in older CF patients
      (b) Stasis of thickened bile
      (c) Common bile duct obstruction (15–20%)

CF: defective CFTR Cl⁻ is degraded in Golgi apparatus

CF: loss of NaCl in sweat; loss of NaCl in luminal secretions (dehydrated)

CF: nasal polyps

Respiratory infections: most common cause of death in CF

CF: chronic pancreatitis producing malabsorption and type 1 diabetes

CF: males infertile > females

CF: meconium ileus; rectal prolapse

(12) Secondary biliary cirrhosis
- Due to obstruction of bile ductules by thick secretions

d. Screen infants
- Increased serum immunoreactive trypsin levels

e. Sweat test findings diagnostic for CF
(1) Sweat chloride > 60 mmol/L in children
(2) Sweat chloride > 80 mmol/L in adult

f. Treatment
(1) Antibiotics for documented respiratory infections
(2) Bronchodilators
(3) Pancreatic enzyme replacement
(4) Corticosteroids in children (alternate day)
(5) Vitamin supplements
- Fat-soluble vitamins important
(6) Recombinant human deoxyribonuclease aerosol
- Improves mucociliary clearance of viscid sputum

X. **Lung Tumors**
- Primary lung cancer is the most common fatal cancer in both men and women.

A. **Epidemiology**
1. Incidence of lung cancer is declining in men but increasing in women.
2. Peak incidence is at 55 to 65 years of age.
3. Most common cancer-related death in both men and women
4. Causes
a. Cigarette smoking most common cause
- Risk increases with quantity and duration of smoking
b. Radon gas (uranium mining)
c. Asbestos
d. Certain metals
- Chromium, cadmium, beryllium, arsenic
e. Secondhand smoke
f. Ionizing radiation
g. Air pollution
h. History of tuberculosis
5. Classified as small cell (13%) or non–small cell (87%) cancers
a. Primary lung cancer by specific type in decreasing incidence
(1) Adenocarcinoma
(2) Squamous cell carcinoma (Fig. 16-30A)
(3) Small cell lung carcinoma (Fig. 16-30B)
(4) Large cell carcinoma
(5) Bronchial carcinoid
6. Squamous and small cell lung carcinomas
a. Greatest smoking association
b. Tend to be centrally located (i.e., main stem bronchus) (Fig. 16-30C and D)
7. Adenocarcinomas
a. Weakest smoking association
b. Tend to be more peripherally located (Fig. 16-30E and F)
- Filters in cigarettes remove large carcinogens leaving small ones to move peripherally.
8. Common sites for metastasis
a. Hilar lymph nodes most common site
b. Adrenal gland (50%)
c. Liver (30%)
d. Brain (20%)
e. Bone (osteolytic)

B. **Tumors and tumor-like disorders** (Table 16-6)

A **solitary pulmonary nodule** or coin lesion (e.g., see Fig. 16-10G) is the term applied to a peripheral lung nodule < 5 cm. Causes of a solitary pulmonary nodule in descending order include granulomas (e.g., TB, histoplasmosis), malignancy (usually primary cancer), and a bronchial (chondroid) hamartoma. Patients < 35 years old have a 1% risk of a solitary coin lesion representing a malignancy, but patients ≥ 50 years old have a 50% to 60% risk of malignancy, usually a primary cancer. In evaluating solitary coin lesions, comparing previous chest x-rays for changes in size of the nodule is the most important initial step.

Margin notes:

CF: serum immunoreactive trypsin excellent screen at birth

Sweat test: diagnostic test for CF

Primary lung cancer: declining in men, increasing in women

Cigarette smoking: most common cause of lung cancer

Squamous cell and small cell carcinoma: centrally located

Adenocarcinoma: peripherally located

Solitary pulmonary nodule: most often granulomas

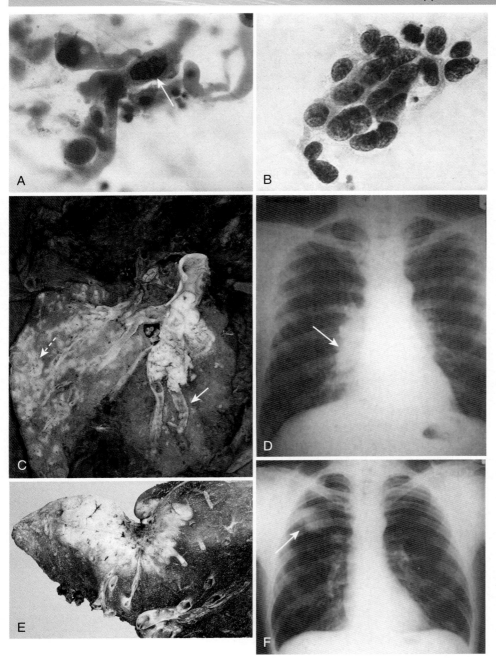

16-30: A, Sputum cytology in squamous cell carcinoma. Note the orange-staining, keratinized squamous carcinoma cells with irregular, hyperchromatic nuclei (*arrow*). **B,** Fine needle aspirate of a lymph node with metastatic small cell carcinoma of lung. Note the cluster of cells with hyperchromatic nuclei and scant cytoplasm. **C,** Primary lung cancer arising in a central bronchus and extending into the lumen. Note that the lumen is obstructed by gray-white tumor causing distal bronchiectasis (*solid arrow*) and obstructive pneumonia (*interrupted arrow*). **D,** Chest radiograph of bronchogenic carcinoma presenting as a central right hilar mass (*arrow*). **E,** Peripheral adenocarcinoma with scar retracting the pleural surface (scar carcinoma). The black pigment is anthracotic pigment. **F,** Chest radiograph of bronchogenic carcinoma presenting as a mass in the periphery of the right upper lobe (*arrow*). (*A and B from Kumar V, Fausto N, Abbas A: Robbins and Cotran's Pathologic Basis of Disease, 7th ed. Philadelphia, WB Saunders, 2004, p 760, Figs. 15-43A, 15-43B, respectively; C and E from Corrin B: Pathology of the Lungs. London, Churchill Livingstone, 1999, pp 463, 472, Figs. 13-1.5, 13-1.13B, respectively; D and F from Grieg JD: Color Atlas of Surgical Diagnosis. London, Mosby-Wolfe, 1996, pp 90, 89, Figs. 13-7, 13-6, respectively.*)

C. Metastatic cancer
  1. Epidemiology
     a. Most common lung cancer
     b. Cancers most often responsible for metastasis
        (1) Primary breast cancer most common cause
        (2) Colon cancer, renal cell carcinoma
  2. Sites of lung metastasis
     a. Parenchyma (Figs. 16-31 and 16-32)
     b. Pleura and pleural space (malignant effusions)
     c. Lymphatics (causes severe dyspnea)
  3. Dyspnea is the most common symptom.
D. Clinical findings in primary lung cancer
  1. Cough
     • Most common symptom (75%)
  2. Weight loss (40%)

Metastasis: most common lung cancer; breast cancer most common primary cancer

Cough: most common symptom

TABLE 16-6. **TUMORS AND TUMOR-LIKE DISORDERS OF THE LUNG**

TYPE OF TUMOR OR DISORDER	LOCATION IN LUNG	COMMENTS
Adenocarcinoma (see Fig. 16-30E and F)	Peripheral	More common in women Some types are associated with cigarette smoking Scar carcinomas: develop in scars (e.g., old tuberculous granuloma); no relationship to smoking Bronchioloalveolar carcinoma: derives from Clara cells (nonciliated epithelium); malignant cells spread along alveolar walls (look like pegs); radiologically mimic lobar pneumonia; no relationship to smoking
Squamous cell carcinoma (see Fig. 16-30A)	Central	More common in men Strong association with cigarette smoking Tend to cavitate May ectopically secrete PTH-related protein (peptide)
Small cell carcinoma (see Fig. 16-30B)	Central	More common in men Strong association with cigarette smoking Arise from neuroendocrine cells (Kulchitsky cells) Rapidly growing cancer that metastasizes early May ectopically secrete ADH or ACTH
Large cell carcinoma	Peripheral	Undifferentiated cancer that metastasizes early; no relationship to smoking
Bronchial carcinoid	Central	Low-grade cancer of neuroendocrine origin; no association with smoking; present at a mean age of 55 years old; most common primary lung tumor in children; ~20% locally metastasize; present with hemoptysis (most common), cough, carcinoid syndrome (<1%)
Carcinoma metastatic to the lung (see Figs. 16-31 and 16-32)	Multifocal	More common than primary cancer Sites of metastasis: parenchyma (most common), pleura/pleural space, endobronchial mucosa, lymphatics (causes dyspnea)
Bronchial hamartoma	Peripheral (90%) Central (10%)	Non-neoplastic proliferation of cartilage and adipose tissue Appears as solitary "coin" lesion on chest radiograph; popcorn calcifications

ACTH, adrenocorticotropic hormone; ADH, antidiuretic hormone; PTH, parathyroid hormone.

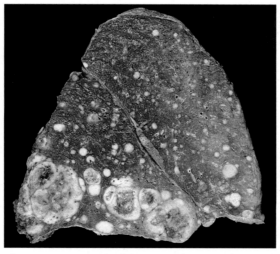

16-31: Metastatic renal cell carcinoma showing multiple nodular lesions scattered throughout the lung parenchyma. *(From Kumar V, Fausto N, Abbas A: Robbins and Cotran's Pathologic Basis of Disease, 7th ed. Philadelphia, WB Saunders, 2004, p 766, Fig. 15-47.)*

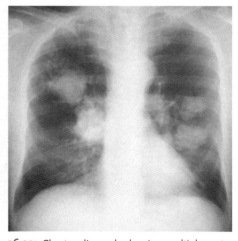

16-32: Chest radiograph showing multiple metastatic nodules throughout both lung fields. *(From Goldman L, Ausiello D: Cecil's Textbook of Medicine, 23rd ed. Philadelphia, Saunders Elsevier, 2008, p 600, Fig. 84-9.)*

3. Chest pain (30%)
4. Hemoptysis (25–30%)
5. Dyspnea
6. Pancoast tumor (superior sulcus tumor)
   a. Usually a primary squamous cancer located at the extreme apex of lung
   b. Destruction of superior cervical sympathetic ganglion produces Horner syndrome (Fig.16-33)
      (1) Ipsilateral lid lag

Horner syndrome: lid lag, miosis, anhydrosis

(2) Miosis (pinpoint pupil)

(3) Ipsilateral anhydrosis (lack of sweating)

7. Superior vena cava syndrome (refer to Chapter 9; Fig. 16-34)

8. Paraneoplastic syndromes

    a. Digital clubbing

      • Due to reactive periosteal changes in the underlying bone

    b. Muscle weakness (Eaton-Lambert syndrome)

      (1) Antibody directed against calcium channel in muscle

      (2) Usually associated with small cell carcinoma

    c. Ectopic hormone secretion (see earlier)

Eaton-Lambert syndrome: muscle weakness; antibody against calcium channel

E. Diagnosis

1. Chest x-ray

    a. Central masses

      (1) Squamous cell carcinoma

      (2) Small cell carcinoma

    b. Peripheral masses

      (1) Adenocarcinoma

      (2) Scar carcinoma

2. Sputum cytologic examination

3. Fine needle aspiration

4. Bronchoscopy with lavage

5. New techniques for early detection

    a. Low-dose spiral (helical) CT scan

    b. Molecular markers in sputum

F. Treatment

1. Surgery

2. Radiation

3. Chemotherapy

4. Targeted biologic therapies

    • Bevacizumab and erlotinib

G. Prognosis

1. Non–small cell cancers fare better than small cell carcinoma.

2. Overall combined 5-year survival rate is ~15%.

XI. Mediastinum Disorders

A. Mediastinal masses

1. Epidemiology

    a. Usually metastatic primary lung cancer in older patients

    b. Usually primary disease in younger patients

    c. Anterior mediastinum is the most common site (>50%).

    d. Most common primary mediastinal masses, in descending order:

      (1) Neurogenic tumors

        (a) Located in the posterior mediastinum

Anterior compartment: most common site for mediastinal masses

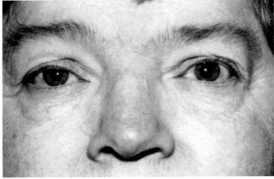

16-33: Horner's syndrome in right eye. Note the mild lid lag and miotic pupil when compared to the left eye. *(Courtesy of Shannath Merbs, MD, The Wilmer Ophthalmological Institute, Johns Hopkins University.)*

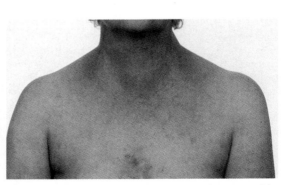

16-34: Superior vena caval syndrome. Note distention of the veins over the front of the chest. *(From Corrin B: Pathology of the Lungs. London, Churchill Livingstone, 1999, p 464, Fig. 13-1–7.)*

(b) Usually malignant in children
- Neuroblastoma

(c) Usually benign in adults
- Ganglioneuroma

(2) Thymomas (see later)

(3) Pericardial cyst
- Located in the middle mediastinum

(4) Malignant lymphomas
(a) Located in the anterior mediastinum
(b) Usually nodular sclerosing Hodgkin's lymphoma in a woman

(5) Teratoma
(a) Located in the anterior mediastinum
(b) Majority are benign cystic teratomas.
(c) Small percentage are malignant teratomas.

2. Thymoma
a. Epidemiology
(1) Located in the anterior mediastinum
(2) Benign (70%), malignant (30%)

b. Epithelium, *not* lymphoid tissue, is the neoplastic component.

c. Majority express systemic symptoms of myasthenia gravis (refer to Chapter 23).
(1) Less than 15% of myasthenia patients have a thymoma.
(2) Majority (65–75%) have follicular B cell hyperplasia in the thymus.
- Site for synthesis of antiacetylcholine receptor antibodies

d. Other thymoma associations
(1) Hypogammaglobulinemia
(2) Pure RBC aplasia
(3) Increased incidence of autoimmune disease (e.g. Graves' disease)

XII. Pleural Disorders

A. Movement of pleural fluid (PF)
1. Fluid moves from parietal pleura to pleural space to lungs.
2. Movement depends upon the balance of Starling pressures (refer to Chapter 4).
a. Parietal capillary hydrostatic pressure > visceral capillary hydrostatic pressure.
b. Parietal capillary oncotic pressure equals visceral capillary hydrostatic pressure.

B. Etiology and pathogenesis of pleural effusions
1. Increased hydrostatic pressure in visceral pleura
- Example—congestive heart failure
2. Decreased oncotic pressure
- Example—nephrotic syndrome
3. Obstruction of lymphatic drainage from the visceral pleura
- Example—lung cancer
4. Increased vessel permeability of visceral pleural capillaries
- Examples—pulmonary infarction, pneumonia
5. Metastasis to the pleura
- Example—metastatic breast cancer

C. Types of pleural effusions
1. Transudates
a. Ultrafiltrate of plasma involving disturbances in Starling pressures
b. Examples
(1) Increased hydrostatic pressure in congestive heart failure
(2) Decreased oncotic pressure in nephrotic syndrome
2. Exudates
a. Protein-rich and cell-rich fluid
- Due to an increased vessel permeability in acute inflammation
b. Examples—pneumonia, tuberculosis, infarction, metastasis
3. Chylous
a. Indicates interruption of the thoracic duct
b. Etiology
(1) Malignancy (most common)
- Blocks lymphatic drainage
(2) Trauma
- Iatrogenic tear during surgery or pathologic
c. Turbid, milky appearance

Neurogenic tumors: most common mediastinal mass; located in posterior mediastinum

Symptoms in thymomas: most often associated with myasthenia gravis

PF movement: parietal pleura to pleural space to lungs

Congestive heart failure: most common overall cause of a pleural effusion

PF exudate: acute inflammation; infarction, pneumonia, metastasis

PF exudate: tuberculosis and malignancy most common cause

Chylous effusion: lymphedema; malignancy most common cause

TABLE 16-7. **PLEURAL FLUID (PF) TRANSUDATES VERSUS EXUDATES**

COMPONENT	TRANSUDATE	EXUDATE
PF protein/serum protein	<0.5	>0.5
PF LDH/serum LDH	<0.6	>0.6
PF LDH	<200 U/L	>200 U/L

LDH, lactate dehydrogenase; PF, pleural fluid.

      (1) Due to chylomicrons (diet-derived triglyceride; refer to Chapter 9)
      (2) Chylomicrons form a supranate in a test tube after refrigeration.
   d. PF triglyceride > 110 mg/dL is diagnostic.
 4. Pseudochylous
   a. Turbid, milky appearance
   b. Caused by inflammation with increased amount of necrotic debris
     • PF cholesterol increased
   c. Most commonly caused by rheumatoid lung disease
 5. Laboratory distinction of transudates versus exudates (Table 16-7)
   a. PF and serum concentrations of lactate dehydrogenase (LDH) and protein are most useful.
     • Ratios of PF protein and LDH to serum protein and LDH increase test sensitivity and specificity.
   b. Test sensitivity is 99% and specificity is 98% if at least one of the three criteria for an exudate is present.
   c. Additional criteria
      (1) pH > 7.4 indicates a transudate.
      (2) pH < 7.4 indicates an exudate.
 6. Clinical findings
   a. Dullness to percussion
   b. Absent breath sounds
   c. Absent vocal tactile fremitus
   d. Contralateral shift of the mediastinum
     • Only large effusions
 7. Imaging (Fig. 16-35)
   a. Blunting of the costophrenic angle
   b. Obscuration of the diaphragm

D. Spontaneous pneumothorax
 1. Epidemiology
   a. More common in men than women
   b. Commonly seen in tall, thin, young men 20 to 40 years of age
   c. Risk increases with smoking
   d. Approximately 25% recurrence rate within 2 years
 2. Causes
   a. Primary (idiopathic; most common)
      (1) Rupture of apical subpleural bleb(s)
      (2) Blebs are secondary to high negative intrapleural pressures.
      (3) Most patients are male smokers between 30 and 40 years old.
      (4) Recurrence in the contralateral lung is common.
   b. Chronic obstructive lung disease
      (1) Most common secondary cause
      (2) Paraseptal emphysema
   c. Marfan syndrome
   d. Scuba diving
   e. Insertion of subclavian catheter
 3. Pathogenesis
   a. Rupture of a subpleural or intrapleural bleb produces a hole in the pleura.
   b. Pleural cavity pressure is the *same* as the atmospheric pressure.
      (1) Loss of the negative intrathoracic pressure
      (2) Causes a portion of lung or the entire lung to collapse
 4. Clinical findings
   a. Sudden onset of dyspnea with pleuritic type of chest pain (90%)
   b. Physical examination
      (1) Tympanitic percussion note
      (2) Absent breath sounds

Margin notes:

Pseudochylous effusion: pleural effusion in RA

Pleural effusion: blunting costophrenic angle; obscure diaphragm

Spontaneous pneumothorax: commonly seen in tall, thin, young men

Spontaneous pneumothorax: rupture of apical subpleural bleb

Spontaneous pneumothorax: emphysema most common secondary cause

Spontaneous pneumothorax: loss of negative intrathoracic pressure

Spontaneous pneumothorax: sudden onset of dyspnea and pleuritic chest pain

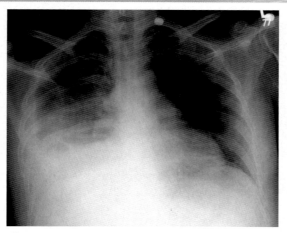

16-35: Frontal chest radiograph showing a right pleural effusion. Note the blunting of the right costophrenic angle and obscuration of the right hemidiaphragm. *(From Pretorius ES, Solomon JA: Radiology Secrets, 2nd ed. St. Louis, Mosby, 2006, p 539, Fig. 66-2A.)*

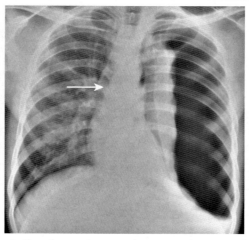

16-36: Left tension pneumothorax. Note the margin of the lung in the left pleural cavity and the tracheal deviation to the right *(arrow)*. *(From Goldman L, Ausiello D: Cecil's Textbook of Medicine, 23rd ed. Philadelphia, Saunders Elsevier, 2008, p 601, Fig. 84-11.)*

(3) Trachea deviated to the side of the collapse if there is total lung collapse
5. Upright chest x-ray
   a. White visceral pleural line
   b. Absence of vessel markings peripheral to line
6. Treatment
   a. Observation alone if asymptomatic and pneumothorax < 15%
   b. One hundred percent oxygen administration
     • Reduces partial pressure of nitrogen; hence, increasing rate of pneumothorax absorption
   c. Chest tube insertion or thoracoscopy may be required.

E. Tension pneumothorax
1. Causes
   a. Penetrating trauma to the lungs (e.g., knife wound)
   b. Rupture of tension pneumatocysts (see section VI)
2. Pathogenesis
   a. Flap-like pleural tear (check valve) allows air into the pleural cavity but prevents its exit.
     • Similar in concept to filling a tire up with air
   b. Increased pleural cavity pressure
   c. Produces compression atelectasis (see section IV)
3. Clinical findings
   a. Sudden onset of severe dyspnea and pleuritic chest pain
   b. Physical examination
     (1) Tympanitic percussion note and absent breath sounds
     (2) Trachea and mediastinal structures deviate to contralateral side if large tension pneumothorax (Fig. 16-36).
       • Compromised venous return to the heart, if the pneumothorax is located on the left side
   c. Treatment
     (1) Relieve pressure first.
       • Insert a needle into the second intercostal space on the midclavicular line.
     (2) Insert a chest tube.

Tension pneumothorax: penetrating trauma to lungs; check valve type of pleural tear

Tension pneumothorax: increase in pleural cavity pressure with each breath

Tension pneumothorax: trachea deviates to contralateral side

CHAPTER 17
GASTROINTESTINAL DISORDERS

I. **Oral Cavity and Salivary Gland Disorders**
   A. **Cleft lip and palate**
      1. Epidemiology
         a. Most common congenital disorder of oral cavity
            - ~1:800 live births
         b. Genetic factors involved
            - Recurrence in subsequent siblings (3%)
         c. More common in whites than blacks
         d. Cleft lip and palate (50%)
         e. Cleft lip alone (25%)
            - Male > female
         f. Cleft palate alone (25%; Fig. 17-1)
            - Female > male
         g. Complications
            (1) Malocclusion
            (2) Eustachian tube dysfunction
               - Chronic otitis media
            (3) Speech problems
      2. Pathogenesis
         - Failure of fusion of facial processes
      3. Treatment is surgery.
   B. **Common infections in the oral cavity** (Table 17-1 and Fig. 17-2)
   C. **Oral manifestation of HIV**
      1. Candidiasis (see Fig. 17-2F)
         - Most common oral infection
      2. Apthous ulcers (stomatitis; canker sores)
         a. Unknown origin
            (1) Virus versus immunologic
            (2) Often stress-induced
         b. Painful ulcers covered by a shaggy gray membrane (Fig. 17-3)
      3. Hairy leukoplakia (see Fig. 17-2B)
         - Glossitis due to Epstein-Barr virus (EBV)
      4. Kaposi's sarcoma
         a. Hard palate is the most common location.
         b. Due to human herpesvirus 8
   D. **Dental caries**
      1. *Streptococcus mutans* produces acid from sucrose fermentation.
         - Acid erodes enamel and exposes underlying dentine.
      2. Fluoride prevents dental caries.
         - Excess fluoride causes a chalky discoloration of the teeth.
   E. **Noninfectious ulcerations in the oral cavity**
      1. Pemphigus vulgaris and mucous membrane pemphigoid
         - Both are immunologic skin disorders (refer to Chapter 24).
      2. Erythema multiforme (refer to Chapter 24)
         a. Hypersensitivity reaction against *Mycoplasma* or drugs (e.g., sulfonamides)
         b. Called Stevens-Johnson syndrome when it involves the mouth
      3. Apthous ulcers (stomatitis; see Fig. 17-3)

Cleft lip/palate: most common congenital disorder of oral cavity

Cleft lip/palate: failure of fusion of facial processes

Pre-AIDS–defining lesions: thrush, hairy leukoplakia, apthous ulcers

Kaposi's sarcoma: hard palate; HHV-8

Dental caries: caused by *Streptococcus mutans*

Fluoride: prevents dental caries

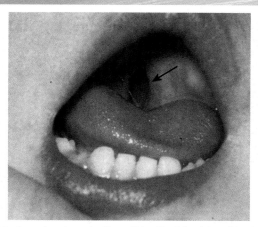

17-1: Cleft palate. Note the defect in the palate *(arrow)*. *(From Grieg JD: Color Atlas of Surgical Diagnosis. London, Mosby-Wolfe, 1996, p 68, Fig. 10-7.)*

TABLE 17-1. INFECTIONS OF THE ORAL CAVITY

INFECTION	PATHOGEN	FEATURES
Viral		
Exudative tonsillitis (see Fig. 17-2A)	Viruses: most cases	Culture is necessary to differentiate bacterial versus viral infection
Hairy leukoplakia (see Fig. 17-2B)	EBV	Glossitis associated with bilateral white excrescences on lateral border of tongue Pre-AIDS-defining lesion (refer to Chapter 3)
Herpes labialis (see Fig. 17-2C)	HSV type 1	Recurrent vesicular lesions on the lips (virus remains dormant in cranial sensory ganglia) Reactivated by stress, sunlight, and menses *Treatment:* oral acyclovir, valacyclovir, famciclovir; topical acyclovir, penciclovir
Mumps	Paramyxovirus	Bilateral parotitis (70%) with increased serum amylase Complications: meningoencephalitis, unilateral orchitis or oophoritis, pancreatitis
Herpangina	Coxsackievirus	Occurs in children Multiple vesicles or ulcers on soft palate and pharynx surrounded by erythema
Hand-foot-mouth disease	Coxsackievirus	Occurs in young children Vesicles located in mouth and distal extremities
Bacterial		
Cervicofacial actinomycosis (see Fig. 17-2D)	*Actinomyces israelii*	Draining sinus tract from facial or cervical area "Sulfur granules" in pus; contain gram-positive, branching filamentous bacteria; anaerobe Often follows after extraction of an abscessed tooth *Treatment:* ampicillin, penicillin G
Diphtheria (see Fig. 16-10C)	*Corynebacterium diphtheriae*	Toxin produces "shaggy" gray pseudomembrane in posterior pharynx and upper airways *Treatment:* erythromycin
Peritonsillar abscess	*Streptococcus pyogenes*	Uvula deviates to contralateral side; "hot potato" voice; foul-smelling breath Complication due to tonsillitis *Treatment:* surgical drainage of pus; penicillin G or V; add clindamycin for serious invasive infections
Ludwig's angina	Aerobic/anaerobic *Streptococcus, Eikenella corrodens*	Cellulitis involving the submaxillary and sublingual space; follows fascial planes and may spread into pharynx, carotid sheath, superior mediastinum Causes: dental extraction (most common), trauma to floor of mouth *Treatment:* surgical drainage; clindamycin + metronidazole
Pharyngitis	*S. pyogenes*	Associated with tonsillitis Potential for acute rheumatic fever and glomerulonephritis *Treatment:* penicillin V
Scarlet fever	*S. pyogenes*	Pharyngitis, tonsillitis, glossitis Erythrogenic toxin produces rash on skin and tongue (initially white and then strawberry colored) Increased risk for glomerulonephritis Nephritogenic strains pose no risk for acute rheumatic fever *Treatment:* penicillin G or V

TABLE 17-1. INFECTIONS OF THE ORAL CAVITY—cont'd

INFECTION	PATHOGEN	FEATURES
Bacterial—cont'd		
Sialadenitis	*Staphylococcus aureus*	Bacterial inflammation of major salivary gland Secondary to a calculus, which obstructs the duct in postoperative patients *Treatment*: oxacillin, nafcillin if methicillin susceptible; TMP/SMX if community-acquired methicillin resistant; vancomycin if methicillin resistant in hospital
Congenital syphilis (see Fig. 17-2E)	*Treponema pallidum* (spirochete)	Abnormalities involving incisors (tapered like a peg) and molar teeth (resemble mulberries) *Treatment*: aqueous crystalline penicillin G
Fungal		
Oral thrush (see Fig. 17-2F)	*Candida albicans* (yeast)	May occur in neonates, immunocompromised patients (common pre-AIDS-defining lesion), diabetes mellitus, and following antibiotic therapy *Treatment*: fluconazole, itraconazole

EBV, Epstein-Barr virus; HSV, herpes simplex virus; TMP/SMX, trimethoprim-sulfamethoxazole.

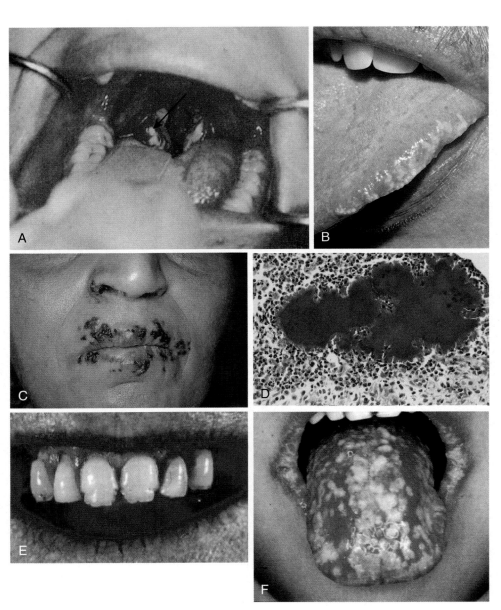

17-2: **A,** Exudative tonsillitis. Note the gray-white pus in the tonsillar crypts (*arrow*). **B,** Hairy leukoplakia along the lateral border of the tongue. It is a glossitis due to Epstein-Barr virus and is a pre-AIDS-defining lesion. **C,** Herpes simplex type 1. Note the clusters of vesicles around the vermilion border of the upper and lower lips. **D,** Actinomycosis. Note the colony of *Actinomyces* (sulfur granule) surrounded by an inflammatory infiltrate. **E,** Notched teeth in congenital syphilis. **F,** Oral thrush. Note the extensive white "curd-like" plaque that can be wiped off leaving an erythematous base. (*A courtesy of Edward L. Applebaum, MD, Department of Otolaryngology, University of Illinois, Urbana, Illinois; B from Lookingbill D, Marks J: Principles of Dermatology, 3rd ed. Philadelphia, WB Saunders, 2000, p 338, Fig. 23-7; C from Swartz MH: Textbook of Physical Diagnosis, 5th ed. Philadelphia, Saunders Elsevier, 2006, p 333, Fig. 12-10; D from Corrin B: Pathology of the Lungs. London, Churchill Livingstone, 2000, p 195, Fig. 5.3.15; E from Bouloux P: Self-Assessment Picture Tests: Medicine, Vol. 1. London, Mosby-Wolfe, 1997, p 11, Fig. 21; F from Grieg JD: Color Atlas of Surgical Diagnosis. London, Mosby-Wolfe, 1996, p 65, Fig. 10-1.*)

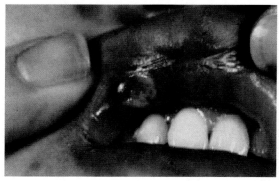

17-3: Apthous ulcer. Note the ulcerated surface on the lip covered by a shaggy gray exudate. *(From Bouloux P: Self-Assessment Picture Tests: Medicine, Vol. 1. London, Mosby-Wolfe, 1997, p 35, Fig. 69.)*

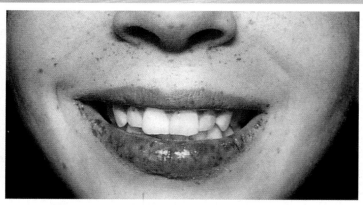

17-4: Peutz-Jeghers syndrome. Note the melanin pigmentation on the lips. *(From Swartz MH: Textbook of Physical Diagnosis, 5th ed. Philadelphia, Saunders Elsevier, 2006, p 334, Fig. 12-12.)*

Behcet's syndrome: recurrent apthous ulcers, uveitis, genital ulcers

    4. Behçet's syndrome
      a. Epidemiology
        (1) Combination of environmental + genetic factors
          • HLA-B51, HLA-B27 associations
        (2) May be precipitated by herpes simplex or parvovirus
        (3) High incidence in Turkey and eastern Mediterranean
      b. Pathophysiology
        • Immune complex small vessel vasculitis
      c. Clinical findings
        (1) Recurrent aphthous ulcers, genital ulcerations
        (2) Uveitis, erythema nodosum
        (3) Attacks last 1 to 4 weeks
      d. Treatment
        (1) Anti-inflammatory medications
        (2) Corticosteroids
        (3) Colchicine
        (4) Thalidomide

F. Pigmentation abnormalities

Melanin pigmentation in oral mucosa: Addison's disease, Peutz-Jeghers syndrome

    1. Peutz-Jeghers syndrome (see section IV)
      • Melanin pigmentation of the lips and oral mucosa (Fig. 17-4)
    2. Addison's disease (see Fig. 22-21)
      a. Increased adrenocorticotropic hormone (ACTH) stimulates melanocytes.
      b. Melanin pigmentation of the buccal mucosa
    3. Lead poisoning
      • Lead deposits along the gingival margins in adults with gingivitis

G. Tooth discoloration

Tooth discoloration: tetracycline, ↑ fluoride, erythropoietic porphyria

    1. Tetracycline
      a. Drug discolors newly formed teeth.
      b. Drug *not* recommended in a child < 12 years of age.
    2. Excess fluoride
      • Mottled, chalky white discoloration
    3. Congenital erythropoietic porphyria
      a. Porphyrins deposit in the teeth
      b. Reddish brown discoloration

H. Macroglossia (enlarged tongue)

Macroglossia: myxedema, Down syndrome, acromegaly, amyloidosis, MENIIb

    1. Myxedema
      • Severe primary hypothyroidism
    2. Down syndrome
    3. Acromegaly
    4. Amyloidosis
    5. Mucosal neuromas in multiple endocrine neoplasia (MEN) syndrome IIb (III)

I. Glossitis (inflammation of tongue)

    1. Sore, beefy red tongue with or without papillary atrophy

2. Causes
   a. Long-standing iron deficiency
   b. Vitamin B$_{12}$ or folate deficiency
   c. Scurvy (vitamin C deficiency)
   d. Pellagra (niacin deficiency)
   e. Scarlet fever
   f. EBV-associated hairy leukoplakia

J. **Leukoplakia and erythroplakia**
   1. Leukoplakia literally means "white patch" (Fig. 17-5).
      • It has an ~30% rate of progression to oral cancer.
   2. Erythroplakia is a red patch (Fig. 17-6).
      • It has an ~60% rate of progression to oral cancer.
   3. Lesion does *not* wipe off.
   4. Both lesions are due to squamous hyperplasia of the epidermis.
      • Increased risk for squamous dysplasia or invasive squamous cancer
   5. Causes
      a. Chronic irritation (e.g., dentures)
      b. All forms of tobacco use
      c. Alcohol abuse
      d. Human papillomavirus (HPV)
   6. Locations
      a. Vermilion border lower lip (most common site)
      b. Buccal mucosa
      c. Hard and soft palates
      d. Floor of the mouth
   7. Always biopsy these lesions because of the high risk for progression to oral cancer.

K. **Lichen planus** (refer to Chapter 24)
   1. Often associated with Wickham's stria on buccal mucosa
      • Fine, white, lacy lesions
   2. May be associated with squamous cell carcinoma

L. **Dentigerous cyst**
   1. Derives from epithelial elements of dental origin (odontogenic origin)
   2. Associated with the crown of an unerupted or impacted third molar tooth
   3. Association with ameloblastomas in 15% to 30% of cases

Glossitis: deficiency of iron, B$_{12}$, folate, vitamin C, niacin; scarlet fever; hairy leukoplakia

Leukoplakia/ erythroplakia: smoking and alcohol are major risk factors

Leukoplakia/ erythroplakia: biopsy to rule out squamous dysplasia or cancer

Wickham's stria: association with squamous dysplasia or cancer

Dentigerous cyst: association with 3rd molar and ameloblastoma

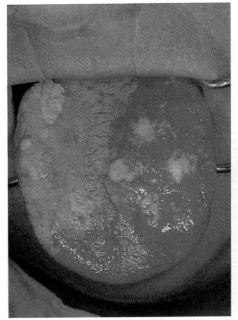

17-5: Leukoplakia of the tongue with invasive squamous cell carcinoma. Discrete raised white patches are evident on both sides of the tongue. *(From Forbes C, Jackson W: Color Atlas and Text of Clinical Medicine, 2nd ed. St. Louis, Mosby, 2003, p 362, Fig. 8-28.)*

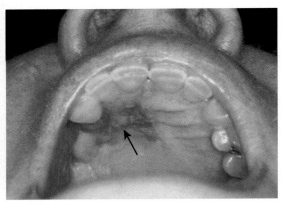

17-6: Erythroplakia. Note the raised erythematous area *(arrow)* on the palate. *(From Goldman L, Ausiello D: Cecil's Textbook of Medicine, 23rd ed. Philadelphia, Saunders Elsevier, 2008, p 1451, Fig. 200-2.)*

M. Benign tumors of the oral cavity (excluding salivary gland)

1. Squamous papillomas

   a. Most common benign tumor in oral cavity

   b. Exophytic tumor with a fibrovascular core

   c. May occur on the tongue, gingiva, palate, or lips

2. Ameloblastoma

   a. Arise from enamel organ epithelium or a dentigerous cyst

   b. Located in the mandible

      (1) Produces a radiolucency in bone that has a "soap bubble" appearance

      (2) Locally invasive but do *not* metastasize

N. Malignant tumors of the oral cavity (excluding salivary gland)

1. Epidemiology

   a. Majority are well-differentiated squamous cell carcinomas

   b. More common in men than women

   c. Risk factors

      (1) Smoking is the most common risk factor.

         • Pipe, cigarettes, chewing tobacco

      (2) Alcohol abuse (synergistic with smoking)

      (3) Synergism between smoking and alcohol excess

         • Increases relative risk 30-fold

      (4) HPV

      (5) Chronic irritation from dentures

      (6) Lichen planus

   d. Cancer sites in descending order

      (1) Lower lip (vermilion border; Fig. 17-7)

      (2) Floor of mouth

      (3) Lateral border of tongue

   e. Metastasis

      • "Tonsillar node" (superior jugular node)

   f. Verrucous carcinoma

      • Associated with smokeless tobacco

   g. Basal cell carcinoma

      (1) Most common cancer of upper lip

      (2) Associated with ultraviolet light B exposure

2. Treatment for squamous cancer

   • Surgery and radiation; chemotherapy in advanced cases

O. Salivary gland disorders

1. Sjögren's syndrome (refer to Chapter 23)

   a. Female dominant autoimmune disease associated with rheumatoid arthritis

   b. Autoimmune destruction of minor salivary glands and lacrimal glands

2. Salivary gland tumors

   a. Epidemiology

      (1) Parotid gland is the most common site.

         • Major salivary gland tumors are more likely to be benign.

      (2) Minor salivary gland tumors are more likely to be malignant.

   b. Pleomorphic adenoma (mixed tumor)

Side notes (left margin):

Squamous papillomas: most common benign tumor in oral cavity

Ameloblastoma: most common odontogenic tumor; "soap bubble" appearance in mandible

Squamous cell carcinoma: smoking products most common risk factor

Squamous cell carcinoma: most common site is lower lip

Basal cell carcinoma: most common oral site is upper lip

Sjögren's syndrome: dry eyes, dry mouth

Parotid gland: most common site for salivary gland tumors

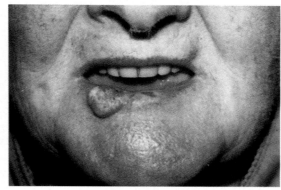

17-7: Squamous cell carcinoma of the lower lip. *(From Grieg JD: Color Atlas of Surgical Diagnosis. London, Mosby-Wolfe, 1996, p 67, Fig. 10-5.)*

(1) Most common benign tumor of major and minor salivary glands
  • Parotid gland is the most common site.
(2) Female dominant
(3) Painless, moveable mass at the angle of the jaw
(4) Epithelial cells intermixed with myxomatous and cartilaginous stroma
  • Tumor projections through capsule increase risk of recurrence
(5) May transform into a malignant tumor
  • Facial nerve involvement is a sign of malignancy.

  c. Warthin's tumor (papillary cystadenoma lymphomatosum)
(1) Benign parotid gland tumor
  • Male dominant
(2) Heterotopic salivary gland tissue trapped in a lymph node
  • Cystic glandular structures are located within benign lymphoid tissue.

  d. Mucoepidermoid carcinoma
(1) Most common malignant salivary gland tumor
(2) Most commonly located in the parotid gland
(3) Mixture of neoplastic squamous and mucus-secreting cells

II. Esophageal Disorders
A. Signs and symptoms of esophageal disease
1. Heartburn
  • Most commonly due to gastroesophageal reflux disease
2. Dysphagia (difficulty swallowing) for solids alone
  a. Symptom of an obstructive lesion
  b. Examples—esophageal cancer, esophageal web, stricture
3. Dysphagia for solids and liquids
  a. Symptom of a motility disorder
  b. Oropharyngeal (upper esophageal) dysphagia
    (1) Striated muscle dysmotility
    (2) Examples—dermatomyositis, myasthenia gravis, stroke
  c. Lower esophageal dysphagia
    (1) Smooth muscle dysmotility
    (2) Examples—systemic sclerosis, CREST syndrome (see page 47), achalasia

B. Tracheoesophageal (TE) fistula
1. Characteristics
  a. Proximal esophagus ends blindly (Fig. 17-8).
  b. Distal esophagus arises from the trachea.
2. Clinical findings
  a. Maternal polyhydramnios (excess amniotic fluid)
  • Swallowed amniotic fluid cannot be reabsorbed in the small intestine.
  b. Abdominal distention in newborn
  • Air in the stomach from tracheal fistula
  c. Difficulty with feeding
    (1) Food regurgitates out of the mouth.
    (2) Chemical pneumonia from aspiration
  d. VATER syndrome
    (1) *V*ertebral abnormalities
    (2) *A*nal atresia
    (3) *TE* fistula
    (4) *R*enal disease and absent *r*adius

Margin notes:

Pleomorphic adenoma: most common salivary gland tumor

Warthin's tumor: heterotopic salivary gland tissue in a lymph node

Mucoepidermoid carcinoma: most common malignant salivary gland tumor

Dysphagia for solids: obstructive lesion

Dysphagia for solids and liquids: motor disorder

TE fistula: proximal esophagus ends blindly; distal esophagus from trachea

TE fistula: polyhydramnios

VATER syndrome: *v*ertebral abnormalities, *a*nal atresia, *TE* fistula, *r*enal disease, and absent *r*adius

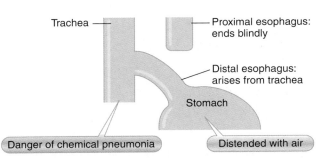

Trachea — Proximal esophagus: ends blindly
Distal esophagus: arises from trachea
Stomach
Danger of chemical pneumonia
Distended with air

17-8: Tracheoesophageal fistula. The proximal esophagus ends blindly, and the distal esophagus arises from the trachea. The stomach is distended with air owing to communication of the esophagus with the trachea.

C. Plummer-Vinson syndrome (refer to Chapter 11)
 1. Due to chronic iron deficiency
 2. Leukoplakia in oral mucosa and esophagus
 3. Intermittent dysphagia for solids
  • Due to an esophageal web or stricture

D. Esophageal diverticulum
 1. Types of diverticulum
  a. True diverticulum
   • Outpouching lined by mucosa, submucosa, muscularis propria, and adventitia
  b. False, or pulsion diverticulum
   (1) Weakness in underlying muscle wall
   (2) Outpouching of mucosa and submucosa into area of weakness

 2. Zenker's diverticulum
  a. Pulsion type located in upper esophagus
   • Area of weakness is cricopharyngeus muscle.
  b. Clinical findings
   (1) Painful swallowing
   (2) Halitosis
    • Entrapped food
   (3) Regurgitate food through mouth
   (4) Diverticulitis
  c. Treatment is surgery.

E. Hiatal hernia
 1. Epidemiology
  a. Found in 50% of persons over 50 years old
   • Increases with age

  b. More common in women than men
  c. Associations
   (1) Sigmoid diverticulosis (25%)
   (2) Esophagitis (25%)
   (3) Duodenal ulcers (20%)
   (4) Gallstones (18%)
 2. Sliding hernia

  a. Most common type of hiatal hernia (99%)
  b. Herniation of proximal stomach into thoracic cavity through the diaphragmatic esophageal hiatus
  c. Clinical findings
   (1) Heartburn

   (2) Nocturnal epigastric distress from acid reflux
   (3) Hematemesis (vomiting blood)
   (4) Ulceration, stricture
   (5) Bowel sounds heard over left lung base
  d. Treatment
   (1) Nonpharmacologic
    (a) Reduce intake of foods/drugs that decrease lower esophageal sphincter tone
     • Examples—coffee, chocolate, calcium channel blockers
    (b) Avoid large quantities of food
    (c) Sleep with head of the bed elevated
   (2) Pharmacologic
    (a) H_2 antagonists
    (b) Proton pump inhibitors
    (c) Prokinetic agents
   (3) Surgery if indicated

 3. Paraesophageal (rolling) hernia (1%)
  a. Gastroesophageal junction remains at the level of the diaphragm.
  b. Part of the stomach bulges into the thoracic cavity.

Pleuroperitoneal diaphragmatic hernias (Bochdalek hernia) are present early in life. The visceral contents extend through the posterolateral part of the diaphragm on the left into the chest cavity causing respiratory distress at birth. Loops of bowel are present in the left pleural cavity on radiograph.

F. Gastroesophageal reflux disease (GERD)
1. Epidemiology
   a. Approximately 10% of adults have GERD daily.
   b. Approximately 80% of pregnant women have GERD.
   c. Hiatal hernia present in ~70% of people with GERD.
   d. Risk factors
      (1) Smoking, alcohol
      (2) Caffeine, fatty foods, chocolate
      (3) Pregnancy, obesity
      (4) Hiatal hernia
2. Pathogenesis
   a. Transient relaxation of lower esophageal sphincter (LES)
      • Reflux of acid and bile into the distal esophagus
   b. Ineffective esophageal clearance of reflux material
3. Clinical findings
   a. Noncardiac chest pain
      • Heartburn, indigestion
   b. Nocturnal cough, nocturnal asthma
   c. Acid injury to enamel
   d. Early satiety, abdominal fullness
   e. Bloating with belching
   f. Barrett's esophagus
4. Diagnostic tests with atypical presentation
   a. Twenty-four–hour esophageal pH monitoring
      • Sensitivity/specificity 80% to 90%
   b. Esophageal endoscopy
   c. Manometry
      • LES pressure < 10 mm Hg
5. Treatment
   a. Nonpharmacologic
      • Similar to hiatal hernia (see earlier)
   b. Pharmacologic
      • Similar to hiatal hernia (see earlier)
   c. Surgery if indicated
      (1) Fundoplication procedure
      (2) Involves putting a gastric wrap around the gastroesophageal junction

G. Barrett's esophagus
1. Complication of GERD
2. Glandular metaplasia in distal esophagus due to acid injury (see Fig. 1-10E)
   • Gastric-type columnar cells and small intestine–type cells (goblet cells)
3. Complications
   a. Ulceration with stricture formation (most common)
   b. Glandular dysplasia with increased risk for distal adenocarcinoma

H. Infectious esophagitis
1. Usually a complication of AIDS
2. Pathogens
   a. Herpes simplex virus (HSV)
      • See multinucleated squamous cells with intranuclear inclusions
   b. Cytomegalovirus (CMV)
      • See basophilic intranuclear inclusions
   c. *Candida*
      • See yeasts and pseudohyphae (extended yeast forms)
3. Presents with painful swallowing (i.e., odynophagia)

I. Corrosive esophagitis
1. Ingestion of strong alkali (e.g., lye) or acid (e.g., HCl)
2. Complications
   a. Stricture formation
   b. Perforation
   c. Squamous cell carcinoma

J. Esophageal varices
1. Epidemiology and pathogenesis
   a. Dilated submucosal left gastric veins (Fig. 17-9)

GERD: relaxed LES causes acid reflux

GERD: nocturnal cough/asthma; acid injury to enamel; Barrett's esophagus

GERD atypical presentation: esophageal pH monitoring, endoscopy, manometry

Barrett's esophagus complications: distal adenocarcinoma, stricture

AIDS-related esophagitis: HSV, CMV, *Candida*

Corrosive esophagitis: strictures, perforation, squamous cancer

Left gastric vein drains blood from distal esophagus and proximal stomach into the portal vein.

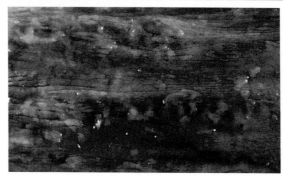

17-9: Esophageal varices, showing many linear-oriented dilated and tortuous veins in the submucosa of the distal esophagus. *(From Damjanov I, Linder J: Pathology: A Color Atlas. St. Louis, Mosby, 2000, p 110, Fig. 6-23A.)*

Esophageal varices: portal hypertension dilates left gastric veins

Ruptured esophageal varices: most common cause of death in cirrhosis

Ruptured esophageal varices: endoscopy most important diagnostic procedure

b. Complication of portal hypertension from cirrhosis
  • Alcohol abuse is the most common cause.
2. Clinical findings
  a. Rupture with massive hematemesis (vomiting blood)
  b. Most common cause of death in cirrhosis
3. Diagnosis
  • Endoscopy
4. Initial management
  a. Endoscopy
    (1) Most important diagnostic procedure
    (2) Value in treatment of the bleed as well
  b. Assess/maintain intravascular volume
  c. Insert nasogastric tube for gastric aspirate/lavage.
    (1) Confirms upper gastrointestinal source of bleeding
    (2) Assesses rate of bleeding
5. Prevention/treatment of bleeds
  a. β-Blockers and isosorbide
    (1) Decrease rate of recurrent bleeding
    (2) Increase survival by 5% to 10%
  b. Transjugular intrahepatic portasystemic stent (TIPS)
    • Used for both treatment of bleeding and intractable ascites
  c. Octreotide intravenous drip (somatostatin analogue) for bleeding
  d. Endoscopic ligation
  e. Endoscopic sclerotherapy
  f. Open surgery with stapling

K. Mallory-Weiss syndrome

Mallory-Weiss syndrome: mucosal tear of distal esophagus

1. Mucosal tear in the proximal stomach and distal esophagus
  • Due to severe retching in alcoholics or bulimia
2. Causes hematemesis

L. Boerhaave's syndrome

Boerhaave's syndrome: rupture of distal esophagus

1. Rupture of the distal esophagus
2. Causes
  a. Endoscopy (~75% of cases)
  b. Retching
  c. Bulimia
3. Complications
  a. Pneumomediastinum

Pneumomediastinum: air in subcutaneous tissue; crunching sound on physical exam

    (1) Air dissects subcutaneously into the anterior mediastinum.
    (2) Crunching sound (Hamman's crunch) is heard on auscultation.
  b. Pleural effusion contains food, acid, amylase.

M. Motor disorders
1. Systemic sclerosis and CREST syndrome (refer to Chapter 3)
2. Achalasia

Achalasia: most common neuromuscular disorder of the esophagus

  a. Epidemiology
    (1) Bimodal

(a) Occurs in those 20 to 40 years old
(b) Occurs after 60 years of age
(2) Men and women affected equally
(3) Risk for esophageal cancer
b. Pathogenesis
(1) Incomplete relaxation of LES
(2) Destruction of ganglion cells in myenteric plexus
(a) Probable autoimmune destruction of myenteric plexus
• HLA-DQw1 association
(b) Decreases proximal smooth muscle contraction
(c) Loss of nitric oxide (NO) synthase producing neurons
• Cause of incomplete relaxation
(3) Dilation of esophagus proximal to LES with absent peristalsis
(4) Acquired cause is Chagas' disease.
• Destruction of ganglion cells by amastigotes (lack flagella)
c. Clinical findings
(1) Nocturnal regurgitation of undigested food
(2) Dysphagia for solids and liquids
(3) Chest pain and heartburn
(4) Frequent hiccups
(5) Nocturnal cough from aspiration
(6) Difficulty belching
d. Diagnosis
(1) Abnormal barium swallow
• Dilated, aperistaltic esophagus with a beak-like tapering at distal end (Fig. 17-10)
(2) Abnormal esophageal manometry
• Detects aperistalsis and failure of LES relaxation
e. Treatment
(1) Nonpharmacologic
(a) Pneumatic dilation
(b) Esophagomyotomy
(2) Pharmacologic (short-term)
(a) Long-acting nitrates
(b) Calcium channel blockers
(c) Botulinum toxin injection

N. Esophageal tumors
1. Leiomyoma
• Most common benign tumor of esophagus

> Achalasia: autoimmune destruction ganglion cells myenteric plexus; loss smooth muscle motility
>
> Achalasia: destruction NO synthase producing neurons causes incomplete relaxation LES
>
> Achalasia: nocturnal regurgitation of undigested food
>
> Achalasia barium swallow: dilated, aperistaltic esophagus; beak-like tapering distal end
>
> Leiomyoma: most common benign tumor of esophagus

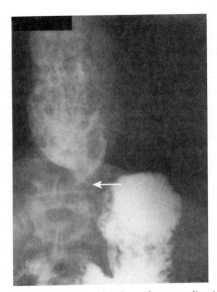

17-10: Barium study of the esophagus in achalasia. Note dilated esophagus ending in a narrowed esophagogastric junction ("birds-beak" appearance) (arrow). (From Grieg JD: Color Atlas of Surgical Diagnosis. London, Mosby-Wolfe, 1996, p 106, Fig. 16-6.)

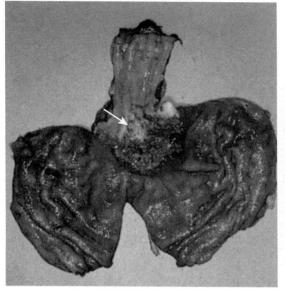

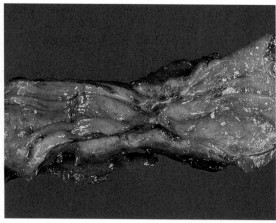

17-11: Distal adenocarcinoma of the esophagus. Note the raised lesion at the junction of the distal esophagus and proximal stomach (*arrow*). *(From Grieg JD: Color Atlas of Surgical Diagnosis. London, Mosby-Wolfe, 1996, p 109, Fig. 16-12 [right].)*

17-12: Midesophagus squamous cell carcinoma. Note the elevated round nodular mass with a central area of ulceration. *(From Rosai J, Ackerman LV: Surgical Pathology, 9th ed. St. Louis, Mosby, 2004, p 626, Fig. 11-14C.)*

2. Adenocarcinoma of distal esophagus (Fig. 17-11)
   a. Most common primary cancer of the esophagus in the United States
   b. Barrett's esophagus is most common predisposing cause.
      • Prevention of GERD decreases risk for developing adenocarcinoma.
3. Squamous cell carcinoma
   a. Epidemiology
      (1) Most common primary cancer in developing countries
         • Caspian Sea to Northern China
      (2) More common in blacks than whites
      (3) Occurs in men more often than women
      (4) Risk factors
         (a) Smoking most common cause
         (b) Alcohol abuse, lye strictures
         (c) Achalasia, Plummer-Vinson syndrome
      (5) Locations
         (a) Upper third (~15%)
         (b) Middle third (~50%) (Fig. 17-12)
         (c) Lower third (~35%)
      (6) Spreads to local nodes first and then to liver and lungs
   b. Clinical findings
      (1) Dysphagia for solids initially
      (2) Weight loss of short duration
      (3) Painless enlargement supraclavicular nodes
      (4) Dry cough and hemoptysis
         • Suggests tracheal invasion
      (5) Hoarseness
         • Probable invasion of recurrent laryngeal nerve
      (6) Odynophagia
      (7) Hypercalcemia
         • Parathyroid harmone–related peptide similar to squamous cancer in lungs
   c. Diagnosis
      (1) Esophagogram
      (2) Endoscopy
   d. Treatment
      • Surgery, radiation therapy, chemotherapy
   e. Prognosis
      • Overall 5-year survival rate is 13%.

Distal adenocarcinoma of esophagus: most common esophageal cancer

Squamous cell carcinoma: smoking cigarettes most common cause

Squamous cell carcinoma: dysphagia for solids + weight loss

Squamous cell carcinoma: symptoms often relate to local invasion

III. Stomach Disorders
A. Signs and symptoms of stomach disease
1. Hematemesis (vomiting blood)
   a. Most commonly due to peptic ulcer disease (PUD)
   b. Other causes—esophageal varices, hemorrhagic gastritis
2. Melena (dark, tarry stools)
   a. Hemoglobin (Hb) is converted into hematin (black pigment) by acid.
   b. Signifies a bleed proximal to duodenojejunal junction (90%)
3. Gastric analysis

B. Congenital pyloric stenosis (CPS)
1. Epidemiology

> **Gastric analysis** includes measurement of basal acid output (BAO), maximal acid output (MAO), and the BAO:MAO ratio. BAO is the acid output of gastric juice collected via a nasogastric tube over a 1-hour period on an empty stomach. It is normally less than 5 mEq/hour. MAO is the acid output of gastric juice that is collected over 1 hour after pentagastrin stimulation. Normally, it is 5 to 20 mEq/hour. The normal BAO:MAO ratio is 0.20:1.

   a. Probable genetic basis
   b. Occurs in males > females
   c. Affected fathers or mothers
      • Increased for child with CPS
   d. Acquired pyloric obstruction
      • Complication of chronic duodenal ulcer disease with pyloric scarring
2. Pathophysiology
   a. Progressive hypertrophy of the circular muscles in the pyloric sphincter
      • *Not* present at birth but occurs over the ensuing 3 to 5 weeks
   b. Deficiency of NO synthase precipitates the disease
3. Clinical findings
   a. Projectile vomiting of non–bile-stained fluid
   b. Hypertrophied pylorus is palpated in the epigastrium (70%).
      • Called an "olive"
   c. Visible hyperperistalsis
4. Treatment
   • Myotomy if it does *not* resolve

C. Gastroparesis
1. Decreased stomach motility
   a. Autonomic neuropathy (e.g., diabetes mellitus)
   b. Previous vagotomy
2. Clinical findings
   a. Early satiety and bloating
   b. Vomiting of undigested food a few hours after eating
3. Treatment
   a. Small volume frequent feeding
   b. Metoclopramide

D. Acute hemorrhagic (erosive) gastritis
1. Terms
   a. Erosions are a breach in the epithelium of the mucosa.
   b. Ulcers are a breach in the mucosa with extension into the submucosa or deeper.
2. Causes
   a. NSAIDs
   b. Alcohol, *Helicobacter pylori* (see below)
   c. CMV (AIDS), smoking
   d. Burns (called Curling's ulcers)
   e. CNS injury (called Cushing's ulcers)
   f. Uremia
   g. *Anisakis*
      • Worm associated with eating raw fish
3. Clinical findings
   a. Hematemesis

PUD: most common cause of hematemesis and melena

Melena: hematin; sign of upper gastrointestinal bleed

Gastric analysis: measures BAO and MAO

CPS: hypertrophy of pyloric sphincter muscles

CPS: vomiting of non–bile-stained fluid

Gastroparesis: sign of autonomic neuropathy; e.g., diabetes mellitus

Gastroparesis: early satiety; vomiting of undigested food

Hemorrhagic gastritis: NSAIDs most common cause; alcohol second

b. Melena

c. Iron deficiency

4. Treatment (excluding *H. pylori*)

   a. Nonpharmacologic

     (1) Avoid mucosal irritants (e.g., NSAIDs, alcohol)

     (2) Cessation of smoking

   b. Pharmacologic

     (1) Misoprostol

     (2) Proton pump inhibitors

E. Chronic atrophic gastritis

1. Type A chronic atrophic gastritis

   a. Involves the body and fundus

   b. Most often due to pernicious anemia (refer to Chapter 11)

   c. Complications

     (1) Achlorhydria with hypergastrinemia (loss of negative feedback)

     (2) Macrocytic anemia due to vitamin B_{12} deficiency

     (3) Increased risk for gastric adenocarcinoma

2. Type B chronic atrophic gastritis

   a. Involves the antrum and pylorus

   b. Epidemiology

     (1) Most common cause is *Helicobacter pylori*.

        • Gram-negative, curved rod

     (2) Present in 30% to 50% of population in United States

     (3) Prevalence increases with age.

     (4) Transmitted by fecal-oral/oral-oral route

        • Common in areas of poor sanitation

   c. Pathophysiology

     (1) Gram-negative, curved rod

     (2) Produces urease, proteases, cytotoxins

        (a) Urease converts amino groups in proteins to ammonia

        (b) Secretion products produce chronic gastritis and PUD.

     (3) Colonizes mucus layer lining (Fig. 17-13)

        (a) Attaches to blood group O receptors on mucosal cells

        (b) *Not* an invasive bacterium

Margin notes:

Type A chronic atrophic gastritis: body and fundus; pernicious anemia

Type B chronic atrophic gastritis: antrum and pylorus; *H. pylori*

H. pylori: urease producer

H. pylori: colonizes mucous layer; noninvasive

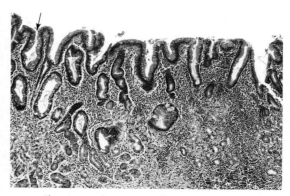

17-13: Silver stain showing *Helicobacter pylori* organisms in the mucus layer lining the gastric epithelial cells. *(From Kumar V, Fausto N, Abbas A: Robbins and Cotran's Pathologic Basis of Disease, 7th ed. Philadelphia, WB Saunders, 2004, p 815, Fig. 17-15.)*

17-14: Chronic atrophic gastritis of the distal stomach secondary to *Helicobacter pylori*. The *arrow* shows clear spaces in the mucosal epithelium representing goblet cells, which are normally present in the intestine. Note the heavy lymphocytic infiltrate throughout all layers of the stomach. *(From Kumar V, Fausto N, Abbas A: Robbins and Cotran's Pathologic Basis of Disease, 7th ed. Philadelphia, WB Saunders, 2004, p 815, Fig. 17-14.)*

    d. Microscopic findings
      (1) Chronic inflammatory infiltrate in the lamina propria
      (2) Intestinal metaplasia (Fig. 17-14)
        • Precursor lesion for adenocarcinoma
    e. Tests to identify *H. pylori* are highly sensitive and specific.
      (1) Urea breath test
        (a) Documents active infection
        (b) Sensitivity and specificity > 90%
      (2) Stool antigen test (excellent screen)
        (a) Positive when there is active infection
        (b) Negative when infection has been eradicated
        (c) Sensitivity and specificity > 90%
      (3) Tests to detect urease in a gastric biopsy
        • Considered gold standard test albeit an invasive test
      (5) Serologic tests
        (a) High sensitivity and specificity
        (b) Do *not* distinguish current from past infection
    f. Treatment
      (1) Bismuth, metronidazole, tetracycline, omeprazole
      (2) Omeprazole, amoxicillin, clarithromycin
      (3) Length of treatment varies from 7 to 14 days
      (4) Test of cure is stool antigen test
        (a) If negative 8 weeks after therapy, infection is cured.
        (b) Does not imply that infection cannot recur
    g. Other disease associations with *H. pylori*
      (1) Duodenal and gastric ulcers (see later)
      (2) Gastric adenocarcinoma (see later)
      (3) Low-grade B-cell malignant lymphoma (see later)
  3. Menetrier's disease (hypertrophic gastropathy)
    a. Giant rugal folds
      (1) Due to hyperplasia of mucus-secreting cells
      (2) Causes hypoproteinemia (protein-losing enteropathy)
    b. Atrophy of parietal cells (achlorhydria)
      • Increased risk for adenocarcinoma

F. Peptic ulcer disease (PUD)
  1. Epidemiology
    a. PUD is most often caused by *H. pylori* (70%).
      • Other parts of the world > 90%
    b. Eradication of *H. pylori* markedly reduces PUD recurrence.
    c. Duodenal ulcers are more common than gastric ulcers.
    d. Locations
      (1) Duodenal ulcer first portion of duodenum (>90%)
      (2) Gastric ulcer in lesser curvature near incisura angularis
    e. Recurrence rate for untreated PUD ~60% (>70% in smokers)
  2. Gross appearance of ulcers
    a. Clean, sharply demarcated, and slightly elevated around the edges
    b. Most gastric ulcers are benign.
      • Small percentage may be malignant (reason for biopsy).
    c. Duodenal ulcers are *never* malignant.
    d. Four layers in sequence are noted in histologic sections of ulcers.
      (1) Necrotic debris
      (2) Inflammation with a predominance of neutrophils
      (3) Granulation tissue (repair tissue)
      (4) Fibrosis
  3. Comparison of gastric and duodenal ulcers (Table 17-2 and Fig. 17-15)

G. Zollinger-Ellison (ZE) syndrome
  1. Epidemiology and pathogenesis
    a. Majority (>60%) are malignant pancreatic islet cell tumors.
    b. Secrete excess gastrin producing hyperacidity
    c. Sporadic in two thirds of cases
    d. Ulcers are usually single and in the usual locations; there may be multiple ulcers.
    e. MEN type I association (20–30% of cases)

Margin notes:

H. pylori: chronic atrophic gastritis; intestinal metaplasia precursor for cancer

Stool antigen test results: + infection; – no infection

Urea breath test/serology: do not distinguish active vs. old infection

Rx of *H. pylori* ↓ risk of gastric cancer and lymphoma

Menetrier's disease: giant rugal folds; ↑ mucus with protein loss; achlorhydria

PUD: *H. pylori* most common cause worldwide

PUD: duodenal > gastric

PUD: duodenal ulcers never malignant; gastric ulcers, small percentage malignant

ZE syndrome: ↑ gastric, ↑ acid

ZE syndrome: malignant islet cell tumor secreting gastrin; single or multiple uclers

TABLE 17-2. **COMPARISON OF GASTRIC ULCERS AND DUODENAL ULCERS**

FEATURE	GASTRIC ULCERS	DUODENAL ULCERS
Percentage of ulcer cases	25%	75%
Epidemiology	Male/female ratio 1:1 Smoking does *not* cause PUD but delays healing	Male/female ratio 2:1 Risk increased with MEN I Increased risk in cirrhosis, COPD, renal failure, hyperparathyroidism
Helicobacter pylori	~ 80% of cases	90–95% of cases
Pathogenesis	Defective mucosal barrier due to *H. pylori* Mucosal ischemia (reduced PGE), bile reflux, delayed gastric emptying BAO and MAO normal to decreased	Defective mucosal barrier due to *H. pylori* Increased acid production (increased parietal cell mass) BAO and MAO both increased
Location	Single ulcer on lesser curvature of antrum (same location for cancer)	Single ulcer on anterior portion of first part of duodenum followed by single ulcer on posterior portion (danger of perforation into pancreas and pancreatitis)
Complications (see Fig. 17-15)	Bleeding (most commonly in left gastric artery) Perforation	Bleeding (most commonly in gastroduodenal artery) Perforation (air under diaphragm, pain radiates to left or right shoulder) Gastric outlet obstruction, pancreatitis
Clinical findings	Epigastric pain exacerbated by eating	Epigastric pain relieved by eating
Diagnosis	Endoscopy: 90–95% accuracy; must biopsy gastric ulcers (1–4% malignant) Upper GI barium study: identify 70–80% PUD	Endoscopy: 90–95% accuracy; no need to biopsy because never malignant Upper GI barium study: identify 70–80% PUD
Treatment	Nonpharmacologic: stop smoking; avoid NSAIDs and alcohol; avoid foods causing symptoms Pharmacologic: eradication of *H. pylori*; H₂ receptor antagonists; proton pump inhibitors; antacids Surgery for resistant cases uncommon: ulcer removal with antrectomy or hemigastrectomy without vagotomy	Nonpharmacologic: stop smoking; avoid NSAIDs and alcohol; avoid foods causing symptoms Pharmacologic: eradication of *H. pylori*; H₂ receptor antagonists; proton pump inhibitors; antacids Surgery for resistant cases uncommon: highly selective vagotomy

BAO, basal acid output; COPD, chronic obstructive pulmonary disease; GI, gastrointestinal; MAO, maximal acid output; MEN, multiple endocrine neoplasia; PGE, prostaglandin E; PUD, peptic ulcer disease.

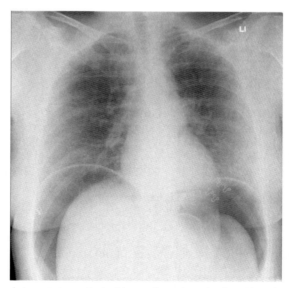

17-15: Plain abdominal radiograph in a supine patient with a perforated peptic ulcer. Note the presence of air under both diaphragms. *(From Goldman L, Ausiello D: Cecil's Textbook of Medicine, 23rd ed. Philadelphia, Saunders Elsevier, 2008, p 1015, Fig. 142-3.)*

 f. Suspicious for ZE syndrome
  (1) Multiple ulcers in usual places
  (2) Ulcers resistant to therapy
  (3) Ulcers distal to first portion of duodenum
  (4) PUD plus diarrhea

ZE syndrome: PUD + diarrhea

(5) Family history of parathyroid or pituitary tumors
(6) PUD without *H. pylori* or history of NSAIDs

2. Clinical findings
   a. Epigastric pain with weight loss
   b. Heartburn from GERD (60%)
   c. Peptic ulceration
      • Most are solitary duodenal ulcers rather than multiple ulcers.
   d. Acid hypersecretion with diarrhea
   e. Maldigestion of food
      • Acid interferes with pancreatic enzyme activity.
3. Laboratory findings
   a. Increased BAO, MAO, and BAO:MAO ratio
   b. Serum gastrin level > 1000 pg/mL
4. Treatment
   • Chemotherapy and proton pump inhibitors

H. Gastric polyps
1. Complication of chronic gastritis and achlorhydria
2. Hyperplastic polyp
   a. Most common type
   b. Hamartoma with no malignant potential
3. Adenomatous polyp
   a. Neoplastic polyp
   b. Potential for malignant transformation

I. Gastric tumors
1. Leiomyoma
   a. Stomach is most common site.
   b. May ulcerate or bleed
2. Primary stomach adenocarcinomas
   a. Epidemiology
      (1) Decreasing incidence in United States
      (2) Increasing incidence in Japan
      (3) Increased incidence in blood group A people
   b. Intestinal type of gastric adenocarcinoma
      • Most common gastric carcinoma
      (1) Risk factors
         (a) Intestinal metaplasia due to *H. pylori* (most important)
         (b) Nitrosamines
         (c) Smoked foods (Japan)
         (d) Diets lacking fruits/vegetables
         (e) Type A chronic atrophic gastritis
         (f) Menetrier's disease
      (2) Polypoid or ulcerated (Fig. 17-16)

Right margin notes:

ZE syndrome: association with MEN I syndrome

Gastric polyps: complication chronic gastritis, achlorhydria

Leiomyoma: most common benign tumor in stomach

Gastric cancer: increased incidence in Japan

Intestinal metaplasia: precursor lesion for gastric adenocarcinoma

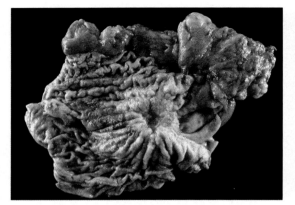

17-16: Gastric adenocarcinoma showing an irregular ulcer crater with piling up of the mucosa around the ulcer. *(From Kumar V, Fausto N, Abbas A: Robbins and Cotran's Pathologic Basis of Disease, 7th ed. Philadelphia, WB Saunders, 2004, p 825, Fig. 17-26.)*

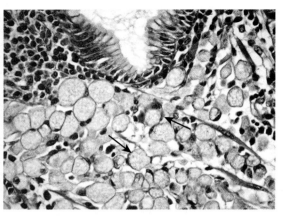

17-17: Diffuse type of gastric adenocarcinoma with signet-ring carcinoma cells *(arrows)*. Mucin produced by the cancer cells pushes the nucleus to the periphery. *(From Kumar V, Fausto N, Abbas A: Robbins and Cotran's Pathologic Basis of Disease, 7th ed. Philadelphia, WB Saunders, 2004, p 825, Fig. 17-27B.)*

Gastric cancer: lesser
curvature pylorus and
antrum most common
site

       (3) Locations
          (a) Lesser curvature of pylorus and antrum (50–60%)
          (b) Cardia (25%), body and fundus
    c. Diffuse type of gastric adenocarcinoma
       (1) Incidence has remained unchanged.
       (2) *Not* associated with *H. pylori*
       (3) Diffuse infiltration of malignant cells in the stomach wall

Diffuse gastric cancer:
"linitis plastica"; *not*
related to *H. pylori*

          (a) Sometimes called "linitis plastica"
          (b) Stomach does *not* peristalse.
          (c) Signet-ring cells infiltrate the stomach wall (Fig. 17-17).

Krukenberg tumor:
metastatic signet-ring
cells to both ovaries

          (d) Produces Krukenberg tumors of the ovaries
            • Hematogenous spread of signet-ring cells to both ovaries
    d. Clinical findings of gastric adenocarcinoma
       (1) Cachexia and weight loss (most common; 60%)
       (2) Epigastric pain (50%)
       (3) Vomiting often with melena (20%)

Gastric cancer: Virchow's
left supraclavicular node
metastasis

       (4) Metastasis to left supraclavicular node (Virchow's node)
       (5) Paraneoplastic skin lesions (refer to Chapter 8)
          (a) Acanthosis nigricans (see Fig. 24-6B)
          (b) Multiple outcroppings of seborrheic keratoses (Leser-Trélat

Gastric cancer: acanthosis
nigricans; Leser-Trélat
sign

             sign; see Fig. 24-6A)
       (6) Metastasis to umbilicus (Sister Mary Joseph sign)
    e. Common metastatic sites
       • Liver, lung, ovaries
    f. Treatment
       • Surgery, local radiation, and chemotherapy
    g. Approximately 10% to 15% overall 5-year survival rate
  3. Primary gastric malignant lymphoma
    a. Stomach is the most common site for extranodal malignant

Gastric lymphoma: most
common cause *H. pylori*

       lymphoma.
    b. Low-grade B-cell lymphoma
       (1) *H. pylori*–related
       (2) MALToma (derives from *m*ucosa-*a*ssociated *l*ymphoid *t*issue)
    c. High-grade B- or T-cell lymphomas
    d. Treatment for *H. pylori* produces 50% cure rate.
IV. Small Bowel and Large Bowel Disorders
  A. Signs and symptoms of small bowel disease
    1. Colicky pain

Colicky pain: symptom of
bowel obstruction

      a. Pain followed by a pain-free interval
        • Accompanied by constipation and inability to pass gas
      b. Symptom of bowel obstruction
        • Example—adhesions from previous surgery
    2. Diarrhea
      a. Sign of
       (1) Infection
       (2) Malabsorption
       (3) Osmotic diarrhea
      b. If bloody, may be a sign of
       (1) Infarction
       (2) Volvulus
       (3) Dysentery
    3. Anemia; malabsorption of
      a. Iron
      b. Folate
      c. Vitamin B_{12}
  B. Signs and symptoms of large bowel disease
    1. Diarrhea
      a. Sign of
       (1) Infection
       (2) Laxative abuse
       (3) Inflammatory bowel disease
      b. If bloody, may be a sign of infarction or dysentery

TABLE 17-3. TYPES OF DIARRHEA

TYPE	CHARACTERISTICS	CAUSES	SCREENING TESTS
Invasive	Pathogens invade enterocytes Low-volume diarrhea Diarrhea with blood and leukocytes (i.e., dysentery)	*Shigella* spp. *Campylobacter jejuni* *Entamoeba histolytica*	Fecal smear for leukocytes: positive in most cases Order stool culture and stool for O&P
Secretory	Loss of isotonic fluid High-volume diarrhea Mechanisms: Laxatives Enterotoxins stimulate Cl⁻ channels regulated by cAMP and cGMP Serotonin increases bowel motility No inflammation in bowel mucosa	Laxatives: danger of melanosis coli (black bowel syndrome) with use of phenanthracene laxatives Production of enterotoxins: *Vibrio cholerae* Enterotoxigenic *E. coli* Increased serotonin: carcinoid syndrome	Fecal smear for leukocytes: negative Increased 5-HIAA: carcinoid syndrome Stool osmotic gap < 50 mOsm/kg
Osmotic	Osmotically active substance is drawing hypotonic salt solution out of bowel High-volume diarrhea No inflammation in bowel mucosa	Disaccharidase deficiency "Stunned gut" in giardiasis Ingestion of poorly absorbable solutes (e.g., magnesium sulfate laxatives)	Fecal smear for leukocytes: negative Stool osmotic gap > 100 mOsm/kg

cAMP, cyclic adenosine monophosphate; cGMP, cyclic guanosine monophosphate; HIAA, hydroxyindoleacetic acid; O&P, ova and parasites.

2. Dysentery
   a. Refers to bloody diarrhea with mucus
   b. Infection
3. Pain
   a. Inflammatory bowel disease
   b. Ischemic colitis
   c. Diverticulitis
   d. Appendicitis
   e. Peritonitis
4. Tenesmus
   a. Painful, ineffective straining at stool
   b. Commonly present in ulcerative colitis
5. Iron deficiency
   • Consider polyps, colorectal cancer
6. Hematochezia
   a. Massive loss of whole blood per rectum)
   b. Causes
      (1) Sigmoid diverticulosis (most common)
      (2) Angiodysplasia
C. **Diarrheal diseases (excluding malabsorption)**
   1. Diarrhea
      a. More than 250 g of stool per day
      b. Acute diarrhea is defined as less than 3 weeks, chronic diarrhea over 4 weeks
      c. Invasive, osmotic, secretory types (Table 17-3)
   2. Important screening tests
      a. Fecal smear for leukocytes (e.g., invasive diarrhea)
      b. Stool osmotic gap
         (1) 300 mOsm/kg (value used to represent normal POsm) – 2 × (random stool Na⁺ + random stool K⁺)
         (2) Gap < 50 mOsm/kg from POsm is a secretory diarrhea.
            • Indicates that diarrheal fluid approximates POsm
         (3) Gap > 100 mOsm/kg from POsm is an osmotic diarrhea.
            • Indicates a hypotonic loss of stool due to presence of osmotically active substances

Lactase deficiency is a common genetic defect in Native Americans, Asians, and blacks. Colon anaerobes degrade undigested lactose into lactic acid and H₂ gas leading to abdominal distention with explosive diarrhea. Treatment is to avoid dairy products.

3. Summary table of microbial pathogens causing diarrhea (Table 17-4 and Fig. 17-18)

Dysentery: bloody diarrhea with mucus

Melanosis coli: black bowel from laxatives

Hematochezia: sigmoid diverticulosis, angiodysplasia

Types of diarrhea: osmotic, secretory, invasive
Fecal smear for leukocytes: screen for invasive diarrhea

Secretory diarrhea: loss of isotonic fluid
Osmotic diarrhea: loss of hypotonic fluid

Stool osmotic gap: distinguishes secretory from osmotic diarrhea

Lactase deficiency: disaccharidase deficiency in brush border; avoid dairy products

TABLE 17-4. **MICROBIAL PATHOGENS CAUSING DIARRHEA**

PATHOGEN	DISCUSSION
Viruses	
Cytomegalovirus	Common cause of diarrhea in AIDS when CD4 T_H cell count < 50–100 cells/mm³ *Treatment*: ganciclovir
Norwalk virus	Most common cause of adult gastroenteritis Nausea, vomiting, diarrhea that resolves in 12–24 hours Occasionally can be fatal Fecal-oral transmission Common infection on cruise ships *Treatment*: supportive
Rotavirus	Most common cause of childhood diarrhea; particularly occurs in winter months Fecal-oral transmission Damages ion transport pump in small intestine; secretory diarrhea Rotazyme test on stool establishes diagnosis Rotavirus vaccine highly effective in prevention; oral vaccine *Treatment*: oral hydration; nitazoxanide
Bacteria	
Bacillus cereus	Gram-positive rod Food poisoning with preformed toxin Associated with reheated fried rice or tacos Self-limited
Campylobacter jejuni	Curved or S-shaped gram-negative rod Animal reservoirs: cattle, chicken, puppies (common source for children) Transmission fecal-oral via contaminated water, poultry, or unpasteurized milk Most common food-borne illness and invasive enterocolitis in United States Invasive and secretory enterocolitis: dysentery (bloody diarrhea) with crypt abscesses and ulcers resembling ulcerative colitis; high fever and cramping abdominal pain; organisms in stool with blood and leukocytes Complications: Guillain-Barré syndrome (antibodies cross-react with neurons); hemolytic uremic syndrome; HLA-B27 positive seronegative spondyloarthropathy *Treatment*: azithromycin
Clostridium botulinum	Gram-positive rod Adult food poisoning with preformed toxin (blocks release of acetylcholine release in presynaptic terminal of neuromuscular junction in autonomic nervous system; causes descending paralysis, mydriasis, dry mouth *Treatment*: trivalent antitoxin Infant food poisoning often contracted by eating spores in honey (lack protective bacteria); floppy baby with constipation
Clostridium difficile (see Figs. 2-8 and 17-18A)	Gram-positive rod Associated with pseudomembranous colitis; the most common cause of nosocomial diarrhea; secretory type of diarrhea Normally present in 3% of people; carrier rate increases to >20% in hospitalized patients (related to contact with spores in environment and fecal-oral contamination) Antibiotic-induced in 65–90% of cases; antibiotics (e.g., ampicillin, quinolones, clindamycin) cause overgrowth of toxin-producing *C. difficile* in colon; toxins A and B release proinflammatory mediators and cytokines that attract neutrophils and stimulate excess fluid secretion (watery diarrhea) Pseudomembrane covers colon mucosa; composed of cellular debris, leukocytes, fibrin, and mucin Person-to-person induced in 30% of cases Nonspecific lab findings: neutrophilic leukocytosis with left shift; fecal leukocytes; and, decreased serum albumin Cytotoxin assay of stool has greater specificity (75–100%) than culture of stool (75–80%) for securing the diagnosis *Treatment*: metronidazole; vancomycin produces resistant strains
Escherichia coli	Gram-negative rod ETEC: certain strains produce toxin that activate adenylate or guanylate cyclase, causing secretory diarrhea (traveler's diarrhea; accounts for 60% of cases); other causes include *Campylobacter, Salmonella, Shigella* *Treatment*: levofloxacin STEC (O157:H7 serotype): contracted by eating undercooked beef Produces hemolytic uremic syndrome (refer to Chapter 14) Antibiotics *not* recommended; may enhance toxin release
Mycobacterium avium-intracellulare complex (MAC)	Acid-fast rods Causes diarrhea with malabsorption in AIDS (CD4 count < 50 cells/mm³) Foamy macrophages in lamina propria simulate Whipple's disease
Mycobacterium tuberculosis	Acid-fast organisms swallowed from primary focus in lung Invade Peyer's patches Circumferential spread in lymphatics leads to stricture formation

TABLE 17-4. MICROBIAL PATHOGENS CAUSING DIARRHEA—cont'd

PATHOGEN	DISCUSSION
Bacteria—cont'd	
Salmonella species	Gram-negative rod Pathogenic *Salmonella*: *S. typhi*, *S. paratyphi*, *S. enteritidis* Animal reservoirs: turtles, hamsters, lizards *Salmonella enteritidis* enterocolitis: 　Second most common food-borne illness in United States; contracted by eating raw 　　or undercooked egg products, raw milk and milk products, and poultry or drinking 　　contaminated water 　*Treatment:* ciprofloxacin or levofloxacin Typhoid fever caused by *S. typhi*: 　Week 1: invades Peyer's patches and produces sepsis (blood culture best for diagnosis) 　Week 2: diarrhea (positive stool culture); classic triad of bradycardia, neutropenia, splenomegaly 　*Treatment:* treat if symptomatic with fluoroquinolone; antibiotics do *not* shorten the 　　illness and may increase frequency of carrier states 　Chronic carrier state due to gallbladder disease: cholecystectomy
Shigella dysenteriae and Shigella sonnei	Gram-negative rod No animal reservoirs Highly infectious; children in day care centers; mental institutions Mucosal ulceration, pseudomembranous inflammation in rectosigmoid, dysentery Association with HLA-B27 positive seronegative spondyloarthropathy *Treatment:* treat if symptomatic with fluoroquinolone or azithromycin
Staphylococcus aureus	Gram-positive coccus Food poisoning with preformed toxin; culture food, *not* stool Gastroenteritis occurs in 1–6 hours after eating Self-limited
Vibrio cholerae	Gram-negative comma-shaped rod Enterotoxin stimulates adenylate cyclase in small bowel Contracted from drinking contaminated water or eating contaminated seafood, especially 　crustacea *Treatment:* fluid replacement; glucose and sodium required in oral supplements 　(cotransport system for reabsorption); doxycycline or fluoroquinolone
Yersinia enterocolitica	Gram-negative coccobacillus with bipolar staining Enterocolitis in children; mesenteric lymphadenitis (granulomatous microabscesses) 　that simulates acute appendicitis Association with HLA-B27 positive seronegative spondyloarthropathy *Treatment:* TMP-SMX
Protozoa	
Balantidium coli	Protozoan (ciliate); largest protozoan Transmitted by ingestion of cysts in food or water Produces colonic ulcers with bloody diarrhea *Treatment:* tetracycline
Cryptosporidium parvum (see Fig. 17-18B)	Protozoan (sporozoa) Transmitted by ingestion of oocysts in food or water Responsible for outbreaks of diarrhea in water supply (e.g., Milwaukee, Wisconsin) Most common cause of diarrhea in AIDS Diagnosis: stool antigen test (sensitivity/specificity 98%); oocysts partially acid-fast *Treatment* if immunocompetent: nitazoxanide (less responsive to drug if 　immunodeficient)
Cyclospora, Microsporidia, Isospora belli	Protozoa (sporozoa) Fecal-oral transmission All are common pathogens in AIDS diarrhea *Cyclospora* can contaminate raspberries *Microsporidia* spores *not* partially acid-fast *Cyclospora* oocysts partially acid-fast *Isospora* oocysts partially acid-fast *Treatment:* *Cyclospora:* TMP-SMX double strength; *Microsporidia:* albendazole; 　*Isospora:* TMP-SMX double strength
Entamoeba histolytica (see Fig. 17-18C)	Protozoa (amoeba) Transmitted by ingestion of cysts in food and water Cysts are nonmotile and are present in formed stool; trophozoites are motile and are 　present in diarrhea Produces dysentery (bloody diarrhea); cysts excyst in the cecum and become 　trophozoites in the cecum; trophozoites release powerful histolytic agents that 　produce flask-shaped ulcers; trophozoites can penetrate portal vein tributaries and 　drain to the liver to produce a liver abscess ("anchovy paste" abscess); trophozoites 　can penetrate hepatic vein tributaries and produce systemic disease Trophozoites characteristically phagocytose red blood cells Diagnosis: stool antigen test (sensitivity/specificity 100%) *Treatment:* metronidazole

Continued

TABLE 17-4. **MICROBIAL PATHOGENS CAUSING DIARRHEA—cont'd**

PATHOGEN	DISCUSSION
Protozoa—cont'd	
Giardia lamblia (see Fig. 17-18D)	Protozoa (flagellate) Most common protozoal cause of diarrhea in United States Transmitted by ingestion of cysts in food and water Common in day care centers, mental hospitals, hikers, water supplies (chlorination does *not* kill the cysts), men who have sex with men (anal-oral contact), IgA deficiency, common variable immunodeficiency Produces acute and chronic diarrhea with malabsorption (cysts in formed stool; trophozoites in loose stools) Diagnosis: stool antigen test (sensitivity/specificity 100%) *Treatment:* tinidazole or nitazoxanide
Helminths	
Anisakis simplex	Intestinal nematode Transmission: eating raw fish dishes (i.e., sushi, sashimi); eating pickled herring Larvae penetrate gastric and intestinal mucosa Produce cramping abdominal pain; epigastric distress with nausea, vomiting, and diarrhea within a few hours after eating Diagnosis: endoscopy; IgE antibody test *Treatment:* removal by endoscope or surgery
Enterobius vermicularis (see Fig. 17-18E)	Intestinal nematode Most common helminth in the United States Transmission: ingestion of eggs Eggs deposited in anus by adult worms cause pruritus ani Other infections: urethritis in girls; acute appendicitis No eosinophilia because adult worms are *not* invasive *Treatment:* albendazole or mebendazole
Trichuris trichiura	Intestinal nematode (whipworm) Transmitted by ingestion of eggs Produces diarrhea; can produce rectal prolapse in children Diagnosis: stool for ova and parasites; eosinophilia *Treatment:* albendazole
Ascaris lumbricoides	Intestinal nematode Largest intestinal nematode Transmitted by ingestion of eggs Larval phase through lungs: cough, pneumonitis, eosinophilia (invasion of tissue) Bowel obstruction in adult phase; no eosinophilia (no invasion of tissue) *Treatment:* albendazole and mebendazole
Necator americanus	Intestinal nematode (hookworm) Adults attach to villi, resulting in blood loss and iron deficiency *Treatment:* albendazole or mebendazole
Strongyloides stercoralis (see Fig. 17-18F)	Intestinal nematode Transmission: filariform larvae in soil penetrate the feet → larval phase through the lungs → swallowed and molt into adults that enter the intestinal mucosa and lay eggs → eggs hatch into rhabditiform larvae which enter the intestinal lumen and are passed in the stool → develop into filariform larvae (infective form) in the soil Autoinfection may occur if filariform larvae in the intestine penetrate the mucosa and migrate to the lungs to repeat the cycle In immunocompromised patients (e.g., AIDS), massive reinfection occurs with dissemination throughout the body Produces abdominal pain and diarrhea *Treatment:* ivermectin
Diphyllobothrium latum	Intestinal cestode (tapeworm) Transmission: ingest larvae in lake trout (Great Lakes) Produce diarrhea with or without vitamin B_{12} deficiency; preferential uptake of vitamin B_{12} by the worm Diagnosis: eggs in the stool *Treatment:* praziquantel

ETEC, enterotoxigenic *Escherichia coli*; STEC, Shiga toxin *E. coli*; TMP-SMX, trimethoprim-sulfamethoxazole.

D. Malabsorption
  1. Definition
    a. Increased fecal excretion of fat plus
    b. Concurrent deficiencies of fat-soluble vitamins, minerals, carbohydrates, and proteins
  2. Pathogenesis
    • Pancreatic insufficiency, bile salt/acid deficiency, small bowel disease

Causes malabsorption: pancreatic insufficiency, bile salt/acid deficiency, small bowel disease

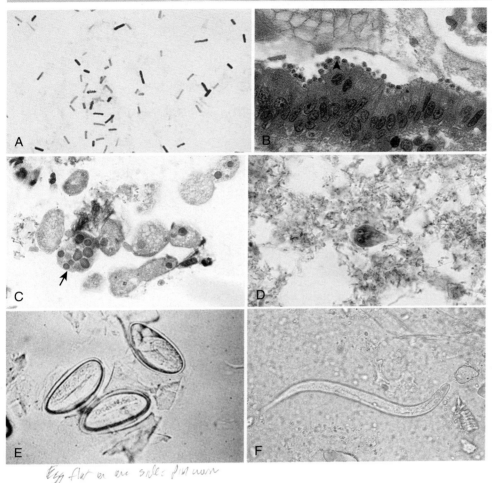

17-18: **A,** *Clostridium* species. Gram-positive rods. **B,** Cryptosporidiosis. Note the small round oocysts of *Cryptosporidium parvum* lining the luminal surface of the small intestine. **C,** *Entamoeba histolytica* trophozoites showing erythrophagocytosis *(arrow).* **D,** *Giardia lamblia* with two nuclei and flagella. **E,** Embryonated eggs of *Enterobius vermicularis.* **F,** *Strongyloides stercoralis.* Larvae in stool sample. (**A** and **F** from Murray PR, Shea YR: *Medical Microbiology,* 2nd ed. St. Louis, Mosby, 2002, pp 402, 887, Figs. 40-1, 84-9, respectively; **B** from Klatt E: *Robbins and Cotran's Atlas of Pathology.* Philadelphia, WB Saunders, 2006, p 175, Fig. 7-69; **C** and **D** from Henry JB: *Clinical Diagnosis and Management by Laboratory Methods,* 20th ed. Philadelphia, WB Saunders, 2001, Plate 55-7C, Plate 55-8C, respectively; **E** from Hart P, Shears CT: *Color Atlas of Medical Microbiology.* St. Louis, Mosby, 1996, p 271, Fig. 446.)

Egg flat on one side: pinworm

3. Pancreatic insufficiency
    a. Most often caused by chronic pancreatitis
       • Most commonly due to alcohol in adults and cystic fibrosis in children
    b. Pathogenesis
      (1) Maldigestion of fats
         (a) Due to diminished lipase activity
         (b) Undigested neutral fats and fat droplets are in stool.
      (2) Maldigestion of proteins
         (a) Due to diminished trypsin
         (b) Undigested meat fibers are in stool.
      (3) Carbohydrate digestion is *not* affected.
         (a) Amylase is present in salivary glands.
         (b) Disaccharidases are present in the brush border of intestinal epithelium.
4. Bile salt/acid deficiency
    a. Bile salts/acid are required to micellarize monoglycerides and fatty acids.
    b. Etiology and pathogenesis
      (1) Inadequate synthesis of bile salts/acids from cholesterol (e.g., cirrhosis)
      (2) Intrahepatic/extrahepatic blockage of bile
        • Examples—primary biliary cirrhosis, stone in common bile duct
      (3) Bacterial overgrowth in small bowel with destruction of bile salts/acids
        • Examples—small bowel diverticula, autonomic neuropathy
      (4) Excess binding of bile salts
        • Example—cholestyramine
      (5) Terminal ileal disease
        (a) Prevents recycling of bile salts/acids
        (b) Examples—Crohn's disease, resection of ileum
5. Small bowel disease

Pancreatic insufficiency: malabsorption of fat and proteins, not carbohydrates

Bile salts/acids: required to micellarize monoglycerides and fatty acids

Small bowel disease: loss of villous absorptive surface

a. Villi are required to reabsorb micelles into enterocytes.
- Villi increase the absorptive surface of the small intestine.
b. Etiology and pathogenesis
  (1) Inability to reabsorb micelles
    (a) Due to loss of villous surface
    (b) Examples—celiac disease (see later), Whipple's disease
  (2) Lymphatic obstruction
    - Examples—Whipple's disease, abetalipoproteinemia (see Chapter 9)

General screening tests for malabsorption: stool for fat, serum beta carotene

6. General screening tests for fat malabsorption
  a. Quantitative stool for fat
    (1) Best screening test
    (2) 72-hour collection of stool
    (3) Positive test > 7 g of fat/24 hours.
  b. Qualitative stool for fat
    (1) Stains are used to identify fat in stool.
    (2) Lacks sensitivity
  c. Decreased serum beta carotene
    - Precursor for fat-soluble retinoic acid (vitamin A)
  d. D-Xylose screening test
    (1) Xylose does *not* require pancreatic enzymes for absorption.
    (2) Lack of reabsorption of orally administered xylose
      - Indicates small bowel disease

D-Xylose: decreased reabsorption indicates small bowel disease

7. Tests to evaluate pancreatic insufficiency
  a. Serum immunoreactive trypsin
    (1) Trypsin is specific for the pancreas.
    (2) Serum immunoreactive trypsin in chronic pancreatitis
      - Decreased concentration; excellent serum for cystic fibrosis

Serum immunoreactive trypsin: excellent newborn screen for cystic fibrosis

Chronic pancreatitis: CT scan dystrophic calcification

  b. CT scan of pancreas shows dystrophic calcification.
    - Sign of chronic pancreatitis
  c. Functional tests
    (1) Secretin stimulation test (requires instrumentation)
      - Tests ability of pancreas to secrete fluids and electrolytes
    (2) Bentiromide test
      - Tests ability of pancreatic chymotrypsin to cleave orally administered bentiromide to para-aminobenzoic acid (measured in urine)

Tests pancreatic insufficiency: secretin stimulation; bentiromide

8. Tests for bile salt/acid deficiency
  a. Total bile acids can be measured.
    - Decreased in liver disease (e.g., cirrhosis)
  b. Bile breath test (oral radioactive test)
    - Decreased amount radioactive cholylglycine in breath indicates bacterial overgrowth or terminal ileal disease

Tests bile salt/acid deficiency: serum bile acids, bile breath test

9. Tests for bacterial overgrowth
  a. ^{14}C-xylose
    (1) Most sensitive/specific test
    (2) Measures $^{14}CO_2$ in the breath
  b. Lactulose-H_2
    - Measures H_2 in the breath

10. Clinical findings in malabsorption
  a. Steatorrhea
    - Excessive, large, sticky, stools that float
  b. Fat-soluble vitamin deficiencies (refer to Chapter 7)
    - Fat-soluble vitamins are A, D, E, K
  c. Water-soluble vitamin deficiencies (refer to Chapter 7)
    - Particularly folate and vitamin B_{12}
  d. Combined anemias (refer to Chapter 11)
    - Example—folate and iron deficiency
  e. Ascites and pitting edema (refer to Chapter 4)
    - Due to hypoproteinemia

Clinical: steatorrhea, fat-/water-soluble vitamin deficiencies, anemia, ascites

11. Celiac disease
  a. Epidemiology
    (1) Inappropriate immune response to gluten in wheat products
      - Also related proteins in rye and barley

Celiac disease: immune disease directed against gluten

(2) Prevalence of 1% in North America

(3) Common in whites; uncommon in blacks and Asians

(4) Occurs at any age

    (a) Highest incidence in infancy

        • First introduction to gluten products

    (b) Third decade

        • Frequent association with pregnancy

    (c) Seventh decade

(5) Associations

    (a) Dermatitis herpetiformis

    (b) Autoimmune disease

        • Hashimoto's thyroiditis, primary biliary cirrhosis

    (c) Type 1 diabetes mellitus

    (d) IgA deficiency

    (e) Down syndrome, Turner's syndrome

> Celiac disease: greatest association with dermatitis herpetiformis

b. Pathogenesis

(1) Multiorgan autoimmune disease

(2) Inappropriate T-cell and IgA-mediated response against gluten in genetically predisposed persons

    • Association with HLA-DQ2 (95%) and HLA-DQ8 (5%)

(3) Timing and dose when gluten introduced in the diet is important.

(4) Tissue transglutaminase (tTG; deamidating enzyme) in the lamina propria has a pivotal role.

    (a) It deaminates mucosally absorbed gluten to produce deaminated and negatively charged gluten peptides.

    (b) It also enhances the immunostimulatory effect of the deaminated gluten peptides.

    (c) These peptides are phagocytosed by antigen-processing cells in the lamina propria.

    (d) They are presented in complex with HLA-DQ2 or -DQ8 to gluten-specific CD4 T-helper cells.

    (e) CD4 T cells produce cytokines that release matrix proteases causing cell death and degradation in the epithelial cells in the villi.

> Celiac disease: tTG has pivotal role

c. Important diagnostic antibodies

(1) Anti-tissue transglutaminase IgA (most important), IgG antibodies

    (a) Sensitivity and specificity 98%

    (b) Excellent screening test

(2) Anti-endomysial (EMA) IgA antibodies

    (a) Sensitivity and specificity 100%

    (b) Excellent screening test

(3) Antigliadin IgA, IgG antibodies

    (a) Sensitivity 80%, specificity 85%

    (b) Moderately good screening test

> Celiac disease: ↑ tTG, EMA, gliadin IgA antibodies

d. Clinical findings

(1) Steatorrhea

(2) Weight loss

(3) Failure to thrive in infants and children

(4) Pallor due to anemia (often combined anemias)

(5) Dermatitis herpetiformis (Fig. 17-19; refer to Chapter 24)

    (a) Considered to be a form of celiac disease

    (b) Villous atrophy in 75% of cases with or without diarrhea

    (c) Low levels of above diagnostic antibodies

(6) Findings related to water-soluble and fat-soluble vitamin deficiencies (refer to Chapter 7)

(7) Other systemic findings

    (a) Bone—osteoporosis, arthritis

    (b) CNS—seizures, depression

    (c) Reproductive—delayed puberty, miscarriages, infertility

> Celiac disease: steatorrhea, weight loss

e. Diagnosis

(1) Above diagnostic antibodies

(2) Endoscopic biopsy (Fig. 17-20)

    (a) Flattened villi, particularly in duodenum and jejunum

> Celiac disease: flattened villi; hyperplastic glands

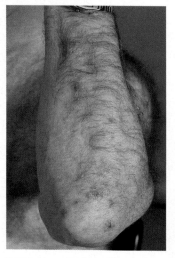

17-19: Dermatitis herpetiformis showing vesicles with erythema on the extensor surface of the forearm. Presence of this lesion has a strong association with underlying celiac disease. *(From Savin JAA, Hunter JAA, Hepburn NC: Diagnosis in Color: Skin Signs in Clinical Medicine. London, Mosby-Wolfe, 1997, p 92, Fig. 3.25.)*

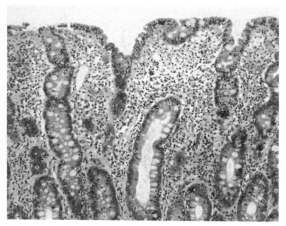

17-20: Celiac disease showing atrophy of the villi, lengthening of the crypts, and a heavy chronic inflammatory infiltrate in the lamina propria. *(From Damjanov I, Linder J: Pathology: A Color Atlas. St. Louis, Mosby, 2000, p 128, Fig. 7-25A.)*

      (b) Hyperplastic glands with intense lymphocytic inflammation
  f. Treatment
     (1) Gluten-free diet
     (2) Correct nutritional deficiencies
        • All fat-soluble vitamins; folate, vitamin B_{12}; calcium
     (3) Corticosteroids in refractory cases
12. Whipple's disease
  a. Epidemiology
     (1) Occurs in men more commonly than women
     (2) Peak incidence in middle age
     (3) Caused by *Tropheryma whippelii*
        • Identified by polymerase chain reaction
     (4) Microscopic
        (a) Blunting of villi
        (b) Foamy PAS-positive macrophages in lamina propria
        (c) Macrophages obstruct lymphatics and reabsorption of chylomicrons
           • Malabsorption of fats
     (5) Clinical findings
        (a) Steatorrhea
        (b) Fever
        (c) Recurrent polyarthritis
        (d) Generalized lymphadenopathy
        (e) Increased skin pigmentation
     (6) Treatment with antibiotics

E. Bowel obstruction
  1. Small bowel (SB) obstruction is the most common site for obstruction.
  2. Radiographic findings
    a. Bowel distention
    b. Air-fluid levels with a step-ladder appearance (Fig. 17-21)
    c. Absence of air distal to obstruction
  3. Causes of obstruction (Table 17-5 and Figs. 17-22 and 17-23)
  4. Clinical findings
    a. Colicky pain
       • Severe pain alternating with pain free intervals

Celiac disease: gluten free diet

Whipple's disease: caused by *Tropheryma whippelii*

Whipple's disease: foamy macrophages

SB obstruction: bowel distention; air/fluid levels

Colicky pain: pain alternating with pain free intervals; sign of bowel obstruction

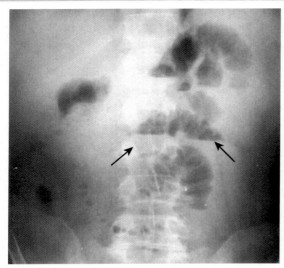

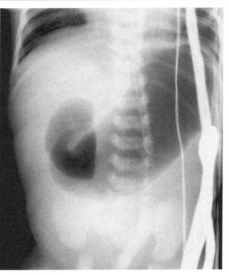

17-21: Radiograph showing small bowel obstruction. Multiple air-fluid levels are present *(arrows)* in dilated small bowel. There is absence of air distal to the obstruction. *(From Katz DS: Radiology Secrets. Philadelphia, Hanley & Belfus, 1998, p 117, Fig. 25-1.)*

17-22: Plain film of the abdomen showing a dilated stomach and duodenal bulb ("double bubble" sign) in a patient with duodenal atresia. *(From Pretorius ES, Solomon JA: Radiology Secrets, 2nd ed. St. Louis, Mosby, 2006, p 467, Fig. 58-2.)*

TABLE 17-5. SMALL AND LARGE BOWEL OBSTRUCTION

ETIOLOGIC DISORDER	DISCUSSION
Adhesions	Most common cause of small bowel obstruction. Adhesions from previous surgery (most common), endometriosis, radiation
Crohn's disease	Lumen in terminal ileum is narrow due to full-thickness inflammation of bowel wall Serosal adhesions from bowel-to-bowel also cause obstruction
Duodenal atresia (see Fig. 17-22)	Atresia is distal to entry of the common bile duct Association with Down syndrome History of maternal polyhydramnios (cannot reabsorb amniotic fluid) Vomiting of bile-stained fluid at birth "Double bubble sign": air in stomach and air in proximal duodenum
Gallstone ileus	Occurs in elderly women with chronic cholecystitis and cholelithiasis Fistula develops between gallbladder and small bowel. Stone passes into small bowel and lodges at the ileocecal valve causing obstruction. Radiograph shows air in biliary tree
Hirschsprung's disease	Absence of ganglion cells in Meissner's submucosal plexus and Auerbach's myenteric plexus causes localized aperistalsis; no sympathetic neurons in aganglionic segment; constant contraction without relaxation, which is necessary for peristalsis, resulting in obstruction Acquired Hirschsprung's disease due to Chagas' disease and destruction of ganglion cells by amastigotes Involves distal sigmoid and rectum; may involve entire rectum and descending colon; proximal uninvolved bowel is dilated but has peristalsis Abdominal pain; chronic constipation without large stools of retentive encopresis; physical exam reveals absent stool on the examining finger, because there is no stool in the rectal vault (very important differential point from other causes of chronic constipation) Association with Down syndrome Alternating signs of obstruction with diarrhea Complication: enterocolitis of dilated bowel (danger of perforation), which is the most common cause of death Diagnose with rectal biopsy *Treatment*: surgical resection of affected segment
Indirect inguinal hernia	Second most common cause of small bowel obstruction (see Table 17-6) Bowel becomes trapped in the inguinal canal
Femoral hernia	Highest rate of bowel incarceration (see Table 17-6)

Continued

TABLE 17-5. **SMALL AND LARGE BOWEL OBSTRUCTION—cont'd**

ETIOLOGIC DISORDER	DISCUSSION
Intussusception (see Fig. 17-23)	Peak incidence ages 1–5 In children, the terminal ileum invaginates into the cecum; mound of hyperplastic lymphoid tissue in Peyer's patches serves as the nidus for the intussusception; combination of obstruction and ischemia; colicky pain with bloody diarrhea; oblong mass palpated in midepigastrium (Dance's sign); usually self-reduces; may require air reduction under fluoroscopy or ultrasound; may occur with rotavirus oral vaccine In adults, a polyp or cancer is the nidus for intussusception
Meconium ileus	Complication of newborn with cystic fibrosis Meconium lacks NaCl and obstructs the bowel lumen
Volvulus (see Fig. 17-23)	Bowel twists around mesenteric root producing obstruction and strangulation Sigmoid colon is most common site in elderly Cecum is the most common site in young adults Risk factors: chronic constipation (most common), pregnancy, laxative abuse

Intussusception   Volvulus

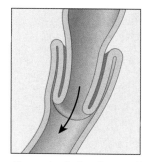 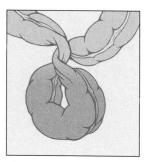

17-23: Schematic of intussusception and volvulus. See text for discussion. *(From Kumar V, Abbas AK, Fausto N, Mitchell RN: Robbins Basic Pathology, 8th ed. Philadelphia, Saunders Elsevier, 2007, p 605, Fig. 15-26.)*

b. Abdominal distention
c. No rebound tenderness
d. Tympanitic to percussion
e. High-pitched tinkling sounds
5. Treatment is surgery.

F. Hernias

1. Mechanisms predisposing to acquired hernias
   a. Increased intra-abdominal pressure (e.g., coughing, heavy weight lifting)
   b. Weakness in abdominal wall
2. Types of hernias (Table 17-6 and Figs. 17-24 and 17-25)

G. Vascular disorders

1. Small bowel is more likely than large bowel to have ischemic damage.
   a. Most of the small bowel is supplied by the superior mesenteric artery (SMA).
   b. Areas supplied by SMA
      (1) Most of the small bowel
      (2) Ascending and transverse colon
      (3) SMA and inferior mesenteric artery (IMA) overlap at the splenic flexure.
         • Splenic flexure is a watershed area (refer to Chapter 1).
2. Types of infarctions
   a. Transmural
      (1) Full-thickness hemorrhagic infarction
         • Usually involves all or part of the small bowel
      (2) Usually due to occlusion of SMA
   b. Mural and mucosal infarctions
      • Usually occur in hypoperfusion states (e.g., shock)
3. Causes of acute ischemia involving small bowel
   a. Acute mesenteric ischemia (50% of cases)
      (1) Embolism from the left side of the heart to the SMA
         • Atrial fibrillation is the most common predisposing arrhythmia.
      (2) Thrombosis of the SMA (Fig. 17-26)

Marginal notes:

Adhesions from previous surgery: most common cause of small bowel obstruction

Indirect inguinal hernia: most common hernia

SMA and IMA: watershed area

Occlusion of SMA: most common cause of small bowel infarction

Atrial fibrillation: most common arrhythmia associated with systemic embolization

TABLE 17-6. **HERNIAS**

HERNIA	DISCUSSION
Direct (see Fig. 17-24)	Single layer of transversalis is stretched in the floor of the triangle of Hesselbach Medial border of triangle is rectus sheath, lateral border is inferior epigastric artery, inferior border is inguinal ligament Hernia bulges through floor of triangle of Hesselbach; bulge disappears when patient reclines. Small bowel cannot enter scrotal sac; therefore, there is no obstruction or incarceration *Treatment*: sutured mesh covering inguinal canal and Hesselbach's triangle
Indirect (see Fig. 17-25)	Most common hernia Pathogenesis in children: persistence of peritoneal connection between inguinal canal and tunica vaginalis Pathogenesis in adults: protrusion of new peritoneal process into inguinal canal Small bowel passes through internal inguinal ring and may enter scrotal sac Bowel directly hits the examining finger within the inguinal canal Complications: entrapped in inguinal canal (incarceration) or strangulated obstruction (hemorrhagic infarction) *Treatment*: 　In children: high ligation of hernia sac at the level of the internal inguinal ring + tightening of the internal inguinal ring 　In adults: sutured mesh covering inguinal canal and Hesselbach's triangle
Femoral	Most common in women Bulge located below inguinal ligament Highest rate of incarceration of small bowel *Treatment*: transversalis fascia and conjoined tendon are sutured to Cooper's ligament
Umbilical	Most common hernia in adults with ascites, pregnancy, or obesity Most common hernia in black newborns Peritoneal protrusion extends into a fascial defect containing remnants of umbilical cord Majority close spontaneously by the second year Incarceration more likely in adults than children *Treatment*: surgery
Ventral	Hernia develops in weakened area of previous surgical excision Obesity most common cause

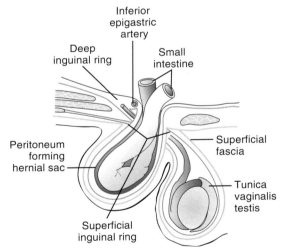

17-24: Schematic of direct inguinal hernia. See text for discussion. *(From Moore NA, Roy WA: Rapid Review Gross and Developmental Anatomy, 2nd ed. St. Louis, Mosby Elsevier, 2007, p 69, Fig. 3-5 A.)*

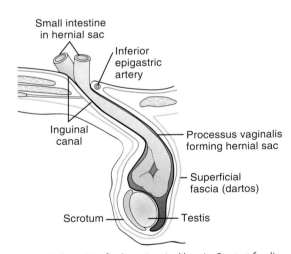

17-25: Schematic of indirect inguinal hernia. See text for discussion. *(From Moore NA, Roy WA: Rapid Review Gross and Developmental Anatomy, 2nd ed. St. Louis, Mosby Elsevier, 2007, p 69, Fig. 3-5B.)*

　　b. Nonocclusive ischemia (25% of cases)
　　　(1) Hypotension secondary to heart failure (most common)
　　　(2) Hypovolemic shock
　　　(3) Patient taking digitalis (? vasospasm)
　　c. Mesenteric vein thrombosis (25% of cases)
　　　(1) Thrombosis states
　　　　(a) Polycythemia vera
　　　　(b) Antiphospholipid syndrome

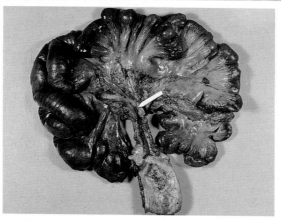

17-26: Hemorrhagic infarction of small bowel, showing the diffuse dark discoloration of the small bowel. Arrow shows a thrombosed superior mesenteric artery attached to the aorta. *(From Damjanov I, Linder J: Pathology: A Color Atlas. St. Louis, Mosby, 2000, p 124, Fig. 7-8.)*

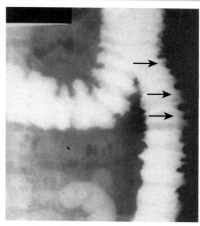

17-27: Single contrast barium enema showing "thumb-printing" of the colonic mucosa *(arrows)* in the region of the splenic flexure in ischemic colitis. *(From Grieg JD: Color Atlas of Surgical Diagnosis. London, Mosby-Wolfe, 1996, p 202, Fig. 26-9.)*

      (2) Extension of renal cell carcinoma into vena cava
  4. Clinical and radiographic findings of small bowel infarction
    a. Sudden onset of diffuse abdominal pain
      • Pain disproportionate to physical findings
    b. Bowel distention
    c. Bloody diarrhea
      • Usually occurs in an elderly patient
    d. Absent bowel sounds (ileus)
    e. *No* rebound tenderness (peritonitis) early in infarction
    f. Profound neutrophilic leukocytosis
    g. Positive stool guaiac
    h. Radiographic findings
      (1) "Thumbprint sign" due to edema in bowel wall
      (2) Bowel distention with air-fluid levels similar to bowel obstruction
    i. Abdominal CT scan has 90% sensitivity.
    j. Treatment
      (1) Surgery for embolic disease
      (2) Thrombotic disease
        • Anticoagulation and surgery if necessary
  5. Ischemic colitis
    a. Involves the splenic flexure of the large bowel
      • Watershed area (refer to Chapter 1)
    b. Atherosclerotic narrowing of SMA causes mesenteric angina.
      (1) Severe pain occurs in splenic flexure shortly after eating.
      (2) Patient loses weight for fear of pain related to eating.
    c. Clinical findings
      (1) History compatible with mesenteric angina
      (2) Pain localized to the splenic flexure
        • Accompanied by bloody diarrhea due to mucosal or mural infarction
      (3) Barium study shows "thumb-printing" of the colonic mucosa (Fig. 17-27).
        • Due to edema of the mucosa
    d. Normal repair of infarction site may result in fibrosis.
      • Common cause of ischemic strictures and obstruction
  6. Angiodysplasia
    a. Dilation of mucosal and submucosal venules in cecum and right colon (Fig. 17-28)
      (1) Usually occurs in elderly individuals
      (2) Vascular ectasias in the cecum increase with age.
    b. Increased wall stress in the cecum stretches the venules.
    c. Clinical findings
      (1) Hematochezia

Small bowel infarction: sudden onset diffuse abdominal pain, bloody diarrhea

Small bowel infarction: distention, absent bowel sounds, no rebound tenderness

Ischemic colitis: mesenteric angina after eating → fear of eating and weight loss

Ischemic colitis with infarction: mesenteric angina + bloody diarrhea

Angiodysplasia: dilation cecal submucosal venules; hematochezia

Angiodysplasia: second most common cause hematochezia

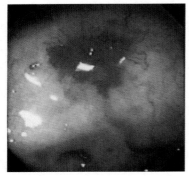

17-28: Colonoscopic view of the cecum showing an area of mucosal bleeding from a ruptured telangiectatic vessel in angiodysplasia. *(From Grieg JD: Color Atlas of Surgical Diagnosis. London, Mosby-Wolfe, 1996, p 202, Fig. 26-8.)*

      (2) Association with von Willebrand disease (vWD) and calcific aortic stenosis

    d. Diagnose with colonoscopy and angiography

    e. Treatment

      (1) Colonoscopy

        (a) Identifies lesions

        (b) Cautery of lesions

      (2) Angiography localizes the disease

      (3) Right hemicolectomy

      (4) Correction of aortic stenosis (if present)

        • Bleeding often abates

H. Small bowel diverticula

  1. Meckel diverticulum

    a. Vitelline (omphalomesenteric) duct remnant

      (1) True diverticulum (Fig. 17-29)

      (2) Mnemonic: 2 inches long, 2 feet from ileocecal valve, 2% of population, 2% symptomatic

    b. Contains pancreatic rests and heterotopic gastric mucosa

      • Increase the risk for bleeding

    c. Clinical findings

      (1) Newborn finding

        • Fecal material in umbilical area due to persistence of vitelline duct

      (2) Bleeding (most common finding)

        • Common cause of iron deficiency in newborns and young children

      (3) Diverticulitis

        • Clinically impossible to distinguish Meckel diverticulitis from appendicitis

    d. Diagnosis

      • ^{99m}Tc nuclear scan identifies parietal cells in ectopic gastric mucosa.

    e. Treatment is surgery.

  2. Small bowel pulsion diverticula

    a. Duodenum is most common site.

      • Wide-mouthed diverticula suggests systemic sclerosis.

Margin notes:

Angiodysplasia: association with vWD and calcific aortic stenosis

Newborn with fecal material in umbilical area: persistence of vitelline duct

Meckel diverticulum: bleeding most common complication

Meckel diverticulitis: mimics acute appendicitis

SB diverticula: duodenum most common site; diverticulitis, bacterial overgrowth

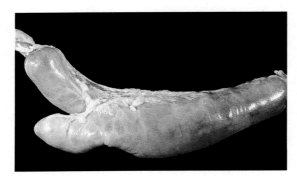

17-29: Meckel diverticulum located on the antimesenteric side of the small intestine. *(From Kumar V, Fausto N, Abbas A: Robbins and Cotran's Pathologic Basis of Disease, 7th ed. Philadelphia, WB Saunders, 2004, p 830, Fig. 17-31.)*

b. Complications
  (1) Diverticulitis (danger of perforation)
  (2) Bacterial overgrowth
    • May produce bile salt deficiency and vitamin B$_{12}$ deficiency

I. Sigmoid colon diverticular disease
  1. Epidemiology
    a. Incidence in general public is 35% to 50%
    b. Incidence increases with age
    c. Most common site for diverticula in entire gastrointestinal tract
  2. Pathogenesis

Sigmoid diverticular disease: constipation most common cause

    a. Due to a low-fiber diet with increased constipation
    b. Sigmoid colon most common site (Figs. 17-30 and 17-31)
    c. Area of weakness is where vasa recta penetrate the muscular propria.
      • Diverticulum is juxtaposed to a blood vessel.
    d. Associations
      (1) Marfan syndrome
      (2) Ehlers-Danlos syndrome
      (3) Adult polycystic kidney disease
  3. Clinical findings

Sigmoid diverticular disease: diverticulitis most common complication

    a. Diverticulitis is the most common complication.
      (1) Caused by stool impacted (fecalith) in diverticulum sac
        • Produces ulceration and ischemia
      (2) Clinical findings
        (a) Fever
        (b) Diarrhea initially followed by constipation
        (c) Left lower quadrant pain ("left-sided appendicitis")
        (d) Tender mass can be palpated in some cases

Sigmoid diverticulitis: "left-sided appendicitis"

Sigmoid diverticulitis: CT scan

      (3) Best diagnosed with CT scan or water-soluble barium study
      (4) Increased risk for perforation and abscess formation
    b. Diverticulosis
      • Painless bleeding; often massive (hematochezia)
  4. Other complications
    a. Most common cause of hematochezia
      (1) Refers to diverticulosis *not* diverticulitis
      (2) Scarring of the vessel in diverticulitis prevents bleeding.

Sigmoid diverticular disease: most common cause hematochezia and fistulas

    b. Most common cause of fistulas (connection between hollow structures)

Colovesical fistula (connection between large bowel and the bladder) is a common fistula in the gastrointestinal tract. It is associated with pneumaturia (air in urine) and recurrent urinary tract infections.

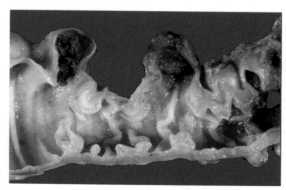

17-30: Gross section of sigmoid colon showing pulsion diverticula with fecal material (fecaliths). *(From Klatt E: Robbins and Cotran's Atlas of Pathology. Philadelphia, WB Saunders, 2006, p 183, Fig. 7-94.)*

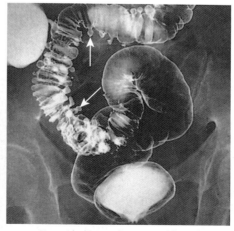

17-31: Sigmoid diverticulosis viewed on barium enema. Multiple diverticula sacs *(arrows)* are outlined by the double-contrast barium technique. *(From Forbes C, Jackson W: Color Atlas and Text of Clinical Medicine, 2nd ed. St. Louis, Mosby, 2003, p 382, Fig. 8-110.)*

5. Treatment
   a. Nonpharmacologic
      • Increase fiber in diet to prevent constipation
   b. Antibiotics for acute disease
   c. Colonic resection in selected cases
      • Examples—repeated episodes diverticulitis; bleeding that does not stop; abscess/fistula formation; obstruction

J. Inflammatory bowel disease
   1. Ulcerative colitis
      a. Most common inflammatory bowel disease
      b. Chronic relapsing ulceroinflammatory disease
      c. Ulcerations are in continuity (Fig. 17-32).
         • Ulcerations are limited to the mucosa and submucosa of rectum and colon (Fig. 17-33).
   2. Crohn's disease
      a. Chronic granulomatous, ulceroconstrictive disease
      b. Transmural inflammation (Fig. 17-34)
      c. Noncaseating granulomas (60% of cases; Fig. 17-35)
         • Discontinuous spread throughout entire gastrointestinal tract
   3. Indeterminate colitis (10%)
      • Features of ulcerative colitis and Crohn's disease
   4. Summary of ulcerative colitis and Crohn's disease (Table 17-7; see Figs. 17-32 to 17-35)

Ulcerative colitis: mucosal/submucosal ulcerations

Crohn's disease: transmural inflammation

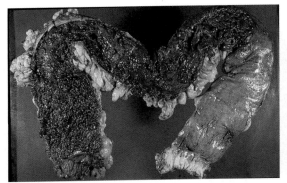

17-32: Ulcerative colitis. The colon shows diffuse ulceration of the mucosal surface and residual islands of inflamed mucosa (pseudopolyps). *(From Damjanov I: Pathology for the Health-Related Professions, 2nd ed. Philadelphia, WB Saunders, 2000, p 271, Fig. 10-10A.)*

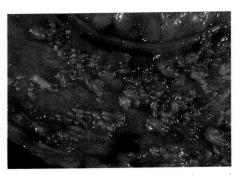

17-33: Ulcerative colitis. Note the linear ulcers and islands of residual mucosa called pseudopolyps. *(From Klatt E: Robbins and Cotran's Atlas of Pathology. Philadelphia, WB Saunders, 2006, p 179, Fig. 7-81.)*

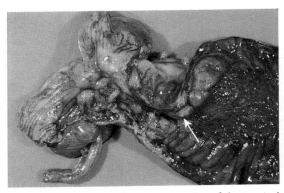

17-34: Crohn's disease, showing a resection of the terminal ileum with attached cecum and appendix; the appendix is to the left. The thickened terminal ileal wall causes the narrowing *(arrow)* at the junction of the ileum and the cecum. The ileal mucosa has a cobblestone appearance due to linear ulcerations (aphthous ulcers) that cut into the underlying submucosa. *(From Damjanov I: Pathology for the Health-Related Professions, 2nd ed. Philadelphia, WB Saunders, 2000, p 271, Fig. 10-10B.)*

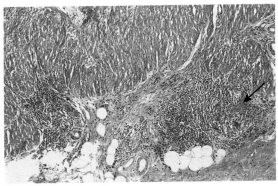

17-35: Crohn's disease. Note the inflammatory infiltrate in the muscle layer of the large intestine with occasional multinucleated giant cells *(arrow)* representing a granuloma. *(From Damjanov I, Linder J: Pathology: A Color Atlas. St. Louis, Mosby, 2000, p 134, Fig. 7-41.)*

K. Irritable bowel syndrome (IBS)
1. Epidemiology
   a. Intrinsic colonic motility disorder
      (1) Possible loss of tolerance to gastrointestinal flora
      (2) Possible genetic factors
      (3) Environmental triggers
   b. Most common functional bowel disorder
   c. Responsible for >50% of referrals to gastroenterologists
   d. Occurs more often in females than males
   e. Small bowel bacterial overgrowth may be present in some cases.
   f. Risk factors
      (1) History of childhood sexual abuse

IBS: intrinsic colonic motility disorder

IBS: most common functional bowel disorder

TABLE 17-7. COMPARISON OF ULCERATIVE COLITIS AND CROHN'S DISEASE

FEATURE	ULCERATIVE COLITIS (UC)	CROHN'S DISEASE (CD)
Epidemiology	More common in whites than blacks No sex predilection Occurs between 14 and 38 years of age Lower incidence in smokers and other nicotine users Lower incidence if previous appendectomy <20 years old	More common in whites than blacks, in Jews than non-Jews No sex predilection Smoking is a risk factor Majority (>75%) of cases occur between 11 and 35 years of age
Extent	Mucosal and submucosal	Transmural
Location	Mainly rectum (usually begins in this location) Extends continuously into left colon (may involve entire colon) Does *not* involve other areas of GI tract	Terminal ileum alone (30% of cases), ileum and colon (50% of cases), colon alone (20% of cases) (see Fig. 17-34) Involves other areas of GI tract (mouth to anus)
Gross features	Inflammatory pseudopolyps (see Figs. 17-32 and 17-33) Areas of friable, bloody residual mucosa Ulceration and hemorrhage	Thick bowel wall and narrow lumen (leads to obstruction) Aphthous ulcers in bowel (early sign) Skip lesions, strictures, fistulas Deep linear ulcers with cobblestone pattern Fat creeping around serosa
Microscopic features	Ulcers and crypt abscesses containing neutrophils Dysplasia or cancer may be present	Noncaseating granulomas (60% of cases), lymphoid aggregates (see Fig. 17-35) Dysplasia or cancer less likely
Clinical findings	Recurrent left-sided abdominal cramping with bloody diarrhea and mucus Fever, tenesmus, weight loss Extragastrointestinal: primary sclerosing cholangitis (UC > CD), erythema nodosum, iritis/uveitis (CD > UC), pyoderma gangrenosum, HLA-B27 positive arthritis. p-ANCA antibodies > 45% of cases	Recurrent right lower quadrant colicky pain (obstruction) with diarrhea Bleeding occurs only with colon or anal involvement (fistulas; abscesses) Apthous ulcers in mouth Extragastrointestinal: erythema nodosum, sacroiliitis (HLA-B27 association), pyoderma gangrenosum, iritis (CD > UC), primary sclerosing cholangitis (UC > CD)
Radiography	"Lead pipe" appearance in chronic disease	"String" sign in terminal ileum from luminal narrowing by inflammation, fistulas
Complications	Toxic megacolon (hypotonic and distended bowel) Adenocarcinoma: greatest risks are pancolitis, early onset, duration of disease > 10 years)	Fistulas, obstruction, colon cancer (UC > CD) Calcium oxalate renal calculi (increased reabsorption of oxalate through inflamed mucosa) Malabsorption due to bile salt deficiency Macrocytic anemia due to vitamin B_{12} deficiency
Treatment	Sulfasalazine or mesalamine (5-ASA active metabolite; O_2 free radical scavenger; inhibits lipoxygenase pathway in arachidonic acid metabolism) Corticosteroids for severe disease (systemically or enemas) Nicotine patch Immunosuppressants: azathioprine or cyclosporine Surgery: colectomy with ileostomy usually cures	Sulfasalazine or mesalamine (5-ASA; oral salicylate) Corticosteroids for moderate to severe disease Steroid analogues that target areas of GI tract (e.g., budesonide) Immunosuppressants: azathioprine or cyclosporine Metronidazole for colonic fistulas TNF inhibitors for enterocutaneous fistulas Surgery for obstruction, fistulas, toxic megacolon, refractory disease

ASA, aminosalicylic acid; GI, gastrointestinal; TNF, tumor necrosis factor.

  (2) Domestic abuse in women
  (3) Increased stress, depression, personality disorder
 2. Alternating bouts of diarrhea and constipation
  a. Abdominal pain and bloating relieved by defecation
  b. Stools accompanied by mucus
  c. Abnormal defecation
   (1) Straining
   (2) Sense of incomplete evacuation
 3. Normal flexible sigmoidoscopy/colonoscopy
 4. Treatment
  a. Nonpharmacologic
   (1) Mainstay is adequate fiber intake.
   (2) Eliminate foods that aggravate
    • Examples—coffee, fatty foods, dairy products
  b. Pharmacologic
   (1) Antispasmodics-anticholinergics
    • Example—dicyclomine
   (2) Loperamide is effective for diarrhea.
    • Serotonin type 3 receptor antagonist
   (3) Lubiprostone (chloride channel activator) is effective for constipation.
   (4) Rifaximin is effective if small bowel bacterial overgrowth is documented.

L. Small bowel malignancy
 • Small bowel is the *least* common site in the gastrointestinal tract for a primary malignancy.
 1. Primary adenocarcinoma
  • Duodenum most common site
 2. Carcinoid tumor
  a. Most common small bowel malignancy
  b. Neuroendocrine tumor
   (1) Contains neurosecretory granules visible on electron microscopy
   (2) Carcinoid tumors are malignant.
   (3) Metastatic potential correlates with size and depth.
    (a) Size > 2 cm
    (b) Depth of invasion (~50% of bowel thickness)
   (4) Foregut (e.g., stomach) and hindgut (e.g., rectum) carcinoid tumors
    • Invade but *rarely* metastasize
   (5) Midgut carcinoid tumors (e.g., terminal ileum)
    • Invade and metastasize
  c. Locations
   (1) Vermiform appendix (Fig. 17-36)
    (a) Most common site (40%)
    (b) Usually <2 cm, which is too small to metastasize to liver
   (2) Small bowel (20%)
    (a) Majority in terminal ileum
    (b) Commonly metastasize to liver
    (c) Tumor produces bioactive compounds (e.g., serotonin)
     • Compounds are delivered to the liver by the portal vein.

Margin notes:

IBS: alternating bouts constipation/diarrhea; increased mucus in stool

IBN: mainstay is adequate fiber intake

Small bowel: least common site for malignancy in GI tract

Carcinoid tumors: malignant neuroendocrine tumors

Vermiform appendix: most common site for carcinoid tumor

Carcinoid tumor terminal ileum: metastasis to liver causes carcinoid syndrome

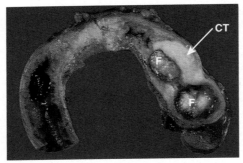

17-36: Carcinoid tumor (CT) of the vermiform appendix. Note the yellow mass in the wall of the appendix (*arrow*). The lumen contains fecaliths (F). *(From Grieg JD: Color Atlas of Surgical Diagnosis. London, Mosby-Wolfe, 1996, p 196, Fig. 25-20.)*

(d) Serotonin is metabolized to 5-hydroxyindoleacetic acid (5-HIAA).
- 5-HIAA is excreted in the urine.

(e) Serotonin is completely metabolized and does *not* enter the systemic circulation.
- No signs or symptoms of carcinoid syndrome

(3) Esophagus, stomach, colon collectively (10%)

d. Bright yellow tumor

e. Carcinoid syndrome

(1) For gut origins (e.g., terminal ileum) of the carcinoid tumor, liver metastasis *must* occur to produce the syndrome.

(a) Serotonin is secreted by metastatic tumor nodules.

(b) Serotonin entering hepatic vein tributaries gains access to the systemic circulation.

(c) May occur without metastasis if located in the bronchus (rare)

(2) Clinical findings

(a) Due to serotonin and other bioactive compounds (e.g., histamine, bradykinin)

(b) Flushing of the skin (75–90%)
- Due to vasodilation; may be triggered by emotion, alcohol, other foods

(c) Diarrhea (>70%)
- Increased bowel motility

(d) Intermittent wheezing and dyspnea (25%)
- Due to bronchospasm

(e) Facial telangiectasia

(f) Tricuspid regurgitation and pulmonary stenosis
- Serotonin increases collagen production in the valves.

(3) Diagnosis

(a) Increase in urine 5-HIAA

(b) CT scan of liver to detect metastasis

(c) Scanning techniques to detect primary location and metastasis

(4) Treatment

(a) Avoid alcohol

(b) Surgical resection of primary tumor

(c) Chemotherapy

(d) Somatostatin analogue
- Effective in controlling diarrhea and flushing

3. Malignant lymphoma

a. Usually occur in Peyer's patches of terminal ileum

b. Usually B-cell origin (e.g., Burkitt's lymphoma)

M. Small and large bowel polyps

1. Non-neoplastic (hamartomatous) polyps

a. Hyperplastic polyp

(1) Most common type in adults

(2) Majority are in the sigmoid colon.

(3) *No* malignant potential or polyposis syndromes

(4) Histologically have a "sawtooth" appearance

b. Juvenile (retention) polyps

(1) Most common polyp in children

(2) Located in the rectum
- Sometimes prolapse out of the rectum and bleed

(3) Solitary polyp
- Smooth surface with enlarged cystic spaces on cut section

(4) Juvenile polyposis
- Autosomal dominant or nonhereditary

(5) Cronkhite-Canada syndrome

(a) Nonhereditary polyposis syndrome

(b) Polyps plus ectodermal abnormalities of the nails

c. Peutz-Jeghers polyposis (PJP)

(1) Autosomal dominant

(2) Hamartomatous polyps predominate in the small bowel
- Less common in stomach and colon

(3) Clinical findings

(a) Mucosal pigmentation of buccal mucosa, lips (see Fig. 17-4)

Carcinoid tumor: bright yellow

Carcinoid syndrome: liver metastasis is necessary

Carcinoid syndrome: flushing, diarrhea, wheezing; ↑ urine 5-HIAA

Bowel primary lymphoma: usually in Peyer's patches in terminal ileum

Sigmoid colon: most common site for gastrointestinal polyps, diverticula, cancer

Hyperplastic polyp: most common polyp in adults

Juvenile polyp: most common polyp in children

Hyperplastic and juvenile polyps: no malignant potential

PJP: predominance small intestine polyps

PJP: ↑ risk colorectal, breast, gynecologic cancers

(b) Increased risk (>50%) for colorectal, breast, gynecologic cancers
- This is true even though the GI polyps are hamartomas.

2. Neoplastic polyps
- Called adenomas
a. Premalignant dysplastic colonic polyps
  (1) Increase with age
  (2) Equal sex incidence
b. Tubular adenoma (adenomatous polyps)
  (1) Most common polyp (60% of polyps)
  (2) Sigmoid colon is most common site.
  (3) Stalked polyp
     (a) Looks like a mushroom (Fig. 17-37)
     (b) Sections show complex branching of glands (adenomatous change) (see Fig. 8-1A).
c. Tubulovillous adenoma (20–30% of polyps)
  (1) Usually stalked polyp
  (2) Adenomatous and villous change (similar to small bowel villi)
d. Villous adenoma (10% of polyps)
  (1) Sessile polyp (no stalk) with primarily a villous component (Fig. 17-38)
  (2) Rectosigmoid location
  (3) Secrete protein and potassium-rich mucus
     - Can produce hypoalbuminemia and hypokalemia
e. Risk factors for malignancy in adenomas
  (1) Adenoma > 2 cm (40% risk of malignancy)
  (2) Multiple polyps
  (3) Polyps with increased villous component
     - Villous adenomas have a 30% to 40% risk for malignancy.
f. Familial polyposis (FP; Fig. 17-39)
  (1) Autosomal dominant (AD)
     (a) All patients develop tubular adenomas and cancer.
     (b) Polyps begin to develop between 10 and 20 years of age.
  (2) Pathogenesis
     - Inactivation of adenomatous polyposis coli (APC) suppressor gene
  (3) Clinical findings
     (a) Malignant transformation usually occurs between 35 and 40 years of age.
        - Prophylactic colectomy is recommended.
     (b) Associated with congenital hypertrophy of retinal pigment epithelium
  (4) Gardner's syndrome
     (a) AD polyposis syndrome
     (b) Additional findings include benign osteomas and desmoid tumors.
  (5) Turcot's polyposis syndrome
     (a) Autosomal recessive (AR) polyposis syndrome

Tubular adenoma: most common neoplastic polyp

Villous adenoma: may cause hypoproteinemia and hypokalemia

Villous adenoma: greatest risk for developing colon cancer

FP: AD; all patients develop colon cancer; complete penetrance

Gardner's syndrome: AD; colon cancer; benign osteomas, desmoid tumors

Turcot's syndrome: AR; colon cancer; brain tumors

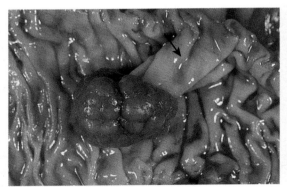

17-37: Tubular adenoma. The head of the stalked polyp has a lobulated, mushroom-like appearance. *Arrow* points to the stalk. *(From Damjanov I, Linder J: Pathology: A Color Atlas. St. Louis, Mosby, 2000, p 138, Fig. 7-55.)*

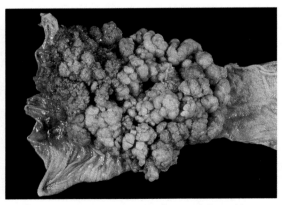

17-38: Villous adenoma. Note the large cauliflower-like mass in the rectosigmoid. These tumors secrete mucus rich in potassium and protein. *(From Rosai J, Ackerman LV: Surgical Pathology, 9th ed. St. Louis, Mosby, 2004, p 803, Fig. 11-197A.)*

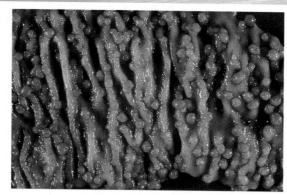

17-39: Familial polyposis. Note the numerous small, sessile polyps. These were present in the entire large bowel. *(From Rosai J, Ackerman LV: Surgical Pathology, 9th ed. St. Louis, Mosby, 2004, p 802, Fig. 11-195.)*

(b) Additional finding of malignant brain tumors
  • Astrocytoma and medulloblastoma

N. Colon cancer
1. Epidemiology
   a. Third most common cancer-related death in adults
   b. Third most common cancer in men and women
   c. Incidence rates have been decreasing.
      • Increase in screening (fecal occult blood test, colonoscopy)
   d. Peak incidence is in the seventh decade.
   e. Rectal cancers
      • Approximately 50% are detected by digital rectal examination.
   f. Colon cancers
      • Approximately 50% are detected by flexible sigmoidoscopy.
   g. Risk factors for colon cancer
      (1) Age > 50 years old
      (2) Cigarette smoking
      (3) Obesity, physical inactivity, heavy alcohol intake
      (4) Hereditary polyposis syndromes (see later)
      (5) Hereditary nonpolyposis colon cancer (refer to Chapter 8)
      (6) Family cancer syndrome (refer to Chapter 8)
      (7) First-degree relatives with colon cancer
      (8) Inflammatory bowel disease
         • Ulcerative colitis > Crohn's disease
      (9) Dietary factors
         • Low-fiber diet; increased saturated fats; reduced vegetable intake
2. Carcinogenesis of colon cancer
   a. Adenoma-carcinoma sequence
      (1) Sequential mutations of different genes
         • *APC, RAS, TP53*
      (2) Accounts for 80% of sporadic colon cancers
   b. Inactivation of DNA mismatch genes (refer to Chapter 8)
3. Locations for colon cancer
   a. Rectosigmoid (50% of cases)
   b. Ascending colon (15% of cases)
   c. Descending colon (15% of cases)
   d. Transverse colon and cecum (each 10% of cases)
4. Screening tests for colon cancer
   a. Fecal occult blood test (FOBT)
      (1) *Not* very sensitive or specific for colon cancer
         • Does *not* distinguish hemoglobin from myoglobin
      (2) Tests are based on the peroxidase activity of heme in Hb.
         • Myoglobin also has peroxidase activity.
      (3) Peroxidase catalyzes the oxidation of a reagent (guaiac) by peroxide.
         • Reaction produces a color change.

Colon cancer: third most common cancer in men and women

Colon cancer: third most common cancer killer in adults

Rectosigmoid: most common site for colon cancer

FOBT: most do not distinguish hemoglobin from myoglobin

b. Varying levels of sensitivity and specificity
   (1) False positive results
       (a) Myoglobin in meat
       (b) Plant peroxidases (e.g., radishes)
   (2) False negative results
   (3) Newer tests detect hemoglobin
c. Colonoscopy (gold standard)
   (1) Start at age 50 if no risk factors
   (2) Every 3 to 5 years if history of polyp removal
   (3) Begin at age 40 if first-degree relative has polyps or colorectal cancer
d. Barium enema

5. Clinical findings in colon cancer
   a. Left-sided cancers
      (1) Tend to obstruct
          (a) Bowel diameter is smaller than right colon.
          (b) Lesions have an annular, "napkin-ring" appearance (Figs. 17-40 and 17-41).
      (2) Change in bowel habits
          (a) Constipation and diarrhea with or without bleeding
          (b) Bright red blood coats the stool
      (3) *Streptococcus bovis* endocarditis (refer to Chapter 10)
   b. Right-sided cancers
      (1) Tend to bleed
          (a) Bowel diameter is greater than left colon.
          (b) Tumors are more polypoid in appearance.
      (2) Blood is mixed in with stool.
      (3) Iron deficiency is more likely than in left-sided cancer.

6. Sites of metastasis for colon cancer
   • Liver (most common), lungs, bone, and brain

7. Prevention
   a. Aspirin and other NSAIDs
      • Decreases incidence of colorectal adenomas
   b. Annual fecal occult blood testing
   c. Estrogens and progestins
      • May reduce colorectal cancer risk
   d. Dietary alterations
      (1) Decrease fat intake to 30% of total caloric intake

Left-sided colon cancer: tend to obstruct; small diameter

Right-sided colon cancer: tend to bleed; large diameter; iron deficiency

Prevention: aspirin, FOBT, dietary alterations, stop smoking

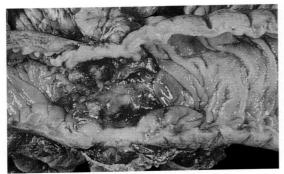

17-40: Adenocarcinoma of the sigmoid colon. Resection of the rectosigmoid shows an annular and ulcerating growth, causing a stricture. *(From Damjanov I, Linder J: Pathology: A Color Atlas. St. Louis, Mosby, 2000, p 139, Fig. 7-61.)*

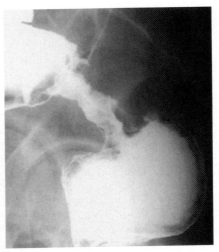

17-41: Spot radiograph from a single contrast phase of a double contrast barium enema showing an adenocarcinoma of the rectum with circumferential narrowing of the lumen ("apple core" lesion). *(From Pretorius ES, Solomon JA. Radiology Secrets, 2nd ed. St. Louis, Mosby, 2006, p 125, Fig. 15-9.)*

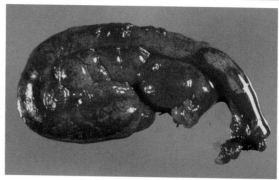

17-42: Acute appendicitis showing erythema and vascular congestion of the serosal surface of the appendix. *(From Damjanov I, Linder J: Pathology: A Color Atlas. St. Louis, Mosby, 2000, p 131, Fig. 7-30.)*

Acute appendicitis: most common abdominal surgical emergency

Acute diverticulitis and appendicitis have the same pathogenesis.

Pain in acute appendicitis: initially periumbilical and then shifts to RLQ

C fibers: refer to midline

Acute appendicitis: pain precedes nausea and vomiting

Aδ fibers: localize pain

      (2) Increase fiber
      (3) Increase intake of fruits and vegetables
    e. ? Statins
      • May inhibit growth of colon cancer lines
    f. Cessation of smoking
  8. Treatment
    • Surgery, chemotherapy, targeted monoclonal antibody therapies
  9. Prognosis
    a. Five-year relative survival rate ~65%
    b. Serum carcinoembryonic antigen (CEA) is used to detect recurrences.

O. Acute appendicitis (Fig. 17-42)
  1. Epidemiology
    a. Occurs in 10% of the population
    b. Most common abdominal surgical emergency
  2. Pathogenesis in children
    a. Lymphoid hyperplasia (60% of cases) often secondary to a viral infection
    b. Examples—adenovirus, measles virus infection or immunization
  3. Pathogenesis in adults
    a. Fecalith obstructs the proximal lumen
      • Increased intraluminal pressure causes mucosal injury and bacterial invasion.
    b. Other causes
      • Seeds (sunflower, persimmons), pinworm infection
    c. Primary pathogens are *Escherichia coli* (most common) and *Bacteroides fragilis.*
  4. Clinical findings in sequence
    a. Initial colicky periumbilical pain (50%)
      (1) Irritation of unmyelinated afferent C fibers on visceral peritoneal surface
      (2) Refer pain to the midline
    b. Fever
      • Very important sign for identifying appendicitis in children with abdominal pain
    c. Nausea, vomiting, and fever
      • Pain *precedes* nausea and vomiting
    d. Cutaneous hyperesthesia at level of T12
    e. Pain shifts to right lower quadrant (RLQ) in 12 to 18 hours.
      (1) Irritation of Aδ fibers on parietal peritoneum
        • Localizes pain to the exact location
      (2) Rebound tenderness at McBurney's point (Blumberg's sign)
      (3) Pain with right thigh extension (psoas sign)
      (4) RLQ pain with palpation of left lower quadrant (Rovsing's sign)
    f. Signs of a lower urinary tract infection may occur.
      (1) Increased frequency
      (2) Dysuria
    g. Laboratory findings
      (1) Neutrophilic leukocytosis with left shift (90%)
      (2) Abnormal urinalysis:
        • Increased protein, hematuria, pyuria

5. Retrocecal appendicitis
   a. Radiograph shows a sentinel loop in the RLQ
   b. Localized ileus (lack of motility) from subjacent appendicitis

6. Complications
   a. Periappendiceal abscess with or without perforation
      (1) Most common complication
      (2) May develop subphrenic abscess
         • Usually due to *Bacteroides fragilis*
   b. Pyelophlebitis
      (1) Infection of the portal vein
      (2) Danger of portal vein thrombosis
      (3) Radiograph shows gas in the portal vein.
   c. Subphrenic abscess
      (1) Persistent fever postoperative
      (2) Diaphragm fixed on the right; right-sided pleural effusion
      (3) Tenderness over lateral seventh and eighth ribs
      (4) Diagnosis
         • Ultrasound, CT scan, gallium scan
      (5) Treatment
         • Extraperitoneal drainage and antibiotics

7. Diagnosis of acute appendicitis
   a. Clinical examination
   b. Spiral CT RLQ after Gastrografin enema
      • Sensitivity 90% and specificity 94%
   c. Plain CT scan with rectal contrast agent
   d. Ultrasonography
      • Sensitivity 75% and specificity 90%

8. Treatment
   a. Appendectomy
   b. Cefoxitin
      • Given prophylactically perioperatively if perforation suspected

Many disorders mimic appendicitis. These disorders include viral gastroenteritis, ruptured follicular cyst, ruptured ectopic pregnancy, mesenteric lymphadenitis, and Meckel's diverticulitis.

V. **Anorectal Disorders**
   A. **Signs and symptoms of anorectal disease**
      1. Bleeding
         a. Internal hemorrhoids (painless)
         b. Anorectal cancer
         c. Infection
         d. Fissure
      2. Pain
         a. Anal fissure
         b. Thrombosed external hemorrhoids
      3. Pruritus (e.g., pinworms)
      4. Anal fistula (e.g., Crohn's disease)
   B. **Disorders**
      1. Internal hemorrhoids
         a. Dilated superior hemorrhoidal veins in mucosa and submucosa
            • Located above the pectinate line (superior plexus)
         b. Causes
            (1) Straining at stool (most common)
               • Often associated with constipation, low-fiber diet
            (2) Pregnancy
            (3) Obesity
            (4) Anal intercourse
            (5) Portal hypertension
         c. Clinical findings
            (1) Often prolapse out of the rectum (Fig. 17-43)

Retrocecal appendicitis: sentinel loop

Acute appendicitis: periappendiceal abscess most common complication

Pyelophlebitis: inflammation of portal vein

Subphrenic abscess: persistent fever postoperative

Acute appendicitis diagnosis: spiral CT or plain CT with rectal contrast

Anorectal bleeding: internal hemorrhoids most common cause

Internal hemorrhoids: straining at stool; painless bleeding

Internal hemorrhoids: commonly prolapse out of the rectum

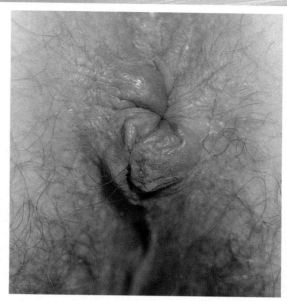

17-43: Prolapsed internal hemorrhoids. *(From Swartz MH: Textbook of Physical Diagnosis, 5th ed. Philadelphia, Saunders Elsevier, 2006, p 510, Fig. 17-33.)*

      (2) Commonly pass bright red blood with stool
        (a) Blood coats the stool.
        (b) Painless bleeding

> In an adult, never assume that blood coating stool is always due to an internal hemorrhoid. Other causes include colorectal and anal cancer; therefore, further investigation is necessary.

Internal hemorrhoids: anal pruritus, soiling of underwear

      (3) Anal pruritus and soiling of underwear
    d. Treatment
      (1) Nonpharmacologic
        • High-fiber diet; warm soaks/sitz baths; avoid prolonged sitting or stooling
      (2) Pharmacologic
        (a) Topical hydrocortisone
        (b) Stool softeners
    e. Surgical
      (1) Rubber-band ligation (best overall), sclerotherapy, infrared photocoagulation
      (2) Hemorrhoidectomy
        • Overall most effective, but most painful

External hemorrhoids: painful thrombosis inferior hemorrhoidal veins

  2. External hemorrhoids
    a. Dilated inferior hemorrhoidal veins
      • Located below the pectinate line (inferior plexus)
    b. Painful thrombosis
    c. Causes and treatment
      • See preceding internal hemorrhoid discussion
  3. Rectal prolapse
    a. Intussusception of the rectum through the anus
      • Due to weak rectal support mechanisms

Rectal prolapse in children < 2 years old: whooping cough, trichuriasis, cystic fibrosis

    b. Causes in children < 2 years old
      (1) Whooping cough
      (2) Trichuriasis
      (3) Common sign of cystic fibrosis

Rectal prolapse in elderly: straining at stool

    c. Common in the elderly
      • Due to straining at stool
    d. May occur with heavy squats in power lifters

Pilonidal sinus/abscess: painful mass in deep gluteal fold

  4. Pilonidal sinus and abscess
    a. Excess hair in a deep gluteal fold
      • Becomes traumatically buried into a sinus

b. Painful sacrococcygeal mass with purulent drainage
c. Treatment
    (1) Incision and drainage first episode
    (2) Chronic disease
        • Marsupialization—wide excision and wound left open
5. Pruritus ani
  a. Epidemiology
    (1) More common in males than females
    (2) Occurs in 1% to 5% of population
  b. Numerous causes
    (1) Anorectal diseases
        • Internal hemorrhoids (common), fissures, anal incontinence, diarrhea, cancer
    (2) Infections
        • Pinworm, *Candida*, venereal diseases
    (3) Local irritants
        • Soap, underwear, obesity, coffee, beer, acidic foods
    (4) Dermatologic disease
        • Psoriasis, atopic dermatitis
    (5) Diabetes mellitus

> Pruritus ani: internal hemorrhoids, diabetes, pinworm

6. Anorectal fistulas
  a. Epidemiology
    (1) Common in all ages
    (2) Associated with constipation
    (3) Pediatric population
      (a) More common in infants
      (b) Boys > girls
    (4) Etiology
      (a) Nonspecific cryptoglandular infection most common
      (b) Inflammatory bowel disease
        • Crohn's disease > ulcerative colitis
      (c) Trauma
        • Episiotomy, prostatectomy, anal intercourse
      (d) Malignancy
        • Anal carcinoma, treatment for anal carcinoma
  b. Treatment is surgery.

> Anorectal fistula: Crohn's disease, cryptoglandular infection

7. Anal fissures
  a. Epidemiology
    • Accounts for >10% of anal complaints
  b. Pathophysiology
    (1) Firm bowel movements
        • Once formed, perpetuated by bowel movements
    (2) Associated and perpetuated by spasm of the internal sphincter
  c. Clinical
    (1) Posterior (90%) fissure and/or ulcer between anal verge and dentate line
        • Consider Crohn's disease if not in this location
    (2) Anal tag at anal verge marks its location.
    (3) Prominent proximal papilla
  d. Treatment
    (1) Nitroglycerin ointment
    (2) Botulinum toxin injection of anal sphincter
    (3) Surgery

> Anal fissure: most posteriorly located; anal tag marks location

8. Anal carcinoma
  a. Basaloid (epidermoid or cloacogenic) carcinoma
    (1) Most common type
    (2) Located in the transitional zone above the dentate line
    (3) Female dominant
    (4) Treatment is surgery.
  b. Squamous cell carcinoma
    (1) Located in the anal canal
    (2) Majority occur in men who have sex with men.
        • HPV 16 and 18 association
    (3) Treatment is surgery.

> Anal carcinoma: basaloid carcinoma most common

> Anal carcinoma: squamous cancer has HPV 16 and 18 relationship

I. Laboratory Evaluation of Liver Cell Injury

A. Bilirubin metabolism and jaundice

1. Bilirubin metabolism (Fig. 18-1)
   a. Unconjugated bilirubin (UCB)
      (1) Senescent RBCs are phagocytosed by splenic macrophages.
      (2) UCB is the end-product of heme degradation.
         • UCB is lipid-soluble (indirect bilirubin).
   b. UCB combines with albumin in the blood.
      (1) UCB is taken up by hepatocytes.
      (2) UCB is conjugated to glucuronic acid to produce conjugated bilirubin (CB).
         • CB is water soluble (direct bilirubin).
   c. CB is secreted into the intrahepatic bile ducts.
      (1) Temporarily stored in the gallbladder
      (2) Enters the duodenum via the common bile duct
   d. Intestinal bacteria convert CB to urobilinogen (UBG).
      (1) UBG is spontaneously oxidized to urobilin.
      (2) Urobilin produces the brown color of stool.
   e. Approximately 20% of UBG is recycled to the liver (90%) and kidneys (10%).
      • Color of urine is due to urobilin.
2. Jaundice
   a. Jaundice is due to an increase in UCB and/or CB.
      (1) Jaundice is first noticed in the sclera (Fig. 18-2).
      (2) Sclera has a high affinity for bilirubin.
   b. Classification of causes of jaundice is based on the percentage of CB (Table 18-1).
      • Percent CB = CB/total bilirubin
   c. Common causes of jaundice (Box 18-1)

B. Summary of liver function tests (Table 18-2)

C. Summary of laboratory findings in selective liver disorders (Table 18-3)

II. Viral Hepatitis

A. Phases of acute viral hepatitis

1. Prodrome
   a. Fever
   b. Painful hepatomegaly; distaste for alcohol/cigarettes
   c. Serum transaminases increase steadily.
      • Peak just *before* jaundice occurs
   d. Atypical lymphocytosis
2. Jaundice
   a. Variable finding depending on the type of hepatitis
   b. Increased urine bilirubin and urine UBG
3. Recovery
   • Jaundice resolves.

B. Microscopic findings in acute viral hepatitis

1. Lymphocytic infiltrate with destruction of hepatocytes (see Fig. 2-9)
   • Apoptosis of hepatocytes (Councilman bodies; see Fig. 1-12)

Margin notes:

UCB: end-product of heme degradation in splenic macrophages

UCB: lipid soluble

CB: glucuronic acid makes bilirubin water soluble

Intestinal bacteria: convert CB → UBG

UBG: 20% recycled to liver and kidneys

Urobilin: color of stool and urine

Viral hepatitis: most common cause of jaundice

Gilbert's disease: 2nd most common cause of jaundice; fasting unconjugated hyperbilirubinemia

Phases acute hepatitis: prodrome, jaundice, recovery

Transaminases: peak before jaundice

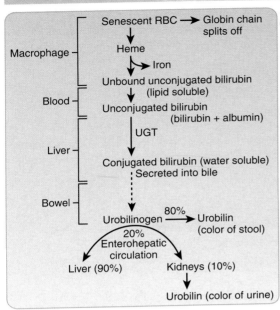

18-1: Bilirubin metabolism. Refer to the text for discussion. RBC, red blood cell; UGT, uridine glucuronosyltransferase.

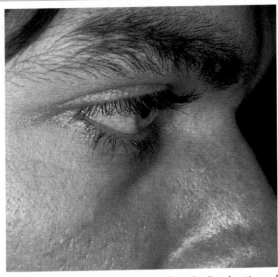

18-2: Scleral icterus. Note the yellowish discoloration of the sclera. *(From Savin J, Hunter JA, Hepburn NC: Diagnosis in Color: Skin Signs in Clinical Medicine. London, Mosby-Wolfe, 1997, Fig. 6.28.)*

TABLE 18-1. **CAUSES OF JAUNDICE**

TYPE OF HYPERBILIRUBINEMIA	URINE BILIRUBIN	URINE UBG	EXAMPLES OF DISORDERS
UCB < 20%			
Increased production of UCB	Absent	↑	Extravascular hemolytic anemias: e.g., spherocytosis, Rh and ABO HDN, warm AIHA
Decreased uptake or conjugation of UCB	Absent	Normal	Gilbert's syndrome (familial nonhemolytic jaundice): common AR or AD defect (depends on the type of mutation); occurs in >5% of population); second most common jaundice (hepatitis most common); most common hereditary cause of jaundice; males > females; impaired glucuronyl transferase activity (70–75% decrease in activity); jaundice occurs with fasting or increase in alcohol or phenobarbital intake; serum UCB rarely >5 mg/dL; all other liver function tests are normal; liver biopsy *not* necessary; no treatment required Crigler-Najjar syndromes: genetic disorders with decreased to absent glucuronyl transferase enzyme; type with no enzymes is incompatible with life (liver transplantation necessary) Physiologic jaundice of newborn: begins on day 3 of life; caused by normal macrophage destruction of fetal RBCs and inability of newborn liver to handle excess load Breast milk jaundice: due to pregnane-3α,20α-diol; does *not* require treatment
Mixed			
CB 20–50%	↑	↑	Viral hepatitis: defect in uptake, conjugation of UCB, and secretion of CB
Obstructive			

CB > 50%	↑	Absent	Decreased intrahepatic bile flow
			  Drug-induced (e.g., OCP)
			  Primary biliary cirrhosis
			  Dubin-Johnson syndrome: AR disorder in secretion into intrahepatic bile ducts; black pigment in hepatocytes
			  Rotor's syndrome: AR disorder similar to Dubin-Johnson syndrome but without black pigment in hepatocytes
			Decreased extrahepatic bile flow
			  Gallstone in common bile duct
			  Carcinoma of head of pancreas

AD, autosomal dominant; AIHA, autoimmune hemolytic anemia; AR, autosomal recessive; CB, conjugated bilirubin; HDN, hemolytic disease of newborn; OCP, oral contraceptive pill; UBG, urobilinogen; UCB, unconjugated bilirubin.

BOX 18-1   COMMON CAUSES OF JAUNDICE

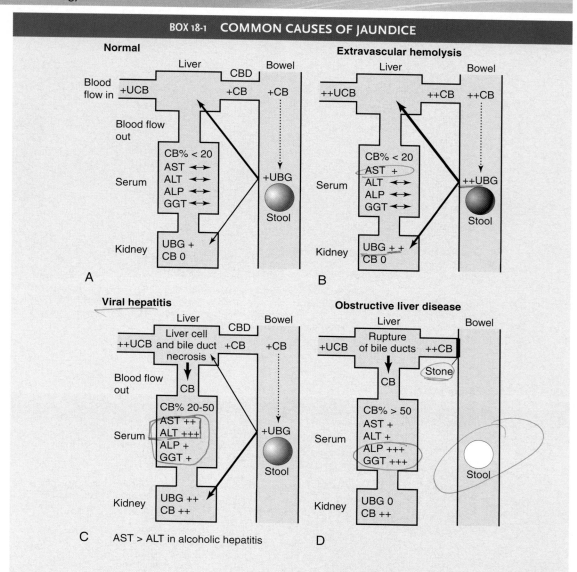

Normal

Extravascular hemolysis

Viral hepatitis

AST > ALT in alcoholic hepatitis

Obstructive liver disease

In this discussion, the symbol (+) is used to indicate degrees of magnitude. **Normal bilirubin metabolism (A)** shows liver uptake of lipid-soluble unconjugated bilirubin (UCB) and its conjugation with glucuronic acid to produce water-soluble conjugated bilirubin (CB). CB is secreted into the common bile duct (CBD) and is emptied into the bowel. Intestinal bacteria convert CB to urobilinogen (UBG), which spontaneously oxidizes to the pigment urobilin. Urobilin is responsible for the color of stool. A small percentage of UBG is reabsorbed into the blood. Most of it enters the liver (*larger arrow*) and a small percentage (*smaller arrow*) enters the urine (UBG). Urobilin is responsible for the color of urine. All of the normal bilirubin in blood is UCB (CB% < 20%) primarily derived from macrophage destruction of senescent RBCs. UCB does *not* enter urine, because it is attached to albumin in the blood and is lipid, *not* water, soluble. CB is *never* a normal finding in urine because it does *not* have contact with blood in its metabolism.

In **extravascular hemolysis (B)** (e.g., hereditary spherocytosis), there is increased macrophage production of UCB causing an increase in serum UCB (++) (CB% < 20%). There is a corresponding increase in uptake and conjugation of UCB, conjugation to CB (++), and conversion of CB in the bowel to UBG (++). This causes darkening of the stool. There is a greater percentage of UBG recycled back to the liver (*wider arrow*) and urine (*wider arrow*). The increase in urine UBG (++), darkens the color of urine. Because RBCs contain the enzyme aspartate aminotransferase (AST), hemolysis of RBCs causes an increase in serum AST. Alanine aminotransferase (ALT), alkaline phosphatase (ALP), and γ-glutamyltransferase (GGT) levels are normal.

In **viral hepatitis (C)**, there is generalized liver dysfunction involving uptake and conjugation of UCB, secretion of CB into bile ducts, and recycling of UBG. Serum UCB is increased (++) owing to a decrease in uptake and conjugation. Serum and urine CB are increased (++) because of liver cell necrosis and disruption of bile ductules between hepatocytes. Urine UBG is increased (++) because UBG is redirected from the liver (*smaller arrow*) to the kidneys (*larger arrow*). Because there is an increase in serum UCB and CB, there is a

BOX 18-1   COMMON CAUSES OF JAUNDICE—cont'd

mixed hyperbilirubinemia with a CB% of 20% to 50%. In viral hepatitis, aLT is higher (+++) than AST (++) and there is a slight increase in ALP and GGT (+). In alcoholic hepatitis, AST is greater than ALT, because alcohol damages mitochondria, which is where AST is normally located.

In **obstructive liver disease (D)**, an increase in serum and urine CB (++) is due to obstruction of intrahepatic or extrahepatic bile flow (stone in the CBD in this case). This causes increased pressure in the intrahepatic bile ductules leading to rupture and egress of CB into sinusoidal blood. There is absence of UBG in the stool (light-colored) and urine. CB% > 50% and there is a marked increase in serum ALP and GGT (+++) and only a slight increase in serum AST and ALT (+).

TABLE 18-2. LIVER FUNCTION TESTS

TEST	DISCUSSION
Liver Cell Necrosis	
Serum alanine transaminase (ALT)	Specific enzyme for liver cell necrosis Present in the cytosol ALT > AST: viral hepatitis
Serum aspartate transaminase (AST)	Present in mitochondria Alcohol damages mitochondria: AST > ALT indicates alcoholic hepatitis
Cholestasis	
Serum γ-glutamyltransferase (GGT)	Intra- or extrahepatic obstruction to bile flow Induction of cytochrome P-450 system (e.g., alcohol): increases GGT
Serum alkaline phosphatase (ALP)	Normal GGT and increased ALP: source of ALP other than liver (e.g., osteoblastic activity in bone) Increased GGT and ALP: liver cholestasis
Bilirubin Excretion	
CB < 20%	Unconjugated hyperbilirubinemia: e.g., extravascular hemolytic anemias
CB 20–50%	Mixed hyperbilirubinemia (e.g., viral hepatitis)
CB > 50%	Conjugated hyperbilirubinemia (e.g., liver cholestasis)
Urine bilirubin	Bilirubinuria: viral hepatitis, intra- or extrahepatic obstruction of bile ducts
Urine UBG	Increased urine UBG: extravascular hemolytic anemias, viral hepatitis Absent urine UBG: liver cholestasis
Hepatocyte Function	
Serum albumin	Albumin is synthesized by the liver Hypoalbuminemia: severe liver disease (e.g., cirrhosis)
Prothrombin time (PT)	Majority of coagulation factors are synthesized in the liver Increased PT: severe liver disease
Blood urea nitrogen (BUN)	Urea cycle is present in the liver Decreased serum BUN: cirrhosis
Serum ammonia	Ammonia is metabolized in the urea cycle in the liver Derives from large bowel and amino acid degradation Increased serum ammonia: cirrhosis, Reye syndrome
Immune Function	
Serum IgM	Increased in primary biliary cirrhosis
Antimitochondrial antibody	Primary biliary cirrhosis
Anti–smooth muscle antibody	Autoimmune hepatitis
Antinuclear antibody (ANA)	Autoimmune hepatitis
Tumor Marker	
α-Fetoprotein (AFP)	Hepatocellular carcinoma

CB, conjugated bilirubin; UBG, urobilinogen.

2. Persistent inflammation and fibrosis is an unfavorable sign.
   • Sign of chronic hepatitis progressing to postnecrotic cirrhosis
C. Epidemiology of viral hepatitis (Table 18-4)
D. Serologic studies in viral hepatitis
   1. Hepatitis A virus (HAV)
      a. Anti-HAV-IgM indicates active infection.

Hepatitis A: most common viral cause of jaundice

HAV: anti-HAV-IgM indicates infection; anti-HAV-IgG indicates recovery/vaccination

TABLE 18-3. SUMMARY OF LABORATORY FINDINGS IN SELECTED LIVER DISORDERS

DISEASE	% CB	AST	ALT	ALP	GGT	UB	URINE UBG
Normal						Absent	↑
Viral hepatitis	20–50%	↑↑↑	↑↑↑↑	↑	↑	↑↑	↑↑
Alcoholic hepatitis	20–50%	↑↑	↑	↑	↑↑↑	↑↑	↑↑
Cholestasis	>50%	↑	↑↑	↑↑↑	↑↑↑	↑↑↑	Absent
Extravascular hemolysis	<20%	↑↑ RBCs	N	N	N	Absent	↑↑

Arrows represent degree of magnitude.
ALP, alkaline phosphatase; ALT, alanine aminotransferase; AST, aspartate aminotransferase; CB, conjugated bilirubin; GGT, γ-glutamyltransferase; UB, urine bilirubin; UBG, urobilinogen.
From Goljan EF, Sloka KI: Rapid Review Laboratory Testing in Clinical Medicine. St. Louis, Mosby, 2008, Table 9-20, p 312.

Extravascular hemolysis: ↑↑ UBG, no UB

HBsAg: first antigen to arrive and last one to leave with recovery

HBeAg and HBV-DNA: infective particles

Anti-HBc-IgM: only marker present during window phase

Anti-HBc-IgG: present after 6 months

Anti-HBs: protective antibody; immunization or recovery from past infection

HBsAg > 6 months defines chronic HBV

"Healthy" carrier: HBsAg, anti-HBc-IgG

Infective carrier: HBsAg, HBeAg, HBV-DNA, anti-HBc-IgG

  b. Anti-HAV-IgG indicates recovery from infection or vaccination.
    • Protective antibody
2. Hepatitis B virus (HBV) (Fig. 18-3 and Table 18-5)
  a. Hepatitis B surface antigen (HBsAg)
    (1) Appears within 2 to 8 weeks after exposure
      • First marker of infection
    (2) Persists up to 4 months in acute hepatitis
      • HBsAg longer than 6 months defines chronic HBV.
  b. Hepatitis B e antigen (HBeAg) and HBV-DNA
    (1) Infective particles
    (2) Appear *after* HBsAg and disappear *before* HBsAg
  c. Anti-HBV core antibody IgM (anti-HBc-IgM)
    (1) Nonprotective antibody
      • Remains positive in acute infections
    (2) Persists during "window phase" or "serologic gap"
      • HBsAg, HBV DNA, and HBeAg are absent.
    (3) Converts entirely to anti-HBc-IgG by 6 months
  d. Anti-HBV surface antibody (anti-HBs)
    (1) Protective antibody
    (2) Marker of immunization after HBV vaccination
  e. Chronic HBV
    (1) Persistence of HBsAg longer than 6 months
      • Anti-HBc-IgM converts to anti-HBc-IgG.
    (2) "Healthy" chronic carrier
      (a) Presence of HBsAg and anti-HBc-IgG
      (b) Absence of DNA and e antigen
      (c) Still contagious but at a much lower risk
    (3) Infective chronic carrier
      (a) Presence of HBsAg, anti-HBc-IgG, and infective particles (DNA and e antigen)
      (b) Increased risk for postnecrotic cirrhosis and hepatocellular carcinoma

TABLE 18-4. VIRAL HEPATITIS: TRANSMISSION AND CLINICAL FINDINGS

VIRUS	TRANSMISSION	DISCUSSION
Hepatitis A (HAV)	Fecal-oral	Infectious hepatitis Incubation 15–50 days (average 30 days) Accounts for 37% of acute hepatitis in U.S. Most preventable infection in travelers Increased incidence in children/employees in day care centers, prisons, travelers to developing countries, males who have sex with males (anal intercourse), parents adopting children from other countries Clinical: jaundice > 70%; fever; nausea/vomiting; abdominal pain Majority recover; no carrier state; no chronic hepatitis Serology: see text Passive immunization: immunoglobulin (passive transfer of antibodies) for pre-exposure prophylaxis and postexposure prophylaxis Active immunization: protective antibodies in 1 month

TABLE 18-4. VIRAL HEPATITIS: TRANSMISSION AND CLINICAL FINDINGS—cont'd

VIRUS	TRANSMISSION	DISCUSSION
Hepatitis B (HBV) *Hepadnovirus*	Parenteral, orally, sexual, vertical (pregnancy, breast feeding)	Incubation 30–180 days Primarily spread via blood (IVDA) and sexually Accounts for 45% of acute hepatitis in U.S. Clinical: variable fever; profound malaise; painful hepatomegaly (87%); serum sickness prodrome (15–20%): immunocomplex disease (HBsAg + antibody); vasculitis (PAN), urticaria, polyarthritis, membranous glomerulopathy Recovery in >90% of immunocompetent patients; 1–2% develop chronic hepatitis Newborns and immunodeficient patients more likely to develop chronic hepatitis (>90%) Complications: fulminant hepatitis <1% especially if coinfected with hepatitis D; hepatocellular carcinoma secondary to postnecrotic cirrhosis Serology: see text Prevention: immunization with recombinant vaccine *Treatment* of chronic hepatitis: pegylated IFN-α; nucleoside analogues that block viral replication (e.g., lamivudine; entecavir); liver transplant
Hepatitis C (HCV) *Flavivirus*	Parenteral, sexual	Incubation 2–26 weeks (average, 6–7 weeks) Most common blood-borne infection in the U.S. Accounts for 18% of acute hepatitis in U.S. Most common main indication for liver transplantation in U.S. Most cases due to IVDA (60%); hemophiliacs transfused before 1987 Post-transfusion hepatitis rare due to screening Maternal-fetal transmission is infrequent (estimated 5%) Clinical: mild hepatitis (70–80% subclinical); jaundice uncommon (80% anicteric) Chronic hepatitis in >70% of cases Other clinical associations: type I MPGN, alcohol excess, PCT, lichen planus, B cell lymphoma Complications: hepatocellular carcinoma secondary to postnecrotic cirrhosis Prevention: no preventive vaccine available *Treatment*: early treatment of acute infection with pegylated IFN-α may prevent chronic infection; pegylated IFN-α also used in treating chronic HCV; liver transplant
Hepatitis D (HDV) *Hepadeno*	Parenteral, sexual	Incomplete RNA virus that requires HBsAg to replicate Accounts for <1% of acute hepatitis in U.S. Chronic state less likely with coinfection (HBV and HDV exposure at same time) than superinfection (HBV carrier exposed to blood containing HBV and HDV) Chronic infection develops in 60–85% of people infected Serology: see text Prevention: immunization with recombinant vaccine for HBV
Hepatitis E *Calicivirus*	Fecal-oral (water-borne)	Occurs in developing countries Only produces acute hepatitis Fulminant hepatitis may develop in pregnant women

HBsAg, surface antigen; IFN, interferon; IVDA, intravenous drug abuse; MPGN, membranoproliferative glomerulonephritis; PAN, polyarteritis nodosa; PCT, porphyria cutanea tarda.

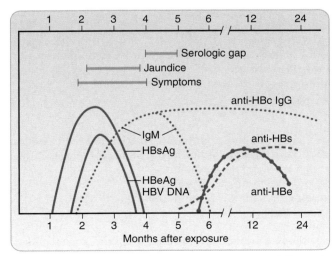

18-3: Serologic markers in hepatitis B. Anti-HBc, anti-HBV core antigen; anti-HBe, anti-HBV e antigen; anti-HBs, anti-HBV surface antibody; HBsAg, hepatitis B surface antigen; HBeAg, hepatitis B e antigen; HBV, hepatitis B virus; IgG, immunoglobulin G; IgM, immunoglobulin M.

TABLE 18-5. SEROLOGIC STUDIES IN HEPATITIS B VIRUS (HBV)

HBsAg	HBeAg HBV DNA	Anti-HBc-IgM	Anti-HBc-IgG	Anti-HBs	INTERPRETATION
+	−	−	−	−	Earliest phase of acute HBV
+	+	+	−	−	Acute infection
−	−	+	−	−	Window phase, or serologic gap
−	−	−	+	+	Recovered from HBV
−	−	−	−	+	Immunized
+	−	+	+	−	"Healthy" carrier
+	+	−	+	−	Infective carrier

Anti-HBc, core antibody; anti-HBs, surface antibody; HBeAg, e antigen; HBsAg, surface antigen.

3. Hepatitis C virus (HCV)
   a. Screen with enzyme immunoassay (EIA)
      (1) Presence of anti-HCV-IgG indicates active infection or recovery.
         • Sensitivity > 97%
      (2) It does *not* differentiate among acute, chronic, or resolved infection.
      (3) It is *not* a protective antibody.
   b. Confirmatory tests
      (1) Recombinant immunoblot assay (RIBA)
         (a) Supplemental test if EIA is positive
         (b) More specific but less sensitive than EIA
      (2) HCV RNA using polymerase chain reaction
         (a) Gold standard test for diagnosing HCV
         (b) Detects virus as early as 1 to 2 weeks after infection
         (c) Used to monitor patients on antiviral therapy
      (3) Positive RIBA and HCV RNA indicate active infection.
      (4) Positive RIBA and negative HCV RNA indicate recent recovery.
4. Hepatitis D virus (HDV)
   a. Presence of anti-HDV-IgM or IgG indicates active infection.
   b. IgG is *not* a protective antibody.
5. Hepatitis E virus (HEV)
   a. Presence of anti-HEV-IgM indicates active infection.
   b. Anti-HEV-IgG indicates recovery (protective antibody).
E. **Other laboratory test findings** (see Box 18-1C)
   1. CB 20% to 50% (mixed hyperbilirubinemia)
      a. Decreased uptake/conjugation of UCB
      b. CB gains access to blood via damaged bile ductules.
   2. Increased urine UBG and urine bilirubin
      a. CB is water soluble and is filtered in the kidneys.
      b. UBG recycled back to inflamed liver is redirected to the kidneys.
   3. Increased serum transaminases
      a. Serum ALT is greater than AST.
      b. Serum ALT is the last liver enzyme to return to normal.
III. **Other Inflammatory Disorders**
   A. **Summary of important infectious diseases** (Table 18-6 and Fig. 18-4)
   B. **Autoimmune hepatitis**
      1. Epidemiology
         a. Two types
            (1) Type 1 is the predominant form in the United States and worldwide (80%).
            (2) Type 2 is uncommon in the United States (not discussed).
         b. Occurs most often in young women
         c. Range of presentations
            (1) Symptomatic with increased transaminases
            (2) Fulminant hepatitis
            (3) Cirrhosis
         d. Human leukocyte antigen (HLA) DR3 and DR4 association
         e. Other autoimmune associations
            • Examples—Hashimoto's thyroiditis, Graves' disease
      2. Clinical findings
         a. Fever

HCV testing: screen with EIA; confirm with RIBA and HCV RNA

HCV RNA: gold standard test

HCV, HDV: no protective antibodies

Viral hepatitis: urine UBG ++, urine bilirubin ++

Serum ALT: last enzyme to return to normal

Autoimmune hepatitis: type 1 most common in the United States

TABLE 18-6. INFECTIOUS DISEASES OF THE LIVER

DISEASE	PATHOGEN(S)	CHARACTERISTICS
Ascending cholangitis	Escherichia coli	Inflammation of bile ducts (cholangitis) from concurrent biliary infection and duct obstruction (e.g., stone) Life-threatening disease Triad of fever, jaundice, RUQ pain Most common cause of multiple liver abscesses *Treatment*: decompression and drainage; piperacillin-tazobactam
Liver abscess	Escherichia coli, Bacteroides fragilis, Streptococcus faecalis	Majority are in the right lobe; majority are solitary Causes: ascending cholangitis (most common); intra-abdominal infection (e.g., spread via the portal vein, diverticulitis, bowel perforation); direct extension (e.g., empyema of gallbladder, subphrenic abscess); hematogenous spread (e.g., bacterial endocarditis) Clinical: spiking, intermittent fever; RUQ or right costovertebral angle tenderness; jaundice is uncommon Diagnosis: ultrasound (least expensive); CT scan *Treatment*: percutaneous drainage; metronidazole + ceftriaxone
Granulomatous hepatitis	Mycobacterium tuberculosis, Histoplasma capsulatum	Sign of miliary spread (refer to Chapter 16)
Spontaneous peritonitis	Escherichia coli in adults, Streptococcus pneumoniae in children	Develops in ascites (e.g., cirrhosis, nephrotic syndrome) *Treatment*: cefotaxime
Leptospirosis	Leptospira interrogans	Gram-negative; tightly wound spirochetes; crook at the end resembles a shepherd's staff Reservoirs: rats, dogs (most common); spirochetes excreted in urine Transmission: swimming in contaminated water (ponds on farms); farmers, miners, people who work with sewage Biphasic disease (Weil's disease): Septicemic phase: fever, jaundice, hemorrhagic diathesis, renal failure (interstitial nephritis), conjunctivitis and photophobia, meningitis; phase terminated by the appearance of antibodies (beginning of immune phase) Immune phase: presence of numerous organisms in the urine; urine best examined by darkfield microscopy to confirm the diagnosis *Treatment*: penicillin G
Amebiasis	Entamoeba histolytica	Protozoan (ameba) Most common cause of a liver abscess worldwide (*not* in the United States) Usually produces a right lobe abscess (refer to Chapter 17) *Treatment*: metronidazole followed by paromomycin
Clonorchiasis	Clonorchis sinensis (Chinese liver fluke)	Intestinal fluke (trematode) Nonschistosomal life cycle: egg (human) → ciliated miracidial larva → infects snail (1st intermediate host) → produce fork-tailed cercarial larvae → infect a 2nd intermediate host (fish in clonorchiasis) → form infective metacercariae → man ingests the 2nd intermediate host → develops disease Contracted by ingesting encysted larvae in fish; larvae enter CBD and become adults. May produce cholangiocarcinoma *Treatment*: praziquantel
Schistosomiasis	Schistosoma mansoni	Fluke (trematode) Schistosomal life cycle: egg (human) → ciliated miracidial larva → infects snail (1st intermediate host) → produce fork-tailed cercarial larvae → penetrate skin in human → produce disease *Schistosoma mansoni*: larvae in the superior mesenteric vein enter into the portal vein, where they develop into adult worms that deposit eggs to which the host develops an inflammatory response marked by concentric fibrosis ("pipestem cirrhosis") in the vessel wall Complications of cirrhosis: portal hypertension, ascites, esophageal varices *Treatment*: praziquantel

Continued

TABLE 18-6. INFECTIOUS DISEASES OF THE LIVER—cont'd

DISEASE	PATHOGEN(S)	CHARACTERISTICS
Echinococcosis (see Fig. 18-4)	*Echinococcus granulosus* (sheepherder's disease)	Intestinal tapeworm (cestode) Single or multiple cysts containing larval forms; cysts can be in the liver (most common site), lungs, and brain Eggs develop into a larval form only; larval form only develops into an adult, which can lay eggs Infected sheep is intermediate host (larval form in liver cyst); dog that eats the sheep liver is the definitive host (larva develops into adults, which produce eggs); human who eats the eggs from the dog becomes the intermediate host (eggs develop into larvae, which penetrate the bowel and enter the liver to produce the hydatid cyst) Can be contracted by children eating grass contaminated with dog excreta Inner germinal layer of hydatid cysts has protoscolices (larva) in brood capsules Rupture of cysts can produce anaphylaxis *Treatment:* percutaneous drainage + albendazole

CBD, common bile duct; RUQ, right upper quadrant.

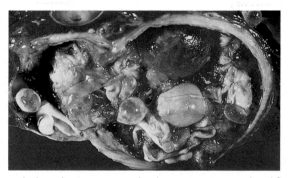

18-4: Hydatid cyst. A single cyst in the liver shows numerous daughter cysts containing larval forms. *(From MacSween R, Burt A, Portmann B, et al: Pathology of the Liver, 4th ed. London, Churchill Livingstone, 2002, p 388, Fig. 8-35.)*

Autoimmune hepatitis: + serum ANA, + anti–smooth muscle antibodies

Neonatal hepatitis: multifactorial; biopsy shows multinucleated giant cells

    b. Jaundice
    c. Hepatosplenomegaly
  3. Laboratory findings for type 1
    a. Positive serum antinuclear antibody (ANA) test (>60%)
    b. Anti–smooth muscle antibodies (>85%)
    c. Increased serum transaminases
    d. Decreased serum albumin in severe disease
    e. Prolonged prothrombin time in severe disease
  4. Treatment
    a. Initial treatment with corticosteroids + azathioprine
    b. Liver transplantation if resistant to therapy
C. Neonatal hepatitis
  1. Epidemiology
    a. Idiopathic
    b. Associated with congenital infections
      • Example—cytomegalovirus
    c. Associated with inborn errors of metabolism
      • Example—α_1-antitrypsin deficiency
  2. Biopsy shows multinucleated giant cells.
    • "Giant cell" hepatitis
D. Reye syndrome
  1. Epidemiology
    a. Postinfectious triad:
      (1) Encephalopathy

(2) Microvesicular fatty change

(3) Transaminase elevation

b. Uncommon since the role of aspirin was elucidated

c. Usually develops in children < 4 years old

- Often follows a chickenpox or influenza infection

2. Pathogenesis

a. Mitochondrial damage (? virus, salicylates)

b. Disruption of the urea cycle

- Increase in serum ammonia

c. Defective β-oxidation of fatty acids

3. Microvesicular fatty change (? salicylate effect)

a. Small cytoplasmic globules *without* nuclear displacement

b. No inflammatory infiltrate

4. Clinical findings

a. Initially afebrile, quiet, lethargic, sleepy, and vomiting

- Hepatomegaly and liver dysfunction present

b. Encephalopathy findings in progression

- Signs and symptoms related to cerebral edema and increasing pressure

(1) Sleepy but respond; vomiting

(2) Stuporous, seizures, decorticate rigidity, intact papillary reflexes

(3) Deepening coma, decerebrate rigidity, fixed pupils

(4) Coma, loss of deep tendon reflexes, fixed dilated pupils, flaccidity/decerebrate

(5) Death

5. Laboratory findings

a. Transaminasemia

b. Normal to slight increase in total bilirubin

c. Increased serum ammonia and prothrombin time (PT)

- Levels predict degree of severity

d. Hypoglycemia

e. Cerebrospinal fluid usually normal

6. Treatment

a. Supportive

b. Mannitol, glycerol, or hyperventilation to reduce cerebral edema

7. Approximately 25% to 50% mortality rate

E. Acute fatty liver of pregnancy

1. Abnormality in β-oxidation of fatty acids (FAs)

2. Fatal to mother and fetus unless the baby is delivered

F. Preeclampsia (refer to Chapter 21)

1. Hypertension, proteinuria, dependent pitting edema in third trimester

2. Liver cell necrosis around portal triads (zone 1)

- Increased serum transaminases

3. HELLP syndrome

a. *H*emolytic anemia with schistocytes (refer to Chapter 11)

b. *EL*evated serum transaminases

c. *L*ow *p*latelets

- Due to disseminated intravascular coagulation (refer to Chapter 14)

G. Fulminant hepatic failure

- Acute liver failure with encephalopathy within 8 weeks of hepatic dysfunction

1. Causes

a. Viral hepatitis (most common overall cause)

b. Drugs (e.g., acetaminophen most common cause)

c. Reye syndrome

2. Gross and microscopic findings

a. Wrinkled capsular surface due to loss of hepatic parenchyma

b. Dull red to yellow necrotic parenchyma with blotches of green (bile)

3. Clinical findings

- Hepatic encephalopathy (see section VII), jaundice

4. Laboratory findings

a. Decrease in transaminases

- Liver parenchyma is destroyed.

b. Increase in PT and ammonia

5. Treatment (refer to section VII, Cirrhosis)

Margin notes:

Reye syndrome: association with aspirin and infection (chickenpox, influenza)

Reye syndrome: encephalopathy, fatty change in liver, ↑ transaminases

Reye syndrome: sleepy but respond → stuporous → obtundation → coma

Reye syndrome: ↑ transaminasemia, bilirubin, PT, ammonia; ↓ glucose

Fatty liver of pregnancy: dysfunction in β-oxidation FAs; deliver baby

Preeclampsia: periportal triad liver cell necrosis; HELLP syndrome

Fulminant hepatic failure: viral hepatitis most common overall cause

Fulminant hepatitis: acetaminophen most common drug cause

Fulminant hepatic failure: ↓ transaminases, ↑ PT and ammonia

IV. **Circulatory Disorders**
   A. **Prehepatic obstruction to blood flow**
     • Obstruction of blood flow to the liver (i.e., hepatic artery, portal vein)
    1. Hepatic artery thrombosis with infarction
      a. Liver infarction is uncommon because of a dual blood supply.
       • Hepatic artery and portal vein tributaries normally empty blood into the sinusoids.
      b. Causes
       (1) Liver transplant rejection
       (2) Vasculitis due to polyarteritis nodosa (PAN)
    2. Portal vein thrombosis
      a. Causes
       (1) Pylephlebitis (inflammation of portal vein)
        (a) Most often due to acute appendicitis
        (b) Air in portal vein from bacterial gas
       (2) Polycythemia vera
       (3) Hepatocellular carcinoma
        • Tumor invasion of the portal vein
      b. Clinical findings
       (1) Portal hypertension, ascites, splenomegaly
       (2) *No* hepatomegaly
   B. **Intrahepatic obstruction to blood flow**
     • Intrahepatic obstruction to sinusoidal blood flow
    1. Causes
      a. Cirrhosis (see section VII)
      b. Centrilobular hemorrhagic necrosis
      c. Peliosis hepatis
      d. Sickle cell disease (see Chapter 11)
    2. Centrilobular hemorrhagic necrosis
      a. Most often due to left-sided heart failure (LHF) and right-sided heart failure (RHF)
       (1) LHF decreases cardiac output causing hypoperfusion of the liver.
        • Causes ischemic necrosis of hepatocytes located around central vein (refer to Chapter 1)
       (2) RHF causes a backup of systemic venous blood into the central veins and sinusoids.
      b. Enlarged liver with a mottled red appearance ("nutmeg" liver) (Fig. 18-5)
       (1) Congestion of central veins and sinusoids
       (2) Necrosis of hepatocytes around the central vein
      c. Clinical findings
       (1) Painful hepatomegaly with or without jaundice
       (2) Increased transaminases caused by ischemic necrosis
       (3) May progress to cardiac cirrhosis
        • Fibrosis around central veins
      d. Treatment
       • Treat heart failure

Marginal notes:

Hepatic artery infarction: uncommon due to dual blood supply

Hepatic artery infarction: liver transplant rejection, PAN

Portal vein thrombosis: ascites, portal hypertension, no hepatomegaly; air in portal vein

Intrahepatic obstruction to blood flow: cirrhosis most common cause

Centrilobular necrosis: combined LHF and RHF; "nutmeg" liver

Centrilobular necrosis: may progress to cardiac cirrhosis

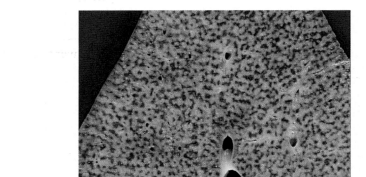

18-5: Centrilobular hemorrhagic necrosis ("nutmeg" liver). The liver has a mottled cut surface. Dark areas represent congested central veins and sinusoids. *(From Damjanov I, Linder J: Pathology: A Color Atlas. St. Louis, Mosby, 2000, p 146, Fig. 8-8.)*

3. Peliosis hepatis
   a. Sinusoidal dilation due to blood
   b. Causes
      (1) Anabolic steroids
      (2) *Bartonella henselae* causing bacillary angiomatosis (refer to Chapter 9)
         • Occurs in AIDS
   c. Potential for intraperitoneal hemorrhage

C. **Posthepatic obstruction to blood flow**
   • Obstruction of blood flow out of the liver (e.g., hepatic vein)
   1. Causes
      a. Hepatic vein thrombosis
      b. Veno-occlusive disease
   2. Hepatic vein thrombosis
      a. Causes
         (1) Polycythemia vera
            • Most common cause (up to 40% of cases)
         (2) Hypercoagulable state (20% of cases)
            (a) Oral contraceptive pills
            (b) Protein C/S deficiency
            (c) Antiphospholipid syndrome
         (3) Hepatocellular carcinoma (<5% of cases)
            • Invades hepatic vein
      b. Clinical findings
         (1) Enlarged, painful liver
         (2) Portal hypertension, ascites, splenomegaly
         (3) High mortality rate
      c. Laboratory findings
         (1) Increased transaminases
         (2) Increased PT
      d. Diagnosis
         (1) Ultrasound with pulsed Doppler first-line test
         (2) MRI
      e. Treatment
         (1) Anticoagulation
         (2) In situ thrombolysis
         (3) Stenting, various shunts
      f. Prognosis
         • Approximately 75% mortality rate in first year
   3. Veno-occlusive disease
      a. Complication of bone marrow transplantation
      b. Collagen develops around the central veins.

D. **Hematobilia**
   • Blood in the bile in patients with trauma to the liver

V. **Alcohol-Related and Drug- and Chemical-Induced Liver Disorders**
   A. **Alcohol-related disorders**
      1. Risk factors for alcohol-related liver disease (refer to Chapter 6)
      2. Pathways for alcohol metabolism (refer to Chapter 6)
      3. Types of liver disease
         a. Fatty change is the most common type of disease (see Fig. 1-8).
            (1) Substrates of alcohol metabolism are used to synthesize liver triglyceride.
            (2) Clinical findings
               • Tender hepatomegaly *without* fever or neutrophilic leukocytosis
            (3) Treatment
               • Alcohol rehabilitation
         b. Alcoholic hepatitis
            (1) Pathogenesis
               (a) Genetic predisposition is likely.
               (b) Due to acetaldehyde damage to hepatocytes
               (c) Stimulation of collagen synthesis around the central vein
                  • Perivenular fibrosis
            (2) Microscopic findings
               (a) Fatty change with neutrophil infiltration

Margin notes:

Peliosis hepatis: anabolic steroids, *Bartonella henselae*

Polycythemia vera: most common cause of hepatic vein thrombosis

Hepatic vein thrombosis: hepatomegaly, portal hypertension, ascites

Veno-occlusive disease: complication of bone marrow transplantation

Hematobilia: blood in bile from liver trauma

Alcohol liver disease: fatty change, hepatitis, cirrhosis

Alcoholic hepatitis: acetaldehyde damages hepatocytes

(b) Mallory bodies
- Damaged cytokeratin intermediate filaments in hepatocytes (see Fig. 1-7)

(c) Perivenular fibrosis

(3) Clinical findings
  (a) Painful hepatomegaly
  (b) Fever, neutrophilic leukocytosis, ascites, hepatic encephalopathy
  (c) May progress to alcoholic cirrhosis

(4) Laboratory findings
  (a) Absolute neutrophilic leukocytosis
  (b) Serum aspartate aminotransferase (AST) > alanine aminotransferase (ALT)
  (c) Increased serum alkaline phosphatase (ALP) and γ-glutamyltransferase (GGT)
    - Serum GGT disproportionately increase to ALP (see Table 18-2)
  (d) Thrombocytopenia in some cases
  (e) Hypoglycemia in some cases

(5) Treatment
  (a) Mandatory to stop drinking
  (b) Corticosteroids helpful in some cases

c. Cirrhosis (see section VII)

4. Laboratory findings (refer to Chapter 6; see Fig. 6-1)

B. Chemical- and drug-induced liver disease (Table 18-7)

VI. **Obstructive (Cholestatic) Liver Disease**

A. Types of cholestatic liver disease

1. Intrahepatic cholestasis
   a. Blockage of the intrahepatic bile ducts
   b. Causes
      (1) Drugs (e.g., oral contraceptive pills [OCPs], anabolic steroids)
      (2) Neonatal hepatitis
      (3) Pregnancy-induced cholestasis (estrogen)

2. Extrahepatic cholestasis
   a. Blockage of common bile duct (CBD)
   b. Causes
      (1) Stone usually originating from the gallbladder
      (2) Primary sclerosing cholangitis
      (3) Extrahepatic biliary atresia
      (4) Carcinoma head of pancreas

B. Gross and microscopic

1. Enlarged, greenish liver
2. Bile ducts distended with bile (Fig. 18-6), bile lakes, bile infarcts

C. Clinical findings

1. Jaundice with pruritus
   - Pruritus due to bile salts deposited in skin
2. Malabsorption
   - Bile salts do *not* enter the small intestine.

Margin notes (left column):

Alcoholic hepatitis: fatty change, neutrophil infiltration, Mallory bodies

Alcoholic hepatitis: acetaldehyde damages hepatocytes

Intrahepatic fibrosis: methotrexate, amiodarone

Intrahepatic cholestasis: OCP, anabolic steroids

Extrahepatic cholestasis: most commonly caused by a stone in CBD

TABLE 18-7. DRUG- AND CHEMICAL-INDUCED LIVER DISEASES

DISEASE	CAUSE
Tumors	
Angiosarcoma	Vinyl chloride, arsenic, thorium dioxide (radioactive contrast material)
Cholangiocarcinoma	Thorium dioxide
Hepatocellular carcinoma	Vinyl chloride, aflatoxin (due to *Aspergillus* mold)
Liver cell adenoma	Oral contraceptive pills
Other Liver Diseases	
Acute hepatitis	Isoniazid (caused by toxic metabolite), halothane, acetaminophen, methyldopa
Cholestasis	Oral contraceptive pills (OCPs; estrogen interferes with intrahepatic bile secretion), anabolic steroids (same mechanism as OCPs)
Fatty change	Amiodarone (resembles alcoholic hepatitis; Mallory bodies and progression to cirrhosis), methotrexate
Fibrosis	Methotrexate, retinoic acid, amiodarone

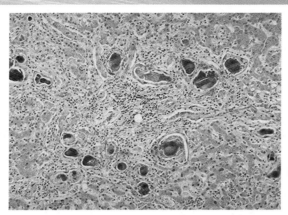

18-6: Cholestasis. Note the dilated bile ductules filled with yellowish-green bile. *(From Klatt E: Robbins and Cotran's Atlas of Pathology. Philadelphia, WB Saunders, 2006, p 199, Fig. 8-11.)*

  3. Cholesterol deposits in skin
   a. Due to cholesterol in bile
   b. Example—xanthelasma (see Fig. 9-2B)
  4. Light-colored stools
   • Due to a lack of urobilin
 D. Laboratory findings (see Box 18-1D)
  1. CB > 50%
  2. Bilirubinuria
  3. Absent urine UBG
  4. Increase in serum ALP and GGT
 E. Benign intrahepatic cholestasis of pregnancy
  1. Due to estrogen inhibition of intrahepatic bile secretion
  2. *Not* dangerous to the fetus or mother
 F. Extrahepatic biliary atresia
  1. Cause of jaundice in newborns
  2. Inflammatory destruction of all or part of the extrahepatic bile ducts
  3. Bile duct proliferation in the triads
  4. Common indication for liver transplantation in a child
 G. Primary sclerosing cholangitis (PSC)
  1. Epidemiology
   a. Obliterative fibrosis of intrahepatic and extrahepatic bile ducts
   b. Primary disease
    (1) Genetic predisposition
     • Association with HLA-DR52a (100%) and HLA-Cw7 (86%)
    (2) Male dominant (70%); usually <45 years old
    (3) Associations
     (a) Inflammatory bowel disease (70%)
      • Ulcerative colitis > Crohn's disease
     (b) Other sclerosing disorders
      • Retroperitoneal and mediastinal sclerosing fibrosis
    (4) Complications
     (a) Cirrhosis
     (b) Cholangiocarcinoma
  2. Clinical findings
   a. Jaundice
   b. Pruritus
    • Deposition of bile salts/acids in skin
   c. Hepatosplenomegaly
  3. Laboratory findings
   a. CB > 50%
   b. Bilirubinuria
   c. Absent urine UBG
   d. Increase in serum ALP and GGT

Cholestasis: urine UBG 0, urine bilirubin ++

Cholestasis in pregnancy: effect of estrogen on intrahepatic bile secretion

Extrahepatic biliary atresia: jaundice in newborn

PSC: obliterative fibrosis intrahepatic and extrahepatic bile ducts

PSC: strong association with ulcerative colitis > Crohn's disease

PSC: cirrhosis, cholangiocarcinoma

4. Diagnosis
   a. Endoscopic retrograde cholangiopancreatography (ERCP)
   b. Dye study shows narrowing and dilation of bile ducts ("beading")
5. Treatment
   a. Immunosuppressants
      • Corticosteroids, azathioprine, methotrexate
   b. Invariably require a liver transplant

VII. Cirrhosis
   • Irreversible diffuse fibrosis of the liver with formation of regenerative nodules

A. Regenerative nodules
   1. Hepatocyte reaction to injury (Fig. 18-7)
   2. Lack normal liver architecture (Fig 18-8)
      • Lack of portal triads and sinusoids
   3. Surrounded by bands of fibrosis
   4. Compress sinusoids and central veins

      a. Intrasinusoidal hypertension
      b. Reduction in the number of functional sinusoids
      c. Increase in hydrostatic pressure in portal vein

B. Causes

   1. Alcoholic liver disease (most common)
   2. Postnecrotic cirrhosis (HBV, HCV)
   3. Autoimmune disease
      a. Primary biliary cirrhosis
      b. Autoimmune hepatitis (see section III)
   4. Metabolic diseases
      a. Hemochromatosis
      b. Wilson's disease
      c. α_1-Antitrypsin deficiency
      d. Galactosemia

C. Complications associated with cirrhosis
   1. Hepatic failure
      • End-point of progressive damage to the liver
      a. Multiple coagulation defects
         (1) Due to inability to synthesize coagulation factors
         (2) Produces a hemorrhagic diathesis
      b. Hypoalbuminemia from decreased synthesis of albumin
         • Produces dependent pitting edema and ascites

      c. Hepatic encephalopathy
         (1) Reversible metabolic disorder
         (2) Increase in aromatic amino acids (e.g., phenylalanine, tyrosine, tryptophan)
            • Converted into false neurotransmitters (e.g., γ-aminobutyric acid)
         (3) Increase in serum ammonia
            • Due to a defective urea cycle that cannot metabolize ammonia

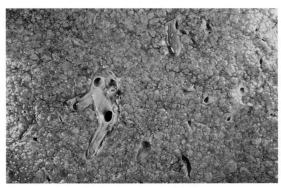

18-7: Alcoholic cirrhosis, showing diffuse micronodular surface of the liver. The regenerative nodules are surrounded by collagen. *(From Damjanov I, Linder J: Pathology: A Color Atlas. St. Louis, Mosby, 2000, p 154, Fig. 8-42.)*

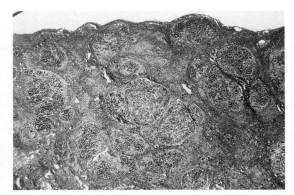

18-8: Micronodular cirrhosis with regenerative nodules (red) surrounded by dense binds of fibrous tissue (blue). *(From MacSween R, Burt A, Portmann B, et al: Pathology of the Liver, 4th ed. London, Churchill Livingstone, 2002, p 599, Fig. 13-20.)*

Ammonia derives from metabolism of amino acids and from the release of ammonia from amino acids by bacterial ureases in the bowel. Ammonia (NH_3) is diffusible and is reabsorbed into the portal vein for delivery to the urea cycle where it is metabolized into urea. Ammonium (NH_4) is *not* reabsorbed in the bowel and is excreted in stool. Methods for reducing ammonia in the colon include restriction of protein intake (most cost effective) and the use of oral neomycin, which destroys the colonic bacteria. Oral administration of lactulose results in the release of hydrogen ions, causing NH_3 to be converted to NH_4, which is excreted in the feces.

> Ammonia: derives from amino acid metabolism and urease-producing bacteria in bowel
>
> ↓ Ammonia: ↓ protein intake; antibiotics; lactulose

    (4) Factors precipitating encephalopathy
        (a) Increased protein (most important)
          • Dietary or blood in gastrointestinal tract; increases bacterial conversion of urea into ammonia
        (b) Alkalosis keeps ammonia in NH_3 state (see earlier).
          • Diuretics (loop and thiazide) produce metabolic alkalosis.
        (c) Sedatives
        (d) Portasystemic shunts
          • Shunt ammonia away from the liver, which normally metabolizes ammonia in the urea cycle

> Precipitating factors: ↑ protein, alkalosis, sedatives, portasystemic shunts

    (5) Clinical findings
        (a) Alterations in the mental status
        (b) Somnolence and disordered sleep rhythms
        (c) Asterixis (i.e., inability to sustain posture, flapping tremor)
        (d) Coma and death in late stages

> Hepatic encephalopathy: alterations mental status, somnolence, asterixis

    (6) Treatment (see ammonia discussion)
  2. Portal hypertension (PH)
    a. Pathogenesis
      (1) Resistance to intrahepatic blood flow due to intrasinusoidal hypertension
      (2) Anastomoses between portal vein tributaries and the arterial system

> Portal vein: splenic vein superior mesenteric vein
>
> Portal vein hypertension: due to intrasinusoidal hypertension from regenerative nodule compression

    b. Complications
      (1) Ascites (see later)
      (2) Congestive splenomegaly
        (a) Increased hydrostatic pressure in splenic vein
        (b) Hypersplenism with various cytopenias may occur (refer to Chapter 13)
      (3) Esophageal varices (refer to Chapter 17; see Fig. 17-9)
      (4) Hemorrhoids
      (5) Periumbilical venous collaterals (caput medusae)
    c. Shunts used in treating PH
      (1) Portacaval shunt
        • Connects the portal vein with the vena cava
      (2) Mesocaval shunt
        • Connects the superior mesenteric vein with the portal vein.
      (3) Splenorenal
        (a) Most physiologic shunt
        (b) Connects the splenic vein with the renal vein
        (c) Reduces PH and bleeding from varices without bypassing the liver

> PH and shunts: shunts that bypass the liver can precipitate encephalopathy
>
> Splenorenal shunt: does *not* bypass liver; most physiologic shunt

      (4) Transjugular intrahepatic portosystemic shunt (TIPS)
        (a) Metal stent connects portal vein with hepatic vein.
        (b) Reduces portal vein pressure
        (c) Increases risk for encephalopathy
        (d) Used in treatment of acute esophageal bleeds (refer to Chapter 17)
        (e) Used in treating patients awaiting liver transplantation

> TIPS: ↓ portal vein pressure; connects portal vein with hepatic vein

  3. Ascites (Fig. 18-9)
    a. Pathogenesis
      (1) Portal hypertension
        • Increase in portal vein hydrostatic pressure
      (2) Hypoalbuminemia
        • Decreases oncotic pressure
      (3) Secondary hyperaldosteronism; causes:
        (a) Decreased cardiac output
          • Activates the renin-angiotensin-aldosterone system (retention of Na^+ and water)
        (b) Liver is unable to metabolize aldosterone.

> Ascites: transudate due to alterations in Starling pressures; secondary aldosteronism

b. Clinical findings
(1) Abdominal distention with a fluid wave
(2) Increased risk for spontaneous bacterial peritonitis

> **Peritoneal fluid analysis** is useful in distinguishing ascites of liver origin from ascites of peritoneal origin. The gradient between serum albumin and ascitic fluid albumin (serum albumin – ascitic fluid albumin) is very helpful in making this distinction. A difference > 1.1 g/dL is ascites of liver origin, while a difference < 1.1 g/dL is of peritoneal origin (e.g., peritonitis). Recall that ascites of liver origin is a transudate, which is a protein-poor and cell-poor fluid; hence, the expected difference between serum albumin and ascitic albumin is increased. However, ascitic fluid from peritonitis is an exudate, which is a protein-rich and cell-rich fluid; hence, the difference between serum and ascitic fluid is much less. Peritoneal fluid protein concentration and cell count are also useful. A total peritoneal fluid protein concentration < 2.5 g/dL and WBC count < 300 cells/mm^3 + neutrophils < 25% of the total count is consistent with a transudate, while a concentration > 2.5 g/dL and a WBC count > 300 cells/mm^3 + neutrophils > 25% of the total count indicates an exudate.

4. Hepatorenal syndrome
   a. Reversible renal failure *without* renal parenchymal disease
      • Creatinine clearance < 40 mL/minute (refer to Chapter 19)
   b. Approximately 20% of people with hepatic failure die of this syndrome.
   c. Absence of
      (1) Shock
      (2) Volume depletion
      (3) Infection
      (4) Obstructive or parenchymal renal disease
   d. Preservation of renal tubular function
      (1) Random urine Na$^+$ < 20 mEq/L (refer to Chapter 19)
      (2) Absence of significant proteinuria (<500 mg/day) or hematuria
   e. ? Due to decreased renal blood flow
      • Serum blood urea nitrogen and creatinine are increased (refer to Chapter 19)
   f. Treatment
      (1) Supportive care including dialysis
      (2) Vasopressin analogues
      (3) Vasoconstrictors (e.g., norepinephrine, midodrine)
      (4) Albumin for volume expansion
      (5) Liver transplantation is the only curative treatment.
   g. Mortality rate > 80%

5. Hyperestrinism in males
   a. Pathogenesis
      (1) Liver cannot degrade estrogen and 17-ketosteroids (e.g., androstenedione).
      (2) Androstenedione is aromatized into estrogen in the adipose cells.
   b. Clinical findings
      (1) Gynecomastia (see Fig. 18-9)
      (2) Spider telangiectasia (refer to Chapter 9) (Fig. 18-10)
      (3) Female distribution of hair (see Fig. 18-9)
D. Postnecrotic cirrhosis

1. Most often caused by chronic hepatitis due to HBV and HCV
2. Increased incidence of hepatocellular carcinoma
   • Incidence of which virus is most common varies around the world
E. Primary biliary cirrhosis (PBC)
1. Epidemiology
   a. Granulomatous destruction of bile ducts in portal triads
   b. Autoimmune disorder
      • Association with other autoimmune diseases (e.g., Sjögren's syndrome)
   c. Occurs in women (>90%) between 40 and 50 years of age
   d. Progresses from a chronic inflammatory reaction to cirrhosis with PH
   e. Increased risk for hepatocellular carcinoma
2. Pathogenesis
   a. ? Environmental insult affecting mitochondrial proteins triggering CD8 T-cell destruction of intralobular bile duct epithelium

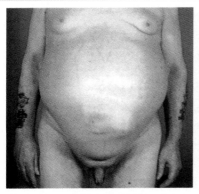

18-9: Patient with cirrhosis. Note abdominal distention due to ascites. Signs of hyperestrinism include gynecomastia and a female distribution of hair (hair does not extend to umbilicus). *(From Grieg JD: Color Atlas of Surgical Diagnosis. London, Mosby-Wolfe, 1996, p 133, Fig. 20-2.)*

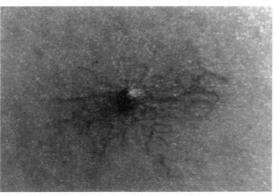

18-10: Spider angioma (telangiectasia) showing a single central arteriole and numerous radiating capillaries. *(From Gitlin M, Strauss R: Atlas of Clinical Hepatology. Philadelphia, WB Saunders, 1995, p 3, Fig. 1.4.)*

    b. Enzyme complex subunit in mitochondrial membrane is the autoantigen recognized by CD8 T cells

    c. Autoantibodies (antimitochondrial antibodies) develop against the mitochondria
- Do *not* correlate with disease activity

  3. Clinical findings

    a. Pruritus (20–70%)

      (1) Unknown etiology (*not* bile salts in skin)

      (2) Early finding well *before* jaundice appears

    b. Painful hepatosplenomegaly

    c. Jaundice (60%)
- Late finding *after* most of the bile ducts have been destroyed

    d. Inflammatory arthropathy (40–70%)

    e. Xanthelasma (40%)

      (1) Late finding

      (2) Due to cholesterol in bile

    f. Kayser-Fleischer ring in cornea
- Due to retention of copper

  4. Laboratory findings

    a. Antimitochondrial antibodies (AMA; >90%)

    b. Serum ANA positive (50%)

    c. Increase in serum IgM

    d. Increased serum ALP and GGT

    e. Increased serum cholesterol
- Component of bile

  5. Treatment

    a. Budesonide + ursodeoxycholic acid

    b. Cholestyramine for pruritus

    c. Liver transplantation
- Improves survival; 70% survive 10 years

F. Secondary biliary cirrhosis

  1. Complication of chronic extrahepatic bile duct obstruction
- Example—cystic fibrosis, where bile is dehydrated (refer to Chapter 16)

  2. *No* increase in serum AMA or IgM

G. Hereditary hemochromatosis

  1. Epidemiology

    a. Autosomal recessive disorder

      (1) Linked to short arm of chromosome 6

      (2) HLA-A3 association

    b. Most common genetic disorder in North European ancestry

Margin notes:

PBC: antimitochondrial antibodies

PBC: pruritus before jaundice

PBC: jaundice is a late finding

PBC: ↑ serum ANA, AMA, IgM

Secondary biliary cirrhosis: cystic fibrosis

c. Male dominant disorder
  • Diagnosis usually made in fifth decade
d. In women, diagnosis usually made 10 to 20 years *after* menopause
  • Due to menses causing loss of iron
2. Pathogenesis
  a. Unrestricted reabsorption of iron in the small intestine
  b. Mutations involving hereditary hemochromatosis gene (*HFE*)
    (1) Two missense mutations (*C282Y* and *H63D*)
    (2) There is a 1:10 carrier rate in the population.
  c. Iron stimulates the production of hydroxyl free radicals (refer to Chapter 1).
    • Free radicals damage tissue and cause fibrosis.

The **normal function of the *HFE* gene product** is to facilitate the binding of plasma transferrin (binding protein of iron) with its mucosal cell transferrin receptor so that transferrin can be endocytosed by intestinal cells. The amount of endocytosed transferrin iron determines how much mucosal cell iron is released into the plasma. In hemochromatosis, when there is a mutated *HFE* gene, mucosal cell transfer of iron to plasma transferrin is always at a maximum resulting in iron overload.

3. Iron deposits in multiple organs
  • Liver (target organ), pancreas, heart, joints, skin, pituitary

Hemosiderosis (secondary hemochromatosis) is caused by multiple blood transfusions (e.g., sickle cell anemia, thalassemia major), alcohol abuse (alcohol increases iron reabsorption), and well water (iron pipes). Iron deposits are more prevalent in macrophages than in parenchymal tissue.

4. Clinical findings
  a. Cirrhosis (60%)
    (1) Iron deposits primarily in hepatocytes (Fig. 18-11).
    (2) Increased risk of hepatocellular carcinoma
  b. "Bronze diabetes"
    (1) Type I diabetes mellitus (60%)
      • Destruction of β-islet cells
    (2) Hyperpigmentation (75%)
      • Iron deposits in skin and increases melanin production
  c. Malabsorption
    • Destruction of exocrine pancreas
  d. Restrictive cardiomyopathy
  e. Hypogonadism
    (1) Amenorrhea in women (25%)
    (2) Testicular atrophy; loss of libido in men (50%)

Marginal notes (left column):

Hemochromatosis: unrestricted reabsorption of iron

Hemochromatosis: missense mutations *HFE* gene on chromosome 6

Iron initiates synthesis hydroxyl free radicals

Hemosiderosis: acquired iron overload disease

Hemochromatosis: "bronze diabetes"

Hemochromatosis: malabsorption, restrictive cardiomyopathy, infertility

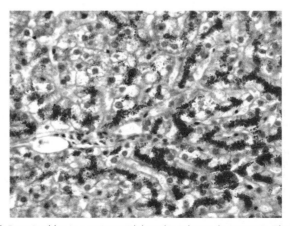

18-11: Liver biopsy stained with Prussian blue in a patient with hereditary hemochromatosis. The hepatocytes are filled with blue iron granules. This is an early stage before parenchymal damage and fibrosis develop. *(From Kumar V, Fausto N, Abbas A: Robbins and Cotran's Pathologic Basis of Disease, 7th ed. Philadelphia, WB Saunders, 2004, p 910, Fig. 18-28.)*

f. Degenerative joint disease (>40%)
  • Chondrocalcinosis (refer to Chapter 23)
5. Laboratory findings
  a. Increased serum iron, percent saturation, and ferritin
    (1) Transferrin saturation is the best screening test.
    (2) Values > 45% indicate further evaluation is necessary.
    (3) Decreased total iron-binding capacity (TIBC)
      • Transferrin synthesis is decreased when iron stores are increased (refer to Chapter 11).
    (4) Serum ferritin is primarily used to follow therapy.
  b. Liver biopsy confirmatory test
  c. Decreased serum luteinizing hormone and follicle-stimulating hormone
6. Screening test for relatives
  • *HFE* gene testing for *C282Y* mutation
7. Treatment
  a. Phlebotomy until serum ferritin < 50 μg/mL, saturation < 30%
  b. Deferoxamine (iron chelator)
8. Normal life expectancy if no cirrhosis

H. Wilson's disease (hepatolenticular degeneration)
1. Epidemiology
  a. Autosomal recessive disorder
  b. Affects men and women equally
  c. Onset of symptoms from 3 to 40 years of age
    • Usually late childhood
  d. Liver disease progresses from acute hepatitis to cirrhosis.
2. Pathogenesis
  a. Gene mutation
    (1) Defective hepatocyte transport of copper into bile for excretion
    (2) Defective incorporation of copper into ceruloplasmin (binding protein for copper in blood)
  b. Unbound copper eventually accumulates in blood.
    (1) Loosely attached to albumin
    (2) Copper deposits in other tissues cause a toxic effect.

Ceruloplasmin is an enzyme that is synthesized in the liver. It contains 6 atoms of copper in its structure. Ceruloplasmin is secreted into the plasma where it represents 90% to 95% of the total serum copper concentration. The remaining 5% to 10% of copper is free copper that is loosely bound to albumin. Ceruloplasmin is eventually taken up and degraded by the liver. The copper that was bound to ceruloplasmin is excreted into the bile. The gene defect in Wilson's disease affects a copper transport system that produces a dual defect—decreased incorporation of copper into ceruloplasmin in the liver and decreased excretion of copper into bile. Accumulation of copper in the liver increases the formation of hydroxyl free radicals causing damage to hepatocytes. Liver disease progresses from acute hepatitis to cirrhosis. In a few years, unbound copper is released from the liver into the circulation (increased in blood and urine) where it damages the brain, kidneys, cornea, and other tissues.

3. Clinical findings
  a. Kayser-Fleischer ring (~70%)
    (1) Due to free copper deposits in Descemet's membrane in the cornea (Fig. 18-12)
    (2) *Not* pathognomonic of Wilson's disease; can be seen in primary biliary cirrhosis
  b. Central nervous system disease (>50%)
    (1) Copper deposits in the putamen
      • Produces a movement disorder resembling parkinsonism
    (2) Copper deposits in the subthalamic nucleus
      • Produces hemiballismus
    (3) Copper is toxic to neurons in the cerebral cortex
      • Produces dementia
  c. Hepatosplenomegaly (50%)
    • Liver biopsy shows increased copper.
  d. Hemolytic anemia
  e. Renal disease
    • Proximal tubule damage produces Fanconi syndrome (refer to Chapter 4).

Hemochromatosis: ↑ serum iron, % saturation, ferritin; ↓ TIBC

Hemochromatosis: % saturation best screen

Serum ferritin: used to follow therapy

Wilson's disease: ↓ incorporation copper into ceruloplasmin, ↓ excretion copper into bile

Ceruloplasmin: enzyme synthesized in the liver that contains copper

Kayser-Fleischer ring: excess copper in Descemet's membrane of cornea

Wilson's disease: lenticular degeneration in CNS; movement disorder; dementia

Wilson's disease: hemolytic anemia; renal disease

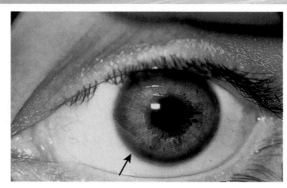

18-12: Kayser-Fleischer ring. The *arrow* depicts deposition of a copper-colored pigment in Descemet's membrane in the cornea. *(From Perkin GD: Mosby's Color Atlas and Text of Neurology. St. Louis, Mosby, 2002, p 151, Fig. 8-15.)*

4. Laboratory findings
   a. Decreased total serum copper
      • Due to decreased ceruloplasmin
   b. Decreased serum ceruloplasmin
      • Useful in diagnosing Wilson's disease in its early stages
   c. Increased serum and urine free copper
      • Useful in diagnosing Wilson's disease in the later stages
5. Treatment
   a. Penicillamine (copper chelator)
   b. Zinc
      • Inhibits copper reabsorption in intestine
   c. Ammonium tetrathiomolybdate
      (1) Competes for copper reabsorption in bowel
      (2) Increases copper excretion in urine
   d. Liver transplantation
I. α₁-Antitrypsin (AAT) deficiency
1. Epidemiology
   a. Autosomal dominant (codominant)
   b. Pathogenesis
      (1) Alleles are inherited codominantly (each allele expresses itself).
      (2) Normal allele is M (95% frequency in the United States).
         • MM is normal genotype with AAT in normal range.
      (3) Deficient variant (decreased AAT) Z allele (1–2% frequency)
      (4) Deficient variant (decreased AAT) S allele (2–3% frequency)
      (5) Severe deficiency most commonly occurs in homozygous ZZ variant.
         (a) Decreased (<15% of normal) AAT levels in serum
         (b) Associated with panacinar emphysema (refer to Chapter 16)
         (c) Associated with cirrhosis of the liver (see later)
      (6) Risk of lung disease in heterozygotes (e.g., MZ) is uncertain.
   c. Most common cause of cirrhosis in children
2. Children with accumulation of AAT in hepatocytes
   a. In ~50% of homozygous ZZ patients, AAT is *not* secreted properly from hepatocytes.
   b. Pathologic accumulation of AAT in hepatocytes causes liver damage.
      • Periodic acid–Schiff stains show red cytoplasmic granules (Fig. 18-13).
   c. Presents as neonatal hepatitis with intrahepatic cholestasis
   d. Hepatitis progresses into cirrhosis.
      • AAT deficiency is the most common cause of cirrhosis in children.
   e. Increased risk for hepatocellular carcinoma
3. Treatment for AAT deficiency
   a. Pooled AAT given intravenously
   b. Liver and lung transplantation
J. Laboratory test abnormalities in cirrhosis
1. Decreased serum blood urea nitrogen (BUN) and increased serum ammonia
   • Due to disruption of the urea cycle

Wilson's disease: ↓ total serum copper, ceruloplasmin; ↓ serum/urine free copper

Rx Wilson's disease: penicillamine (copper chelator)

AAT deficiency: M is the normal allele; Z and S are deficiency variant alleles

Cirrhosis in AAT deficiency: homozygous ZZ variant; AAT not secreted properly and accumulates in the liver

Cirrhosis: ↓ serum BUN, ↑ serum ammonia

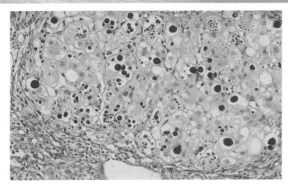

18-13: α_1-Antitrypsin deficiency. The globules are periodic acid–Schiff positive. *(From MacSween R, Burt A, Portmann B, et al: Pathology of the Liver, 4th ed. London, Churchill Livingstone, 2002, p 176, Fig. 4-21.)*

2. Fasting hypoglycemia
    - Defective gluconeogenesis and decreased glycogen stores (see Fig. 6-1)
3. Chronic respiratory alkalosis
    - Toxic products from hepatic dysfunction overstimulate respiratory center (refer to Chapter 4)
4. Lactic acidosis
    - Liver dysfunction in converting lactic acid to pyruvate (see Fig. 6-1)
5. Hyponatremia (refer to Chapter 4)
    a. Decreased cardiac output
    b. Kidney reabsorbs slightly hypotonic solution ($\uparrow$ TBNa$^+$/$\uparrow\uparrow$ TBW)
6. Hypokalemia
    - Secondary aldosteronism increases renal exchange of Na$^+$ for K$^+$ (refer to Chapter 4)
7. Increased PT
    - Decreased synthesis of coagulation factors
8. Hypoalbuminemia
    - Decreased synthesis of albumin
9. Hypocalcemia
    a. Hypoalbuminemia decreases the total serum calcium.
        - Approximately 40% of the total calcium is calcium bound to albumin.
    b. Vitamin D deficiency
        - Decreased liver 25-hydroxylation of vitamin D.
10. Mild transaminasemia
    - Enzymes are *not* markedly increased due to the loss of parenchymal cells.

VIII. Liver Tumors
A. Focal nodular hyperplasia (FNH)
1. Epidemiology
    a. Tumor-like condition
    b. More common in women than men
    c. Cause is unknown
        - Probable reaction to injury
    d. Usually an incidental finding
2. Gross findings
    a. Poorly encapsulated nodule
    b. Central depressed stellate scar
        - Contains large blood vessels
    c. Fibrous septae radiate to the periphery.
3. CT scan
    - Hypervascular mass with arteriovenous connections
4. Treatment
    - Leave it alone unless associated with pain
B. Benign tumors
1. Cavernous hemangioma
    a. Most common benign tumor
    b. Best diagnosed with enhanced CT scan
    c. Rare cause of intraperitoneal hemorrhage

Hypoglycemia in cirrhosis: $\downarrow$ gluconeogenesis, $\downarrow$ glycogen stores

Cirrhosis: lactic acidosis, hyponatremia, hypokalemia

Severe liver dysfunction: $\downarrow$ serum albumin, $\uparrow$ PT

Hypocalcemia in cirrhosis: $\downarrow$ serum albumin, $\downarrow$ 25(OH)-vitamin D

FNH: central stellate scar with radiating fibrous septae

Cavernous hemangioma: most common benign tumor; potential for intraperitoneal hemorrhage

2. Liver (hepatic) cell adenoma
   a. Benign tumor of hepatocytes
   b. Occurs in women more often than men
   c. Causes
      (1) OCPs (most common)
      (2) Anabolic steroids
      (3) Von Gierke's glycogenosis
   d. Highly vascular tumors

      (1) Tendency to rupture during pregnancy
      (2) Produce intraperitoneal hemorrhage
   e. Tend to regress if off OCP and anabolics
3. Treatment is surgery if symptomatic.

C. Malignant tumors
   1. Metastasis
      a. Most common liver cancer (see Fig. 8-2E)

      b. Primary cancers of lung (most common), gastrointestinal tract, breast
      c. Multiple nodular masses
   2. Hepatocellular carcinoma (HCC)
      a. Epidemiology
         (1) Most common primary liver cancer
         (2) Rapidly increasing in the United States due to increase in HCV infection
         (3) Occurs in males more than females
            • Peaks around fifth and sixth decades
         (4) Causes

            (a) Postnecrotic cirrhosis due to chronic HBV and HCV
            (b) Alcoholic cirrhosis
            (c) Aflatoxins (from *Aspergillus* mold in grains and peanuts)
            (d) Hereditary hemochromatosis, Wilson's disease
            (e) PBC, AAT deficiency, tyrosinemia
      b. Pathogenesis
         (1) Most often associated with pre-existing cirrhosis

         (2) Postnecrotic cirrhosis HBV/HCV most common risk factors
      c. Gross findings
         (1) Focal, multifocal, or diffusely infiltrating cancer (Fig. 18-14)
            • With or without pre-existing cirrhosis (usually with pre-existing cirrhosis)
         (2) Portal and hepatic vein invasion is common.
      d. Microscopic findings

         • Characteristic finding is the presence of bile in neoplastic cells.
      e. Clinical findings
         (1) Over one third are asymptomatic.
         (2) Abdominal pain is a common initial presentation.
         (3) Fever
            • Due to liver cell necrosis

         (4) Rapid enlargement of the liver in a patient with cirrhosis
            • Increased ascites; blood present in ascitic fluid

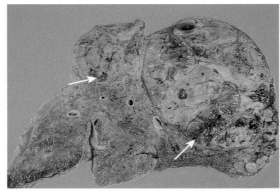

18-14: Hepatocellular carcinoma. Multiple large, hemorrhagic tumor masses are present in the liver (*arrows*). There is also diffuse infiltration of tumor blending in with the remaining liver. (*From Damjanov I, Linder J: Pathology: A Color Atlas. St. Louis, Mosby, 2000, p 161, Fig. 8-70.*)

f. Laboratory findings
   (1) Increased α-fetoprotein (AFP; 70%)
       • Sensitivity 40% to 60%, specificity 80% to 94%
   (2) Increased serum ALP and GGT
       • Sudden increase is a characteristic finding.
   (3) Production of ectopic hormones
       (a) Erythropoietin (EPO; secondary polycythemia)
       (b) Insulin-like factor (hypoglycemia)
       (c) Parathyroid hormone (PTH)-related protein (hypercalcemia)
g. Lung most common metastatic site
h. Diagnosis
   (1) CT scan and ultrasound localize HCC.
   (2) Angiography shows pooling and increased vascularity.
i. Treatment
   (1) Surgery (<20% are surgical candidates)
   (2) Liver transplantation
   (3) Radiation and chemotherapy are usually not helpful.
j. Prognosis
   (1) If unresectable, most die within 6 months.
   (2) If resectable, 5-year survival rate is 30% to 50%.
3. Angiosarcoma
   • Exposure to vinyl chloride (most common cause), arsenic, or thorium dioxide

IX. **Gallbladder and Biliary Tract Disease**
A. **Cystic diseases**
   1. Choledochal cyst
      a. Most common cyst in biliary tract in children younger than 10 years old
      b. Clinical findings
         (1) Abdominal pain with persistent or intermittent jaundice
         (2) Increased incidence of cholelithiasis, cholangiocarcinoma, and cirrhosis
      c. Diagnosis
         (1) Ultrasound is screening test of choice
         (2) Endoscopic retrograde cholangiopancreatography (ERCP) or transhepatic cholangiography
            (a) Useful in identifying intra- and extrahepatic cysts
            (b) Useful in identifying sites of obstruction
      d. Treatment is surgery.
   2. Caroli disease
      a. Autosomal dominant and recessive types
      b. Segmental dilatation of intrahepatic bile ducts
      c. Portal tract fibrosis
      d. Clinical findings
         (1) Association with polycystic kidney disease
            • Autosomal recessive types in children or autosomal dominant in adults
         (2) Increased incidence of cholangiocarcinoma
         (3) Increased incidence of the following:
            • Intrahepatic cholelithiasis, cholangitis, hepatic abscesses, portal hypertension
      e. Treatment
         (1) Surgical resection of an involved lobe
         (2) Liver transplantation
B. **Cholangiocarcinoma**
   1. Most common malignancy of bile ducts
   2. Causes of cholangiocarcinoma
      a. Primary sclerosing cholangitis (see section VI)
         • Most common cause in the United States
      b. *Clonorchis sinensis* (Chinese liver fluke)
      c. Thorotrast (thorium dioxide)
      d. Choledochal cyst, Caroli disease
   3. Locations
      a. Ampulla or common bile duct (most common sites)
      b. Junction of right/left hepatic duct (Klatskin tumor)
      c. Intrahepatic

HCC: ↑ serum AFP; rapidly increasing bloody ascites

Ectopic hormones: PTH-related protein, insulin-like factor; EPO

Liver angiosarcoma: exposure to vinyl chloride (plastic pipes)

Choledochal cyst: most common biliary tract cyst in children; pain with intermittent jaundice

Cystic diseases: increased risk for cholangiocarcinoma

Caroli disease: association with juvenile polycystic kidney disease

Primary sclerosing cholangitis: most common cause of cholangiocarcinoma

4. Clinical findings
   a. Obstructive jaundice
   b. Palpable gallbladder (Courvoisier's sign)
      • Only mid–common bile duct or ampulla locations
   c. Hepatomegaly
5. Diagnosis
   • Ultrasound, ERCP
6. Treatment is surgery.

C. **Gallstones (cholelithiasis)**
1. Components of bile
   a. Bile salts/acids (~67%)
      (1) Hepatic product of cholesterol (CH) metabolism
      (2) Water soluble
      (3) Detergent action renders CH soluble in bile.
   b. Phospholipid (22%)
      (1) Mainly lecithin
      (2) Hydrophobic
      (3) Solubilizes CH in bile
   c. Protein (4.5%), free CH (4%), conjugated bilirubin (0.3%)
   d. Water, electrolytes, bicarbonate
2. Types
   a. Cholesterol stones (75%) (Fig. 18-15)
      (1) Usually stones are of mixed composition.
      (2) Stones contain CH, calcium carbonate, some bilirubin pigment.
         • Can be radiopaque if they contain calcium carbonate
      (3) Rarely are stones purely CH.
      (4) CH stones are radiolucent.
   b. Pigment stones
      (1) Black pigment stones (Fig. 18-16)
         (a) Sign of chronic extravascular hemolytic anemia
            • Examples—sickle cell anemia, hereditary spherocytosis
         (b) Excess bilirubin in bile produces calcium bilirubinate
      (2) Brown pigment stones
         (a) Sign of infection in the common bile duct (CBD)
         (b) Commonly seen in Asians
3. Pathogenesis
   a. Cholesterol stones
      (1) Supersaturation of bile with cholesterol
      (2) Decreased bile salts/acids (refer to Chapter 17) and lecithin
         • Both normally solubilize cholesterol in bile
      (3) Risk factors
         (a) Female > 40 years old

Bile: bile salts/acid, phospholipid, protein, CB, free CH, electrolytes, biocarbonate

Cholesterol gallstones: most common stone

Black pigment gallstone: sign of extravascular hemolysis; calcium bilirubinate

Brown pigment gallstones: sign of CBD infection

CH gallstones: ↑ CH in bile, ↓ bile salts and lecithin

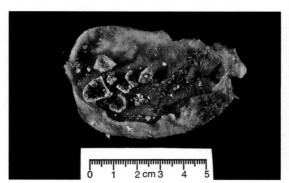

18-15: Yellow cholesterol stones with centers containing entrapped bile pigments. The wall of the gallbladder is scarred. *(From Kumar V, Fausto N, Abbas A: Robbins and Cotran's Pathologic Basis of Disease, 7th ed. Philadelphia, WB Saunders, 2004, p 930, Fig. 18-50.)*

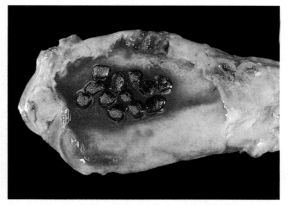

18-16: Black pigmented stones. These types of stones are usually a sign of a chronic extravascular hemolytic anemia where there is an increase in calcium bilirubinate in bile. *(From Kumar V, Fausto N, Abbas A: Robbins and Cotran's Pathologic Basis of Disease, 7th ed. Philadelphia, WB Saunders, 2004, p 931, Fig. 18-51.)*

(b) Obesity
  • Cholesterol is increased in bile.
(c) Use of oral contraceptive pills

Estrogen increases CH stone formation by a number of different mechanisms. Estrogen increases the synthesis of high-density lipoprotein (HDL), which transports cholesterol from peripheral tissue to the liver for excretion in bile. Estrogen also upregulates low-density lipoprotein (LDL) receptor synthesis in hepatocytes and increases HMG-CoA reductase activity, the rate-limiting enzyme in CH synthesis.

Estrogen: ↑ HDL and delivery CH to liver; ↑ LDL receptors and HMG-CoA reductase activity

(d) Rapid weight loss; use of lipid-lowering drugs
(e) Native Americans (e.g., Pima and Navajo Indians)
4. Complications associated with stones
  a. Cholecystitis (most common)
  b. CBD obstruction
  c. Gallbladder cancer
  d. Acute pancreatitis

Stone complications: cholecystitis, CBD obstruction, cancer, acute pancreatitis

D. Acute cholecystitis
1. Epidemiology
  a. More common in women than in men
  b. Occurs most often during fifth and sixth decades
  c. High incidence in Native Americans (see above)
  d. Associated with gallstones in >95% of cases

CH gallstones: ↑ CH in bile, ↓ bile salts and lecithin

2. Stages of development of acute cholecystitis
  a. Stage 1
    (1) Stone lodges in the cystic duct
      (a) Stimulus of food causes gallbladder (GB) contraction.
      (b) Stone is forced into the cystic duct.
    (2) Midepigastric colicky pain occurs.
      • Due to GB contraction against obstructed cystic duct
    (3) Nausea and vomiting *without* pain relief

Stage 1: stone lodges in cystic duct; midepigastric colicky pain

  b. Stage 2
    (1) Stone becomes impacted in the cystic duct.
    (2) Mucus accumulates behind the obstruction.
    (3) Chemical irritation of mucosa
    (4) Bacterial overgrowth (no invasion)
      (a) Most commonly *Escherichia coli*
      (b) Less commonly—*Enterococci, Bacteroides fragilis, Clostridium* sp
    (5) Pain shifts to right upper quadrant (RUQ)
      (a) Dull, continuous aching pain
      (b) Pain radiation to right scapular/shoulder

Stage 2: stone impacts in cystic duct; pain shift to RUQ; radiation to right scapular shoulder

  c. Stage 3
    (1) Bacterial invasion of GB wall
    (2) Localized peritonitis with rebound tenderness
    (3) Positive Murphy sign (see below)
    (4) Absolute neutrophilic leukocytosis
    (5) Attack subsides if the stone falls out of the cystic duct
      (a) Approximately 90% subside over 37 days
      (b) If not, it perforates (next stage)

Stage 3: bacterial invasion GB wall; + Murphy sign; subsides if stone falls out

  d. Stage 4
    (1) Perforation
      • Wall tension from GB distention compresses lumens of intramural vessels → gangrenous necrosis

Stage 4: perforation

3. Other causes *not* associated with stones
  a. AIDS
    • Infection with cytomegalovirus (CMV) or *Cryptosporidium*
  b. Severe volume depletion
4. Clinical findings
  a. Fever
  b. See stages of acute cholecystitis
  c. Vomiting (75%)

d. Radiation of pain to the right scapula/shoulder

Pain radiation: right scapula/shoulder

e. Murphy sign
- Pain when the GB hits the examiner's finger on patient inspiration

f. Jaundice (25%)
   (1) Usually indicates CBD stone
   (2) Indication for CBD exploration

g. Palpable gallbladder (15%)

5. Laboratory findings
   a. Absolute neutrophilic leukocytosis with left shift
   - WBC counts > 12,000 cells/mm^3 (>70%)
   b. Increased serum AST/ALP
   c. Increased serum amylase suggests associated pancreatitis
   d. Increased serum bilirubin > 4 mg/dL unusual
   - Usually indicates stone in CBD

6. Tests to identify stones

Ultrasound: gold standard for diagnosis

   a. Ultrasound is the preferred initial test (Fig. 18-17)
   (1) Gold standard test (>98% sensitivity)
   (2) Detects stones > 12 mm in diameter
   (3) Detects sludge; evaluates GB wall thickness
   (4) *Not* effective in identifying CBD stones (<30% sensitivity)
   b. Plain film
   - Only 20% are radiopaque
   c. Hepatobiliary iminodiacetic acid (HIDA) radionuclide scan

HIDA scan: identifies stone in cystic duct and CBD

   (1) Identifies stone(s) in cystic duct
   - No visualization of GB
   (2) No tracer in duodenum
   - Indicates CBD stone

7. Indications for CBD exploration

Jaundice: indication for CBD exploration

   a. Jaundice
   b. CBD dilatation > 12 mm
   c. No stones in GB
   d. Acute pancreatitis

8. Treatment
   a. Cholecystectomy (laparoscope preferred)
   b. ERCP with sphincterotomy to extract stone in CBD

Treatment cholecystitis: surgery via laparoscope

   c. Meperidine for pain
   (1) Do *not* use morphine
   (2) Contracts the sphincter of Oddi and worsens pain

Pain in cholecystitis: meperidine *not* morphine

   d. Piperacillin-tazobactam

E. Chronic cholecystitis
1. Epidemiology
   - Most common symptomatic disorder of GB

Chronic cholecystitis: most common symptomatic disorder of the GB

2. Pathogenesis
   a. Cholelithiasis with repeated attacks of minor inflammation

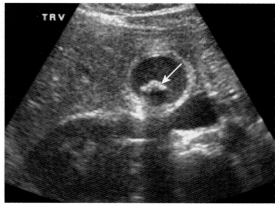

18-17: Ultrasound showing gallstones (*arrow*). (*From Goldman L, Ausiello D: Cecil's Textbook of Medicine, 23rd ed. Philadelphia, Saunders Elsevier, 2008, p 1158, Fig. 159-5.*)

b. Chemical inflammation (infection is uncommon)

3. Clinical findings

   a. Severe, persistent pain 12 hours postprandially in the evening

   b. Pain radiates into the right scapular area.

   c. Recurrent epigastric distress, belching, and bloating

4. Treatment is laparoscopic cholecystectomy.

F. Cholesterolosis

1. Excess cholesterol in bile

   a. Cholesterol deposits in macrophages

   b. Produces a yellow, speckled mucosal surface

2. *No* clinical significance

G. Hydrops of gallbladder

1. Chronic obstruction of cystic duct

2. Distended GB with atrophy of the mucosa/muscle

3. Clear secretions

4. Treatment is surgery.

H. Gallbladder adenocarcinoma

1. Epidemiology

   a. Dominant in elderly women

   b. Poor prognosis

2. Pathogenesis

   a. Cholelithiasis (95% of cases)

   b. Porcelain gallbladder

      (1) Gallbladder with dystrophic calcification

      (2) Mandatory removal of GB

         (a) Approximately 50% risk for progression to cancer

         (b) Immediate surgical removal is warranted.

3. Treatment is surgery.

   a. Majority have already locally invaded liver or porta hepatis at discovery.

   b. Five-year survival rate < 2%

X. Pancreatic Disorders

A. Embryologic abnormalities of the pancreas

1. Annular pancreas

   a. Dorsal and ventral buds form a ring around the duodenum.

   b. Associated with small bowel obstruction

2. Aberrant pancreatic tissue (i.e., heterotopic rest, choristoma)

   • Locations—wall of stomach, duodenum, jejunum, or Meckel diverticulum

3. Major pancreatic duct

   a. Major pancreatic duct and CBD are confluent in their terminal part.

      • Both empty their contents into the duodenum via the ampulla of Vater.

   b. Important in the pathogenesis of acute pancreatitis

      (1) Stone(s) obstruct terminal part of the CBD →

      (2) Increased back-pressure refluxes bile into the major pancreatic duct →

      (3) Bile activates pancreatic proenzymes causing acute pancreatitis

B. Acute pancreatitis

1. Epidemiology and pathogenesis

   a. Alcohol abuse and gallstones are the major causes.

   b. Must be activation of pancreatic proenzymes (inactive enzymes)

      • Activation leads to autodigestion of the pancreas.

   c. Mechanisms of activation of proenzymes

      (1) Obstruction of the main pancreatic duct or terminal CBD

         (a) Gallstones (see section IX)

         (b) Alcohol thickens ductal secretions.

           • Also increases duct permeability to enzymes

      (2) Chemical injury of acinar cells

         • Examples—thiazides, alcohol, triglyceride (>1000 mg/dL)

      (3) Infectious injury of acinar cells

         • Examples—CMV, mumps, coxsackievirus

      (4) Mechanical injury of acinar cells

         • Examples—seat belt trauma, posterior penetration of duodenal ulcer

      (5) Metabolic activation of proenzymes (e.g., hypercalcemia, ischemia, shock)

Margin notes:

Chronic cholecystitis: chemical inflammation

Cholesterolosis: excess CH in bile; speckled yellow mucosal surface

Hydrops: chronic obstruction of cystic duct

GB cancer: association with GB stones; porcelain GB

Porcelain gallbladder: ↑ risk for gallbladder cancer; immediate surgery

Major pancreatic duct: empties into terminal part of CBD; stone blocking CBD causes acute pancreatitis

Alcohol abuse: most common cause of acute pancreatitis

Seat belt trauma: most common cause of pancreatitis in children

d. Trypsin is important in the activation of proenzymes.
   (1) Proteases damage acinar cell structure.
   (2) Lipases and phospholipases produce enzymatic fat necrosis.
   (3) Elastases damage vessel walls and produce hemorrhage (see Fig. 1-11H).
   (4) Activated enzymes also circulate in the blood.
2. Clinical findings
   a. Fever, nausea, and vomiting
   b. Severe, boring (knife-like) midepigastric pain with radiation into the back
      • Radiation into back is due to its retroperitoneal location.
   c. Hypovolemic shock

> **Third space fluid** is sequestered fluid that is unavailable for maintenance of volume in the vascular compartment (nonfunctional extracellular fluid). In acute pancreatitis, it refers to the peripancreatic collection of fluid that commonly occurs as the pancreas autodigests itself. If conditions improve, the third space fluid gains entry back into the vascular compartment and may cause fluid overload.

      • Due to third space loss of fluids
   d. Hypoxemia
      (1) Circulating pancreatic phospholipase destroys surfactant.
         • Loss of surfactant produces atelectasis and intrapulmonary shunting.
      (2) Acute respiratory distress syndrome (ARDS) may occur.
   e. Grey-Turner sign (flank hemorrhage; Fig. 18-18)
   f. Cullen's sign (periumbilical hemorrhage; Fig. 18-19)
   g. Disseminated intravascular coagulation
      • Due to activation of prothrombin by trypsin
   h. Tetany
      (1) Hypocalcemia is caused by enzymatic fat necrosis.
      (2) Calcium binds to fatty acids leading to a decrease in ionized calcium.
3. Complications
   a. Pancreatic necrosis
      (1) Systemic signs occur earlier than usual.
      (2) Higher fever than usual; sinus tachycardia
      (3) Greater degree of neutrophilic leukocytosis
      (4) Peripancreatic infections occur in 40% to 70% of cases.
   b. Pancreatic pseudocyst (20%)
      (1) Collection of digested pancreatic tissue around pancreas
      (2) Abdominal mass with persistence of serum amylase longer than 10 days
         • Amount of amylase in the fluid surpasses renal clearance of amylase.
      (3) Treatment
         (a) If <5 cm, observe and follow with CT scan.
            • Most resolve without surgical intervention.
         (b) If >5 cm, percutaneous drainage with CT or ultrasound guidance

Margin notes:

Pancreatitis: pain radiates into the back; described as a knife-like pain

Third space fluid: fluid unavailable for maintenance of volume in vascular compartment

Hypoxemia: circulating phospholipase destroys surfactant

Grey-Turner sign: flank hemorrhage

Cullen's sign: periumbilical hemorrhage

Persistent increase in serum amylase: consider pancreatic pseudocyst

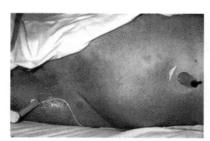

18-18: Grey-Turner sign. Note the purplish discoloration in the loins due to tracking of hemorrhagic necrotic pancreatic material along the retroperitoneal planes. *(From Grieg JD: Color Atlas of Surgical Diagnosis. London, Mosby-Wolfe, 1996, p 162, Fig. 22-5.)*

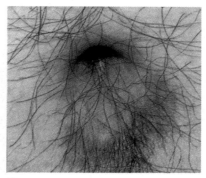

18-19: Cullen's sign. Note the hemorrhagic discoloration around the umbilicus. It is due to tracking of hemorrhagic necrotic pancreatic tissue around the falciform and umbilical ligaments. *(From Grieg JD: Color Atlas of Surgical Diagnosis. London, Mosby-Wolfe, 1996, p 162, Fig. 22-4.)*

c. Pancreatic abscess
  (1) Clinical and laboratory findings
    (a) Abdominal pain
    (b) High fever due to sepsis
      • Usually gram-negative infections such as *E. coli* or *Pseudomonas* spp.
    (c) Neutrophilic leukocytosis
    (d) Persistent hyperamylasemia
  (2) Diagnosis
    (a) CT scan shows multiple radiolucent bubbles in the retroperitoneum.
    (b) CT-guided aspiration of abscess identifies organisms.
  (3) Treatment
    (a) Surgical drainage
    (b) Imipenem-cilastin
d. Pancreatic ascites
  (1) Usually caused by leaking of a pseudocyst
  (2) Peritoneal fluid has high amylase level.
  (3) Usually resolves spontaneously
4. Laboratory findings
  a. Serum amylase
    (1) *Not* specific for pancreatitis
    (2) Also present in salivary glands
      • Increased in mumps
    (3) Amylase in acute pancreatitis
      (a) Sensitivity 85%, specificity 70%
      (b) Initial increase at 2 to 12 hours; peaks over 12 to 30 hours; returns to normal in 2 to 4 days
        • Increased renal clearance
      (c) Present in urine for 1 to 14 days
      (d) Persistent increase in serum amylase > 7 days
        • Suggests pancreatic pseudocyst; collection of amylase-rich fluid around pancreas
      (e) Urine amylase
        • Initial increase over 4 to 8 hours; peaks at 18 to 36 hours; returns to normal over 7 to 10 days
    (4) Amylase in chronic pancreatitis
      (a) Less reliable than in acute disease
      (b) Values either normal, borderline, or slightly increased
  b. Serum lipase
    (1) More specific for pancreatitis
      • Is *not* excreted in urine
    (2) Lipase in acute pancreatitis
      (a) Sensitivity 80%, specificity 75%
      (b) Initial increase in 3 to 6 hours; peaks in 12 to 30 hours; returns to normal over 7 to 14 days
    (3) Lipase in chronic pancreatitis
      • *Not* clinically useful
  c. Serum immunoreactive trypsin
    (1) Trypsin is specific for the pancreas.
    (2) Excellent newborn screen for cystic fibrosis
    (3) Serum immunoreactive trypsin in acute pancreatitis
      (a) Sensitivity 95% to 100%
      (b) Increases 5 to 10 times normal
      (c) Remains increased for 4 to 5 days
    (4) Serum immunoreactive trypsin in chronic pancreatitis
      • Decreased concentration
  d. Neutrophilic leukocytosis
  e. Hypocalcemia, hyperglycemia (destruction of β-islet cells)
5. Imaging studies
  a. CT scan is the gold standard for pancreatic imaging.
  b. Plain abdominal radiograph
    (1) Sentinel loop in subjacent duodenum or transverse colon (cut-off sign)
      • Localized ileus, where the bowel does *not* demonstrate peristalsis

---

Pancreatic abscess: higher fever from gram-negative sepsis; ↑ amylase; CT shows bubbles

Pancreatic ascites: leaking pseudocyst

Amylase: not specific for pancreatitis

Acute pancreatitis: increased clearance of amylase in urine

Serum lipase: more specific and lasts longer than amylase in acute pancreatitis; excellent screen for acute pancreatitis

Serum immunoreactive trypsin: excellent newborn screen for cystic fibrosis

CT scan: gold standard for pancreatic imaging

Plain radiograph: sentinel loop; left-sided pleural effusion

(2) Left-sided pleural effusion containing amylase (10% of cases)
6. Ranson criteria are used to determine prognosis in acute pancreatitis.

Admission (first 24 hours): age > 55 years old, WBC count > 16,000 cells/mm³, serum glucose > 200 mg/dL, serum LDH > 350 IU/L, serum AST > 250 U/L. Subsequent 48 hours: hematocrit drop > 10% with hydration, serum BUN rise > 5 mg/dL, Pao₂ < 60 mm Hg (respiratory failure), base deficit > 4 mEq/L (metabolic acidosis), calcium < 8 mg/dL, fluid sequestration > 6 L. Prognosis: <3 signs = 0.9% mortality rate; 3–4 signs = 11% to 16% mortality rate; 5–6 signs = 33 to 40% mortality rate; >6 signs = 100% mortality rate.

7. Treatment
   a. NPO until clinically improved
   b. Crystalloid solutions
   c. Meperidine or fentanyl for pain
   d. Nasogastric suction if vomiting severe
   e. Oxygen
C. **Chronic pancreatitis**
   1. Epidemiology

Chronic pancreatitis adults: alcohol abuse most common known cause

   a. Occurs in men more commonly than women
   b. Majority are idiopathic.
   c. Known causes

Chronic pancreatitis in children: cystic fibrosis most common cause

      (1) Alcohol abuse is the most common known cause.
      (2) Cystic fibrosis is the most common cause in children.
      (3) Malnutrition is the most common cause in developing countries.
      (4) Autoimmune

Chronic pancreatitis in developing countries: malnutrition

   2. Pathogenesis
      a. Repeated attacks of acute pancreatitis produce duct obstruction.
      b. Calcified concretions occur as well as dilation of the ducts.
         • Radiographic dyes show a "chain of lakes" appearance in the major duct.

Chronic pancreatitis: dyes show "chain of lakes" in major duct

   3. Clinical findings
      a. Severe pain radiating into the back
      b. Malabsorption
         • Indicates >90% exocrine function destroyed

Chronic pancreatitis: malabsorption, type 1 diabetes mellitus

      c. Type 1 diabetes mellitus (70%)
         • Brittle diabetes due to loss of insulin and glucagon
      d. Pancreatic pseudocyst
   4. Laboratory and radiographic findings
      a. Increased amylase and lipase (neither are reliable)
      b. Increased serum immunoreactive trypsin
      c. Tests for pancreatic insufficiency

Chronic pancreatitis: CT scan dystrophic calcification

         (1) CT scan of pancreas shows dystrophic calcification (see Fig. 1-9).
            • Sign of chronic pancreatitis
         (2) Functional tests
            (a) Secretin stimulation test (requires instrumentation)
               • Tests ability of pancreas to secrete fluids and electrolytes
            (b) Bentiromide test

Tests pancreatic insufficiency: secretin stimulation; bentiromide

               • Tests ability of pancreatic chymotrypsin to cleave orally administered bentiromide to para-aminobenzoic acid (measured in urine)
   5. Treatment
      a. Abstain from alcohol.
      b. Addiction is common.
         • Try simple analgesics or NSAIDs
      c. Pancreatic enzymes
      d. Fat-soluble vitamins
      e. Octreotide for pain if idiopathic
   6. Approximately 50% of patients die within 10 years.
D. **Exocrine pancreatic cancer**
   1. Epidemiology
      a. Slightly more common in men than women
      b. Incidence rate is stable in men and women.

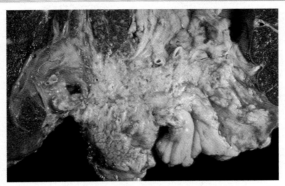

18-20: Pancreatic adenocarcinoma. Yellow tumor has extensively replaced the pancreas. *(From Klatt E: Robbins and Cotran's Atlas of Pathology. Philadelphia, WB Saunders, 2006, p 226, Fig. 9-14.)*

    c. Usually occurs in seventh and eighth decades of life
    d. Adenocarcinoma with varying degrees of differentiation
    e. Causes
        (1) Smoking (most common cause)
          • Includes smokeless tobacco
        (2) Chronic pancreatitis
        (3) Hereditary pancreatitis
        (4) Diabetes mellitus
          • Particularly in women
        (5) High saturated fat diet; obesity; cirrhosis
  2. Pathogenesis
    a. Association with *K-RAS* gene mutation
    b. Mutation of suppressor genes (*TP16* and *TP53*)
  3. Location
    a. Most occur in the pancreatic head (65% of cases) (Fig. 18-20)
      • Often blocks CBD causing jaundice
    b. Remainder occur in the body and tail.
  4. Clinical and laboratory findings
    a. Epigastric pain with weight loss (>90%)
    b. Signs of CBD obstruction (carcinoma of head of pancreas)
        (1) Jaundice (>90%; CB > 50%)
        (2) Light-colored stools (absent UBG)
        (3) Palpable gallbladder (Courvoisier's sign; 30%)
    c. Superficial migratory thrombophlebitis (refer to Chapter 8)
    d. Metastasis to left supraclavicular node (Virchow's node)
      • Also occurs in stomach cancer
    e. Periumbilical metastasis (Sister Mary Joseph's sign)
      • Also occurs in stomach cancer
    f. Increased CA19–9
      • Gold standard tumor marker
  5. Diagnosis
    a. Helical CT scan is best test.
        (1) Shows C sign in cancer of head of pancreas
          • Cancer indents duodenum; looks like the letter C
        (2) CT guided percutaneous biopsy for diagnosis
  6. Treatment
    • Surgery (Whipple's procedure), radiation, chemotherapy

Whipple's procedure is an en bloc resection of the pancreatic head and neck (distal pancreas remains to prevent diabetes mellitus) and resection of part of the CBD. In some cases, there is resection of the antrum with vagotomy.

  7. Five-year survival rate is 20%.

Margin notes:
Pancreatic carcinoma: smoking most common cause; chronic pancreatitis

Carcinoma in head of pancreas: jaundice, light-colored stools, palpable gallbladder

Pancreatic cancer: metastasis left supraclavicular node

Pancreatic cancer: CA19–9 gold standard tumor marker

Pancreas carcinoma: CT scan best test

CHAPTER 19
KIDNEY DISORDERS

I. **Renal Function Overview**
   A. **Excretes harmful waste products**
      • Examples—urea, creatinine, uric acid
   B. **Maintains acid–base homeostasis** (refer to Chapter 4)
      • Controls the synthesis and excretion of bicarbonate and hydrogen ions
   C. **Reabsorbs essential substances**
      • Examples—sodium, glucose, amino acids
   D. **Regulates water and sodium metabolism** (refer to Chapter 4)
      1. Controls water by concentrating and diluting urine
      2. Controls sodium reabsorption in the proximal and distal collecting tubules
   E. **Maintains vascular tone** (refer to Chapter 4)
      1. Angiotensin II (ATII)
         a. Vasoconstricts peripheral resistance arterioles and efferent arterioles
         b. Stimulates the synthesis and release of aldosterone
      2. Renal-derived prostaglandin (PGE_2)
         • Vasodilates the afferent arterioles
   F. **Produces erythropoietin** (refer to Chapter 11)
      • Synthesized in the renal cortex by interstitial cells in peritubular capillary bed
   G. **Maintains calcium homeostasis** (refer to Chapter 22)
      1. Second hydroxylation of vitamin D
         a. 1-α-Hydroxylase is synthesized in the proximal renal tubule cells.
         b. Converts 25-hydroxycholecalciferol to 1,25-dihydroxycholecalciferol.
      2. Functions of vitamin D
         a. Increases gastrointestinal reabsorption of calcium and phosphorus
         b. Promotes bone mineralization; maintains serum calcium level

Second hydroxylation of vitamin D: 1-α-hydroxylase in proximal tubule

Vitamin D promotes bone mineralization by stimulating the release of alkaline phosphatase from osteoblasts. Alkaline phosphatase hydrolyzes pyrophosphate and other inhibitors of calcium-phosphate crystallization.

Renal stone: most common upper urinary tract cause of hematuria

Infection: most common cause of lower urinary tract hematuria

Transitional cell carcinoma bladder: most common noninfectious cause of lower urinary tract hematuria

Benign prostatic hyperplasia: most common cause of microscopic hematuria in adult males

         c. Increases monocytic stem cells to become osteoclasts
II. **Important Laboratory Findings in Renal Disease**
   A. **Hematuria**
      1. Upper urinary tract (kidneys, ureter) causes of hematuria
         a. Renal stone
         b. Glomerulonephritis
            • Characterized by dysmorphic RBCs (irregular membrane)
         c. Renal cell carcinoma
      2. Lower urinary tract (bladder, urethra, prostate) causes of hematuria
         a. Infection
         b. Transitional cell carcinoma
            • Most common cause of gross hematuria in the absence of infection
         c. Benign prostatic hyperplasia
            • Most common cause of microscopic hematuria in adult males

3. Drugs associated with hematuria
   a. Anticoagulants (warfarin, heparin)
   b. Cyclophosphamide
      (1) Hemorrhagic cystitis
      (2) Risk factor for transitional cell carcinoma

B. **Proteinuria**
   1. General
      a. Protein > 150 mg/24 hours or >30 mg/dL (dipstick)
      b. Persistent proteinuria usually indicates renal disease.
      c. Qualitative tests include dipsticks and sulfosalicylic acid (SSA).
         (1) Dipsticks are specific for albumin.
         (2) SSA detects albumin and globulins.
      d. Quantitative test is a 24-hour urine collection.
   2. Types of proteinuria (Table 19-1)

III. **Renal Function Tests**
   A. **Serum blood urea nitrogen (BUN)**
      • Normal serum BUN is 7 to 18 mg/dL.
      1. End-product of amino acid and pyrimidine metabolism
         • Produced by the liver urea cycle
         a. Filtered in the kidneys
            (1) Partly reabsorbed in the proximal tubule
            (2) Amount reabsorbed is flow dependent.
               (a) Decreased glomerular filtration rate, more reabsorbed
               (b) Increased glomerular filtration rate, less reabsorbed
         b. Extrarenal loss with very high serum concentration
         c. Serum levels depend on the following:
            (1) Glomerular filtration rate (GFR)
            (2) Protein content in the diet
            (3) Proximal tubule reabsorption
            (4) Functional status of the urea cycle
      2. Causes of increased and decreased serum BUN (Table 19-2)
   B. **Serum creatinine**
      • Normal serum creatinine is 0.6 to 1.2 mg/dL.

Anticoagulants: most common drugs causing hematuria

Persistent proteinuria: usually indicates intrinsic renal disease

Urea: some extrarenal loss (e.g., skin) with high serum concentration

Congestive heart failure: most common cause of increased serum BUN

TABLE 19-1. TYPES OF PROTEINURIA

TYPE	DEFINITION	CAUSES
Functional	Protein < 2 g/24 hr *Not* associated with renal disease	Fever, exercise, congestive heart failure Orthostatic (postural): occurs with standing and is absent in the recumbent state; urine protein is absent in the first morning void; *no* progression to renal disease
Overflow	Protein loss is variable LMW proteinuria Amount filtered > tubular reabsorption	Multiple myeloma with BJ proteinuria Hemoglobinuria: e.g., intravascular hemolysis Myoglobinuria: crush injuries, McArdle's glycogenosis (deficient muscle phosphorylase); increase in serum creatine kinase
Glomerular	Nephritic syndrome: protein > 150 mg/24 hr, but <3.5 g/24 hr Nephrotic syndrome: protein > 3.5 g/24 hr	Damage of GBM: nonselective proteinuria with loss of albumin and globulins; example is post-streptococcal glomerulonephritis Loss of negative charge on GBM: selective proteinuria with loss of albumin and *not* globulins; example is minimal change disease (lipoid nephrosis)
Tubular	Protein < 2 g/24 hr Defect in proximal tubule reabsorption of LMW proteins (e.g., amino acids at normal filtered loads)	Heavy metal poisoning: e.g., lead and mercury poisoning Fanconi syndrome: inability to reabsorb glucose, amino acids, uric acid, phosphate, and bicarbonate Hartnup disease: defect in reabsorption of neutral amino acids (e.g., tryptophan) in the gastrointestinal tract and kidneys

BJ, Bence Jones protein; GBM, glomerular basement membrane; LMW, low molecular weight.

TABLE 19-2. CAUSES OF INCREASED AND DECREASED SERUM BUN

CAUSE	DISCUSSION
Increased Serum BUN	
Decreased cardiac output	CHF, shock (e.g., hemorrhage) ↓ Cardiac output → ↓ GFR → ↑ proximal tubule reabsorption of urea → ↑ serum BUN
Increased protein intake	High-protein diet, blood in gastrointestinal tract ↑ Amino acid degradation → ↑ serum BUN
Increased tissue catabolism	Third-degree burns, postoperative state ↑ Amino acid degradation → ↑ serum BUN
Acute glomerulonephritis	Poststreptococcal glomerulonephritis ↓ GFR → ↑ serum BUN
Acute or chronic renal failure	Acute tubular necrosis, diabetic glomerulopathy ↓ GFR → ↑ serum BUN
Postrenal disease	Urinary tract obstruction (e.g., urinary stone, BPH) ↓ GFR back-diffusion of urea → ↑ serum BUN
Decreased Serum BUN	
Increased plasma volume	Normal pregnancy, SIADH ↑ Plasma volume → ↑ GFR → ↓ serum BUN
Decreased urea synthesis	Cirrhosis, Reye syndrome, fulminant liver failure Dysfunctional urea cycle → ↓ serum BUN
Decreased protein intake	Kwashiorkor (↑ CHO is protein sparer), starvation gluconeogenesis in kidneys ↓ Amino acid degradation → ↓ serum BUN

BPH, benign prostatic hyperplasia; BUN, blood urea nitrogen; CHF, congestive heart failure; CHO, carbohydrate; GFR, glomerular filtration rate; SIADH, syndrome of inappropriate antidiuretic hormone.

Creatinine: end-product of creatine metabolism

Creatinine: filtered; not reabsorbed or secreted

1. Metabolic end-product of creatine in muscle
   - Creatine binds phosphate in muscle for ATP synthesis.
2. Creatinine is filtered in the kidneys and *not* reabsorbed or secreted.
   - Excellent metabolite for renal clearance testing
3. Serum concentration varies with age and muscle mass.
   - Increased with age, decreased in muscle wasting
4. Increase in serum BUN and creatinine is called azotemia.
5. Causes of increased and decreased serum creatinine
   - Similar to those for serum BUN

Creatine supplements: ↑ serum creatinine

Azotemia: ↑ serum BUN and creatinine

Urea: filtered; partly reabsorbed

C. Serum BUN:creatinine (Cr) ratio
1. Using normal values, the normal ratio is 15 (Fig. 19-1A).
   a. Creatinine is filtered and is neither reabsorbed nor secreted.
   b. Urea is filtered and partly reabsorbed in the proximal tubule.
   c. BUN:Cr ratio depends on changes at several times:
      (1) Before the kidneys (prerenal)
      (2) Within the kidney parenchyma (renal)
      (3) After the kidneys (postrenal)
2. Prerenal, renal, and postrenal azotemia
   a. Azotemia refers to an increase in serum BUN and creatinine.
   b. Prerenal azotemia
      (1) Caused by a decrease in cardiac output
         (a) Hypoperfusion of the kidneys decreases GFR.
         (b) There is *no* intrinsic renal parenchymal disease.
      (2) Examples—blood loss, congestive heart failure

Prerenal azotemia: ↓ cardiac output, ↓ GFR; ratio > 15

      (3) Serum BUN:Cr ratio > 15 (Fig. 19-1B)
         (a) Decreased GFR causes creatinine and urea to back up in blood.
            - Ratio remains unchanged, because of proportionate increase.
         (b) After filtration, proportionately more urea is reabsorbed back into the blood due to the decreased flow rate ($P_O > P_H$; refer to Chapter 4).
            - All of the creatinine is excreted in the urine.
         (c) Addition of proportionately more urea to blood increases the ratio to >15.
         (d) Example—serum BUN 80 mg/dL, serum creatinine 4 mg/dL
            - BUN:Cr ratio is 20.

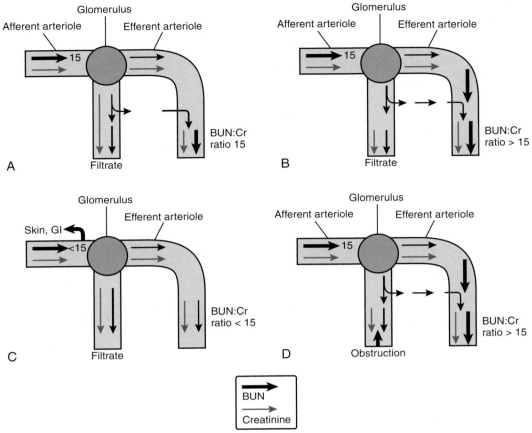

19-1: Blood urea nitrogen (BUN) and creatinine (Cr) ratios in normal persons (**A**), and in prerenal (**B**), renal (**C**), and postrenal azotemia (**D**). See text for discussion. *(From Goljan EF, Sloka KI: Rapid Review Laboratory Testing in Clinical Medicine. St. Louis, Mosby Elsevier, 2008, p 102, Fig. 4-15.)*

   c. Renal azotemia (uremia)
      (1) Caused by parenchymal damage to the kidneys
      (2) Examples—acute tubular necrosis, chronic renal failure
      (3) Serum BUN:Cr ratio ≤15 (Fig. 19-1C).
         (a) Decreased GFR causes creatinine and urea to back up in blood; increased extrarenal loss of urea
            • Ratio is already <15 due to extrarenal loss of urea
         (b) After filtration, both urea and creatinine are lost in the urine.
            • Proximal tubule cells are sloughed off in renal failure.
         (c) Serum BUN:Cr ratio remains ≤15.
         (d) Example—serum BUN 80 mg/dL, serum creatinine 8 mg/dL
            • BUN:Cr ratio is 10.
   d. Postrenal azotemia
      (1) Caused by urinary tract obstruction below the kidneys
        • *No* intrinsic parenchymal disease
      (2) Examples—prostate hyperplasia; blockage of ureters by stones/cancer
      (3) Serum BUN:Cr ratio > 15 (Fig. 19-1D)
         (a) Obstruction to urine flow decreases the GFR.
         (b) Backup of urea and creatinine in the blood
            • Proportionate increase at this point; ratio unchanged
         (c) Increased tubular pressure causes back-diffusion of urea (*not* creatinine) into blood.
            • Disproportionate increase in urea increases ratio to >15.
      (4) Persistent obstruction damages tubular epithelium causing renal azotemia (ratio ≤ 15).

Renal azotemia: intrinsic renal disease; extrarenal loss of urea; ratio ≤ 15

Postrenal azotemia: obstruction behind kidneys; initially ratio > 15; ≤15 if obstruction persists

D. Creatinine clearance (CCr)
1. Correlates with GFR

> **Elderly patients** normally have a decrease in CCr. Therefore, it is important to calculate the dose and dose interval for drugs that are nephrotoxic (e.g., aminoglycosides) in order to avoid precipitating acute renal failure due to nephrotoxic acute tubular necrosis.

   a. Annual decrease in CCr of 1 mL/minute after age 50 years
   b. Useful in detecting renal dysfunction
2. Creatinine clearance (CCr) formula
   a. Measured CCr = UCr (mg/dL) × V (mL/min) ÷ PCr (mg/dL)
      (1) V = volume of a 24-hour urine collection in mL/minute, and UCr and PCr are the creatinine concentration of urine and plasma, respectively.
      (2) CCr results are dependent on a correct 24-hour urine collection.
   b. Normal adult CCr is 97 to 137 mL/minute.
      (1) In general, CCr < 100 mL/minute is abnormal.
      (2) CCr < 10 mL/minute indicates renal failure.
3. Causes of increased and decreased CCr (Table 19-3)

E. Urinalysis (Table 19-4 and Fig. 19-2)
   • Gold standard test in the initial workup of renal disease

TABLE 19-3. CAUSES OF INCREASED AND DECREASED CREATININE CLEARANCE (CCr)

CAUSE	DISCUSSION
Increased CCr	
Normal pregnancy	Normal increase in plasma volume causes an increase in the GFR leading to an increase in CCr; highest at the end of the first trimester
Early diabetic glomerulopathy	Efferent arteriole becomes constricted due to hyaline arteriolosclerosis causing an increase in the GFR and CCr
	Increased GFR damages the glomerulus (hyperfiltration injury)
Decreased CCr	
Elderly people	GFR normally decreases with age causing a corresponding decrease in the CCr; danger when using nephrotoxic drugs
Acute and chronic renal disease	ARF due to acute tubular necrosis, CRF due to diabetic glomerulopathy

ARF, acute renal failure; CRF, chronic renal failure; GFR, glomerular filtration rate.

TABLE 19-4. URINALYSIS

COMPONENTS	DISCUSSION
General Examination	
Color	Dark yellow: concentrated urine, bilirubinuria, ↑ UBG, vitamins
	Red or pink: hematuria, hemoglobinuria, myoglobinuria, drugs (e.g., phenazopyridine, a urinary anesthetic), porphyria
	Smoky-colored urine: acid pH urine converts Hb to hematin; common finding in nephritic type of glomerulonephritis
	Black urine after exposure to light: alkaptonuria (AR disease with deficiency of homogentisate oxidase) with an increase in homogentisic acid in the urine; turns black when exposed to light
Clarity	Cloudy urine with alkaline pH: normal finding most often due to phosphates
	Cloudy urine with acid pH: normal finding most often due to uric acid
	Other: bacteria, WBCs, Hb, myoglobin also decrease clarity
Specific gravity	Evaluates urine concentration and dilution
	Specific gravity > 1.023 (UOsm 900 mOsm/kg) indicates urine concentration and *excludes* intrinsic renal disease
	Hypotonic urine has a specific gravity <1.015 (~UOsm 220 mOsm/kg)
	UOsm is the best indicator of urine concentration/dilution
	Fixed specific gravity (1.008–1.010): correlates with UOsm; lack of concentration and dilution (e.g., chronic renal failure)
Chemical Dipsticks	
pH	Determined by diet and acid-base status of the patient; pure vegan usually has alkaline pH (citrate converted into bicarbonate); meat eater usually has acid pH (organic acids in meat)
	Alkaline pH + smell of ammonia: urease-producing pathogen (e.g., *Proteus*)
Protein	Detects albumin (*not* globulins)
	SSA: detects albumin and globulins (e.g., BJ protein)
	Albuminuria: reagent strip and SSA have the *same* results
	BJ protein: SSA *greater than* reagent strip result; always confirm BJ protein with urine immunoelectrophoresis

TABLE 19-4. **URINALYSIS—cont'd**

COMPONENTS	DISCUSSION
Glucose	Specific for glucose; will not detect fructose or other sugars Detect glucose in urine as low as 30 mg/dL ↑ Serum glucose + glucosuria: diabetes mellitus Normal serum glucose + glucosuria: normal pregnancy (normally have a low renal threshold for glucose), benign glucosuria (low renal threshold for glucose) Microalbuminuria dipsticks: more sensitive than standard dipstick; sensitive to 1.5–8 mg/dL; microalbuminuria is the first sign of diabetic nephropathy
Ketones	Detects acetone, acetoacetic acid (*not* β-OHB); nitroprusside in the test system only reacts with AcAc and acetone, *not* β-OHB. Ketonuria: DKA, starvation, ketogenic diets, pregnancy (normal finding), isopropyl alcohol poisoning
Bilirubin	Detects conjugated (water-soluble) bilirubin Bilirubinuria: viral hepatitis, obstructive jaundice
Urobilinogen	Normal to have trace amounts (normal urine color is due to urobilin) Absent urine UBG, ↑ urine bilirubin: obstructive jaundice ↑ Urine UBG, absent urine bilirubin: extravascular hemolytic anemia (e.g., hereditary spherocytosis) ↑ Urine UBG, ↑ urine bilirubin: hepatitis
Blood	Detects RBCs, Hb, and myoglobin Hematuria: e.g., renal stone Hemoglobinuria: e.g., intravascular hemolytic anemia Myoglobinuria: e.g., crush injuries; ↑ serum creatine kinase
Nitrites	Detects nitrites produced by nitrate reducing uropathogens (e.g., *E. coli*); test sensitivity and specificity is 30% and 90%, respectively; requires ~4 hr for nitrate reducing uropathogens to convert nitrates to nitrites and patients with UTI frequently have increased frequency of urination, which explains the tests poor sensitivity
Leukocyte esterase	Detects esterase in neutrophils (pyuria); ~ 80% sensitivity Infections: urethritis, cystitis, pyelonephritis Sterile pyuria (neutrophils present but *negative standard urine culture*): *Chlamydia trachomatis* urethritis, tuberculosis, drug-induced interstitial nephritis
Sediment	
Cells	Bacteria: usually a sign of a urinary tract infection Red blood cells (hematuria): renal stone, cancer (bladder, renal), glomerulonephritis; hematuria is >2–3 RBCs per HPF Dysmorphic RBCs: indicates hematuria of glomerular origin (see Fig. 19-2A) Neutrophils (pyuria; see Fig. 19-2B): urinary tract infection, sterile pyuria; pyuria refers to ≥10 WBCs/HPF in a centrifuged specimen or ≥5 WBCs/HPF in an uncentrifuged specimen Oval fat bodies (see Fig. 19-2C): renal tubular cells with lipid (nephrotic syndrome)
Casts	Casts are formed in tubular lumens in the kidney; they are composed of a protein matrix (Tamm-Horsfall protein) within which are entrapped cells, debris, or protein leaking through the glomeruli; their presence proves a renal origin of the disease Hyaline cast (see Fig. 19-2D): acellular, ghost-like cast containing protein; no significance in the absence of proteinuria RBC cast (see Fig. 19-2E): nephritic type of glomerulonephritis (e.g., post-streptococcal glomerulonephritis) WBC cast (see Fig. 19-2F): acute pyelonephritis, acute tubulointerstitial nephritis Renal tubular cell cast (see Fig. 19-2G): acute tubular necrosis Fatty cast: contains lipid (e.g., cholesterol); sign of nephrotic syndrome (e.g., lipoid nephrosis) Waxy (broad) cast (see Fig. 19-2H): refractile, acellular cast; sign of chronic renal failure
Crystals	Calcium oxalate: pure vegan diet, ethylene glycol poisoning, calcium oxalate stone Uric acid: hyperuricemia associated with gout or massive destruction of cells after chemotherapy Triple phosphate: may be a sign of urinary tract infection due to urease producing uropathogens (e.g., *Proteus* species) Cystine: hexagonal crystal seen in cystinuria

AcAc, acetoacetic acid; AR, autosomal recessive; BJ, Bence Jones; DKA, diabetic ketoacidosis; Hb, hemoglobin; HPF, high-powered field; β-OHB, hydroxybutyric acid; SSA, sulfosalicylic acid; UBG, urobilinogen; UTI, urinary tract infection.

IV. Clinical Anatomy of the Kidney

A. Blood supply of the kidney

1. Renal cortex receives ~90% of the blood supply.
2. Renal medulla is relatively ischemic due to reduced blood supply.
3. Renal vessels are end-arteries.
   a. *No* collateral circulation
   b. Occlusion of any branch of a renal artery produces infarction.
4. Afferent arterioles
   a. Contain the juxtaglomerular apparatus
      • Produces the enzyme renin
   b. Blood flow is controlled by renal-derived PGE_2 (vasodilator).

Renal medulla: relatively ischemic

Renal PGE_2: vasodilation afferent arteriole

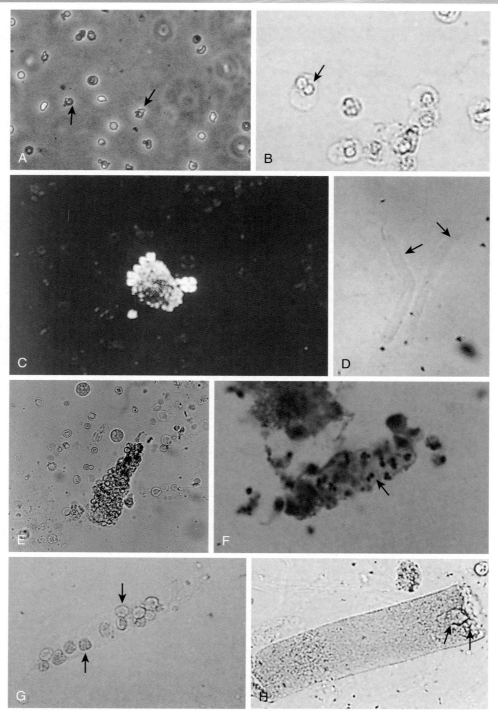

19-2: **A,** Dysmorphic RBCs. This phase-contrast microscopy of urine sediment shows dysmorphic RBCs (*arrows*) with protrusions from the RBC membrane related to damage from glomerular inflammation. They are a sign of hematuria of glomerular origin. **B,** Sediment with neutrophils. The *arrow* points to a bilobed neutrophil. **C,** Oval fat body under polarization showing classic Maltese crosses. The Maltese crosses are due to cholesterol, which is always increased in the nephrotic syndrome. **D,** Hyaline casts. The *arrows* show two hyaline casts that are acellular and have smooth borders. **E,** RBC cast in the urine. Note the cylindrical cast composed of red-staining cells. **F,** White blood cell cast. The cast is filled with multilobed cells (*arrow*) representing neutrophils. These casts are seen in acute pyelonephritis and acute drug-induced tubulointerstitial nephritis. **G,** Renal tubular cell cast. The cast has numerous renal tubular cells with round nuclei (*arrows*). These casts are a sign of acute tubular necrosis. **H,** Waxy/broad cast in the urine sediment. The diameter of the cast is increased due to tubular atrophy. It has a refractile quality, with distinct margins. *Arrows* show degenerating renal tubular cells. (*A and E from Forbes C, Jackson W: Color Atlas and Text of Clinical Medicine, 2nd ed. St. Louis, Mosby, 2003, p 276, Figs. 6.10, 6.11, respectively; **B, C, D, F, G**, and **H** from Henry JB: Clinical Diagnosis and Management by Laboratory Methods, 20th ed. Philadelphia, WB Saunders, 2001, Plates 18-4, 18-12, 18-13A, 18-17, 18-11, 18-14, respectively.*)

c. Direct blood into the glomerular capillaries
5. Efferent arterioles
   a. Drain the glomerular capillaries
   b. Blood flow controlled by ATII (vasoconstrictor).
   c. Eventually become the peritubular capillaries

ATII: vasoconstrictor of efferent arterioles

> **Nonsteroidal anti-inflammatory drugs** inhibit production of PGE_2; therefore, intrarenal blood flow is controlled by the efferent arterioles, whose blood flow is maintained by ATII, a vasoconstrictor. This increases the risk of ischemic damage to the medulla.

B. Structure of the glomerulus (Fig. 19-3)
1. Glomerular capillaries contain fenestrated epithelium.
   • Holes in the endothelial surface are important in the filtration process.
2. Glomerular basement membrane (GBM)
   a. Composed of type IV collagen
   b. Size and charge are the primary determinants of protein filtration.
      (1) Heparan sulfate produces the negative charge of the GBM.
      (2) Cationic proteins of low molecular weight (LMW) are permeable.
      (3) Albumin has a strong negative charge and is *not* permeable.
         (a) Loss of the negative charge causes loss of albumin in the urine.
         (b) Called selective proteinuria (e.g., minimal change disease)
      (4) GBM is permeable to water and LMW (<70,000 daltons) proteins (e.g., amino acids).
   c. Causes of GBM thickening
      (1) Deposition of immunocomplexes
         • Example—membranous glomerulopathy
      (2) Increased synthesis of type IV collagen
         • Example—diabetes mellitus
3. Visceral epithelial cells (VEC)
   a. Primarily responsible for production of the GBM
   b. Contain podocytes (foot-like processes) and slit pores between the podocytes
      • Serve as a distal barrier for preventing protein loss in the urine
   c. Fusion of the podocytes is present in any cause of the nephrotic syndrome.

GBM: size and charge determine protein filtration

Albumin: negative charge; repelled by negatively charged GBM

Fusion of the podocytes: sign of nephrotic syndrome

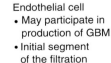

Endothelial cell
• May participate in production of GBM
• Initial segment of the filtration barrier; fenestrated

Glomerular basement membrane (GBM)
• The microskeleton of the glomerulus
• Participates in filtration barrier

Fenestra

Visceral epithelial cell with podocytes
• Produces GBM
• Intercellular junctions are the final filtration barrier

Parietal epithelial cell

Mesangial cell
• Contractile
• Produces matrix
• Phagocytic

Mesangial matrix
• Supporting framework for mesangial cells and peripheral GBM

19-3: Schematic of a normal glomerulus. See text for discussion. *(Modified and reproduced with permission from Striker LJ, Olson JL, Striker GL: The Renal Biopsy, 2nd ed. Philadelphia, WB Saunders, 1990.)*

4. Mesangial cells
   a. Support the glomerular capillaries
   b. Can release inflammatory mediators and proliferate
      • Example—IgA glomerulopathy has mesangial immunocomplex deposits.

5. Parietal epithelial cells

   a. Lining cells of Bowman's capsule
   b. Proliferation causes "crescents" that encroach upon and destroy the glomerulus.

V. **Congenital Disorders and Cystic Diseases of the Kidneys**
   A. **Horseshoe kidney**
      1. Most common congenital kidney disorder
      2. Majority (90% of cases) are fused at the lower pole (Fig. 19-4).
         • Kidney is trapped behind the root of the inferior mesenteric artery.

      3. Clinical findings
         a. Increased incidence with Turner's syndrome
         b. Danger of infection and stone formation

   B. **Cystic diseases of the kidney** (Table 19-5 and Figs. 19-5 and 19-6)

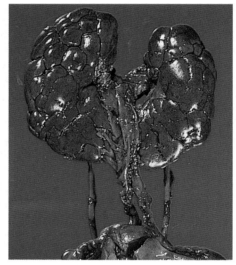

19-4: Horseshoe kidney. Note that the lower poles of the kidneys are fused. *(From Damjanov I, Linder J: Pathology: A Color Atlas. St. Louis, Mosby, 2000, p 211, Fig. 11-3.)*

TABLE 19-5. CYSTIC DISEASES OF THE KIDNEYS

CYSTIC DISEASE	DISCUSSION
Renal dysplasia (see Fig. 19-5)	Most common cystic disease in children No inheritance pattern Abnormal development of one or both kidneys; abnormal structures persist in the kidneys (e.g., cartilage, immature collecting ductules). Present as an enlarged, irregular, cystic, unilateral (bilateral) flank mass Bilateral dysplastic kidneys may lead to renal failure; accounts for ~20% of cases of CRF in children
Juvenile polycystic kidney disease	AR inheritance Bilateral cystic disease; cysts in the cortex and medulla Cysts also occur in the liver Association with congenital hepatic fibrosis leading to portal hypertension Enlarged kidneys at birth; most serious types are incompatible with life Maternal oligohydramnios (decreased amniotic fluid); newborns have Potter's facies, a deformation due to oligohydramnios; findings include low-set ears, parrot beak nose, and lung hypoplasia
Adult polycystic kidney disease (see Fig. 19-6)	AD inheritance; defect on chromosome 16 Bilateral cystic disease develops by 20–25 years of age; bilaterally palpable kidneys; cysts involve all parts of the nephron in the cortex and medulla Cysts are present in the liver (50%), pancreas (10%), spleen (5%) Hypertension (>80% of cases); associated with stroke due to rupture of intracranial berry aneurysms (aneurysms in 10–30% of cases), intracerebral hemorrhage, lacunar infarcts CRF begins at age 40–60; due to destruction of kidneys by slowly expanding cysts; accounts for ~10% of cases of CRF; it is the most common cause of death Other associations: sigmoid diverticulosis, hematuria, mitral valve prolapse, slight risk for developing renal cell carcinoma Treatment: renal transplantation

TABLE 19-5. CYSTIC DISEASES OF THE KIDNEYS—cont'd

CYSTIC DISEASE	DISCUSSION
Medullary sponge kidney	No inheritance pattern Most commonly discovered with an IVP; striations are present in the papillary ducts of the medulla ("Swiss-cheese" appearance); multiple cysts of the collecting ducts are present in the medulla Recurrent UTIs, hematuria, and renal stones
Acquired polycystic kidney disease	Most common cause is renal dialysis; occurs in ~50% of patients on long-term dialysis Tubules are obstructed by interstitial fibrosis or oxalate crystals Small risk for developing renal cell carcinoma
Simple retention cysts	Most common adult renal cyst Derived from tubular obstruction May produce hematuria Requires needle aspiration to distinguish it from renal cell carcinoma

AD, autosomal dominant; AR, autosomal recessive; CRF, chronic renal failure; IVP, intravenous pyelogram; UTIs, urinary tract infections.

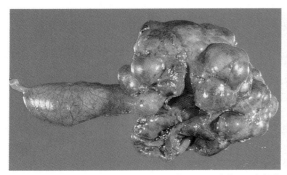

19-5: Renal dysplasia. Note the multicystic deformed kidney and dilated ureter. *(From Damjanov I, Linder J: Pathology: A Color Atlas. St. Louis, Mosby, 2000, p 213, Fig. 11-11.)*

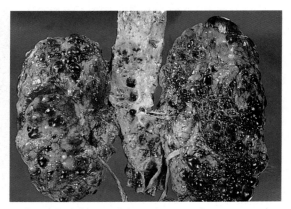

19-6: Adult polycystic kidney disease. There is complete effacement of normal kidney architecture by cysts within the cortex and medulla of both kidneys. *(From Damjanov I, Linder J: Pathology: A Color Atlas. St. Louis, Mosby, 2000, p 212, Fig. 11-7.)*

VI. Glomerular Disorders
A. Terminology of glomerular disease (Table 19-6)
- Normal glomerulus (Fig. 19-7A)
B. Routine studies on biopsy specimens
1. H&E (hematoxylin and eosin) and other special stains
   - Used to help classify the type of glomerular disease
2. Immunofluorescence (IF) stain
   a. Identifies patterns and type of protein deposition
   b. Linear pattern (Fig. 19-7B)
      (1) It is a characteristic finding in anti-GBM disease.
         - Example—Goodpasture syndrome

Linear IF: anti-GBM disease (e.g., Goodpasture syndrome)

TABLE 19-6. NOMENCLATURE AND DESCRIPTION OF GLOMERULAR DISORDERS

TERM	DESCRIPTION
Focal glomerulonephritis	Only a few glomeruli are abnormal
Diffuse glomerulonephritis	All glomeruli are abnormal
Proliferative glomerulonephritis	>100 nuclei in affected glomeruli
Membranous glomerulopathy	Thick GBM, no proliferative change
Membranoproliferative glomerulonephritis	Thick GBM, hypercellular glomeruli
Focal segmental glomerulosclerosis	Fibrosis involving only a segment of the involved glomerulus
Crescentic glomerulonephritis	Proliferation of parietal epithelial cells around glomerulus
Primary glomerular disease	Involves only glomeruli and no other target organs (e.g., minimal change disease)
Secondary glomerular disease	Involves glomeruli and other target organs (e.g., SLE)

GBM, glomerular basement membrane; SLE, systemic lupus erythematosus.

19-7: **A,** Normal glomerulus. **B,** Linear immunofluorescence. The uninterrupted smooth immunofluorescence along the glomerular basement membrane is caused by deposition of IgG antibodies directed against the membrane (e.g., Goodpasture syndrome). **C,** Granular immunofluorescence. Granular irregular deposits in the capillaries are caused by immunocomplex deposition (e.g., poststreptococcal glomerulonephritis). **D,** Fusion of the podocytes. *Arrow* shows fusion of the podocytes. This finding occurs in all glomerular diseases that present with the nephrotic syndrome (e.g., minimal change disease). **E,** Subendothelial immunocomplex deposits viewed with electron microscopy. The band of electron-dense material extends around the glomerular basement membrane and hugs the interface of the membrane with the capillary lumen. The *arrow* points to immune deposits directly beneath the nucleus of the endothelial cell. A thin rim of normal basement membrane (light gray) separates the deposits from the epithelial side of the membrane. The patient had diffuse proliferative glomerulonephritis due to systemic lupus erythematosus. **F,** Subepithelial immunocomplex deposits viewed with electron microscopy. *Arrows* point to electron-dense deposits directly beneath the visceral epithelial cells in a patient with poststreptococcal glomerulonephritis. The normal basement membrane has a light gray appearance. **G,** Poststreptococcal diffuse proliferative glomerulonephritis. The glomerulus is hypercellular due to an increase in neutrophils and mesangial cells. **H,** Crescentic glomerulonephritis. *Arrows* point to a proliferation of parietal epithelial cells in Bowman's capsule, occupying approximately 50% of the entire urinary space. The cells encase and compress the glomerular tuft. **I,** Diffuse membranous glomerulopathy. The H&E (hematoxylin and eosin)-stained biopsy shows glomerular basement membranes that are uniformly thickened. There is no proliferative component. **J,** Diabetic glomerulosclerosis. *Broken arrow* points to an afferent or efferent arteriole that has hyaline arteriolosclerosis, with an increase in proteinaceous material in the wall of the vessel. *Solid arrow* shows a mesangial nodule containing type IV collagen and trapped protein. *(**A, F,** and **G** from Damjanov I: Pathology for the Health-Related Professions, 2nd ed. Philadelphia, WB Saunders, 2000, pp 329, 341, 329, Figs. 13-5A, 13-8C, 13-5B, respectively; **B, H** from Kumar V, Fausto N, Abbas A: Robbins and Cotran's Pathologic Basis of Disease, 7th ed. Philadelphia, WB Saunders, 2004, pp 969, 977, Figs. 20-10E, 20-17, respectively; **C, E, J** from Damjanov I, Linder J: Pathology: A Color Atlas. St. Louis, Mosby, 2000, p 224, 229, Figs. 11-54, 11-64, respectively; **D** from Laszik ZG, Lajoie G, Nadasky T, Silva FG: Medical diseases of the kidney. In Silverberg SG, Delellis RA, Frable WJ [eds]: Principles and Practice of Surgical Pathology and Cytopathology, 3rd ed. New York, Churchill Livingstone, 1997, p 2079; **I** from Kern WF, Silva FG, Laszik ZG, et al [eds]: Atlas of Renal Pathology. Philadelphia, WB Saunders, 1999, p 53, Fig. 5-30.)*

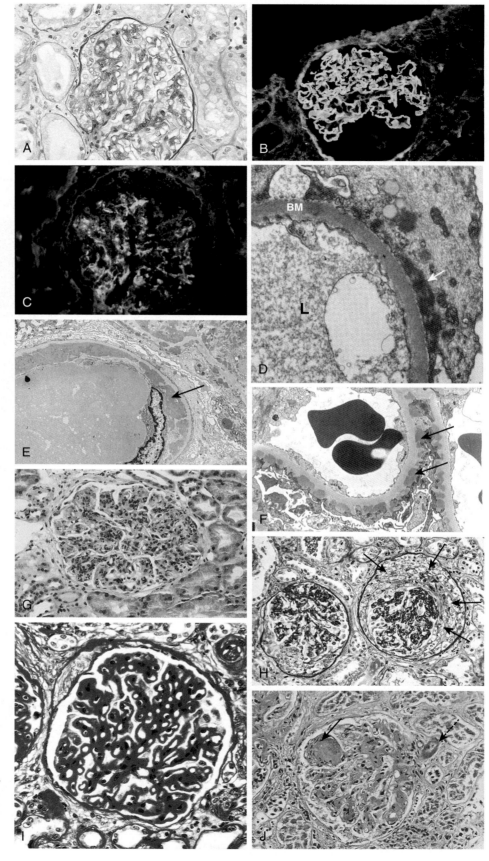

      (2) Antibodies line up against evenly distributed antigens in the GBM.
- Cannot be detected by electron microscopy

    c. Granular ("lumpy-bumpy") pattern (Fig. 19-7C)
- Usually indicates immunocomplex (IC) deposition in the glomerulus

Granular pattern: immunocomplex type of glomerulonephritis

  3. Electron microscopy (EM)

    a. Detects submicroscopic defects in the glomerulus; examples:

      (1) Fusion of podocytes in the nephrotic syndrome (Fig. 19-7D)

      (2) Damage to visceral epithelial cells

    b. Detects the site(s) of IC deposition

      (1) Deposits are electron-dense (dark color)

      (2) Sites are designated

EM: immunocomplex deposits are electron-dense

        (a) Subendothelial (Fig. 19-7E)
- Trapped between the endothelial cell and GBM

        (b) Subepithelial (Fig. 19-7F)
- Passed through the GBM but caught beneath the podocytes

        (c) Intramembranous
- Within the GBM

        (d) Mesangial

C. Mechanisms producing glomerular disease

  1. Immunocomplexes (type III hypersensitivity)

    a. Circulate and deposit in glomeruli or they develop in situ
- Example: DNA–anti-DNA complexes in SLE

    b. ICs activate the complement system.

      (1) C5a is produced, which is chemotactic to neutrophils.

      (2) Neutrophils damage the glomeruli.
- Damage to the glomeruli by neutrophils, which occurs in nephritic types of glomerulonephritis.

Immunocomplexes: most common mechanism causing glomerulonephritis

Immunocomplexes: activate complement → C5a produced → attracts neutrophils

  2. Antibodies directed against GBM antigens
- Example—Goodpasture syndrome

  3. T-cell production of cytokines

    a. Cytokines cause the GBM to lose its negative charge.

    b. Cytokines damage podocytes causing them to fuse.

    c. Example—minimal change disease in the nephrotic syndrome

D. Clinical manifestations of glomerular diseases

  1. Nephritic syndrome

  2. Nephrotic syndrome

  3. Chronic glomerulonephritis

E. Nephritic syndrome

  1. Glomerular injury is primarily due to neutrophils.

  2. Clinical and laboratory findings

    a. Hypertension
- Due to salt retention

Nephritic syndrome: neutrophil-related injury to glomeruli

    b. Periorbital puffiness

      (1) Due to salt retention in the loose skin in that area

      (2) In some cases, edema can be more generalized.
- Sodium retention increases plasma hydrostatic pressure.

Pitting edema: does *not* distinguish nephritic from nephrotic syndrome

    c. Oliguria (~400 mL urine/day)

      (1) Due to decreased GFR from inflamed glomeruli

      (2) Tubular function is intact.

    d. Hematuria

      (1) Dysmorphic RBCs with irregular membranes (see Fig. 19-2A)

      (2) Due to inflamed glomeruli from IC deposition

    e. Neutrophils in the sediment (see Fig. 19-2B)
- Particularly in IC types

    f. RBC casts are a key finding (see Fig. 19-2E).
- Occasionally, WBC casts are also present.

    g. Proteinuria > 150 mg/day, but <3.5 g/day

    h. Azotemia with a BUN:Cr ratio > 15
- Tubular function is intact in acute glomerulonephritis.

Nephritic syndrome: moderate proteinuria; dysmorphic RBCs, RBC casts

  3. Primarily nephritic types of glomerular disease (Table 19-7; see also Fig. 19-7B to H)

TABLE 19-7. **PRIMARILY NEPHRITIC TYPES OF GLOMERULAR DISEASE**

GLOMERULAR DISEASE	CLINICOPATHOLOGIC FINDINGS
IgA glomerulopathy (Berger's disease)	Most common nephropathy; majority are nephritic (5% nephrotic) Affects children and adults Increased mucosal synthesis and decreased clearance of IgA; increased serum IgA (50%) Focal proliferative glomerulopathy Mesangial IgA IC deposits with granular IF; ICs activate alternative complement pathway Overlapping features with HSP may occur Episodic bouts of hematuria (microscopic or gross) usually following an upper respiratory infection; hypertension Slow progression to CRF (40–50%) *Treatment*: corticosteroids decrease proteinuria; treat hypertension
Post-streptococcal glomerulonephritis (see Fig. 19-7C, F, and G)	Most common type of postinfectious GN Usually follows group A streptococcal infection of skin (e.g., scarlet fever) or pharynx Subepithelial IC deposits with granular IF; ICs activate alternative complement pathway Diffuse proliferative pattern with neutrophil infiltration Hematuria 1–3 weeks following group A streptococcal infection by a nephritogenic strain (never produces acute rheumatic fever); periorbital edema (sodium retention); edema can occasionally be more extensive but is related to sodium retention *not* hypoalbuminemia; hypertension (usually transient; sometimes severe) Increased anti-DNase B titers; ASO is degraded by oil in the skin and is *not* increased; streptozyme test is positive (can detect anti-DNase B, ASO, anti-AH, and anti-NAD antibodies) Usually resolves; CRF is uncommon *Treatment*: supportive; penicillin G or V if cultures are positive for *Streptococcus pyogenes*; treat hypertension
Diffuse proliferative glomerulonephritis (SLE) (see Fig. 19-7C and E)	Diffuse proliferative GN is most common subtype of glomerular disease in SLE; other types can have a nephrotic presentation Subendothelial IC deposits with granular IF; DNA–anti-DNA ICs activate classical complement pathway "Wire looping" of capillaries (corresponds with subendothelial ICs); neutrophil infiltration with hyaline thrombi in capillary lumens Kidneys are major target organ in SLE (~90%) Serum ANA test usually has a rim pattern, which corresponds with the presence of anti-dsDNA antibodies Evolves into CRF in most cases; common cause of death in SLE *Treatment*: corticosteroids + cyclophosphamide

Rapidly progressive crescentic glomerulonephritis (see Fig. 19-7B and H)	Clinical syndrome that may be primary or secondary type of glomerular disease
	Rapid loss of renal function progresses to ARF over days to weeks; very poor prognosis
	May or may not be associated with crescent formation (crescentic GN)
	Clinical associations: Goodpasture's syndrome, microscopic polyarteritis (p-ANCA), Wegener's granulomatosis (c-ANCA)
	Goodpasture syndrome:
	  Male dominant disease; 80% HLA-BR2 positive
	  Anti–basement membrane antibodies against collagen in glomerular and pulmonary capillaries
	  Linear IF; EM has *no* electron-dense deposits; crescentic GN (accounts for 5% of all cases)
	Begins with hemoptysis and ends with renal failure
	Treatment: plasma exchange; immunosuppressive therapy with corticosteroids and cyclophosphamide; renal transplantation

AH, antihyaluronidase; ANA, antinuclear antibody; ANCA, antineutrophil cytoplasmic antibody; ARF, acute renal failure; ASO, antistreptolysin O; CRF, chronic renal failure; ds, double-stranded; EM, electron microscopy; GN, glomerulonephritis; HSP, Henoch-Schönlein purpura; IC, immunocomplex; IF, immunofluorescence; NAD, nicotinamide adenine dinucleotidase; SLE, systemic lupus erythematosus.

F. Nephrotic syndrome
1. Glomerular injury is due to cytokines *not* neutrophils.
   a. Cytokines damage podocytes causing them to fuse together.
   b. Cytokines destroy the negative charge of the GBM.
2. Clinical and laboratory findings
   a. Key finding is proteinuria > 3.5 g/24 hours.
   b. Generalized pitting edema and ascites
      (1) Due to hypoalbuminemia
         • Pitting edema in nephritic syndrome is due to sodium retention.
      (2) Increased risk for developing spontaneous peritonitis (refer to Chapter 18)
         • Due to *Streptococcus pneumoniae*

Nephrotic syndrome: cytokine injury to podocytes; loss of negative charge on GBM

Nephrotic syndrome: proteinuria > 3.5 g/24 hours; fatty casts

c. Hypertension in some types
- Due to sodium retention
d. Hypercoagulable state due to loss of antithrombin III
- Potential for renal vein thrombosis
e. Hypercholesterolemia
- Hypoalbuminemia increases synthesis of cholesterol (unknown mechanism).
f. Hypogammaglobulinemia
- Due to the loss of γ-globulins in the urine
g. Fatty casts with maltese crosses and oval fat bodies (see Fig. 19-2C)
- Key finding of the nephrotic syndrome
3. Primarily nephrotic types of glomerular disease (Table 19-8; see Fig. 19-7D, F, and I)

G. **Systemic diseases with nephrotic syndrome**
1. Diabetic glomerulopathy
- Nodular glomerulosclerosis (Kimmelstiel-Wilson disease)
a. Epidemiology
(1) Glomerulopathy occurs in type 1 and 2 diabetes.
- Occurs more often in type 1 (35–45%) than type 2 diabetes (20%)
(2) Most common cause of chronic renal failure in United States
- Type 1 > type 2 diabetes mellitus

> Nephrotic syndrome: less glomerular inflammation than nephritic syndrome

> Diabetic glomerulopathy: type 1 > type 2 diabetes

TABLE 19-8. PRIMARILY NEPHROTIC TYPES OF GLOMERULAR DISEASE

GLOMERULAR DISEASE	CLINICOPATHOLOGIC FINDINGS
Minimal change disease (lipoid nephrosis) (see Fig. 19-7D)	Most common cause of nephrotic syndrome in children; more common in girls than boys; occurs in ~15% of adults with nephrotic syndrome T-cell cytokines cause the GBM to lose its negative charge; selective proteinuria (albumin *not* globulins) Secondary causes: Hodgkin's lymphoma Structurally normal glomeruli; positive fat stains in glomerulus and tubules Negative IF; EM shows fusion of podocytes and *no* deposits Often preceded by respiratory infection or routine immunization Usually normotensive (90%), unlike other types of nephrotic syndrome *Treatment*: children respond well to steroid therapy; CRF is rare
Focal segmental glomerulosclerosis	Primary or secondary disease; secondary causes—HIV (most common glomerular disease) and intravenous heroin abuse Negative IF; EM focal damage of VECs Nonselective proteinuria, microscopic hematuria (60–80%) Hypertension early (20%) Poor prognosis; commonly progresses to CRF *Treatment*: corticosteroids (only 15–20% response)

Diffuse membranous glomerulopathy (see Fig. 19-7I)	Most common cause of nephrotic syndrome in adults
	Primary and secondary types; secondary causes:
	   Drugs: e.g., captopril, gold therapy
	   Infections: HBV, *Plasmodium malariae*, syphilis
	   Malignancy: carcinomas, Hodgkin's lymphoma
	   Autoimmune disease: SLE (nephrotic presentation)
	Diffuse thickening of membranes; silver stains show "spike and dome" pattern beneath VECs (subepithelial deposits)
	Subepithelial ICs with granular IF
	Treatment: corticosteroids may slow progression

Type I MPGN	Most common type of MPGN; nephrotic presentation (60%); some cases have a nephritic presentation Associated with HBV, HCV (more common), or cryoglobulinemia Subendothelial ICs with granular IF; ICs activate classical and alternative complement pathways; EM shows tram tracks caused by splitting of the GBM by an ingrowth of mesangium Hypertension (35%); majority have hematuria Majority progress to CRF *Treatment*: response to corticosteroids *not* established
Type II MPGN	Associated with the C3 nephritic factor (C3NeF), an autoantibody that binds to C3 convertase (C3bBb); prevents degradation of C3 convertase causing sustained activation of C3 resulting in very low C3 levels Diffuse intramembranous deposits ("dense deposit disease"); EM shows tram tracks Hypertension (35%); majority have hematuria Majority progress to CRF *Treatment*: response to corticosteroids *not* established

CRF, chronic renal failure; EM, electron microscopy; GBM, glomerular basement membrane; HBV, hepatitis B; HCV, hepatitis C; ICs, immuno-complexes; IF, immunofluorescence; MPGN, membranoproliferative glomerulonephritis; SLE, systemic lupus erythematosus; VECs, visceral epithelial cells.

Diabetic glomerulopathy: poor glycemic control is the most common cause

(3) Risk factors
    (a) Poor glycemic control
    (b) Hypertension
    (c) Diabetic retinopathy
      • High correlation with coexisting glomerulopathy
b. Pathogenesis
  (1) Nonenzymatic glycosylation (NEG) of the GBM
    • Also affects tubule basement membranes

NEG: ↑ vessel/tubular permeability to protein

    (a) Glycosylation refers to glucose attaching to amino acids.
    (b) Increases vessel and tubular cell permeability to proteins
  (2) NEG of the afferent and efferent arterioles
    (a) Produces hyaline arteriolosclerosis (refer to Chapter 9)
    (b) Involves efferent arterioles *before* afferent arterioles
  (3) Osmotic damage to glomerular capillary endothelial cells

Osmotic damage: ↑ sorbitol

    (a) Glucose is converted by aldose reductase into sorbitol.
    (b) Sorbitol is osmotically active.
    (c) Water enters the cells causing damage.

Hyaline arteriolosclerosis of efferent arteriole: ↑ GFR producing hyperfiltration injury

  (4) Hyperfiltration damage to the mesangium
    (a) Selective hyaline arteriolosclerosis of efferent arterioles
    (b) Increases the GFR, which damages mesangial cells
  (5) Diabetic microangiopathy; increased deposition of type IV collagen
    • GBM, tubular cell basement membranes, mesangium
c. Nonspecific immunofluorescence
d. Electron microscope shows fusion of podocytes (see Fig. 19-7D).
e. Microscopic findings (see Fig. 19-7J)
  (1) Afferent and efferent hyaline arteriolosclerosis
    • When the afferent arteriole becomes hyalinized, the GFR decreases.

Microangiopathy: ↑ deposition type IV collagen

  (2) Nodular masses develop in the mesangial matrix.
    • Due to increased type IV collagen synthesis and trapped proteins
f. Clinical and laboratory findings
  (1) Microalbuminuria

Microalbuminuria: first laboratory sign of diabetic glomerulopathy

    (a) Initial laboratory manifestation of diabetic glomerulopathy
      • Usually begins after ~10 years of poor glycemic control
    (b) Microalbuminuria dipsticks detect albumin levels in the range of 1.5 to 8 mg/dL.

ACE inhibitor/ receptor blockers: slow progression of nephropathy in type 1/type 2 diabetes

An **angiotensin-converting enzyme (ACE) inhibitor** is prescribed when microalbuminuria is first detected. It slows the progression of diabetic glomerulopathy and retinopathy in both types of diabetes mellitus. One possible mechanism is by reducing pressure in the glomerular capillaries by decreasing ATII vasoconstriction of the hyalinized efferent arterioles. Angiotensin receptor blockers are also useful, particularly in type 2 diabetes mellitus. These changes are independent of the blood pressure lowering capabilities of both drugs.

  (2) Other renal diseases associated with diabetes mellitus
    • Renal papillary necrosis, acute and chronic pyelonephritis
2. Renal amyloidosis (refer to Chapter 3, see Figs. 3-6 and 3-7)
  • Associated with primary and secondary amyloidosis
H. Hereditary glomerular diseases
  1. Alport's syndrome
    a. Autosomal dominant disease; perhaps X-linked recessive
      • Autoantibodies to type IV collagen in GBM
    b. *No* specific immunofluorescence or electron microscopic findings
    c. Microscopic findings

Alport's syndrome: hereditary nephritis, sensorineural hearing loss, ocular defects

      • Lipid accumulation in VECs producing foam cells
    d. Sensorineural hearing loss and ocular abnormalities
  2. Thin basement membrane disease
    • "Benign familial hematuria"
    a. Autosomal dominant disorder
    b. Extremely thin GBMs

Thin basement membrane disease: persistent hematuria

      • Normal renal function
    c. Mild proteinuria, persistent microscopic hematuria

I. Chronic glomerulonephritis
1. Causes in descending order of incidence:
   a. Rapidly progressive glomerulonephritis (RPGN; 90%)
   b. Focal segmental glomerulosclerosis (80%)
   c. Type I membranoproliferative glomerulonephritis (40%)
   d. Membranous glomerulopathy (20–30%)
   e. Type IV diffuse proliferative glomerulonephritis in SLE (20%)
   f. IgA glomerulopathy (10%)
2. Gross and microscopic findings
   a. Shrunken kidneys
   b. Glomerular sclerosis and tubular atrophy

> RPGN: most common cause of chronic glomerulonephritis

VII. Disorders Affecting Tubules and Interstitium
A. Acute tubular necrosis (ATN)
1. Epidemiology
   a. Greater than 10% of intensive care unit patients develop acute renal failure (ARF).
   b. Greater than 40% of hospital ARF is iatrogenic (doctor-induced).
   c. ARF occurs in 20% of patients with sepsis.
   d. ARF develops in >50% of patients with septic shock.
   e. Acute renal failure (ARF)
      (1) Acute suppression of renal function developing in 24 hours
      (2) Accompanied by anuria or oliguria (~400 mL/24 hours)
      (3) ATN is the most common cause of ARF.
         • Subdivided into ischemic and nephrotoxic types
   f. Other causes of ARF
      (1) Postrenal obstruction
         • Examples—prostate hyperplasia; invasive cervical cancer
      (2) Vascular disease
         • Example—malignant hypertension
      (3) RPGN, drugs, disseminated intravascular coagulation (DIC), urate nephropathy
2. Ischemic ATN
   a. Most often caused by prerenal azotemia due to hypovolemia
   b. Ischemia damages endothelial cells.
      (1) Causes decrease in vasodilators
         • Examples—nitric oxide, PGI_2
      (2) Increase in vasoconstrictors
         • Example—endothelin
      (3) Net effect is vasoconstriction of afferent arterioles, which decreases GFR.
   c. Ischemia damages tubule cells
      (1) Causes detachment of tubular cells into the lumen causing obstruction (Fig. 19-8)
         • Produces pigmented renal tubular cell casts (see Fig. 19-2G)
      (2) Casts obstruct the lumen causing an increase in intratubular pressure.
         (a) Decreases GFR
         (b) Pushes fluid into the interstitium
         (c) Net effect is oliguria.

> ATN: most common cause of ARF
>
> Ischemic ATN: most common type of ATN

> Prerenal azotemia: most common cause of ischemic ATN

> Renal tubular cell cast: key cast of ATN

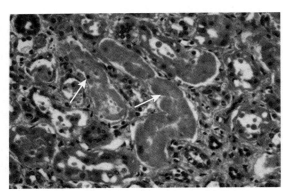

19-8: Acute tubular necrosis. Coagulation necrosis of proximal renal tubule cells (*arrows*) is evident with some detachment from the basement membrane. This will form renal tubular cell casts. (*From Kern WF, Silva FG, Laszik ZG, et al [eds]: Atlas of Renal Pathology. Philadelphia, WB Saunders, 1999, p 129, Fig. 12-3.*)

d. Sites of tubular damage
    (1) Straight segment of proximal tubule
        • Part of the nephron most susceptible to hypoxia
    (2) Medullary segment of the thick ascending limb (TAL)
        • Location of the Na^+-K^+-2 Cl^- cotransporter
    (3) Tubular basement membranes are disrupted at these sites.
        • Interferes with renal tubular cell regeneration

3. Nephrotoxic type

  a. Causes

> Aminoglycosides: most common cause of nephrotoxic ATN

    (1) Aminoglycosides most common cause (e.g., gentamicin)
    (2) Radiocontrast agents
    (3) Heavy metals (e.g., lead and mercury)

  b. Microscopic findings
    (1) Primarily damages the proximal tubule cells
    (2) Tubular basement membrane is intact.

4. Clinical and laboratory findings in ATN

  a. Oliguria, in most cases
    • Some cases have polyuria (~800 mL/24 hours).

> ATN: renal tubular cell casts

  b. Pigmented renal tubular cell casts (see Fig. 19-2G)
  c. Hyperkalemia, increased anion gap metabolic acidosis (refer to Chapter 4)

> BUN: creatinine ratio ≤ 15; hyperkalemia, metabolic acidosis

  d. Increased serum BUN and creatinine (ratio ≤ 15)
  e. Hypokalemia (diuresis phase) and infection are common problems

5. Treatment

  a. Treat prerenal azotemia
    • Volume expansion if hypovolemic; increase renal blood flow
  b. Low dose dopamine
  c. Fenoldopam (dopamine α-1-receptor agonist)
  d. Dialysis

6. Differential diagnosis of oliguria (Box 19-1)

B. Tubulointerstitial nephritis (TIN)

1. Overview
  • Acute or chronic inflammation of tubules and interstitium
  a. Causes of TIN

> APN: most common cause of TIN

    • Acute pyelonephritis (APN; most common)
  b. Drugs
  c. Infections
    • Examples—legionnaires' disease, leptospirosis
  d. SLE, lead poisoning
  e. Urate nephropathy, multiple myeloma

2. Acute pyelonephritis

  a. Epidemiology

> APN: most common cause of TIN
>
> APN: women > men

    (1) More common in women than men
        • Women have a short urethra.
    (2) *Escherichia coli* most common cause

> APN: *E. coli* most common cause

        • *Enterococcus* second in frequency
    (3) Risk factors
        (a) Indwelling urinary catheter
        (b) Urinary tract obstruction
        (c) Medullary sponge kidney
        (d) Diabetes mellitus, pregnancy
        (e) Sickle cell trait/disease

  b. Pathogenesis
    (1) Vesicoureteral reflux (VUR) with ascending infection (most common)
        (a) Intravesical portion of the ureter is normally compressed with micturition.
            • Prevents reflux of urine into the ureter(s)

> VUR: urine refluxes into the ureters during micturition

        (b) In VUR, the intravesical portion of the ureter is *not* compressed during micturition.
            • Urine refluxes into the ureter(s).
        (c) Should be corrected by reimplantation of the ureters/stents

BOX 19-1   DIFFERENTIAL DIAGNOSIS OF OLIGURIA

Oliguria is defined as a urine output < 400 mL/day or <20 mL/hour. The major causes of oliguria include prerenal azotemia (most common cause), acute glomerulonephritis (nephritic type), acute tubular necrosis (renal azotemia), and postrenal azotemia. Laboratory tests that are commonly used in differentiating the types of oliguria include urine osmolality (UOsm), fractional excretion of sodium (FENa$^+$), random urine sodium (UNa$^+$), and the serum BUN:Cr (blood urea nitrogen/creatinine) ratio (see section III). These tests evaluate tubular function. A UOsm > 500 mOsm/kg indicates good concentrating ability and intact tubular function, but a UOsm < 350 mOsm/kg indicates poor concentrating ability and tubular dysfunction. The FENa$^+$ represents the amount of sodium excreted in the urine divided by the amount of sodium that is filtered by the kidneys. The calculation is as follows:

$$FENa^+ = [(UNa^+ \times PCr) \div (PNa^+ \times UCr)] \times 100$$

where UNa$^+$ is a random urine sodium, PNa$^+$ is serum sodium, UCr is random urine creatinine, and PCr is plasma creatinine. Creatinine is used in the formula, because the amount of sodium filtered is dependent on the glomerular filtration rate (GFR), which closely approximates the creatinine clearance (CCr). An FENa$^+$ < 1% indicates good tubular function and *excludes* acute tubular necrosis (ATN) as a cause of oliguria. An FENa$^+$ > 2% indicates tubular dysfunction and is highly predictive of ATN as the cause of oliguria. A random UNa$^+$ < 20 mEq/L indicates intact tubular function, while a random UNa$^+$ > 40 mEq/L indicates tubular dysfunction. A serum BUN:Cr ratio > 15 indicates intact tubular function, but a serum BUN:Cr ratio ≤ 15 indicates tubular dysfunction. In prerenal azotemia and acute glomerulonephritis (nephritic type) tubular function is preserved. In order to distinguish the two, the urine sediment examination is most useful. In prerenal azotemia, the urine sediment has *no* abnormal findings or may have a few hyaline casts. The sediment in acute glomerulonephritis (nephritic type) has hematuria and RBC casts. ATN and postrenal azotemia (long-standing obstruction) both have tubular dysfunction. Postrenal azotemia of short duration has normal tubular function and has laboratory findings similar to prerenal azotemia. In order to distinguish ATN from postrenal azotemia as a cause of tubular dysfunction and oliguria, the urine sediment is most useful. In ATN, the sediment has pigmented renal tubular cell casts, but in postrenal azotemia, the sediment is usually normal. In addition, the patient will likely have a history of a renal stone, benign prostatic hyperplasia, or cervical cancer, which commonly obstructs the ureters where they enter the urinary bladder.

Disorder	FENa$^+$ %	BUN:Cr	UNa$^+$	UOsm	Urinalysis
Prerenal azotemia	<1	>15	<20	>500	Normal sediment or hyaline casts
Acute glomerulonephritis	<1	>15	<20	>500	RBC casts, hematuria
Acute tubular necrosis	>2	≤ 15	>40	<350	Renal tubular cell casts
Postrenal azotemia (prolonged obstruction)	>2	≤15	>40	<350	Normal sediment

(2) Ascending infection
   (a) Most common mechanism for lower and upper UTIs in females
   (b) Distal urethra and vaginal introitus are normally colonized by *Escherichia coli*.
   (c) Organisms ascend into the urethra and bladder.
     • Causes urethritis and cystitis
   (d) If VUR is present, infected urine ascends to the renal pelvis and renal parenchyma.
     • Causes APN
(3) Hematogenous spread to kidneys
   (a) Uncommon cause of APN
   (b) Suspect if *Staphylococcus aureus* is cultured in urine
c. Gross and microscopic findings
  (1) Grayish white areas of abscess formation are in the cortex and medulla.
  (2) Microabscess formation occurs in the tubular lumens and interstitium (Fig. 19-9).
d. Clinical findings
  (1) Spiking fever, flank pain
  (2) Increased frequency of urination
  (3) Painful urination (dysuria)
e. Laboratory findings
  (1) WBC casts (key finding; see Fig. 19-2F)
  (2) Pyuria, bacteriuria (usually *E. coli*)
  (3) Hematuria

Ascending infection: most common mechanism for upper/lower UTIs in females

Findings in APN and *not* lower UTIs: fever, flank pain, WBC casts in urine

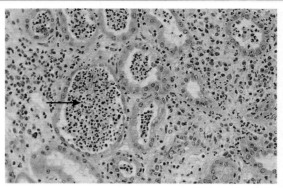

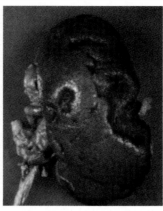

19-9: Acute pyelonephritis showing a neutrophil-dominant infiltrate in the tubular lumens *(arrow)* and interstitium. The neutrophils in the lumens are molded into white blood cell (WBC) casts, which are passed in the urine along with free neutrophils and bacteria (pyuria). *(From Kern WF, Silva FG, Laszik ZG, et al [eds]: Atlas of Renal Pathology. Philadelphia, WB Saunders, 1999, p 149, Fig. 13-15B.)*

19-10: Chronic pyelonephritis. The renal cortex shows deep U-shaped scars. Sections through this scar would have revealed a blunt calyx. *(From Kern WF, Silva FG, Kern W [eds]: Atlas of Renal Pathology. Philadelphia, WB Saunders, 1999, p 149, Fig. 13-16.)*

f. Complications
   (1) Chronic pyelonephritis
   (2) Perinephric abscess
   (3) Renal papillary necrosis
   (4) Septicemia with endotoxic shock
g. Treatment
   (1) Ciprofloxacin given orally if uncomplicated
   (2) Ciprofloxacin IV if hospitalized
   (3) Repair VUR
3. Chronic pyelonephritis (CPN)
   a. Pathogenesis

Causes of CPN: VUR in young girls, chronic hydronephrosis

   (1) VUR starting in young girls
   (2) Lower urinary tract obstruction
       (a) Produces hydronephrosis
       (b) Examples—prostate hyperplasia, renal stones
   b. Gross and microscopic findings
      (1) Reflux type of CPN

CPN: cortical scars overlie blunt calyces; visible with IVP

          (a) U-shaped cortical scars (Fig. 19-10) overlying a blunt calyx
          (b) Visible with an intravenous pyelogram (IVP)
      (2) Obstructive type CPN
          (a) Uniform dilation of the calyces
          (b) Diffuse thinning of cortical tissue
      (3) Microscopic findings

CPN: glomerular scarring; tubular atrophy ("thyroidization")

          (a) Chronic inflammation
              • Secondary scarring of the glomeruli
          (b) Tubular atrophy
              • Tubules contain eosinophilic material resembling thyroid tissue ("thyroidization").
   c. Clinical and laboratory findings
      (1) Usually a history of recurrent APN
      (2) May cause hypertension

Reflux nephropathy: hypertension in children

          • Reflux nephropathy is a cause of hypertension in children.
      (3) May cause chronic renal failure (CRF)
4. Acute drug-induced TIN

Drugs: methicillin, NSAIDs, rifampin, sulfonamides

   a. Common drug associations
      (1) Penicillin, particularly methicillin
      (2) Rifampin, sulfonamides
      (3) NSAIDs, diuretics

  b. Pathogenesis
   (1) Combination of type I and type IV hypersensitivity
   (2) Occurs ~2 weeks after beginning a drug
  c. Clinical and laboratory findings
   (1) Abrupt onset of fever, oliguria, and rash
    • Withdrawal of the drug causes reversal of the disease.
   (2) Laboratory findings
    (a) BUN:Cr ratio ≤ 15
    (b) Eosinophilia and eosinophiluria (highly predictive)
  d. Treatment is to withdraw the drug.
5. Analgesic nephropathy
  a. Epidemiology
   (1) Common cause of chronic drug-induced TIN
   (2) More common in women than men
   (3) Usually occurs in patients with chronic pain
  b. Pathogenesis
   (1) Chronic use of acetaminophen plus aspirin for 3 or more years
   (2) Acetaminophen free radicals damage renal tubules in medulla (refer to Chapter 1).
   (3) Aspirin inhibits renal synthesis of PGE_2 leaving ATII unopposed.
    • Decreased blood flow to the renal medulla
  c. Complications
   (1) Renal papillary necrosis (Fig. 19-11)
    (a) Sloughing of renal papillae
     • Produces gross hematuria, proteinuria, and colicky flank pain
    (b) An IVP shows a "ring defect" where one or more papillae used to reside.
    (c) Other causes of renal papillary necrosis
     • Diabetes, sickle cell trait/disease, APN
   (2) Hypertension, CRF
   (3) Renal pelvic and bladder transitional cell carcinomas
6. Urate nephropathy
  a. Deposition of urate crystals in the tubules and interstitium
  b. Causes
   (1) Massive release of purines (precursor of uric acid)
    • Usually following aggressive treatment of disseminated cancer (e.g., leukemia)
   (2) Lead poisoning, gout
  c. May produce ARF

Patients with disseminated cancers should receive allopurinol, an xanthine oxidase inhibitor, *before* being treated with chemotherapy. This prevents urate nephropathy (tumor lysis syndrome) and acute renal failure.

7. Chronic lead poisoning
  a. Pathogenesis
   (1) Decreases excretion of uric acid (urate nephropathy)
    • Can also decrease uric acid secretion producing gout
   (2) Direct toxic effect produces TIN

Margin notes:

Acute drug-induced TIN: abrupt onset fever, oliguria, rash

Analgesic nephropathy: acetaminophen + aspirin; renal papillary necrosis

Renal papillary necrosis: "ring defect" on IVP from sloughing of papilla

Prevention of urate nephropathy: allopurinol *before* aggressive cancer therapy

Chronic Pb poisoning: proximal tubules with nuclear acid-fast inclusions

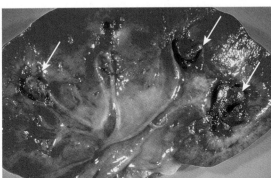

19-11: Analgesic nephropathy showing multiple brownish necrotic papillae (*arrows*). (From Kumar V, Fausto N, Abbas A: *Robbins and Cotran's Pathologic Basis of Disease*, 7th ed. Philadelphia, WB Saunders, 2004, p 1003, Fig. 20-45.)

b. Proximal tubule cells contain characteristic nuclear acid-fast inclusions.
   8. Multiple myeloma: mechanisms for renal disease
      a. Bence Jones (BJ) proteinuria (refer to Chapter 13)
         (1) BJ protein produces tubular casts.
            • Light chains are toxic to renal tubular epithelium.
         (2) Casts obstruct the lumen and incite a foreign body giant cell reaction.
            • Reaction involves tubules and interstitium leading to renal failure.
      b. Nephrocalcinosis (refer to Chapter 1)
         (1) Due to hypercalcemia
            • Metastatic calcification of the basement membrane of collecting tubules
         (2) Causes polyuria and renal failure
      c. Primary amyloidosis producing nephrotic syndrome (refer to Chapter 3)
         • Light chains are converted to amyloid (see Figs. 3-6 and 3-7).

VIII. Chronic Renal Failure
   A. Epidemiology and pathogenesis
      1. Progressive irreversible azotemia that develops over months to years
      2. Culminates in end-stage renal disease
         a. Kidneys no longer function well enough to sustain life.
         b. GFR < 10 mL/minute.
      3. Primary causes, in descending order
         a. Diabetic mellitus (37%)
         b. Hypertension (30%)
         c. Chronic glomerulonephritis (12%)
            • Particularly due to RPGN and focal segmental glomerulosclerosis
         d. Cystic renal disease
            • Renal dysplasia in children, adult polycystic kidney disease
   B. Gross appearance
      • Bilateral, small shrunken kidneys
   C. Hematologic findings
      1. Normocytic anemia with corrected reticulocyte count < 3% (refer to Chapter 11)
         • Primarily due to decreased erythropoietin
      2. Qualitative platelet defects (refer to Chapter 14)
   D. Renal osteodystrophy
      1. Osteitis fibrosa cystica
         a. Due to hypovitaminosis D (refer to Chapter 7)
            (1) Causes hypocalcemia, which stimulates production of parathyroid hormone (PTH)
            (2) Called secondary hyperparathyroidism (HPTH) (refer to Chapter 22)
         b. Secondary HPTH increases bone resorption.
            (1) Causes cystic lesions in bone (e.g., jaw)
            (2) Hemorrhage into cysts causes a brown discoloration.
      2. Osteomalacia
         a. Decreased mineralization of the organic bone matrix (osteoid)
         b. In CRF, it is due to hypovitaminosis D.
            • Causes hypocalcemia, leading to decreased bone mineralization
         c. Produces fractures and bone pain
      3. Osteoporosis (refer to Chapter 23)
         a. Loss of organic bone matrix and minerals
            • Causes an overall reduction in bone mass
         b. In CRF, it is due to chronic metabolic acidosis.
            • Excess H^+ ions are buffered by bone.
         c. Produces fractures and bone pain
   E. Cardiovascular findings
      1. Hypertension from salt retention
      2. Hemorrhagic fibrinous pericarditis
      3. Congestive heart failure, accelerated atherosclerosis
   F. Miscellaneous findings
      1. Hemorrhagic gastritis
      2. Uremic frost (urea crystals deposit on skin)
   G. Laboratory findings
      1. Acid–base and electrolyte abnormalities
         a. Hyperkalemia and increased anion gap metabolic acidosis (refer to Chapter 4)
         b. Sodium is usually normal *except* in salt-losing types of CRF.

BJ proteinuria: casts with foreign body giant cell reaction

CRF: normocytic anemia; qualitative platelet defect

Renal osteodystrophy: due to secondary HPTH, osteomalacia, osteoporosis

CRF: hypertension, pericarditis, CHF, atherosclerosis

2. Hypocalcemia; causes:
   a. Hypovitaminosis D
      (1) Due to decreased synthesis of 1-α-hydroxylase
      (2) Decreased reabsorption of calcium from the small intestine
   b. Hyperphosphatemia
      (1) Due to decreased renal excretion
      (2) Drives calcium into bone and soft tissue
         • Metastatic calcification (refer to Chapter 1)
3. Normocytic anemia; prolonged bleeding time
4. Increased serum cystatin C
   a. Cysteine protease inhibitor produced by all nucleated cells
   b. Filtered by glomerulus but *not* secreted
   c. Less dependent on age, sex, race, and muscle mass than creatinine
   d. May be superior to creatinine in assessing severity of renal function
      • Biomarker of kidney function
5. Urinalysis findings
   a. Fixed specific gravity
      (1) Tubular dysfunction causes lack of concentration and dilution.
      (2) Free water clearance is zero (refer to Chapter 4).
   b. Waxy/broad casts (see Fig. 19-2H)

H. Treatment
1. Nonpharmacologic
   a. Restrict sodium
   b. Low-protein diet (refer to Chapter 7)
   c. Adjust drug doses to renal clearance
   d. Kidney transplantation
2. General
   a. ACE inhibitors
      (1) Reduce proteinuria and disease progression
      (2) Treat hypertension
   b. Dialysis
   c. Erythropoiesis stimulating agents
   d. Calcium supplementation and vitamin D (calcitriol)
      • Treat renal osteodystrophy
   e. Phosphate binder (e.g., sevelamer)

IX. Vascular Disorders
A. Benign nephrosclerosis (BNS)
1. Most common renal disease in essential hypertension
2. Pathogenesis
   a. Hyaline arteriolosclerosis of arterioles in the renal cortex.
   b. Causes tubular atrophy, interstitial fibrosis, glomerular sclerosis
3. Small kidneys with a finely granular cortical surface (Fig. 19-12)
4. Laboratory findings
   a. Mild proteinuria
   b. Hematuria (no RBC casts)
   c. Renal azotemia

B. Malignant hypertension
1. Epidemiology
   a. Sudden onset of accelerated hypertension
      (1) May occur in normotensive individuals
      (2) May occur in those with BNS (most common)
      (3) May occur as a complication of various disorders
   b. Risk factors
      (1) Pre-existing BNS (most common)
      (2) Hemolytic-uremic syndrome
      (3) Thrombotic thrombocytopenic purpura
      (4) Systemic sclerosis
2. Pathogenesis
   a. Vascular damage to arterioles and small arteries
   b. Gross and microscopic changes

CRF: ↑ anion gap metabolic acidosis; ↑ serum phosphorus/potassium; ↓ serum calcium

Cystatin C: biomarker of kidney function

Free water clearance in CRF: zero

Waxy casts: sign of CRF

BNS: kidney of essential hypertension; due to hyaline arteriolosclerosis

Malignant hypertension: pre-existing BNS most common cause

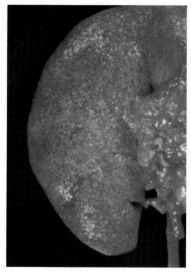

19-12: Benign nephrosclerosis showing a finely granular cortical surface due to atrophy of tubules, glomerular sclerosis, and interstitial fibrosis in the renal cortex. *(From Kern WF, Silva FG, Laszik ZG, et al [eds]: Atlas of Renal Pathology. Philadelphia, WB Saunders, 1999, p 166, Fig. 14-10.)*

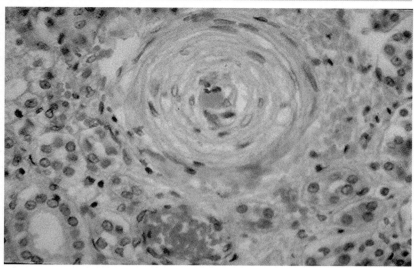

19-13: Malignant hypertension. A feature of malignant hypertension is hyperplastic arteriolosclerosis due to smooth muscle hyperplasia and basement membrane reduplication giving the vessel an "onion skin" appearance. *(From Klatt E: Robbins and Cotran's Atlas of Pathology. Philadelpha, WB Saunders, 2006, p 7, Fig. 1-17.)*

         (1) Fibrinoid necrosis and necrotizing arteriolitis and glomerulitis
            • Pinpoint hemorrhages on the cortical surface ("flea-bitten" kidneys)
         (2) Hyperplastic arteriolosclerosis ("onion skin" lesion; refer to Chapter 9) (Fig. 19-13)
            • Smooth muscle hyperplasia and reduplication of basement membrane

Malignant hypertension: ≥ 210/120 mm Hg, encephalopathy, renal failure

3. Clinical findings
   a. Rapid increase in blood pressure to ≥210/120 mm Hg
   b. Hypertensive encephalopathy
      (1) Cerebral edema
      (2) Papilledema
         • Loss of the normal optic nerve disk margin
      (3) Retinopathy
         • Flame hemorrhages, exudates
      (4) Potential for an intracerebral bleed
   c. Oliguric acute renal failure
4. Laboratory findings
   a. Azotemia with BUN:Cr ratios ≤ 15
   b. Hematuria with RBC casts

Malignant hypertension: IV nitroprusside

   c. Proteinuria
5. Initial treatment is intravenous sodium nitroprusside.

C. Renal infarction

Renal infarction: embolization most common

1. Causes
   a. Embolization from thrombi in the left side of the heart (most common)
   b. Atheroembolic renal disease
   c. Vasculitis, particularly polyarteritis nodosa
2. Gross and microscopic appearance
   a. Irregular, wedge-shaped pale infarctions in the cortex

Renal infarction: hematuria and flank pain

   b. Old infarcts have a V-shaped appearance due to scar tissue.
3. Sudden onset of flank pain and hematuria

D. Sickle cell nephropathy

Sickle cell trait/ disease: hematuria; loss concentration; renal papillary necrosis, APN

1. Occurs with sickle cell trait or disease
2. Clinical presentations
   a. Asymptomatic hematuria (most common) (refer to Chapter 11)
      • Due to infarctions in the medulla

b. Loss of concentrating ability
c. Renal papillary necrosis
d. Pyelonephritis

E. Diffuse cortical necrosis
1. Complication of an obstetric emergency
    • Examples—preeclampsia, abruptio placentae
2. Due to DIC limited to the renal cortex
    a. Fibrin clots in arterioles and glomerular capillaries
    b. Bilateral, diffuse, pale infarct of the renal cortex
3. Anuria (no urine) in a pregnant woman followed by ARF

> Diffuse cortical necrosis: anuria followed by ARF in pregnant woman

X.   Obstructive Disorders
A. Hydronephrosis
1. Epidemiology
    a. Children usually have congenital malformation.
        • Examples—bladder neck obstruction; urethral valve
    b. Adults usually have acquired disease.
        • Examples—stone (most common); prostate hyperplasia
2. Causes
    a. Renal stone (most common)
    b. Retroperitoneal fibrosis
    c. Cervical cancer, benign prostatic hyperplasia
3. Gross findings
    a. Dilated ureter and renal pelvis (Fig. 19-14)
    b. Compression atrophy of the renal medulla and cortex
4. May produce postrenal azotemia
5. Treatment is to relieve the obstruction.
    • Catheter (most often); nephrostomy tube; cystoscopy

> Hydronephrosis: most common complication of upper urinary tract obstruction

B. Renal stones (urolithiasis)
1. Epidemiology
    a. Stones occur in males more often than females.
    b. Incidence is greater during the summer.
        • Insufficient fluid intake
2. Causes
    a. Hypercalciuria in the absence of hypercalcemia
        (1) Most common metabolic abnormality

> Renal stone: most common cause of upper urinary tract obstruction

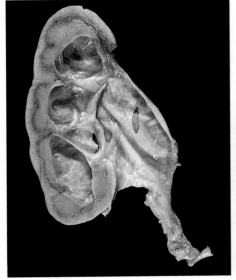

19-14: Hydronephrosis of the kidney. There is marked dilation of the renal pelvis and calyces with thinning of the overlying cortex and medulla due to compression atrophy. (*From Kumar V, Fausto N, Abbas A: Robbins and Cotran's Pathologic Basis of Disease, 7th ed. Philadelphia, WB Saunders, 2004, p 1013, Fig. 20-56.*)

19-15: Staghorn calculi. Note the staghorn calculi in the renal calyces and the renal pelvis. (*From Kern WF, Silva FG, Laszik ZG, et al [eds]: Atlas of Renal Pathology. Philadelphia, WB Saunders, 1999, p 155, Fig. 13-30.*)

Hypercalciuria: most common metabolic abnormality causing calcium stones

Thiazides: increase reabsorption of calcium out of urine

Renal stone: calcium oxalate most common; calcium phosphate

Struvite stone: MAP; urease producers; alkaline urine pH

Renal stone: ipsilateral colicky pain in flank radiating to groin; hematuria

Plain film: 80% stones radiopaque

Spiral CT: best overall sensitivity and specificity; expensive

Ultrasound: detects hydronephrosis, not stone

Stone prevention: hydration is very important

Rx for calcium stones: hydrochlorothiazide

      (2) Due to increased gastrointestinal reabsorption of calcium
- Called absorptive hypercalciuria

    b. Decreased urine volume concentrates the urine.
- Hydration is essential in preventing stone formation.

    c. Reduced urine citrate
- Citrate normally chelates calcium.

    d. Primary HPTH (10% of cases)

    e. Diets high in dairy products (contain phosphate) or oxalates

    f. Urinary infections due to urease producers (e.g., *Proteus*)

  3. Types of renal stones

    a. Calcium stones (~80%)

      (1) Calcium oxalate stone (>50%) is the most common type in adults.
- Increased incidence in pure vegans and those with Crohn's disease

      (2) Calcium phosphate stones (10–20%) are the most common type in children.
- Associated with dairy products and distal renal tubular acidosis

    b. Magnesium ammonium phosphate (MAP)

      (1) "Staghorn calculus" or struvite stone (15%; Fig. 19-15)

      (2) Associated with urease producers (e.g., *Proteus*)

      (3) Urine is alkaline and smells like ammonia.

    c. Uric acid (8%), cystine (3%)

  4. Clinical findings

    a. Sudden onset of flank tenderness

    b. Nausea and vomiting

    c. Colicky pain radiating into groin

    d. Patient constantly moving to try to relieve pain

    e. Gross hematuria may be evident.

  5. Laboratory findings

    a. Hematuria

    b. May find crystals in urine

    c. Hypercalcemia
- Consider primary HPTH

  6. Diagnosis

    a. Plain film (kidney-ureter-bladder [KUB])
- Approximately 80% of stones are radiopaque.

    b. Unenhanced spiral (helical) CT
- Sensitivity 96%, specificity 100%

    c. Ultrasound (sensitivity 15%, specificity 90%)

    d. Strain urine to collect stone

      (1) Always send for analysis

      (2) Greater than 50% pass stone within 48 hours.

      (3) Recurrence occurs in ~50% of patients.

  7. Treatment is tailored to type of stone.

    a. Calcium stone

      (1) Hydrochlorothiazide
- Increases renal tubule reabsorption of calcium (refer to Chapter 4)

      (2) Cellulose phosphate
- Binds calcium in intestine

    b. Uric acid stone

      (1) Allopurinol

      (2) Increase urinary pH
- Makes uric acid soluble in urine

    c. Struvite stone

      (1) Surgical removal because of size

      (2) Antibiotic to eliminate urease producer

    d. Surgical removal

      (1) Extracorporeal shock wave lithotripsy

      (2) Ureteroscopic stone extraction

XI. Tumors of the Kidney and Renal Pelvis

  A. Angiomyolipoma

    1. Hamartoma composed of blood vessels, smooth muscle, and adipose cells

2. Associated with tuberous sclerosis (refer to Chapter 25)
   a. Mental retardation
   b. Multisystem hamartomas

B. Renal cell carcinoma
- Alias Grawitz tumor, clear cell carcinoma, hypernephroma
1. Epidemiology
   a. Sporadic (most common) and hereditary types
   b. Occurs in men more frequently than women
     - Occurs in the sixth to seventh decades
   c. Risk factors
     (1) Smoking (most common)
     (2) Von Hippel–Lindau disease (VHL)
       (a) Autosomal dominant
       (b) Chromosome 3 relationship
       (c) Hemangioblastomas of cerebellum and retina
       (d) Bilateral renal cell carcinoma (50–60%)
     (3) Adult polycystic kidney disease
     (4) Obesity, asbestos exposure, exposure to lead
     (5) Exposure to gasoline and petroleum products
2. Pathogenesis
   a. Cytogenetic abnormalities occur in sporadic and hereditary cancers
     - Translocations with loss of von Hippel–Lindau suppressor gene
   b. Cancer derives from proximal tubule cells
3. Gross and microscopic findings
   a. Clear cell carcinoma
     (1) Most common type (70–80%)
     (2) Most are sporadic.
      - Remainder are associated with VHL.
     (3) Upper pole mass with cysts and hemorrhage (Fig. 19-16)
      - Tumor is a bright yellow mass larger than 3 cm (75–80%).
     (4) Composed of clear cells that contain lipid and glycogen (Fig. 19-17)
     (5) Tendency for renal vein invasion (15–20%)
      - Yellow tumor may invade inferior vena cava and extend to right side of heart.
     (6) Metastasis
       (a) Lungs are the most common site (50–60%)
        - Often hemorrhagic, "cannonball" appearance on radiographs
       (b) Bone (lytic lesions; 30–40%)
       (c) Regional nodes (15–30%)
       (d) Hemorrhagic nodules in the skin
        - Due to increased vascularity in the tumor

Angiomyolipoma: hamartoma associated with tuberous sclerosis

Renal cell carcinoma: yellow tumor with renal vein invasion

Renal cell carcinoma: derives from proximal tubule cell

Renal cell carcinoma: smoking most common cause

Renal cell carcinoma: invades renal vein; poor prognosis

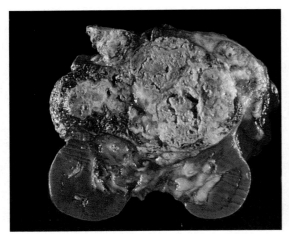

19-16: Renal cell carcinoma. The large, yellow upper pole mass with multifocal areas of hemorrhage extends into the renal pelvis. *(From Damjanov I, Linder J: Pathology: A Color Atlas. St. Louis, Mosby, 2000, p 234, Fig. 11-79.)*

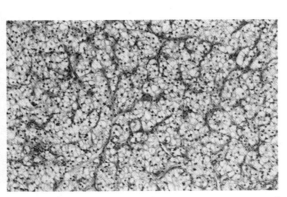

19-17: Renal cell carcinoma: This microscopic section of a renal cell carcinoma shows cells with a clear cytoplasm. *(From Kern WF, Silva FG, Laszik ZG, et al [eds]: Atlas of Renal Pathology. Philadelphia, WB Saunders, 1999, p 281, Fig. 23-5.)*

Triad: hematuria, flank pain, abdominal mass

4. Clinical findings
   a. Hematuria (50–60%)
   b. Abdominal mass (25–45%)
   c. Flank pain (35–40%)
   d. Hypertension (20–40%)
   e. Triad—hematuria, abdominal mass, flank pain (5–10%)
   f. Weight loss (30–35%)
   g. Fever (5–15%)
   h. Left-sided varicocele (2–3%; refer to Chapter 20)
      • Relates to invasion of left renal vein blocking left spermatic vein drainage
5. Laboratory findings
   a. Elevated erythrocyte sedimentation rate (50–60%)
   b. Normocytic anemia (20–40%)

Renal cell carcinoma: ectopic secretion EPO and PTH-related peptide

   c. Ectopic secretion of hormones
      (1) Erythropoietin (EPO)
         • Produces secondary polycythemia (4%)
      (2) PTH-related protein
         • Produces hypercalcemia (3–6%)
6. Diagnosis
   • Ultrasound; abdominal CT; MRI
7. Treatment is nephrectomy.
8. Prognosis
   a. Characteristically has late metastases
      • May recur 10 to 20 years after the tumor has been removed
   b. Average 5-year survival rate is 45% with metastasis.
      • Up to 70% of cases do not have metastasis.
   c. Extension into the renal vein or through the renal capsule has a poor prognosis
      • 10% to 15% 5-year survival rate

C. Renal pelvic cancer
1. Transitional cell carcinoma (TCC)
   a. Most common type
      • Approximately 50% have similar tumors elsewhere in the urinary tract.
   b. Risk factors

TCC renal pelvis: smoking most common cause

      (1) Smoking (most common)
      (2) Phenacetin abuse
      (3) Aromatic amines (aniline dyes)
      (4) Cyclophosphamide
2. Squamous cell carcinoma
   • Risk factors include renal stones and chronic infection.

D. Wilms' tumor
1. Epidemiology
   a. Accounts for ~5% of childhood cancer
   b. Most common primary renal tumor in children
   c. Occurs between 2 and 5 years of age
   d. Sporadic type (most common)

Wilms' tumor: most common primary renal tumor in children

   e. Genetic type
      (1) Autosomal dominant inheritance (chromosome 11)
      (2) WAGR syndrome
         • *W*ilms' tumor, *a*niridia (absent iris), *g*enital abnormalities, *r*etardation
      (3) Beckwith-Wiedemann syndrome
         • Wilms' tumor, enlarged body organs, hemihypertrophy of extremities
2. Large, necrotic, gray-tan tumor
   a. Derived from mesonephric mesoderm
   b. Contains abortive glomeruli and tubules, primitive blastemal cells, and rhabdomyoblasts

Wilms' tumor: child with unilateral flank mass and hypertension

Wilms' tumor: hypertension due to renin secretion

3. Clinical findings
   a. Unilateral palpable mass in a child with hypertension
      • Hypertension due to renin secretion
   b. Lungs are the most common site of metastasis.
   c. With combined therapies 2-year survival rate is >90%.

CHAPTER 20
LOWER URINARY TRACT AND MALE REPRODUCTIVE DISORDERS

I. **Common Ureteral Disorders**
   A. **Congenital megaloureter**
      - May be associated with Hirschsprung's disease
   B. **Ureteritis cystica**
      1. Manifestation of chronic inflammation
      2. Smooth cysts project from the mucosa into the lumen.
         - Similar findings may be present in the bladder.
      3. May undergo glandular metaplasia and predispose to adenocarcinoma
   C. **Ureteral stones**
      - Ureters are the most common site for stones to cause obstruction.
   D. **Retroperitoneal fibrosis**
      1. Causes
         a. Majority are idiopathic.
         b. Ergot derivatives used in the treatment of migraines
         c. Association with other sclerosing conditions
            (1) Primary sclerosing cholangitis
            (2) Sclerosing mediastinitis, Reidel's fibrosing thyroiditis
         d. Retroperitoneal malignant lymphoma
      2. Complications
         a. Hydronephrosis is the most common complication.
         b. May cause right scrotal varicocele (see section V)
            - Blocks the drainage of the right spermatic vein into the vena cava
   E. **Ureteral cancers**
      - Transitional cell carcinoma (TCC) is the most common cancer.
II. **Urinary Bladder Disorders**
   A. **Congenital disorders**
      1. Exstrophy of the bladder (Fig. 20-1)
         a. Developmental failure of the anterior abdominal wall and bladder
            (1) Bladder mucosa is exposed to the body surface.
            (2) Often associated with epispadias (see section IV)
         b. Complications
            (1) Inflammation predisposes to glandular metaplasia.
            (2) Predisposition for adenocarcinoma of the bladder
      2. Urachal cyst remnants
         a. Drainage of urine from umbilicus in a newborn; midline urachal cyst
         b. Predispose to adenocarcinoma of the bladder
            - Most common cause of bladder adenocarcinoma
   B. **Acute and chronic cystitis**
      1. Risk factors for lower urinary tract (LUT) infection
         a. Female sex
            (1) Short urethra
            (2) Ascending infection (refer to Chapter 19)
         b. Indwelling urinary catheter
            (1) Most common cause of sepsis in hospitalized patients

Congenital megaloureter: association with Hirschsprung's disease

Ureteritis cystica: risk factor bladder adenocarcinoma

Hydronephrosis: most common complication of retroperitoneal fibrosis

TCC: most common cancer of ureter

Exstrophy: developmental failure anterior abdominal wall and bladder

Exstrophy: risk factor for bladder adenocarcinoma

Urachal cyst remnants: most common cause of bladder adenocarcinoma; drainage of urine from umbilicus

Indwelling catheters: most common cause sepsis/urinary tract infections in a hospital

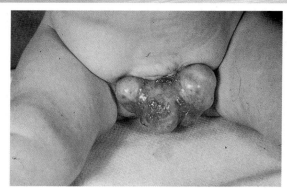

20-1: Exstrophy of the bladder. Red mucosa of the urinary bladder is seen protruding through the defect in the anterior abdominal wall. *(Courtesy of Dr. Roger D. Smith, Cincinnati, Ohio, and GRIPE.)*

(2) Account for 50% of nosocomial urinary tract infections

  c. Sexual intercourse

    (1) "Honeymoon cystitis" from trauma to the urethra

    (2) Voiding after intercourse reduces the risk for infection

  d. Diabetes mellitus, neurogenic bladder

  e. Cyclophosphamide

    (1) Produces hemorrhagic cystitis

    (2) Prevented with mesna

  f. *Schistosoma hematobium*

    (1) Transmission

      (a) Penetration of the skin by the fork-tailed cercariae

      (b) Larvae enter veins in urinary bladder wall.

      (c) Larvae develop into adult worms that deposit eggs.

      (d) Host develops an intense inflammatory response.

      (e) Produce squamous metaplasia of bladder epithelium

    (2) Eggs have a large terminal spine.

    (3) Treatment is praziquantel.

2. Causes of acute cystitis

  a. *Escherichia coli*

    (1) Most common uropathogen (80–90%)

    (2) Gram-negative rod (Fig. 20-2)

    (3) Most common cause of sepsis in a hospitalized patient

    (4) Treatment is trimethoprim-sulfamethoxazole

  b. Adenovirus

    • Causes hemorrhagic cystitis

  c. *Staphylococcus saprophyticus*

    (1) Causes acute cystitis in young sexually active women

      • Accounts for ~10% to 20% of LUT infections

    (2) Coagulase negative

Margin notes:

Cyclophosphamide: hemorrhagic cystitis; prevented with mesna

Schistosoma hematobium: egg with large terminal spine

E. coli: most common uropathogen; sepsis in hospital

S. saprophyticus: LUT in young, sexually active female; coagulase negative

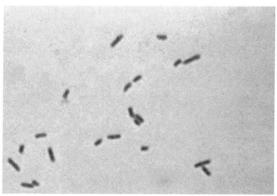

20-2: Gram stain of *Escherichia coli*: Note the gram-negative rods. *(From McPherson R, Pincus M: Henry's Clinical Diagnosis and Management by Laboratory Methods, 21st ed. Philadelphia, Saunders, 2006, Fig. 56-14.)*

(3) Treatment is trimethoprim-sulfamethoxazole
  d. Acute urethral syndrome in women
  - Female counterpart to nonspecific urethritis (NSU) in men
  e. *Chlamydia trachomatis*
    (1) Most common cause of acute urethral syndrome
    (2) Identification of *Chlamydia*
    - Polymerase chain reaction (PCR) testing of voided urine
    (3) Treatment is azithromycin 1 g orally
  f. Other pathogens
    - *Mycoplasma hominis, Ureaplasma urealyticum, Neisseria gonorrhoeae*
3. Clinical findings in LUT infections
  a. Dysuria (painful urination)
  b. Increased frequency, urgency, nocturia
  c. Suprapubic discomfort
  d. Gross hematuria
4. Laboratory findings in LUT infections
  a. Pyuria at or above 10 WBCs per high-power field (HPF) in a centrifuged specimen
    - More than 2 WBCs/HPF in an uncentrifuged specimen
  b. Bacteriuria, hematuria
  c. Positive dipstick for leukocyte esterase and nitrite (refer to Chapter 19)
  d. At or above 10^5 colony-forming units (CFUs)/mL
    - Gold standard criterion of infection
5. Asymptomatic bacteriuria in women
  a. Two successive cultures with 10^5 or more CFUs/mL in an asymptomatic patient
  b. Causes
    (1) Pregnancy
    - Acute pyelonephritis may occur in 1% to 2% of cases.
    (2) Elderly women in nursing homes
  c. Treatment
    (1) Pregnant women
    - Amoxicillin
    (2) Asymptomatic, healthy elderly women
    - No treatment necessary
6. Sterile pyuria
  a. Neutrophils in the urine and negative standard culture after 24 hours
    - Positive leukocyte esterase, negative nitrite
  b. Causes
    (1) *Chlamydia trachomatis*
    (2) Renal tuberculosis
    (3) Acute tubulointerstitial nephritis (refer to Chapter 19)
7. Malacoplakia
  a. Associated with a chronic *E. coli* infection of the bladder
  b. Microscopic findings
    (1) Yellow, raised mucosal plaques
    (2) Foamy macrophages filled with laminated mineralized concretions
      (a) Called Michaelis-Gutmann bodies
      (b) Defective phagosomes that cannot degrade bacterial products

C. Miscellaneous disorders
1. Acquired diverticula
  a. Most are due to benign prostatic hyperplasia (BPH)
  b. Causes obstruction of urine outflow and increased intravesical pressure
  c. Diverticulitis and stone formation are common complications
2. Cystocele
  a. Common in middle-aged to elderly women
  b. Mechanism
    (1) Relaxation of pelvic support causes descent of the uterus
    (2) Bladder wall protrudes into the vagina
    - Creates a pouch that collects residual urine
3. Cystitis cystica and glandularis
  a. Bladder rendition of ureteritis cystica
  b. Increased risk for developing bladder adenocarcinoma

C. trachomatis: most common cause of acute urethral syndrome in women and NSU in men

LUT signs: dysuria, ↑ frequency, urgency

$\geq 10^5$ CFUs/mL: gold standard for LUT infection

Asymptomatic bacteriuria: treat pregnant woman with amoxicillin; no treatment for healthy elderly women

Sterile pyuria: neutrophils in the urine, negative standard culture

Malacoplakia: Michaelis-Gutmann bodies

Acquired bladder diverticula: most common cause is BPH; chronic *E. coli* infection

Cystocele: bladder wall protrudes into vagina

Cystitis cystica/glandularis: risk of bladder adenocarcinoma

Urinary bladder control and incontinence disorders: Relaxation of the detrusor muscle is involved in the storage of urine, while contraction of the muscle is important in emptying the bladder. The sympathetic nervous system relaxes the detrusor muscle and contracts the internal sphincter; hence, it is important in the retention of urine in the bladder. In contradistinction, the parasympathetic nervous system is involved in emptying the bladder. It accomplishes this function by contracting the detrusor muscle and relaxing the internal sphincter muscle. There are four types of urinary incontinence: urge incontinence (40–70% of cases), overflow incontinence, stress incontinence, and functional incontinence. Urge incontinence is caused by overactivity of the detrusor muscle resulting in the production of low volumes of urine. Symptoms include increased urinary frequency, urgency, small volume voids, and nocturia. The most common causes are bladder irritation due to BPH, atrophic urethritis, and infection. Treatment is with anticholinergics, which inhibit parasympathetic stimulation of detrusor contraction. The mechanisms for outflow incontinence are outflow obstruction (e.g., BPH) or detrusor underactivity related to autonomic neuropathy (e.g., diabetes mellitus). Symptoms include dribbling and low urine flow. Treatment involves the use of cholinergic drugs to enhance muscle tone (i.e., increase detrusor contraction) or, if obstruction is the cause (e.g., BPH), α-adrenergic blockers to relax smooth muscles in the bladder neck. The mechanism for stress incontinence is laxity of pelvic floor muscles with a concomitant lack of bladder support. This may be the result of not maintaining the posterior urethrovesical angle of 90–100 degrees or a lack of estrogen; hence, this type of incontinence primarily occurs in women. Symptoms relate to the loss of urine when there is an increase in intra-abdominal pressure (e.g., laughing, cough, sneezing). Treatment is to increase internal sphincter tone with α-adrenergic agonists (contract smooth muscle cells at the bladder neck); using topical estrogen therapy; and encouraging the patient to do Kegel pelvic floor muscle exercises. If these treatments do not control the incontinence, then surgery is the final option. The mechanism for functional incontinence is inability to reach toilet facilities in time. Patients are normally continent; however, if they are taking diuretics or drinking too many caffeinated beverages incontinence may occur.

Retain urine: ↑ sympathetic activity—relax detrusor muscle, contract internal sphincter muscle

Void urine: ↑ parasympathetic activity—contract detrusor muscle, relax internal sphincter muscle

D. Bladder tumors
1. Bladder papilloma
   - Very uncommon benign tumor
2. Transitional cell carcinoma (TCC)
   a. Epidemiology

TCC: most common bladder cancer

   (1) Most common bladder cancer (>95% of cases)
   (2) More common in men than women
   (3) Incidence increases with age.
   (4) Causes

TCC: most common cause is smoking cigarettes

      (a) Smoking cigarettes (most common cause)
         - Less risk for other tobacco products
      (b) Workers in dye, rubber, or leather industries
      (c) Cyclophosphamide
      (d) Arsenic exposure
      (e) Beer consumption
         - Due to nitrosamines in beer

Squamous cell carcinoma of bladder: *S. hematobium* infection

      (f) *Schistosoma hematobium*
         - 70% produce squamous cell carcinoma, 30% TCC
   b. Pathogenesis
      (1) Genetic factors
         (a) Numerous chromosomes implicated
         (b) Genes implicated: *TP53* and *RB* suppressor genes: *HRAS* protooncogene
         (c) Alteration in epidermal derived growth factor receptor
      (2) Environmental factors (see earlier discussion)

TCC: multifocal tumor; recurrences are the rule

      (3) Multifocality ("field effect") and recurrence are the rule.
         (a) Common malignant stem cell abnormality
         (b) Reimplantation of the tumor from another site
   c. Gross and microscopic findings
      (1) Low-grade cancers
         - Usually papillary and are *not* usually invasive (Fig. 20-3)
      (2) High-grade cancers
         - Papillary or flat and are usually invasive
      (3) Most common sites
         - Lateral or posterior walls at the base of the bladder

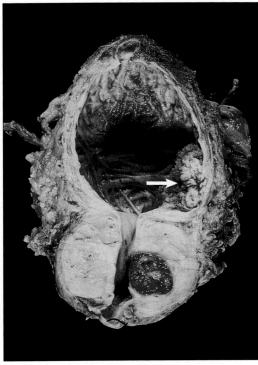

20-3: Transitional cell carcinoma of urinary bladder. The *arrow* shows a papillary exophytic mass arising from the mucosal surface of the bladder. The red lesion in the prostate gland is an infarction. *(From Rosai J, Ackerman LV: Surgical Pathology, 9th ed. St. Louis, Mosby, 2004, p 1328, Fig. 17-175.)*

(4) Significance of blood group antigens (A, B, or H)
- Better prognosis if the tumor has the antigens

d. Clinical findings
(1) Painless gross/microscopic hematuria
- Most common sign (70–90%)
(2) Dysuria, increased frequency of urination

e. Treatment
(1) Surgical resection
(2) Intravesical chemotherapy
(3) Radiotherapy

f. Prognosis
- Five-year survival rate for all stages combined is 80%.

3. Squamous cell carcinoma of the bladder
a. Epidemiology
(1) Association with *Schistosoma hematobium*
- Eggs are located in the urinary bladder venous plexus.
(2) Common cancer in Egypt
(3) 70% of cancers are squamous cell carcinoma, 30% are TCC

b. Pathogenesis of squamous cell carcinoma
(1) Eggs are surrounded by eosinophils.
(2) IgE antibodies are attached to the eggs.
(3) Eosinophils have Fc receptors for IgE.
(4) Eosinophils attach to receptors and release major basic protein, which destroys the egg.
- Type II hypersensitivity reaction
(5) Chronic bladder irritation/infection produces squamous metaplasia.
- Metaplasia can progress to dysplasia and squamous cell carcinoma.

4. Causes of adenocarcinoma of the bladder
a. Urachal remnants (most common cause)
b. Cystitis glandularis
c. Exstrophy of the bladder

TCC: painless hematuria most common sign

Bladder squamous cancer: *S. hematobium*

Killing helminth eggs: type II hypersensitivity reaction involving eosinophils

5. Embryonal rhabdomyosarcoma (sarcoma botryoides)

Embryonal sarcoma: most common sarcoma in children; in boys, protrudes from urethra

   a. Most common sarcoma in children
      • Accounts for ~3% of childhood cancer
   b. Most common site for boys is urinary system.
      • Presents as grape-like masses protruding from the urethral orifice
   c. Most common site in girls is the vagina.

Cancers invading bladder: cervical and prostate cancer

6. Cancers invading the bladder
   a. Invasive cervical cancer and prostate cancer
   b. Produce obstruction of the urethra and the ureters
   c. Produce hydronephrosis, postrenal azotemia, and death by renal failure

III. **Urethral Disorders**
      A. Infections
         1. Chlamydial and gonococcal infections in men and women

STD urethritis: *Chlamydia* and *Neisseria gonorrhoeae*

            • Urethra is the most common site for these sexually transmitted diseases.
         2. Nonvenereal diseases causing urethritis
            a. Most commonly due to *E. coli*
            b. Complications
               (1) Cystitis in women
               (2) Prostatitis in men

Reiter's syndrome: *Chlamydial* urethritis, conjunctivitis, HLA-B27 arthritis

         3. *Chlamydial* urethritis is a common component of Reiter's syndrome in men.
            a. Urethritis
            b. Sterile conjunctivitis
            c. HLA-B27–associated arthritis (refer to Chapter 23)
      B. Urethral caruncle
         1. Female dominant disease
         2. Friable, red painful mass is present at the urethral orifice.
         3. Chronically inflamed granulation tissue causes bleeding.

Urethra: squamous cell carcinoma most common cause

      C. Squamous cell carcinoma
         • Most common cancer of the urethra

IV.   **Penis Disorders**
      A. Malformations of the urethral groove
         1. Hypospadias

Hypospadias: abnormal opening on ventral surface of penis

            a. Abnormal opening on the ventral surface of the penis (Fig. 20-4)
            b. Most common malformation of urethral groove

Hypospadias: most common malformation of urethral grove

            c. Risk factors
               (1) Father or previous male sibling had defect
               (2) Monozygotic twins
                  • ? Insufficient production of human chorionic gonadotropin by single placenta

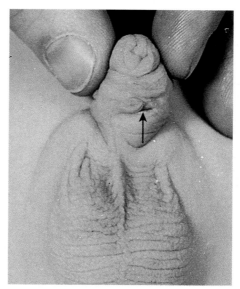

20-4: Hypospadias. The *arrow* shows the urethral opening on the ventral surface of the penis. *(From Damjanov I, Linder J: Pathology: A Color Atlas. St. Louis, Mosby, 2000, p 211, Fig. 11-6.)*

       d. Frequently associated with ventral curvature of penis
- Called chordee

       e. Pathogenesis
          (1) Due to faulty closure of the urethral folds
          (2) Possibly related to abnormal androgen production

    2. Epispadias
       a. Abnormal opening on the dorsal surface of the penis
       b. Due to a defect in the genital tubercle

B. Phimosis
    1. Orifice of the prepuce is too small to retract over the head of the penis
    2. Commonly associated with infections

C. Balanoposthitis
    1. Infection of the glans and prepuce
       a. Usually occurs in uncircumcised males with poor hygiene
       b. Accumulation of smegma leads to infection.
- *Candida*, pyogenic bacteria, and anaerobes

    2. Inflammatory scarring may produce an acquired phimosis.

D. Miscellaneous disorders
    1. Peyronie's disease
       a. Type of fibromatosis (refer to Chapter 23)
       b. Painful contractures of the penis
- Causes lateral curvature of the penis

       c. May cause infertility
    2. Priapism
       a. Persistent and painful erection
       b. Causes include sickle cell disease, penile trauma

E. Carcinoma in situ (CIS)
    1. Bowen's disease
       a. Leukoplakia involving the shaft of the penis and scrotum
          (1) Patients usually >35 years old
          (2) Association with human papillomavirus (HPV) type 16
       b. Precursor for invasive squamous cell carcinoma (~10% of cases)
       c. Association with other types of visceral cancer
    2. Erythroplasia of Queyrat
       a. Erythroplakia located on the mucosal surface of the glans and prepuce
       b. HPV type 16 association
       c. Precursor for invasive squamous cell carcinoma
    3. Bowenoid papulosis
       a. Multiple pigmented reddish brown papules on the external genitalia
       b. Association with HPV type 16
       c. Does *not* develop into invasive squamous cell carcinoma
- Only CIS with no predisposition for invasion

F. Squamous cell carcinoma
    1. Most common cancer of the penis
       a. Usually affects men 40 to 70 years old
       b. Most common sites
- Glans or mucosal surface of prepuce

    2. HPV type 16, 18 association in two thirds of cases
- Smoking may act as a cocarcinogen with HPV.

    3. Risk factors
       a. Lack of circumcision
- Greatest risk factor

       b. Bowen's disease, erythroplasia of Queyrat
    4. Metastasizes to inguinal and iliac nodes

V. Testis, Scrotal Sac, Epididymis Disorders
A. Cryptorchidism
    1. Normal descent of testes
       a. Transabdominal phase
          (1) Testes descend to lower abdomen or pelvic brim
          (2) Müllerian inhibitory factor (anti-müllerian hormone) is responsible for this phase
       b. Inguinoscrotal phase
          (1) Descent through the inguinal canal into the scrotum

---

Margin notes:

Hypospadias: faulty closure urethral folds; androgen dysfunction

Epispadias: abnormal opening on dorsal surface of penis; defect of genital tubercle

Phimosis: orifice of prepuce cannot retract over head of penis

Balanoposthitis: infection of glans and prepuce

Peyronie's disease: fibromatosis; lateral curvature of penis; infertility

Priapism: persistent painful erection

Risk factors for invasive squamous cell carcinoma: Bowen's disease, erythroplasia of Queyrat

Bowenoid papulosis: HPV 16; no invasive cancer

Penis cancer: squamous cell carcinoma

Circumcision: protects against developing cancer of the penis; HPV 16, 18 relationship

Testes transabdominal phase: müllerian inhibitory factor

    (2) Androgen- and human chorionic gonadotropin (hCG)–dependent

2. Cryptorchidism
  a. Epidemiology
    (1) Incomplete or improper descent of the testis into the scrotal sac
    (2) Most common genitourinary disorder in male children
    (3) Occurs 30% premature and 5% of full-term males
    (4) Associations
       • Testicular feminization, Kallmann's syndrome, cystic fibrosis
    (5) Locations
      (a) Inguinal canal most common site (80%)
         • Palpable mass; majority are unilateral (90%)
      (b) Intra-abdominal (5–10% of cases)
    (6) Many will spontaneously descend by 3 months of age
      (a) Due to combination of androgens and hCG
      (b) Spontaneous descent uncommon after 3 months
  b. Complications if uncorrected
    (1) Potential for infertility
      (a) Arrest in germ cell maturation
      (b) Testicular atrophy
      (c) Similar changes occur in the normally descended contralateral testis.
      (d) Greatest risk if intra-abdominal or long duration in inguinal canal

    (2) Increased risk for developing a seminoma
      (a) Five- to tenfold increased risk for cancer in cryptorchid testis
      (b) Risk also applies to the normally descended testicle
    (3) Increased risk for undescended testis to undergo torsion
  c. Treatment
    (1) Orchiopexy as early as 6 months; should be completed by 2 years of age
    (2) Hormonal therapy with hCG produces variable results
    (3) Administration gonadotropin-releasing hormone (GnRH) prior to orchiopexy may improve fertility in adult.

B. Orchitis
1. Mumps
  a. Infertility is uncommon.
  b. Most cases are unilateral.
  c. Orchitis is more likely in an older child or adult.

2. Congenital or acquired syphilis
3. HIV
4. Extension of acute epididymitis

C. Epididymitis
1. Causes
  a. Pathogens in patients < 35 years old
    (1) *Neisseria gonorrhoeae*
    (2) *Chlamydia trachomatis*
  b. Pathogens in patients > 35 years old
    (1) *E. coli*
    (2) *Pseudomonas aeruginosa*
  c. Tuberculosis

    (1) Begins in the epididymis
      • Spreads to the seminal vesicles, prostate, and testicles
    (2) Caseating granulomatous inflammation
  d. AIDS
    • Association with cytomegalovirus, *Toxoplasma*, *Salmonella*
2. Signs and symptoms of acute epididymitis
  a. Usually unilateral scrotal pain with radiation into spermatic cord or flank
  b. Scrotal swelling, epididymal tenderness
  c. Urethral discharge
    • If it is sexually transmitted

  d. Prehn's sign
    • Elevation of the scrotum decreases pain.

3. Treatment
  a. If <35 years old, ceftriaxone + doxycycline (STD treatment)
  b. If >35 years old, ciprofloxacin extended release

D. Varicocele
1. Epidemiology
    a. Occurs in 15% to 20% of all males
        (1) Usually between 15 and 25 years of age
        (2) Rarely occurs after 40 years old
    b. Occurs in 40% of infertile males
    c. Most common cause of left-sided scrotal enlargement in an adult
        • "Bag of worms" appearance (Fig. 20-5)
    d. Left spermatic vein drains into the left renal vein
        (1) Increased resistance to blood flow
        (2) Blockage of left renal vein can also produce a varicocele.
            • Examples—renal cell carcinoma invading renal vein; superior mesenteric artery compressing left renal vein
    e. Right spermatic vein drains into the vena cava
        (1) Blockage of right spermatic vein produces right-sided varicocele.
        (2) Examples—retroperitoneal fibrosis; thrombosis inferior vena cava
2. Pathogenesis
    • Incompetent valves in left spermatic vein from increased pressure
3. Clinical
    a. Aching pain in scrotum
    b. Dragging sensation in testicle
    c. Visible "bag of worms"
    d. Infertility (controversial)
        • Heat decreases spermatogenesis.
4. Diagnosis by ultrasound
5. Treatment
    a. Varicocelectomy
    b. Embolization by intervention radiologist
E. Torsion of the testicle
1. Epidemiology
    a. Majority occur between 12 and 18 years old.
    b. Predisposing factors
        (1) Violent movement or physical trauma
            • Most common causes
        (2) Cryptorchid testis
        (3) Atrophy of testis
    c. Twisting of spermatic cord cuts off the venous/arterial blood supply
        • Danger for hemorrhagic infarction of the testicle

> Varicocele: most often left-sided; spermatic vein empties into left renal vein

> Varicocele: smoker with sudden onset of left varicocele; consider renal carcinoma invading renal vein

> Varicocele: "bag of worms" appearance

> Torsion of testicle: violent movement or trauma most common cause

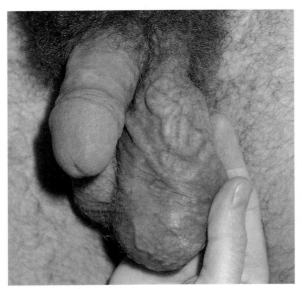

20-5: Varicocele in the left scrotal sac. Note the "bag of worms" appearance. See text for the discussion. *(From Swartz MH: Textbook of Physical Diagnosis, 5th ed. Philadelphia, Saunders Elsevier, 2006, p 545, Fig. 18-27.)*

2. Clinical findings
   a. Sudden onset of testicular pain
   b. Absent cremasteric reflex (key diagnostic finding)
      • Stroking the inner thigh with a tongue blade normally causes the scrotum to retract.
   c. Testicle is drawn up into the inguinal canal.
3. Diagnosis is by ultrasound.
4. Treatment
   a. One third spontaneously remit.
   b. Surgery is imperative within 12 hours for those that do not remit.

F. Hydrocele
1. Most common cause of scrotal enlargement
   a. Due to a failure of closure of the tunica vaginalis
   b. Fluid accumulates in serous space between the layers of the tunica vaginalis.
   c. Invariably associated with an indirect inguinal hernia
2. Diagnosis
   • Ultrasound distinguishes fluid versus a testicular mass causing scrotal enlargement.
3. Other fluid accumulations
   a. Hematocele contains blood.
   b. Spermatocele contains sperm.
4. Treatment is surgery.

G. Testicular tumors
1. Epidemiology
   a. Most common malignancy between ages 15 and 35
   b. Occurs more often in whites than blacks
2. Types of testicular tumors
   a. Malignant testicular tumors are most often germ cell in origin (95% of cases).
   b. Benign testicular tumors are usually sex-cord stromal tumors (5% of cases).
   c. Classification of germ cell tumors
      (1) 40% are of one cell type
         • Seminoma is the most common type (40%).
      (2) 60% are mixtures of two or more patterns.
         • Most common mixture is embryonal carcinoma, teratoma, choriocarcinoma, yolk sac tumor.
      (3) Best classified as seminomas or nonseminomatous
3. Risk factors
   a. Cryptorchid testicle
      (1) Overall most common risk factor
      (2) Greatest risk is an intra-abdominal cryptorchid testis.
   b. Testicular feminization (refer to Chapter 5)
   c. Klinefelter's syndrome (XXY) (refer to Chapter 5)
   d. Inguinal hernia, mumps orchitis
4. Clinical finding
   • Unilateral, painless enlargement of the testis
5. Tumor markers
   a. α-Fetoprotein (AFP)
      • Yolk sac (endodermal sinus) tumor origin
   b. Human chorionic gonadotropin (hCG)
      • Choriocarcinoma
   c. Lactate dehydrogenase
      (1) Nonspecific cancer enzyme
      (2) Degree of elevation correlates with tumor mass
6. Summary of testicular tumors (Table 20-1 and Figs. 20-6 and 20-7)
7. Diagnosis
   a. Ultrasound
   b. CT scan or MRI of pelvis and abdomen
      • Testicular cancer most often involves para-aortic lymph nodes
8. Treatment
   a. Inguinal orchiectomy
   b. Adjuvant chemotherapy

VI. Prostate Disorders
A. Clinical anatomy
1. Dihydrotestosterone (DHT) is responsible for developing the prostate.

Margin notes (left column):

Torsion of testicle: absent cremasteric reflex, testis high in inguinal canal

Hydrocele: most common cause of scrotal enlargement

Hydrocele: persistent tunica vaginalis; inguinal hernia also present

Seminoma: most common testicular cancer

Testicular cancers: seminomas and nonseminomas

Testicular cancer: cryptorchidism most common risk factor

Unilateral, painless testicular mass: testicular cancer

Testicular cancer markers: AFP, hCG

Testicular cancer: para-aortic nodes *not* inguinal nodes

DHT: embryologic development of prostate

TABLE 20-1. **TESTICULAR TUMORS***

TUMOR	AGE (YEARS)	MORPHOLOGIC/CLINICAL FINDINGS	TUMOR MARKER(S)	PROGNOSIS
Seminoma (see Figs. 20-6 and 20-7)	30–35; >65	Most common germ cell tumor (40%) Gray tumor *without* hemorrhage or necrosis. Large cells with centrally located nucleus containing prominent nucleoli. Lymphocytic infiltrate Metastasis: lymphatic (para-aortic lymph nodes) *before* hematogenous (lungs) Spermatocytic variant occurs in older individuals and rarely metastasizes	↑ hCG in 10%	Excellent Extremely radiosensitive
Embryonal carcinoma	20–25	Bulky tumor with hemorrhage and necrosis. Other tumor types often present Metastasis: hematogenous before lymphatic	↑AFP and/or hCG in 90%	Intermediate Less radiosensitive than seminomas
Yolk sac (endodermal sinus) tumor	Most common testicular tumor in children < 4 years old	Characteristic Schiller-Duval bodies resemble primitive glomeruli	↑AFP in all cases	Good
Choriocarcinoma	20–30	Most commonly mixed with other tumor types Contains trophoblastic tissue (syncytiotrophoblast and cytotrophoblast) May produce gynecomastia (hCG is an LH analogue)	↑ hCG in all cases	Poor Most aggressive tumor; hematogenous spread to lungs
Teratoma	Affects males of all ages	Contains derivatives from ectoderm, endoderm, mesoderm Mixed with embryonal carcinoma (teratocarcinoma)	↑ AFP and/or hCG in 50%	Good Usually benign in children and malignant in adults (usually squamous cell carcinoma)
Malignant lymphoma	Most common testicular cancer in men > 60 years of age	Secondary involvement of both testes by diffuse large cell lymphoma	None	Poor

* Listed in order of prognosis.
AFP, α-fetoprotein; hCG, human chorionic gonadotropin; LH, luteinizing hormone.

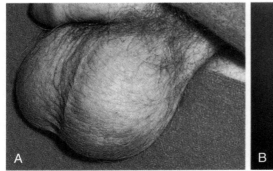
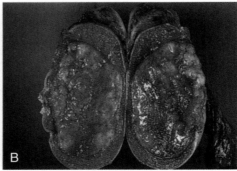

20-6: Seminoma of the testicle showing the scrotal mass (**A**) and the excised mass (**B**). Note the tumor replaces most of the testicle. *(From Grieg JD: Color Atlas of Surgical Diagnosis. London, Mosby-Wolfe, 1996, p 307, Fig. 38-8.)*

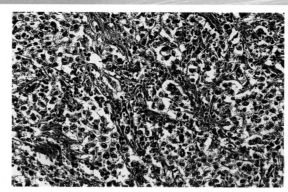

20-7: Microscopic section of a seminoma. Note the large tumor cells with fibrous septa infiltrated by numerous lymphocytes. *(From Rosai J, Ackerman LV: Surgical Pathology, 9th ed. St. Louis, Mosby, 2004, p 1421, Fig. 18-57.)*

2. Zones of the prostate
   a. Peripheral zone
     (1) Palpated during a digital rectal examination (DRE)
     (2) Primary site for prostate cancer
   b. Transitional zone
     • Primary site for the glandular component of BPH
   c. Periurethral zone
     • Primary site for the fibromuscular (stromal) component of BPH

B. Acute/chronic prostatitis
1. Epidemiology
   a. Approximately 50% of males develop prostatitis in their lifetime.
   b. Chronic prostatitis is more common than acute prostatitis.
   c. Causes
     (1) Acute prostatitis
       (a) Intraprostate reflux of urine from the posterior urethra or urinary bladder
       (b) Often associated with acute cystitis
       (c) Young to middle aged adult males
       (d) Pathogens in patients < 35 years old
         • Consider *Chlamydia trachomatis, Neisseria gonorrhoeae*
       (e) Pathogens in patients > 35 years old
         • *E. coli, Pseudomonas aeruginosa, Klebsiella pneumoniae*
     (2) Chronic prostatitis
       (a) Majority are abacterial
       (b) Common in bicycle riders
       (c) Chronic bacterial infection
         • Due to recurrent acute prostatitis
2. Clinical findings
   a. Dysuria, urgency, increased frequency
   b. Fever occurs in acute prostatitis.
   c. Lower back, perineal, or suprapubic pain
   d. Painful/swollen gland on rectal examination
   e. Hematuria may occur.
3. Fractionated urine culture and examination for WBCs
   a. Specimen collections
     • Some consider this cumbersome and impractical.
     (1) First 10 mL is the urethral component.
     (2) Second midstream sample is the bladder component.
     (3) Third specimen at the end of micturition is the prostate component.
     (4) Fourth specimen is secretions milked out after prostate massage.
       • Contraindicated in acute prostatitis
   b. Diagnosis of prostatitis
     (1) More than 20 WBCs/HPF in the third and fourth samples suggests acute prostatitis.
     (2) Increased bacterial count in third and fourth specimens is confirmatory.

Prostatitis: chronic > acute

Acute prostatitis < 35 years old: consider *Chlamydia, Neisseria*

Chronic prostatitis: majority are abacterial

Chronic prostatitis: can radiate to lower back, perineum, suprapubic area

4. Treatment
   a. If acute prostatitis in men < 35 years old, ceftriaxone + doxycycline (STD treatment)
   b. If acute prostatitis in men > 35 years old, ciprofloxacin extended release of trimethoprim-sulfamethoxazole
   c. If chronic bacterial prostatitis, ciprofloxacin

C. Benign prostatic hyperplasia (BPH)
   1. Epidemiology
      a. Age-dependent change
         (1) Majority of men develop BPH as they age.
         (2) Approximately 80% have BPH at 80 years of age.
      b. More common in blacks than whites
      c. Develops in the transitional and periurethral zones
      d. DRE has a sensitivity of 50% in detecting BPH.
      e. Approximately 30% of men with BPH have occult prostate cancer.
   2. Pathogenesis
      a. DHT is the primary mediator.
         • Causes hyperplasia of glandular and stromal cells (see Fig. 1-14)
      b. Stromal cells are the site of DHT synthesis.
      c. Estrogen is a co-mediator.
         • Increases the synthesis of androgen receptors
   3. Gross and microscopic findings
      a. Hyperplasia of glandular cells and stromal cells
         (1) Leads to nodule formation (Fig. 20-8)
         (2) Nodules are yellow-pink and are soft.
      b. Glandular hyperplasia develops nodules in the transitional zone.
      c. Stromal hyperplasia develops nodules in the periurethral zone.
         • Most responsible for obstruction of the urethra
   4. Clinical and laboratory findings
      a. Signs of obstruction
         (1) Trouble initiating and stopping the urinary stream
         (2) Dribbling, incomplete emptying
         (3) Nocturia, dysuria
      b. Hematuria
      c. Prostate-specific antigen (PSA; see later)
         (1) Proteolytic enzyme
            (a) Increases sperm motility
            (b) Maintains seminal secretions in the liquid state
         (2) PSA is usually normal (0–4 ng/mL) or between 4 and 10 ng/mL (30–50%)
            • Rarely >10 ng/mL
      d. Complications
         (1) Obstructive uropathy
            (a) Most common complication

> BPH: most common cause of enlarged prostate in men > 50 years old

> BPH: periurethral/transitional zones

> DHT: primary mediator for developing BPH; estrogen co-mediator

> Obstructive uropathy: most common complication of BPH; produces bladder diverticula

> BPH: 30% to 50% have ↑ PSA

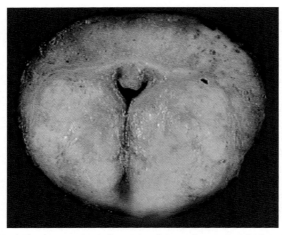

20-8: Benign prostatic hyperplasia. The gross section of prostate shows yellow periurethral nodular masses, causing narrowing of the lumen of the urethra. (*From Damjanov I, Linder J: Pathology: A Color Atlas. St. Louis, Mosby, 2000, p 249, Fig. 12-31.*)

(b) Postrenal azotemia
- Potential for progressing to acute renal failure if left untreated

(c) Bilateral hydronephrosis

(d) Bladder diverticula from increased pressure

(e) Bladder wall smooth muscle hypertrophy

(2) Bladder infections due to residual urine

(3) Prostatic infarcts

(a) Pain on DRE

(b) Enlarged, indurated gland

(c) Increased PSA values due to infarction

(4) *No* risk for progression into carcinoma

5. Diagnosis

a. DRE is insensitive test.

b. Transrectal ultrasound if nodules palpated or increased PSA (see later discussion)

6. Treatment

a. Nonpharmacologic
- Avoid caffeine or any other foods that exacerbate symptoms

b. General

(1) Medications

(a) α-adrenergic blockers
- Relax smooth muscle tone in capsule/bladder neck

(b) 5α-Reductase inhibitors
- Block conversion of testosterone to DHT

(c) ? Usefulness of saw palmetto; 5α-reductase inhibitor

(2) Surgery
- Transurethral resection of the prostate (TURP) is most commonly used.

D. Prostate cancer

1. Epidemiology

a. Most common cancer in adult males
- Second most common cancer-related death in adult males

b. Incidence increases with age

(1) Approximately 65% of all prostate cancers are diagnosed in men ≥ 65 years old.

(2) Average age of diagnosis is 72 years old.

c. More common in blacks than whites
- Rare in Asians

d. Usually asymptomatic until advanced

e. Peripheral in location

f. Risk factors

(1) Advancing age
- Most important risk factor

(2) First-degree relatives (father and brothers)

(3) Black men

(4) Smoking cigarettes, high saturated fat diet

2. Pathogenesis
- DHT-dependent

3. Gross and microscopic findings

a. Develops in the peripheral zone

(1) Palpable by DRE

(2) Obstructive uropathy is *not* an early finding.

b. Prostate intraepithelial neoplasia (PIN)

(1) Foci of atypia/dysplasia

(2) May be a precursor lesion for prostate cancer

c. Invasive cancer has a firm, gritty, yellow appearance (Fig. 20-9).

d. Hallmarks of malignancy

(1) Invasion of the capsule around the prostate

(2) Blood vessel/lymphatic invasion

(3) Perineural invasion

(4) Extension into the seminal vesicles or base of the bladder

4. Clinical findings in symptomatic prostate cancer

a. Generally silent until advanced stage

b. Obstructive uropathy implies extension into the bladder base

c. Low back/pelvic pain

BPH: most common cause of bladder diverticula

Prostate infarct: pain on DRE; ↑ PSA

BPH is *not* a risk factor for prostate cancer.

Rx of BPH: α-adrenergic blockers of smooth muscle

BPH surgery: TURP

Prostate cancer: most common cancer in men

Prostate cancer: peripheral in location

Advancing age: greatest risk factor for prostate cancer

Prostate cancer: DHT-dependent

Prostate cancer: generally silent until advanced stage

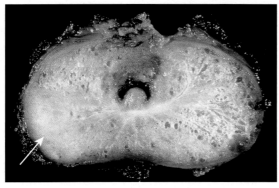

20-9: Prostate cancer. The *arrow* points to a triangular area of prostate cancer located at the periphery of the gland. The remainder of the gland has a normal, spongy appearance. *(From Kumar V, Fausto N, Abbas A: Robbins and Cotran's Pathologic Basis of Disease, 7th ed. Philadelphia, WB Saunders, 2004, p 1052, Fig. 21-34.)*

       (1) Portends bony metastases to vertebra and pelvic bones
          • Due to spread via the Batson venous plexus (refer to Chapter 8)
       (2) Alkaline phosphatase is increased.
          • Due to osteoblastic metastases
    d. Compression of the spinal cord
  5. Diagnosis of prostate cancer
    a. DRE negative in 10% of cases.
    b. Screening
       (1) DRE/PSA annually beginning at 50 years of age
       (2) PSA is sensitive but *not* specific for cancer.
          • BPH and prostatic infarcts can increase PSA, lowering its specificity by increasing false positive results.
       (3) PSA > 10 ng/mL is highly predictive of cancer.
          • 70% positive predictive value
       (4) PSA between 4 and 10 ng/mL is a gray zone.
          • Overlap between early cancer and BPH
       (5) Other more sensitive methods of reporting PSA
         (a) Measurement of free versus bound forms of circulating PSA
           • Increased free levels are seen in BPH, while increased bound levels are seen in prostate cancer.
         (b) PSA doubling time
           • The shorter the doubling time, the more aggressive the tumor
         (c) Rate of change of PSA values with time (PSA velocity)
           • Yearly PSA velocity > 0.75 ng/mL increases likelihood of developing prostate cancer if total serum PSA is normal.
         (d) Age-adjustment of total serum PSA (controversial)
         (e) Ratio between serum PSA and volume of the prostate gland (prostate density)
  6. Spread of prostate cancer
    a. Perineural invasion
    b. Lymphatic spread to regional lymph nodes
    c. Hematogenous spread
       (1) Bone is the most common extranodal site (see Fig. 8-9)
          • In descending order—lumbar spine, proximal femur, and pelvis
       (2) Lungs and liver
  7. Diagnosis
    a. Transrectal needle core biopsies of prostate; indications:
       (1) Abnormal PSA value (see earlier)
       (2) Abnormal DRE
       (3) Previous diagnosis of atypia or carcinoma in situ
  8. Imaging
    a. Radionuclide bone scan
       • Evaluate bone metastasis
    b. CT scan, MRI, transrectal ultrasound
       • Evaluate extent of disease

Margin notes:

Prostate cancer: osteoblastic metastases; lumbar spine, pelvis

PSA: more sensitive than specific in prostate cancer

PSA: ↑ free PSA consider BPH; ↑ bound PSA consider prostate cancer

Diagnosis prostate cancer: transrectal needle core biopsies

9. Treatment
  a. Early disease
     - Surgery, external beam radiation, radioactive seed implants
  b. Advanced disease
     - Hormonal therapy, chemotherapy, radiation, or combination

Prognosis: markedly improved because of early detection and improved treatment

10. Prognosis
  a. Dramatic increase in survival due to early detection and improved therapy
  b. Five-year survival rate for all stages is almost 99%.
  c. Ten-year relative survival rate is 91%.
  d. Fifteen-year relative survival rate is 76%.

VII. **Male Hypogonadism**
   A. **Normal male reproductive physiology**
      1. Follicle-stimulating hormone (FSH)
         a. Stimulates spermatogenesis in the seminiferous tubules
         b. Negative feedback relationship with inhibin
            (1) Inhibin is synthesized in Sertoli cells in seminiferous tubules.
            (2) Decreased inhibin causes an increase in FSH.

FSH: stimulates spermatogenesis

      2. Luteinizing hormone (LH)
         a. Stimulates testosterone synthesis in the Leydig cells.
         b. Testosterone has a negative feedback with LH.
            - Decreased testosterone causes an increase in LH.

LH: stimulates testosterone synthesis in Leydig cells

      3. Testosterone
         a. Maintains male secondary sex characteristics
         b. Enhances spermatogenesis in the seminiferous tubules
         c. Increases libido (sexual desire)
         d. Decreased testosterone causes male hypogonadism and infertility.

Testosterone: enhance spermatogenesis, libido

      4. Sex hormone–binding globulin (SHBG or androgen-binding globulin)
         a. Binding protein for testosterone and estrogen
            (1) In both men and women, SHBG is mainly synthesized in the liver.
            (2) In men, the Sertoli cells also synthesize SHBG.
            (3) Estrogen increases synthesis of SHBG in the liver.
            (4) Androgens, insulin, obesity, and hypothyroidism all cause decreased synthesis of SHBG.

SHBG: synthesized in Sertoli cells and liver

         b. SHBG has a higher binding affinity for testosterone than estrogen.
            - "Estrogen amplifier"
            (1) Increased SHBG decreases free testosterone levels.
            (2) Decreased SHBG increases free testosterone levels.

↑ SHBG causes ↓ free testosterone

↓ SHBG causes ↑ free testosterone

   B. **Pathogenesis of male hypogonadism**
      1. Decreased production of testosterone
         - Examples—hypopituitarism, Leydig cell dysfunction
      2. Resistance to testosterone
         - Example—androgen receptor deficiency in testicular feminization
   C. **Clinical presentations**
      1. Impotence

Impotence: most common manifestation of male hypogonadism

         a. Most common manifestation
         b. Failure to sustain an erection during attempted intercourse or during intercourse

↓ Testosterone causes ↓ libido

Testosterone, per se, does *not* have any role in producing an erection (parasympathetic response) or ejaculation (sympathetic response). However, decreased testosterone decreases libido, which decreases psychic desire.

      2. Loss of male secondary sex characteristics
         a. Estrogen activity is unopposed.
         b. Findings include female hair distribution, gynecomastia
      3. Osteoporosis
         - Testosterone normally inhibits osteoclastic activity and increases osteoblastic activity.

Hypogonadism: impotence, female secondary sex characteristics, osteoporosis

      4. Infertility
         - Decreased spermatogenesis

D. Classification of male hypogonadism
1. Primary hypogonadism
   - Due to Leydig cell dysfunction
   a. LH is increased.
      - Loss of negative feedback imposed by testosterone
   b. Hypergonadotropic (increased LH) hypogonadism
2. Secondary hypogonadism
   - Due to hypothalamic/pituitary dysfunction
   a. Decreased LH
   b. Hypogonadotropic (decreased LH) hypogonadism

E. Primary hypogonadism: Leydig cell dysfunction
1. Causes
   a. Chronic alcoholic liver disease
      - Inhibits binding of LH to Leydig cells (? mechanism)
   b. Chronic renal failure
      - Toxins have a direct toxic effect on Leydig cell
   c. Irradiation, orchitis, trauma
2. Laboratory findings in Leydig cell dysfunction
   a. Decreased testosterone
      - Due to destruction of Leydig cells
   b. Increased LH
      - Due to decreased testosterone
   c. Decreased sperm count
      - Due to testosterone deficiency
   d. Normal FSH
      - Inhibin is present in Sertoli cells.

F. Primary hypogonadism: Leydig cell and seminiferous tubule dysfunction
1. Causes
   - Same causes as Leydig cell dysfunction
2. Laboratory findings
   a. Decreased testosterone
      - Due to destruction of Leydig cells
   b. Increased LH
      - Due to decreased testosterone
   c. Decreased sperm count
      - Due to testosterone deficiency and seminiferous tubule dysfunction
   d. Increased FSH
      - Due to decrease in inhibin

G. Causes of secondary hypogonadism
1. Constitutional delay in puberty
   - A testicular volume > 4 mL indicates puberty has begun.
2. Kallmann's syndrome
   a. Autosomal dominant disorder
   b. Maldevelopment of the olfactory bulbs and GnRH-producing cells
   c. Clinical findings
      (1) Delayed puberty
      (2) Anosmia, color blindness
   d. Laboratory findings
      - Decreased FSH, LH, testosterone, and sperm count
3. Hypopituitarism (refer to Chapter 22)
   a. Causes
      (1) Craniopharyngioma in children
      (2) Nonfunctioning pituitary adenoma in adults
   b. Laboratory findings
      - Decreased FSH, LH, testosterone, and sperm count

H. Summary of causes of male hypogonadism (Table 20-2)

VIII. Male Infertility

A. Epidemiology and pathogenesis
1. Decreased sperm count
   a. Primary testicular dysfunction
      (1) Leydig cell dysfunction (refer to section VII)

Primary hypogonadism: ↑ LH, ↓ testosterone

Secondary hypogonadism: ↓ LH, ↓ testosterone

Primary hypogonadism, Leydig cell dysfunction: alcohol, renal failure, orchitis, radiation

Primary hypogonadism, Leydig cell dysfunction: ↓ testosterone, sperm count; ↑ LH; normal FSH

Primary hypogonadism Leydig cell + seminiferous tubule dysfunction: ↓ testosterone, sperm count; ↑ LH; ↑ FSH

Secondary hypogonadism causes: constitutional, Kallmann's syndrome, hypopituitarism

Secondary hypogonadism Kallmann's syndrome/ hypopituitarism: ↓ testosterone, sperm count; ↓ LH; ↓ FSH

TABLE 20-2. **SUMMARY OF CAUSES OF MALE HYPOGONADISM**

DYSFUNCTION	TESTOSTERONE	SPERM COUNT	LH	FSH
Primary				
Leydig dysfunction	↓	↓	↑	N
Seminiferous tubule dysfunction	N	↓	N	↑
Leydig cell and seminiferous tubule dysfunction	↓	↓	↑	↑
Secondary				
Hypopituitarism	↓	↓	↓	↓

FSH, follicle-stimulating hormone; LH, luteinizing hormone; N, normal.

Seminiferous tubule dysfunction: accounts for ~90% of cases of male infertility

End-organ dysfunction: obstruction of vas deferens

Semen analysis: gold standard test for infertility

Impotence + preserved NPT: psychogenic cause of impotence

Vascular insufficiency: most common cause impotence men > 50 years old

    (2) Seminiferous tubule dysfunction
      (a) Causes
        • Varicocele (refer to section V), Klinefelter's syndrome (refer to Chapter 5), orchitis
      (b) Normal testosterone and LH
        • Leydig cells are intact.
      (c) Decreased sperm count
        • Loss of seminiferous tubules and decreased testosterone
      (d) Increased FSH
        • Inhibin is decreased.
    b. Secondary hypogonadism
      • Pituitary and hypothalamic dysfunction (refer to section VII)
  2. End-organ dysfunction
    a. Causes
      (1) Obstruction of vas deferens
      (2) Disorders involving accessory sex organs or ejaculation
    b. Normal testosterone, FSH, LH, prolactin
    c. Sperm count variable

B. Laboratory tests for male infertility
  1. Semen analysis
    a. Gold standard test for infertility
    b. Components of semen
      (1) Spermatozoa derive from the seminiferous tubules.
      (2) Coagulant derives from the seminal vesicles.
      (3) Enzymes to liquefy semen derive from the prostate gland.
    c. Components evaluated in a standard semen analysis
      (1) Volume
        • Volume does *not* correlate with the number of sperm.
      (2) Sperm count
        • Normal is 20 to 150 million sperm/mL.
      (3) Sperm morphology
        • Morphology is very abnormal in reconnections of a vasectomy.
      (4) Sperm motility
  2. Serum gonadotropins, testosterone, prolactin

IX. **Erectile Dysfunction**
  A. Causes of erectile dysfunction
    1. Psychogenic
      a. Most common cause of impotence in young men
      b. Stress at work, marital conflicts, performance anxiety
      c. Nocturnal penile tumescence (NPT)
        (1) Average male has ~5 erections while sleeping at night.
        (2) NPT is preserved in impotence that is due to psychogenic causes.
        (3) All other causes of impotence have a loss of NPT.
    2. Decreased testosterone
      • Decreased libido (see section VII, Male Hypogonadism)
    3. Vascular insufficiency
      a. Most common cause of impotence in men > 50 years old
      b. Example—Leriche syndrome

(1) Impotence due to vascular insufficiency
(2) Aortoiliac atherosclerosis with decreased penal blood flow
(3) Calf claudication with atrophy
(4) Diminished femoral pulse
4. Neurologic disease
a. Parasympathetic system (S2–S4) is necessary for erection.
b. Sympathetic system (T12–L1) is necessary for ejaculation.
c. Neurogenic causes of impotence
(1) Multiple sclerosis
(2) Autonomic neuropathy due to diabetes mellitus
(3) Radical prostatectomy
5. Drug effects; examples:
a. Leuprolide (GnRH agonist)
b. Methyldopa, psychotropics
6. Endocrine disease
a. Diabetes mellitus
• Autonomic neuropathy + vascular insufficiency
b. Primary hypothyroidism
• Increased prolactin inhibits GnRH release
c. Prolactinoma
• Prolactin inhibits GnRH release
7. Penis disorders
a. Peyronie's disease (fibromatosis)
b. Priapism
B. Drugs used in erectile dysfunction
1. Sildenafil (Viagra)
a. Most common drug used for the treatment of erectile dysfunction
b. Mechanism
(1) Inhibits the breakdown of cyclic guanosine monophosphate (cGMP) by type 5 phosphodiesterase
(2) Increased levels of cGMP cause vasodilation in the corpus cavernosum and the penis.
2. Yohimbe
• Herb that produces vasodilatation of vessels

Parasympathetic for erection: S2–S4

Sympathetic for ejaculation: T12–L1

Neurologic causes erectile dysfunction: multiple sclerosis, diabetes mellitus

Drugs erectile dysfunction: leuprolide, methyldopa, psychotropics

Endocrine disease erectile dysfunction: diabetes, primary hypothyroidism, prolactinoma

Sildenafil: increases cGMP, which causes vasodilation in corpus cavernosum

Yohimbe: vasodilation

I. **Sexually Transmitted Diseases and Other Genital Infections**
- Summary of infections (Table 21-1 and Fig. 21-1)

II. **Vulva Disorders**

A. **Bartholin gland abscess**
- Most often caused by *Neisseria gonorrhoeae*

B. **Non-neoplastic dermatoses**

1. Lichen sclerosis (Fig. 21-2)

a. Usually occurs in postmenopausal women

b. Thinning of the epidermis
- Parchment-like appearance of skin

c. Small risk for developing squamous cell carcinoma

2. Lichen simplex chronicus

a. White plaque-like lesion (leukoplakia)
- Due to squamous cell hyperplasia

b. Small risk for developing squamous cell carcinoma

C. **Benign and malignant tumors**

1. Papillary hidradenoma

a. Benign tumor of the apocrine sweat gland

b. Painful nodule on the labia majora

2. Vulvar intraepithelial neoplasia (VIN)

a. Dysplasia ranges from mild to carcinoma in situ

b. Strong human papillomavirus (HPV) type 16 association

c. Precursor for developing squamous cell carcinoma

3. Squamous cell carcinoma

a. Most common cancer

b. Risk factors

(1) HPV type 16

(2) Smoking cigarettes

(3) Immunodeficiency (e.g., AIDS)

c. Metastasize first to the inguinal nodes

4. Extramammary Paget's disease

a. Red, crusted vulvar lesion

b. Intraepithelial adenocarcinoma

(1) Tumor derives from primitive epithelial progenitor cells.

(2) Malignant Paget's cells contain mucin (Fig. 21-3).
- Mucin is periodic acid–Schiff (PAS) positive.

(3) Spreads along the epithelium
- Rarely invades the dermis

5. Malignant melanoma

a. Melanoma cells are histologically similar to Paget's cells.

b. Unlike Paget's cells, melanoma cells are PAS negative.

Margin notes:

Lichen sclerosis: thin epidermis; parchment-like skin

Lichen simplex: leukoplakia (hyperplasia)

Papillary hidradenoma: painful apocrine gland tumor

VIN: HPV 16 association

Extramammary Paget's disease: intraepithelial adenocarcinoma; PAS positive

Melanoma: PAS negative

TABLE 21-1. SEXUALLY TRANSMITTED DISEASES AND OTHER GENITAL INFECTIONS

PATHOGEN	DESCRIPTION AND TREATMENT
Calymmatobacterium granulomatis	STD; gram-negative coccobacillus that causes granuloma inguinale Organism phagocytized by macrophages (Donovan bodies) Creeping, raised sore that heals by scarring; no lymphadenopathy *Treatment*: doxycycline or trimethoprim-sulfamethoxazole
Candida albicans (see Fig. 21-1A)	Yeasts and pseudohyphae (elongated yeasts); part of normal vaginal flora Second most common vaginitis in the United States Risk factors: diabetes, antibiotics, pregnancy, OCP Pruritic vaginitis with a white discharge and fiery red mucosa *Treatment*: fluconazole (single dose)
Chlamydia trachomatis	STD; often coexists with *Neisseria gonorrhoeae* (45% of cases) Incubation period 7–12 days after exposure; red inclusions (reticulate bodies) in infected metaplastic squamous cells; reticulate bodies divide to form elementary bodies, which are the infective bodies producing infection Infections in males: NSU (sterile pyuria), epididymitis, proctitis Infections in females: urethritis (sterile pyuria), cervicitis, PID, perihepatitis (FHC syndrome—scar tissue between peritoneum and surface of liver from pus from PID), proctitis, Bartholin gland abscess Infections in newborns: conjunctivitis (ophthalmia neonatorum), pneumonia DNA probe test for quick diagnosis *Treatment*: azithromycin 1 g (single dose); doxycycline
C. trachomatis subspecies	STD; lymphogranuloma venereum Papules with no ulceration; inguinal lymphadenitis with granulomatous microabscesses and draining sinuses Lymphedema of scrotum or vulva; women also may develop rectal strictures *Treatment*: doxycycline
Gardnerella vaginalis (see Fig. 21-1B)	Gram-negative rod that causes bacterial vaginosis Most common vaginitis Malodorous vaginal discharge; vaginal pH > 4.5 Organisms adhere to squamous cells producing "clue cells" Increased incidence of preterm delivery and low-birth-weight newborns *Treatment*: metronidazole; same treatment in pregnancy
Haemophilus ducreyi	STD; gram-negative rod that causes chancroid Male dominant disease (10:1); high incidence of HIV Incubation 4–7 days Painful genital and perianal ulcers with suppurative inguinal nodes Diagnosis with Gram stain ("school of fish" appearance) and culture *Treatment*: ceftriaxone or azithromycin 1 g (single dose)
HSV-2 (see Fig. 21-1C and D)	STD; virus remains latent in sensory ganglia Recurrent vesicles that ulcerate; locations—penis, vulva, cervix, perianal area Tzanck preparation: scrapings removed from the base of an ulcer; see multinucleated squamous cells with eosinophilic intranuclear inclusions Pregnancy: if virus is shedding, baby is delivered by cesarean section *Treatment*: acyclovir (decreases recurrences)
HPV (see Fig. 21-1E)	STD; types 6 and 11 (90%; low risk types) associated with condyloma acuminata (venereal warts); fernlike or flat lesions in genital area (e.g., penis, vulva, cervix, perianal) Most common overall STD; 80% of sexually active women will have acquired HPV by age 50 Types 16 and 18 (high risk types) associated with dysplasia and squamous cancer Virus produces koilocytic change in squamous epithelium Cells have wrinkled pyknotic nuclei surrounded by a clear halo Approximately 90% spontaneously clear within 2 years (most within 8 months); older women will more often have persistent disease Vaccine decreases risk for developing cervical cancer *Treatment*: topical podophyllin; α-IFN injection; imiquimod cream
Neisseria gonorrhoeae (see Fig. 21-1F)	STD; gram-negative diplococcus that infects glandular or transitional epithelium; symptoms appear 2–7 days after sexual exposure Infection sites similar to *C. trachomatis* Complications: ectopic pregnancy, male sterility, disseminated gonococcemia (C6–C9 deficiency risk factor), septic arthritis, FHC syndrome Disseminated gonococcemia: septic arthritis (knee), tenosynovitis (hands, feet), pustules (hands, feet); more common in women than men DNA probe test for quick diagnosis *Treatment*: ceftriaxone

Continued

TABLE 21-1. **SEXUALLY TRANSMITTED DISEASES AND OTHER GENITAL INFECTIONS—cont'd**

PATHOGEN	DESCRIPTION AND TREATMENT
Treponema pallidum (see Fig. 21-G, H, and I)	STD; gram-negative spirochete that causes syphilis Primary syphilis: solitary painless, indurated chancre; locations—penis, labia, mouth Secondary syphilis: maculopapular rash on trunk, palms, soles; generalized lymphadenopathy; condylomata lata, which are flat lesions in same area as condylomata acuminata; alopecia Tertiary syphilis: neurosyphilis, aortitis, gummas Congenital syphilis (refer to Chapter 5) Nonspecific screening tests: RPR or VDRL; titers decrease after treatment Confirmatory treponemal test: FTA-ABS; positive with or without treatment Jarisch-Herxheimer reaction: intensification of rash in primary or secondary syphilis may occur due to proteins released from dead organisms after treatment with penicillin *Treatment*: penicillin
Trichomonas vaginalis (see Fig. 21-1J)	STD; flagellated protozoan with jerky motility Produces vaginitis, cervicitis, and urethritis; strawberry-colored cervix and fiery red vaginal mucosa; greenish, frothy discharge *Treatment*: metronidazole (both partners)

FHC, Fitz-Hugh–Curtis; FTA-ABS, fluorescent treponeme antibody-absorption test; HPV, human papillomavirus; HSV, herpes simplex virus; IFN, interferon; NSU, nonspecific urethritis; OCP, oral contraceptive pill; PCR, polymerase chain reaction; PID, pelvic inflammatory disease; RPR, rapid plasma reagin; STD, sexually transmitted disease; VDRL, Venereal Disease Research Laboratory.

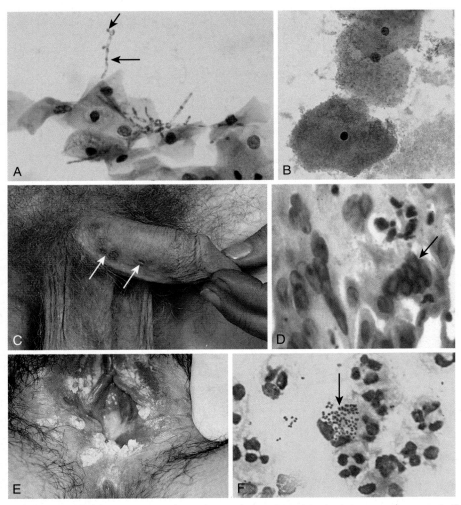

21-1: Genital infections. **A,** *Candida. Bottom arrow* shows elongated yeasts (pseudohyphae), *top arrow* shows yeasts. **B,** *Gardnerella vaginalis.* Superficial squamous cells are covered by granular material representing bacterial organisms attached to the surface. **C,** Herpes type 2. *Arrows* show ulcerated, red lesions on the shaft of the penis. **D,** Herpes type 2. Biopsy showing a multinucleated squamous cell with smudged, "ground glass" nuclei with intranuclear inclusions (*arrow*). **E,** Human papillomavirus. Numerous keratotic papillary processes are present on the surface of the labia. These are called venereal warts or condylomata acuminata. **F,** *Neisseria gonorrhoeae.* Neutrophils (*arrow*) show numerous, phagocytosed gram-negative diplococci.

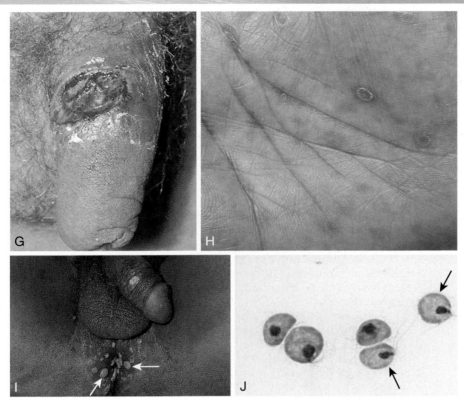

21-1 cont'd: G, *Treponema pallidum.* Note the well-demarcated primary chancre just distal to the glans penis. **H,** *Treponema pallidum.* Note the characteristic palmar papules and plaques of secondary syphilis. **I,** *Treponema pallidum.* Note the flat, plaque-like lesions (*arrows*) of condyloma latum. **J,** *Trichomonas vaginalis.* Note the numerous pear-shaped, flagellated organisms (*arrows*). (***A** and **D** from Atkinson BF: Atlas of Diagnostic Cytopathology. Philadelphia, WB Saunders, 1992, pp 76, 78, and 80, Figs. 2–49B, 2–55, and 2–63, respectively; **B** and **E** from Damjanov I, Linder J: Pathology: A Color Atlas. St. Louis, Mosby, 2000, pp 261 and 260, Figs. 13–10B and 13–8, respectively; **C** from Bouloux P-M: Self-Assessment Picture Tests: Medicine, Vol 1. St. Louis, Mosby, 1996, p 17, Fig. 33; **F** from Greer I, Cameron IT, Kitchener HC, Prentice A: Mosby's Color Atlas and Text of Obstetrics and Gynecology. St. Louis, Mosby, 2000, p 274, Fig. 10–50; **G** from Swartz MH: Textbook of Physical Diagnosis, 5th ed. Philadelphia, Saunders Elsevier, 2006, p 537, Fig. 18–13; **H** from Lookingbill D, Marks J: Principles of Dermatology, 3rd ed. Philadelphia, WB Saunders, 2000, p 124, Fig. 10-17; **I** from Swartz MH: Textbook of Physical Diagnosis, 5th ed. Philadelphia, Saunders Elsevier, 2006, p 553, Fig. 18-13; **J** from Kumar V, Fausto N, Abbas A: Robbins and Cotran's Pathologic Basis of Disease, 7th ed. Philadelphia, WB Saunders, 2004, p 1064, Fig. 22-4.)*

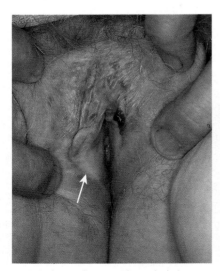

21-2: Lichen sclerosis. The vulva shows a parchment-like appearance (*arrow*). (*From Savin JAA, Hunter JAA, Hepburn NC: Diagnosis in Color: Skin Signs in Clinical Medicine. London, Mosby-Wolfe, 1997, p 124, Fig. 4.81.*)

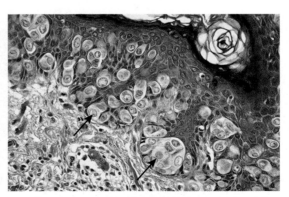

21-3: Extramammary Paget's disease. Large, pink-staining, malignant Paget's cells (*arrows*) are disposed singly and in clusters within the epidermis. (*From Rosai J, Ackerman LV: Surgical Pathology, 9th ed. St. Louis, Mosby, 2004, p 1492, Fig. 19-17B.*)

III. **Vagina Disorders**
  A. **Rokitansky-Kuster-Hauser (RKH) syndrome**
    1. Absence of the upper vagina and uterus
    2. Anatomic cause of primary amenorrhea
  B. **Gartner's duct cyst**
    1. Remnant of the wolffian (mesonephric) duct
    2. Presents as a cyst on the lateral wall of the vagina
  C. **Benign and malignant tumors**
    1. Rhabdomyoma
      a. Benign tumor of skeletal muscle
      b. Other locations are the tongue and heart.
    2. Embryonal rhabdomyosarcoma
      a. Occurs in girls < 5 years old
      b. Necrotic, grape-like mass protrudes from the vagina (Fig. 21-4).
    3. Clear cell adenocarcinoma of the vagina (Fig. 21-5)
      a. Epidemiology
        (1) Occurs in women with intrauterine exposure to diethylstilbestrol (DES)
          • DES was used to prevent a threatened abortion.
        (2) DES inhibits müllerian differentiation.
          • Müllerian structures: tubes, uterus, cervix, upper third of vagina
        (3) Vaginal adenosis
          (a) Remnants of müllerian glands
            • Produces red, superficial ulcerations in the upper portion of the vagina
          (b) Precursor lesion for clear cell adenocarcinoma
        (4) Small risk for developing the cancer (1:1000)
        (5) Cancer may involve upper vagina or cervix.
      b. Other DES abnormalities
        (1) Abnormally shaped uterus that thwarts implantation
        (2) Cervical incompetence
          • Common cause of recurrent abortions
    4. Vaginal squamous cell carcinoma
      a. Primary squamous cell carcinoma has an HPV type 16 association.
      b. Most cancers are an extension of a cervical squamous cancer into the vagina.
IV. **Cervix Disorders**
  A. **Clinical anatomy and histology**
    1. Cervix includes the endocervix + exocervix
      • The exocervix begins at the cervical os.
    2. Exocervix is normally lined by squamous epithelium.
    3. Endocervical glands are normally lined by mucus-secreting columnar cells.

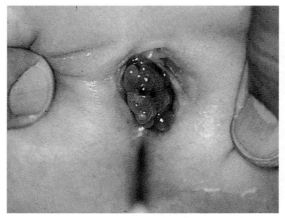

21-4: Embryonal rhabdomyosarcoma of vagina. Note the bloody, necrotic mass protruding out of the vagina. *(From Damjanov I, Linder J: Pathology: A Color Atlas. St. Louis, Mosby, 2000, p 266, Fig. 13-29.)*

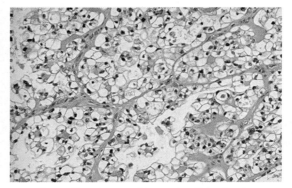

21-5: Clear cell carcinoma of the vagina. Note the clear, vacuolated cells with ill-defined glandular spaces. *(From Klatt E: Robbins and Cotran's Atlas of Pathology. Philadelphia, WB Saunders, 2006, p 295, Fig. 13-12.)*

4. Endocervical epithelium normally migrates down to the exocervix.
    a. Exposure to the acid pH of the vagina produces squamous metaplasia.
    b. The area undergoing metaplasia is called the transformation zone.
        (1) This zone is where squamous dysplasia and cancer develop.
        (2) It must be sampled when performing a cervical Papanicolaou (Pap) smear.
    c. Metaplastic squamous cells block endocervical gland orifices.
        (1) Obstruction of outflow of mucus produces nabothian cysts (see Fig. 21-17).
        (2) Nabothian cysts are a normal finding in adult women.

B. Acute and chronic cervicitis
    1. Epidemiology
        a. Accounts for 20% to 25% of patients presenting with vaginal discharge
        b. Can be found in any sexually active woman
        c. Subdivided into acute and chronic cervicitis
    2. Acute cervicitis
        a. Acute inflammation is normally present in the transformation zone.
        b. Pathologic acute cervicitis; causative agents:
            • *Chlamydia trachomatis, N. gonorrhoeae, Trichomonas vaginalis, Candida,* herpes simplex virus (HSV-2), HPV
        c. Clinical findings
            (1) Vaginal discharge (most common)
            (2) Pelvic pain
            (3) Dyspareunia
            (4) Painful on palpation
            (5) Bleeds easily when obtaining cultures
            (6) Cervical os is erythematous and may be covered by an exudate.
        d. Diagnosis
            (1) DNA probe for *Chlamydi*a and *Neisseria gonorrhoeae*
                • These organisms account for >50% of acute cervicitis.
            (2) Wet mount for *Trichomonas*
            (3) Obtain a cervical Pap smear
        e. Treatment
            (1) If culture or DNA probe positive, treat with appropriate antibiotic.
            (2) If culture negative, cryosurgery is an option.
            (3) Advise safe sex with the use of condoms
    3. Chronic cervicitis
        • Occurs when acute cervicitis persists
    4. Follicular cervicitis
        a. Caused by *C. trachomatis*
        b. Pronounced lymphoid infiltrate with germinal centers
        c. *Chlamydia* infects metaplastic squamous cells.
            (1) Cells contain vacuoles with red inclusions (reticulate bodies).
            (2) Reticulate bodies develop into elementary bodies, which are infective particles.
        d. Cervicitis is the primary source for conjunctivitis and pneumonia in newborns.

C. Cervical Pap smear
    1. Purpose
        a. Screening test to rule out squamous dysplasia and cancer
        b. To evaluate the hormone status of the patient
    2. Sample sites
        • Vagina, exocervix, transformation zone

Because the transformation zone is the site for squamous dysplasia and squamous cancer, it must be adequately sampled. The presence of metaplastic squamous cells or mucus-secreting columnar cells indicates proper sampling. Absence of these cells means that the Pap smear must be repeated.

    3. Interpretation of the Pap smear
        a. Superficial squamous cells indicate adequate estrogen.
        b. Intermediate squamous cells indicate adequate progesterone.
        c. Parabasal cells indicate a lack of estrogen and progesterone.
        d. Normal nonpregnant adult woman
            • 70% superficial squamous cells, 30% intermediate squamous cells

---

Transformation zone: site where squamous dysplasia and cancer develop

Acute cervicitis: vaginal discharge most common complaint

Acute cervicitis: *C. trachomatis* and *N. gonorrhoeae* > 50% of cases

Follicular cervicitis: caused by *C. trachomatis*

Reticulate bodies: produce elementary bodies, the infective particle of *Chlamydia*

Cervical Pap smear: screen for dysplasia/cancer, evaluates hormonal status

Superficial squamous cells: adequate estrogen

Intermediate squamous cells: adequate progesterone

Parabasal cells: lack of estrogen and progesterone

e. Pregnant woman
- 100% intermediate squamous cells from progesterone effect
f. Elderly woman with lack of estrogen and progesterone
- Atrophic smear with parabasal cells and inflammation
g. Woman with continuous exposure to estrogen without progesterone
- 100% superficial squamous cells

D. Cervical (endocervical) polyp

Cervical polyp: non-neoplastic

1. Epidemiology
   a. Non-neoplastic polyp that protrudes from the cervical os
   b. Arises from the endocervix, *not* the cervix
   c. Most commonly present in perimenopausal women and multigravida women
   d. Most commonly occur between 30 and 50 years of age
   e. *Not* precancerous
2. Pathogenesis
   a. Essentially unknown
   b. Inflammation, trauma, pregnancy have been implicated.

Cervical polyp: postcoital bleeding; vaginal discharge

3. Clinical findings
   a. Postcoital bleeding
   b. Vaginal discharge
4. Treatment is surgical excision.

E. Cervical intraepithelial neoplasia (CIN)

CIN: most cases associated with HPV; smoking is risk factor

1. Epidemiology
   a. Majority of cases are associated with HPV.
      (1) Low risk—types 6, 11
      (2) High risk—types 16, 18
      (3) HPV produces koilocytosis in squamous cells (Fig. 21-6).
         - Clear halo containing a wrinkled, pyknotic nucleus

Koilocytosis: HPV effect in squamous cells

   b. Peak incidence is 35 years of age.
   c. False negative rate on detecting dysplasia on a cervical Pap smear is ~40%.
   d. Risk factors
      (1) Early age of onset of sexual intercourse
      (2) Multiple, high-risk partners
      (3) High-risk types of HPV in a biopsy
      (4) Smoking, oral contraceptive pills (OCPs)
      (5) Immunodeficiency
2. Classification of CIN

Cervical dysplasia: precursor for squamous cancer

   a. CIN I
      - Mild dysplasia involving the lower third of the epithelium
   b. CIN II
      - Moderate dysplasia involving the lower two thirds of the epithelium
   c. CIN III (see Fig. 1-17)
      - Severe dysplasia to carcinoma in situ (CIS) involving the full thickness of the epithelium
3. Progression from CIN I to CIN III is *not* inevitable.
   a. Reversal to normal is more likely in CIN I.
   b. Requires ~10 years to progress from CIN I to CIN III

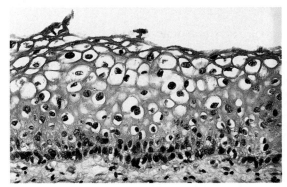

21-6: Koilocytosis caused by human papillomavirus. The squamous cells have wrinkled pyknotic nuclei surrounded by a clear halo. *(From Rosai J, Ackerman LV: Surgical Pathology, 9th ed. St. Louis, Mosby, 2004, p 1530, Fig. 19-74.)*

c. Requires ~10 years to progress from CIN III to invasive cancer
  • Average age for cervical cancer is ~45 years old.
4. Clinical findings
  a. Dysplasia is *not* usually visible to naked eye; colposcopy is required.
    • Occasionally, flat to warty appearing condyloma acuminata are visible.
  b. Colposcopy findings, after application of acetic acid:
    • Acetowhite areas with punctation, mosaic pattern, or abnormal vascularity
5. Treatment
  • Electrocoagulation, cryotherapy, laser ablation, local surgery (conization)

F. Cervical cancer
  1. Epidemiology
    a. Least common gynecologic cancer
      • Due to early detection of CIN with Pap smears
    b. Higher incidence in developing countries
    c. In U.S. population incidence in descending order:
      • Hispanic, black, white
    d. Majority are squamous cell carcinoma (75–80% of cases).
      • Small cell cancer and adenocarcinoma are less common types.
    e. Cause and risk factors
      • Same as those listed for CIN
  2. Clinical findings (Figs. 21-7 and 21-8)
    a. Abnormal vaginal bleeding (most common)
      • Usually postcoital
    b. Malodorous discharge
    c. Postcoital bleeding
  3. Cancer characteristics
    a. Extends down into the vagina
    b. Extends out into the lateral wall of the cervix and vagina
    c. Infiltrates the bladder wall and obstructs the ureters
      • Postrenal azotemia leading to renal failure is a common cause of death.
    d. Distant metastases (e.g., lungs)
  4. Treatment of invasive cancer
    a. Surgery, radiation, or both
    b. Chemotherapy in selected cases
  5. Prognosis
    • The 1- and 5-year relative survival rates are 88% and 72%, respectively.

V. Reproductive Physiology and Selected Hormone Disorders
  A. Sequence to menarche
    1. Breast budding (thelarche)
    2. Growth spurt

Cervical cancer: least common gynecologic cancer; importance of Pap smear

Cervical cancer: abnormal vaginal bleeding most common sign

Cervical cancer: renal failure is a common cause of death.

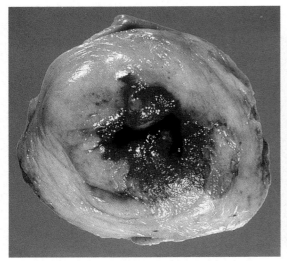

21-7: Squamous cell carcinoma of the cervix. Note the bleeding and ulceration in the cervical os. *(Courtesy of Dr. Hector Rodriguez-Martinez, Mexico City.)*

21-8: Squamous cell carcinoma of cervix with extension down into the vagina, wall of the urinary bladder *(solid arrow)* and wall of the rectum *(interrupted arrow)*. *(Courtesy of Dr. Hector Rodriguez-Martinez, Mexico City.)*

Sequence to menarche: breast budding, growth spurt, pubic hair, axillary hair, menarche

3. Pubic hair
4. Axillary hair
5. Menarche
   a. Mean age of 12.8 years
   b. Anovulatory cycles for 1–1.5 years
B. Summary of the normal menstrual cycle
   • Synthesis of sex hormones in the ovary (Fig. 21-9)
   1. Proliferative (follicular) phase (Fig. 21-10)
      a. Estrogen-mediated proliferation of glands
         • *Most* variable phase of the cycle

Proliferative phase: estrogen-mediated; most variable phase

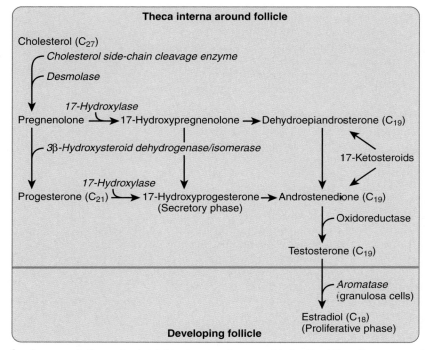

21-9: Synthesis of sex hormones in the ovaries. Luteinizing hormone is responsible for stimulation of hormone synthesis in the theca interna surrounding the developing follicle. Follicle-stimulating hormone increases the synthesis of aromatase in granulosa cells. Aromatase converts testosterone to estradiol. *(From Goljan EF: Star Series: Pathology. Philadelphia, WB Saunders, 1998, Fig. 18-1.)*

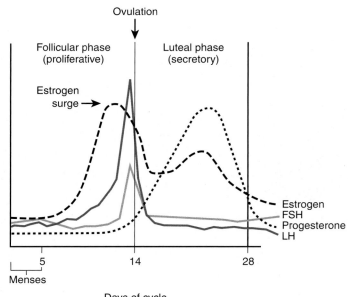

21-10: Menstrual cycle. See text for discussion. FSH, follicle-stimulating hormone; LH, luteinizing hormone. *(From Brown TA: Rapid Review Physiology. St. Louis, Mosby, 2007, p 99, Fig. 3-15.)*

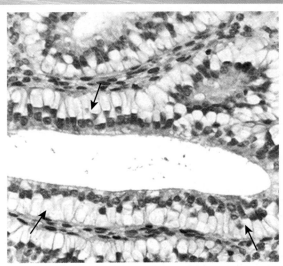

21-11: Subnuclear vacuoles (*arrows*) containing mucin push the nuclei of the endometrial cells toward the apex of the cell. Eventually the mucin passes the nucleus and enters the lumen marking the beginning of the secretory phase. *(From Kumar V, Fausto N, Abbas A: Robbins and Cotran's Pathologic Basis of Disease, 7th ed. Philadelphia, WB Saunders, 2004, p 1081, Fig. 21-5B.)*

    b. Estrogen surge occurs 24 to 36 hours prior to ovulation.
        (1) Stimulates luteinizing hormone (LH) release
            • Positive feedback
        (2) Stimulates follicle-stimulating hormone (FSH) release
           (a) Positive feedback on FSH and LH
           (b) Serum LH > FSH; greatest positive feedback on LH
        (3) LH surge initiates ovulation.
  2. Ovulation
    a. Occurs between days 14 and 16
    b. Ovulation indicators
        (1) Increase in body temperature
            • Effect of progesterone
        (2) Subnuclear vacuoles in endometrial cells (Fig. 21-11)
        (3) Mittelschmerz
            • Peritoneal irritation from blood from the ruptured follicle
  3. Secretory phase (see Fig. 21-10)
    a. Progesterone-mediated
        • *Least* variable phase of the cycle
    b. Increased gland tortuosity and secretion
    c. Edema of stromal cells

> In fertility workups, endometrial biopsies are commonly performed on day 21 to see if ovulation has occurred. Presence of secretory endometrium on day 21 confirms that ovulation has occurred.

    d. Changes occurring after fertilization
        (1) Fertilization usually occurs in the ampullary portion of the fallopian tube.
        (2) Fertilized egg spends 3 days in the fallopian tube.
        (3) Fertilized egg spends 2 days in the uterine cavity.
            • Implants in the endometrial mucosa on day 21
        (4) An exaggerated secretory phase occurs in pregnancy.
            • Called the Arias-Stella phenomenon
  4. Menses
    a. Initiated by drop-off in serum levels of estrogen and progesterone
        (1) Signal for the endometrial cells to undergo apoptosis
        (2) Newborn baby girls commonly have vaginal bleeding.
            • Due to sudden drop of maternal hormones with delivery
    b. Plasmin prevents menstrual blood from clotting.
        • Excess clotting is a sign of menorrhagia.
  5. Functions of FSH
    a. Prepares the follicle of the month

Ovulation: estrogen surge → LH surge → ovulation

Subnuclear vacuoles: sign of ovulation

Secretory phase: progesterone-mediated; least variable phase

Arias-Stella phenomenon: exaggerated secretory phase that occurs in pregnancy

Menses: drop in hormones initiates apoptosis

Newborn girls: may have vaginal bleeding

FSH: prepares follicle, aromatase synthesis, LH receptor synthesis

b. Increases aromatase synthesis in the granulosa cells
c. Increases the synthesis of LH receptors
6. Functions of LH
a. LH in the proliferative phase

LH proliferative phase: synthesize testosterone for conversion by aromatase into estradiol

(1) Increases the synthesis of 17-ketosteroids (KS) in the theca interna (see Fig. 21-9)
   • 17-KS are dehydroepiandrosterone (DHEA) and androstenedione.
(2) DHEA is converted to androstenedione.
(3) An oxidoreductase converts androstenedione to testosterone.
(4) Testosterone enters granulosa cells and is aromatized to estradiol.
b. LH surge is induced by a sudden increase in estrogen.
   • Ovulation occurs when LH > FSH.

LH secretory phase: synthesize 17-OH-progesterone

c. LH in the secretory phase (see Fig. 21-9)
   • Theca interna primarily synthesizes 17-hydroxyprogesterone (17-OH-progesterone).

hCG: LH analogue

7. Hormone changes in pregnancy
a. Human chorionic gonadotropin (hCG)

hCG: maintains corpus luteum of pregnancy for 8–10 weeks

(1) Synthesized in the syncytiotrophoblast lining the chorionic villus
(2) Acts as an LH analogue by maintaining the corpus luteum of pregnancy.
(3) Corpus luteum synthesizes progesterone for ~8 to 10 weeks.
b. Corpus luteum involutes after ~8 to 10 weeks.
(1) Placenta synthesizes progesterone for the remainder of the pregnancy.
(2) Spontaneous abortion may occur if placental production of progesterone is inadequate.

C. Oral contraceptive pills (OCPs)
1. Mixture of estrogen + progestins (progesterone)
a. Baseline levels of estrogen prevent the midcycle estrogen surge.
   • Prevents the LH surge and ovulation

OCP: prevents LH surge and ovulation; progestins cause gland atrophy

b. Progestins arrest the proliferative phase and cause gland atrophy.
c. Progestins inhibit LH, which also prevents the LH surge.
2. OCPs render the cervical mucus hostile to sperm.
3. OCPs alter fallopian tube motility.

D. Sources and types of estrogen
1. Estradiol

Estradiol: estrogen of a nonpregnant woman

a. Primary estrogen in nonpregnant women
b. Derived from aromatization of testosterone in granulosa cells
2. Estrone

Estrone: estrogen of a postmenopausal woman

a. Weak estrogen produced during menopause
b. Derived from adipose cell aromatization of androstenedione
   • Androstenedione is synthesized in the adrenal cortex.

Estrone: androstenedione from adrenal converted by aromatase to estrone

3. Estriol
a. End-product of estradiol metabolism
b. Primary estrogen of pregnancy
   • Derives from fetal adrenal, placenta, and maternal liver (refer section IX)

Estriol: estrogen of pregnancy

E. Sources and types of androgens
1. Androstenedione
   • Equal derivation from ovaries and adrenal cortex
2. DHEA
a. Mainly synthesized in the adrenal cortex (80%)
b. Remainder is synthesized in the ovaries.

DHEA-sulfate: almost exclusively synthesized in adrenal cortex

3. DHEA-sulfate
   • Almost exclusively synthesized in the adrenal cortex
4. Testosterone

Testosterone: ovary and adrenals

a. Derived from conversion of androstenedione to testosterone
b. Testosterone is synthesized in the ovaries and adrenal glands.
   • Testosterone is peripherally converted to dehydroxytestosterone.

SHBG: synthesized in liver

F. Sex hormone–binding globulin (SHBG) (Fig. 21-12)
1. Binding protein for testosterone and estrogen (refer to Chapter 20)
a. In both men and women, SHBG is primarily synthesized in the liver.
b. Estrogen increases synthesis of SHBG in the liver.
c. Androgens, obesity, hypothyroidism all decrease the synthesis of SHBG.

SHBG: higher binding affinity for testosterone than for estrogen

2. SHBG has a greater binding affinity for testosterone than estrogen.
a. Increased SHBG decreases free testosterone (FT) levels.
b. Decreased SHBG increases FT levels.
   • Common cause of hirsutism in women (see later discussion)

SHBG: ↑ SHBG, ↓ FT; ↓ SHBG, ↑ FT

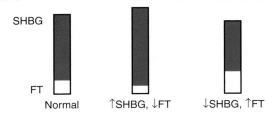

21-12: Schematic of sex hormone–binding globulin (SHBG). See text for discussion. FT, free testosterone. *(From Goljan EF, Sloka KI: Rapid Review Laboratory Testing in Clinical Medicine. St. Louis, Mosby Elsevier, 2008, p 366, Fig. 10-11.)*

G. Normal changes in pregnancy

1. Plasma volume and RBC mass
   a. Both are increased
      - Increase in plasma volume > increase in RBC mass.
   b. Causes a 1-g/dL drop in hemoglobin (Hb) (dilutional effect)
   c. Increases glomerular filtration rate (GFR)
      (1) Creatinine clearance (CCr) is increased.
      (2) Increased clearance of urea and creatinine
         - Serum levels are at the lower limit of normal.
      (3) Increases pressure to pump blood into the maternal lake in the placenta
2. Respiratory alkalosis
   a. Effect of estrogen and progesterone stimulating respiratory center
   b. Decrease in $Paco_2$ causes a corresponding increase in Pao_2.
3. Increased serum thyroxine (T_4) and cortisol
   a. Estrogen stimulates synthesis of thyroid-binding globulin and transcortin.
   b. Increased binding proteins increases total thyroxine and cortisol.
   c. Metabolically active free hormone levels are normal (refer to Chapter 22).
      - *No* clinical signs of overactivity

H. Menopause

1. Epidemiology
   a. Defined as no menses for 1 year after age 40
   b. Causes
      (1) Physiologic
         (a) Waxing and waning of estrogen levels
            - Due to decreased ovarian function
         (b) Depletion of granulosa and thecal cells
         (c) Lack of response to gonadotropins
         (d) Increased LH stimulates androgen production in stromal cells
      (2) Surgical removal/radiation of ovaries
      (3) Turner's syndrome (refer to Chapter 5)
      (4) Family history of early menopause
      (5) Left-handedness
   c. Average age of menopause is 51 years old.
      (1) Age at which it occurs is genetically determined.
      (2) Smokers reach menopause earlier than nonsmokers.
      (3) Onset of perimenopause is mid- to late 40s
2. Clinical findings
   a. Secondary amenorrhea
   b. Hot flushes, night sweats
   c. Atrophic vaginitis
      - Pruritus, burning, bleeding, dyspareunia
   d. Mood swings, anxiety, depression, insomnia
   e. Decreased libido
   f. Urinary incontinence (refer to Chapter 20)
   g. Headaches, tiredness, lethargy
   h. Osteoporosis (refer to Chapter 23)
      - Increased risk for vertebral and Colles fractures
3. Laboratory findings
   a. Increase in FSH and LH
      (1) Due to drop in estrogen and progesterone, respectively
      (2) Serum FSH is the best marker.

Margin notes:

Pregnancy: ↑ RBC mass/↑↑ plasma volume = ↓ Hb and RBC count (dilutional effect)

Pregnancy: ↑↑ plasma volume causes ↑ GFR and CCr

Pregnancy: respiratory alkalosis; estrogen/progesterone stimulation of respiratory center

Pregnancy: ↑ serum T_4/cortisol; due to increase in binding proteins

Menopause: no menses for 1 year after age 40

Menopause: hot flushes, night sweats, mood swings

Menopause: ↑ FSH best marker; absence of menses for 12 months

b. Decreased serum estradiol

c. Serum FSH is the best marker.

4. Treatment

a. Estrogen replacement if symptomatic

b. Progestin added if uterus is still present

• Prevent endometrial adenocarcinoma

c. Risks of long-term combined therapy

(1) Thromboembolism

(2) Coronary heart disease, stroke

(3) Slight risk for breast cancer

(4) Increased risk for dementia in women ≥ 65 years old

• Applies also if only taking estrogen

I. Hirsutism and virilization

1. Epidemiology and pathogenesis

a. Hirsutism is excess hair in normal hair-bearing areas (Fig. 21-13).

• Virilization is hirsutism + male secondary sex characteristics.

b. Male secondary sex characteristics

(1) Increased muscle mass

(2) Acne

(3) Enlarged clitoris (clitoromegaly) (Fig. 21-14)

• Most important finding

Hirsutism: excess hair in normal hair-bearing areas

Virilization: hirsutism + male secondary sex characteristics

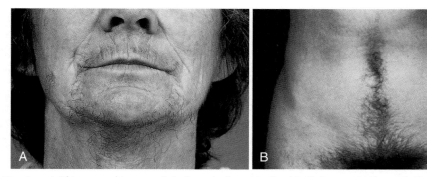

21-13: Hirsutism. **A,** This woman has excess hair above the lip and on the chin. **B,** A woman with a male distribution of hair from the mons pubis to the umbilicus. *(A from Goljan EF, Sloka KI: Rapid Review Laboratory Testing in Clinical Medicine. St. Louis, Mosby Elsevier, 2008, p 369, Fig. 10-12; B from Bouloux P: Self-Assessment Picture Tests: Medicine, Vol. 1. London, Mosby-Wolfe, 1997, p 47, Fig. 93.)*

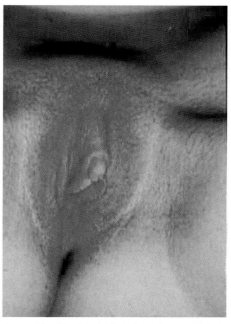

21-14: Clitoromegaly. Note the elongation of the clitoris, which is the gold standard sign of virilization. *(From Bouloux P: Self-Assessment Picture Tests: Medicine, Vol. 1. London, Mosby-Wolfe, 1997, p 4, Fig. 7.)*

c. Both conditions are due to increased androgens of ovarian or adrenal origin
   (1) Ovarian origin—testosterone (free testosterone; sometimes total) is primarily increased
   (2) Adrenal origin—DHEA-sulfate and testosterone increased
d. Causes
   (1) Polycystic ovary syndrome (see later discussion; 75%)
   (2) Idiopathic (5–15%)
   (3) Adrenogenital syndrome (1–8%; refer to Chapter 22)
   (4) Insulin resistance syndrome (3–4%; see section VIII)
   (5) Drugs (<1%)
      • Examples—androgenic progestins, phenytoin, cyclosporin, minoxidil
   (6) Ovarian tumor (<1%; see section VIII)
      • Leydig cell tumor, Sertoli-Leydig cell tumor
   (7) Adrenal tumor (<1%)
      • Adenoma/carcinoma producing Cushing's syndrome
   (8) Obesity
      • Decreased SHBG causes an increase in free testosterone.
   (9) Hypothyroidism
2. Polycystic ovary syndrome (POS)
   a. Epidemiology
      (1) Occurs in 3% of adolescents and adults
      (2) Symptoms begin around menarche.
      (3) Increased risk of endometrial cancer
      (4) Increased pituitary synthesis of LH and decreased synthesis of FSH
         (a) Increased LH increases androgen synthesis.
            • Hirsutism occurs more often than virilization.
         (b) Androgens are aromatized to estrogen in the adipose cells.
            • Increased estrogen increases risk for endometrial carcinoma.
         (c) Increased estrogen has a positive feedback on LH and negative feedback on FSH.
         (d) Suppression of FSH causes follicle degeneration.
         (e) Fluid accumulation produces subcortical cysts that enlarge the ovaries (Figs. 21-15 and 21-16).
   b. Clinical findings
      (1) Menstrual irregularities
         • Oligomenorrhea is the most common complaint.
      (2) Hirsutism, infertility, obesity (40–50%)
   c. Laboratory findings
      (1) LH:FSH ratio > 2
      (2) Increased serum testosterone (free and total) and androstenedione
      (3) Increased serum estrogen

Hirsutism and virilization: hyperandrogenicity of ovarian, adrenal, or drug origin

Hirsutism: polycystic ovary syndrome most common cause

Hirsutism, ovarian cause: ↑ testosterone

Hirsutism, adrenal cause: ↑ DHEA-S, testosterone

POS: increased risk for endometrial cancer

POS: ↑ estrogen and androgens

POS: oligomenorrhea most common complaint

POS: ↑ LH, ↓ FSH; LH:FSH ratio > 2

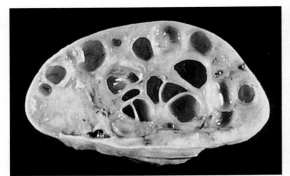

21-15: Polycystic ovary syndrome showing an enlarged ovary with multiple subcortical cysts. *(From Damjanov I, Linder J: Pathology: A Color Atlas. St. Louis, Mosby, 2000, p 262, Fig. 13-17A.)*

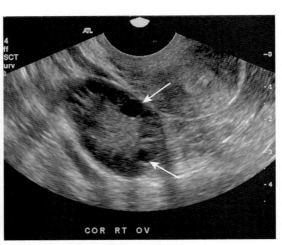

21-16: Polycystic ovary syndrome showing an ultrasound with an enlarged ovary demonstrating multiple subcortical cysts *(arrows)*. *(From Pretorius ES, Solomon JA: Radiology Secrets, 2nd ed. St. Louis, Mosby, 2006, p 204, Fig. 24-7.)*

3. Treatment
   a. Weight reduction in obese women

Rx of POS: low-dose OCPs
or medroxyprogesterone

   b. Low-dose OCPs or medroxyprogesterone
     • Suppress ovarian steroidogenesis and LH
   c. Spironolactone if OCPs unacceptable
     • Block androgen receptors on hair follicle
   d. LH-releasing hormone analogues
     • Inhibit ovarian androgen production

J. Menstrual dysfunction
1. Menorrhagia
   a. Loss of blood > 80 mL per period

Menorrhagia: loss
> 80 mL per period

   b. Menorrhagia likely if:
     (1) Staining of sheets at night with heavy protection
     (2) Excessive passage of clots
      • Indicates plasmin does *not* have enough time to dissolve clot
2. Dysmenorrhea
   a. Epidemiology
     (1) Painful menses
     (2) Approximately 50% of women have dysmenorrhea.
      • Approximately 10% are incapacitated for 1 to 3 days.
     (3) Primary type

Primary dysmenorrhea:
due to PGF$_{2\alpha}$; increases
uterine contractions

      (a) Only occurs in ovulatory cycles
      (b) Due to increased prostaglandin $F_{2\alpha}$ (PGF$_{2\alpha}$)
      (c) Increases uterine contractions
     (4) Secondary type

Secondary dysmenorrhea:
endometriosis most
common cause

      (a) Endometriosis (most common)
      (b) Adenomyosis
      (c) Leiomyomas
      (d) Cervical stenosis
   b. Treatment
     (1) Primary type
      • Nonsteroidals; OCP; nifedipine; magnesium sulfate
     (2) Secondary type
      • Treat the underlying disease
3. Dysfunctional uterine bleeding (DUB)
   a. Epidemiology

DUB: abnormal bleeding
unrelated to an anatomic
cause

     (1) Abnormal uterine bleeding *unrelated* to an anatomic cause
     (2) Diagnosis of exclusion.
     (3) Types of abnormal bleeding in DUB
      (a) Menorrhagia
      (b) Hypomenorrhea
      • Decreased amount of bleeding during normal cycle
      (c) Metrorrhagia
      • Excessive flow and duration at irregular intervals
      (d) Menometrorrhagia
      • Combination of menorrhagia and metrorrhagia
      (e) Oligomenorrhea
      • Intervals > 35 days
      (f) Polymenorrhea
      • Intervals < 21 days

DUB: occurs most often
after menarche and in
perimenopausal period

     (4) Most cases are postmenarchal and perimenopausal (most common).
      • Majority of these are anovulatory DUB.
     (5) Overall, ~90% of abnormal bleeding is caused by anovulation.
     (6) During reproductive age, <10% of abnormal bleeding results from anovulation.
   b. Anovulatory DUB

Anovulatory DUB: most
common type of DUB;
excessive estrogen
stimulation

     (1) Occurs at the extremes of reproductive life
      (a) Menarche to age 20 years
      (b) Perimenopausal period
     (2) Excessive estrogen stimulation relative to progesterone
      (a) Absent secretory phase of the cycle
      (b) Produces endometrial hyperplasia and excessive bleeding

            (3) Treatment
                • OCPs; progestational agents
      c. Inadequate luteal phase
            (1) Ovulatory type of DUB
            (2) Inadequate maturation of the corpus luteum
                  (a) Inadequate synthesis of progesterone
                      • Delay in development of the secretory phase
                  (b) Decreased serum 17-hydroxyprogesterone
                      • Blood drawn 7 days after ovulation: progesterone should be <14 pg/mL.
                  (c) Implicated in infertility and recurrent pregnancy loss
            (3) Treatment
                  (a) If follicle size is normal (ultrasound), progesterone supplementation
                  (b) If follicle size is inadequate, clomiphene sulfate is recommended.
      d. Irregular shedding of the endometrium
            (1) Ovulatory type of DUB
            (2) Persistent luteal phase with continued secretion of progesterone
            (3) Mixture of proliferative and secretory glands in the menstrual effluent
            (4) Treatment
                • OCP; medroxyprogesterone acetate
   4. Causes of abnormal bleeding by age (Table 21-2)
K. Amenorrhea
   1. Epidemiology
      a. Primary amenorrhea
            (1) Absence of menses by 16 years of age
            (2) Most cases are due to constitutional delay.
                • Family history of delayed onset of menses
      b. Secondary amenorrhea
            (1) Absence of menses for 3 months
            (2) Most cases are due to pregnancy.
   2. Pathogenesis
      a. Hypothalamic or pituitary disorder
            (1) Decreased synthesis of FSH and LH
                  (a) Decreased synthesis of estrogen and progesterone
                  (b) Hypogonadotropic (↓ FSH and LH) hypogonadism
            (2) *No* withdrawal bleeding after receiving progesterone
                • Endometrial mucosa is *not* estrogen-stimulated.
            (3) Examples
                  (a) Hypopituitarism, prolactinoma (refer to Chapter 22)
                  (b) Anorexia nervosa (refer to Chapter 7)
      b. Ovarian disorder
            (1) Decreased synthesis of estrogen and progesterone
                  (a) Increase in serum FSH and LH, respectively
                  (b) Hypergonadotropic (↑ FSH and LH) hypogonadism
            (2) *No* withdrawal bleeding after receiving progesterone
                • Endometrial mucosa is *not* estrogen-stimulated.
            (3) Examples
                  (a) Turner's syndrome (refer to Chapter 5)
                  (b) Surgical removal of ovaries

Margin notes:

Ovulatory DUB: inadequate luteal phase; ↓ progesterone

Ovulatory DUB: irregular shedding of endometrium; persistent luteal phase

Primary amenorrhea: most cases due to constitutional delay

Secondary amenorrhea: most cases due to pregnancy

Hypothalamic/pituitary cause: ↓ FSH, LH, estrogen

Ovarian cause: ↑ FSH, LH; ↓ estrogen

Primary amenorrhea + poor female secondary sex characteristics: probable Turner's syndrome

TABLE 21-2. CAUSES OF ABNORMAL BLEEDING BY AGE

AGE BRACKET	CAUSES OF BLEEDING
Prepubertal	Vulvovaginitis: poor hygiene, infection (e.g., gonorrhea), sexual abuse, foreign bodies Embryonal rhabdomyosarcoma
Menarche to 20 years	Anovulatory DUB (most common cause) Von Willebrand's disease (refer to Chapter 14)
20–40 years	Pregnancy and its complications (most common cause) Ovulatory types of DUB PID, hypothyroidism, submucosal leiomyomas, adenomyosis, endometrial polyp, endometriosis
≥40 years	Anovulatory DUB (most common cause in perimenopausal period) Endometrial hyperplasia/cancer (most common cause in menopause)

DUB, dysfunctional uterine bleeding; PID, pelvic inflammatory disease.

TABLE 21-3. DIFFERENTIAL DIAGNOSIS OF AMENORRHEA

DISORDER	FSH/LH	ESTROGEN	EXAMPLES
Hypothalamic/pituitary disorder	↓	↓	Hypopituitarism Anorexia nervosa, prolactinoma
Ovarian disorder	↑	↓	Turner's syndrome
End-organ defect	N	N	Imperforate hymen, Asherman syndrome
Constitutional delay	N	N	Family history of delayed onset of menses

FSH, follicle-stimulating hormone; LH, luteinizing hormone; N, normal.

  c. End-organ defect
   (1) Prevents the normal egress of blood
    • More likely cause of primary amenorrhea
   (2) Normal levels of FSH, LH, estrogen, and progesterone
   (3) *No* withdrawal bleeding after receiving progesterone
   (4) Examples
    (a) Imperforate hymen, Rokitansky-Kuster-Hauser syndrome
    (b) Asherman syndrome
     • Removal of stratum basalis owing to repeated curettage
  d. Summary of amenorrhea (Table 21-3)

VI. Uterine Disorders
 A. Endometritis
  1. Epidemiology
   a. Uterine infection following delivery (vaginal/cesarean section) or abortion
   b. Rate of postpartum endometritis is 1% to 8%.
   c. Most common genital tract infection following delivery
   d. More common in preterm deliveries
  2. Acute endometritis
   a. Most often due to bacterial infection following delivery or miscarriage
   b. Group B streptococcus *(Streptococcus agalactiae)* is a common pathogen.
   c. Other pathogens—group A streptococcus, *Staphylococcus aureus, Bacteroides fragilis, C. trachomatis, N. gonorrhoeae, Escherichia coli*
   d. Clinical findings
    (1) Fever
    (2) Uterine tenderness
    (3) Purulent or foul vaginal discharge (lochia)
    (4) Abdominal pain
   e. Treatment
    • Cefoxitin; ticarcillin-clavulanate; ampicillin-sulbactam
  3. Chronic endometritis
   a. Causes
    (1) Retained placenta
    (2) Gonorrhea, intrauterine device *(Actinomyces israelii)*
   b. Key histologic finding is the presence of plasma cells.
   c. Treatment (see earlier discussion)
 B. Adenomyosis
  1. Epidemiology
   a. Invagination of the stratum basalis into the myometrium (Fig. 21-17)
    (1) Glands and stroma thicken myometrial tissue.
    (2) Produces uterine enlargement
   b. Highest incidence in women in mid- to late 40s
   c. Common finding in hysterectomy specimens
  2. Clinical findings
   • Menorrhagia, dysmenorrhea, pelvic pain
  3. Definitive diagnosis with myometrial biopsy
  4. Treatment is hysterectomy.
 C. Endometriosis
  1. Epidemiology
   a. Functioning glands and stroma are located *outside* the uterus (Fig. 21-18).
    • Cyclic bleeding of gland and stromal implants

Margin notes:

End organ defect: normal FSH, LH, estrogen

Asherman syndrome: removal of stratum basalis by curettage

Acute endometritis: uterine infection following delivery or abortion

Acute endometritis: group B streptococcus common pathogen

Intrauterine device: *Actinomyces* infection

Chronic endometritis: presence of plasma cells in biopsy

Adenomyosis: glands and stroma in myometrium

Endometriosis: functioning glands and stroma outside the confines of the uterus

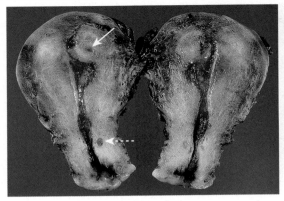

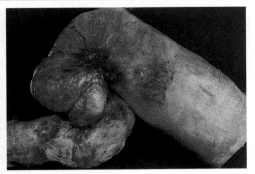

21-17: Adenomyosis. The *solid arrow* shows an area of hemorrhage surrounded by irregularly thickened endometrial stroma. The *interrupted arrow* shows a nabothian cyst in the endocervical canal. *(From Rosai J, Ackerman LV: Surgical Pathology, 9th ed. St. Louis, Mosby, 2004, p 1578, Fig. 19-123.)*

21-18: Endometriosis implants on a loop of intestine. Note the serosal surface has multiple areas of hemorrhage with a "powder burn" appearance. *(From Damjanov I, Linder J: Pathology: A Color Atlas. St. Louis, Mosby, 2000, p 126, Fig. 7-17.)*

   b. Prevalence is highest in women with dysmenorrhea (40–60%)
   c. Average age at time of diagnosis is 25 to 29 years old.
   d. Multifactorial inheritance has been implicated.
      • Approximately 7% occurrence rate in first-degree female relatives
2. Pathogenesis
   a. Reverse menses through fallopian tubes (most common)
      • Implantation of viable endometrial cells
   b. Coelomic metaplasia
   c. Vascular or lymphatic spread
3. Common sites
   • Ovaries (most common), rectal pouch, fallopian tubes, intestine

> The **rectal pouch of Douglas** is anterior to the rectum and posterior to the uterus. It is the most dependent portion of the female pelvis. It can be palpated by digital rectal examination. It is a common site to collect blood (e.g., ruptured tubal pregnancy), malignant cells (e.g., seeding by ovarian cancer), endometrial implants, and pus (e.g., pelvic inflammatory disease).

4. Clinical findings
   a. Dysmenorrhea (most common)
   b. Abnormal bleeding
      • Premenstrual spotting, menorrhagia
   c. Painful stooling during menses
      • Implants located in rectal pouch
   d. Intestinal obstruction and bleeding during menses
   e. Increased risk for ectopic pregnancy
   f. Infertility, dyspareunia
   g. Enlargement of ovaries
      • Blood-filled cysts
5. Diagnosis
   a. Laparoscopy useful for diagnosis and treatment
      • Implants have a "powder burn" appearance
   b. Increased serum cancer antigen 125 (CA125)
      (1) Excellent sensitivity but poor specificity (increased false positive results)
         • It is a cancer antigen that is also increased in surface derived ovarian cancers and other gynecologic disorders.
      (2) More useful in excluding endometriosis when it returns negative
6. Treatment
   a. Combination oral contraceptives
   b. Progestins (e.g., medroxyprogesterone acetate)
   c. Gonadotropin-releasing hormone agonists
   d. Laparoscopic removal of implants

Endometriosis: reverse menses most common cause; coelomic metaplasia; vascular/lymphatic spread

Endometriosis: ovaries most common site of implantation

Rectal pouch of Douglas: site for collection of blood, malignant cells, pus, endometrial implants

Endometriosis triad: dysmenorrhea, dyspareunia, infertility

Endometriosis: laparoscopy useful for diagnosis and treatment

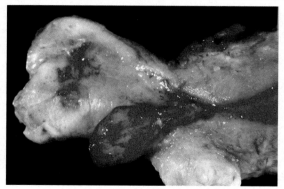

21-19: Endometrial polyp. Note hemorrhagic polyp arising from the endometrial mucosa. It is a common cause of uterine bleeding. *(From Kumar V, Fausto N, Abbas A: Robbins and Cotran's Pathologic Basis of Disease, 7th ed. Philadelphia, WB Saunders, 2004, p 1082, Fig. 22-27C.)*

D. Endometrial polyp (Fig. 21-19)
  1. Epidemiology
     a. Benign polyp that enlarges with estrogen stimulation
     b. Does *not* progress to endometrial carcinoma
     c. Can protrude through the cervix into the vagina
  2. Clinical findings
     a. Common cause of menorrhagia in 20- to 40-year-old age bracket
     b. Spotting between menstrual periods or after menopause
  3. Diagnosis
     a. Vaginal ultrasound
     b. Dilation and curettage (D&C)
  4. Treatment
     a. Dilation and curettage
     b. Hysteroscopy
E. Endometrial hyperplasia
  1. Epidemiology and pathogenesis
     a. Prolonged estrogen stimulation
     b. Risk factors
        (1) Early menarche or late menopause
        (2) Nulliparity
        (3) Obesity
           • Increased aromatization of androgens to estrogen
        (4) Polycystic ovary syndrome
        (5) Taking estrogen without progesterone
        (6) Anovulatory menstrual cycles
        (7) Hereditary nonpolyposis colon cancer (Lynch syndrome; refer to Chapter 8)
     c. Classification
        (1) Simple hyperplasia (Fig. 21-20)
           (a) Increased number of cystically dilated glands
           (b) *No* glandular crowding
        (2) Complex hyperplasia
           (a) Increased number of dilated glands with branching
           (b) Glandular crowding
        (3) Atypical hyperplasia
           (a) Glandular crowding and dysplastic epithelium
           (b) Greatest risk for endometrial cancer
     d. High rate of spontaneous regression
  2. Clinical findings
     a. Menorrhagia, metrorrhagia, menometrorrhagia
     b. Postmenopausal bleeding
  3. Diagnosis
     • Endometrial biopsy
  4. Treatment
     a. OCPs

Endometrial polyp: common cause of menorrhagia; no risk for endometrial cancer

Endometrial hyperplasia: prolonged estrogen stimulation

Endometrial hyperplasia: atypical hyperplasia greatest risk for endometrial cancer

Endometrial hyperplasia: postmenopausal bleeding

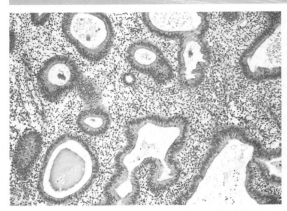

21-20: Simple hyperplasia of endometrial glands showing cystic dilation and focal areas of glandular outpouching. There is no gland crowding or stratification of the epithelial lining. *(From Kumar V, Fausto N, Abbas A: Robbins and Cotran's Pathologic Basis of Disease, 7th ed. Philadelphia, WB Saunders, 2004, p 1086, Fig. 22-31A.)*

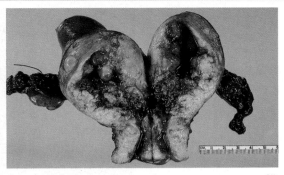

21-21: Endometrial carcinoma showing necrotic tumor filling the uterine cavity and extending completely through the uterine wall and into the endocervical canal. *(From Rosai J, Ackerman LV: Surgical Pathology, 9th ed. St. Louis, Mosby, 2004, p 1586, Fig. 19-136B.)*

  b. Medroxyprogesterone acetate
  c. Hysterectomy if atypia is present

F. Endometrial carcinoma
  1. Epidemiology and pathogenesis
    a. Most common gynecologic tumor
    b. Median age at onset, 60 years old
    c. Prolonged estrogen stimulation
      • Same risk factors as endometrial hyperplasia
    d. OCPs decrease risk.
      • Due to antiestrogen effect of progestins
    e. Increased risk for breast cancer
    f. Types of endometrial cancer
      (1) Well-differentiated adenocarcinoma
        (a) Most common type
        (b) Adenoacanthoma
          • Contains foci of benign squamous tissue (no prognostic significance)
        (c) Adenosquamous carcinoma
          • Contain foci of malignant squamous cancer (worse prognosis)
      (2) Papillary adenocarcinoma
        • Highly aggressive cancer
  2. Cancer characteristics
    a. Spreads down into the endocervix
    b. Spreads out into the uterine wall (Fig. 21-21)
    c. Lungs are the most common site of metastasis
  3. Clinical findings
    • Postmenopausal bleeding (90%)
  4. Diagnosis
    • Endometrial biopsy
  5. Treatment
    • Surgery, radiation, hormones (tamoxifen), or chemotherapy depending on stage

G. Leiomyoma ("fibroids")
  1. Epidemiology
    a. Benign smooth muscle tumor (Fig. 21-22)
    b. Most frequently diagnosed gynecologic tumor
    c. Occurs in 20% to 50% of women > 30 years old
    d. More common in blacks than whites
    e. Estrogen-sensitive tumors
      • May become larger during pregnancy
  2. Tumor characteristics
    a. Commonly undergo the following:
      (1) Degeneration
      (2) Dystrophic calcification

Endometrial carcinoma: most common gynecologic cancer; best prognosis

OCPs: ↓ risk for endometrial cancer

Endometrial cancer: postmenopausal bleeding most common finding

Leiomyoma: most common benign connective tissue tumor in women

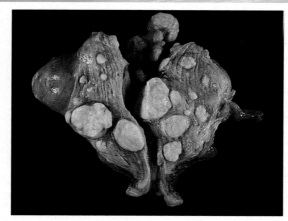

21-22: Leiomyomas. In sagittal section, multiple well-circumscribed, gray-white nodules (leiomyomas) are dispersed through-out the myometrium. Submucosal leiomyomas are a common cause of uterine bleeding. *(From Damjanov I, Linder J: Pathology: A Color Atlas. St. Louis, Mosby, 2000, p 271, Fig. 13-49.)*

          (3) Hyalinization
              • Reason for the term "fibroids"
        b. They rarely transform into leiomyosarcomas (<1%).
     3. Clinical findings
        a. Menorrhagia (when located in submucosa)
        b. Obstructive delivery
        c. Cramping during menses
        d. Pressure on colon (constipation)
        e. Pressure on bladder
          • Increased frequency, urgency, incontinence
     4. Diagnosis
        a. Transabdominal or transvaginal ultrasound
        b. MRI
     5. Treatment
        a. Myotomy if women want to preserve fertility
        b. Hysterectomy
  H. Leiomyosarcoma
     1. Most common sarcoma of the uterus
     2. Tumor characteristics
       • Numerous atypical mitoses and foci of necrosis
     3. Treatment is surgery.
  I. Malignant mixed müllerian tumors (carcinosarcomas)
     1. Endometrial adenocarcinoma + malignant mesenchymal (stromal) tumor
       a. Primarily occur in postmenopausal women
       b. Bulky, necrotic tumors that often protrude through the cervical os
     2. Mesenchymal component may include muscle, cartilage, and bone.
     3. Strong association with previous irradiation
     4. Poor prognosis
     5. Treatment is surgery.
VII. Fallopian Tube Disorders
  A. Hydatid cysts of Morgagni
     1. Cystic müllerian remnants
     2. Most often located around the fimbriated end of the tube
     3. May undergo torsion (>25%), causing abdominal pain
     4. Treatment is surgical removal (laparoscope).
  B. Pelvic inflammatory disease (PID)
     1. Epidemiology
       a. Diagnosed in 2% to 5% of women in STD clinics
       b. Most common cause of female infertility and ectopic pregnancy
       c. Risk factors
         (1) Multiple sexual partners
         (2) Vaginal douching
         (3) Previous episodes of PID
         (4) Unprotected sex

Margin notes:

Clinical: menorrhagia; obstructive delivery

Leiomyosarcoma: most common sarcoma of uterus

Carcinosarcoma: association with previous irradiation

Hydatid cysts: cystic müllerian remnant; may undergo torsion

PID: most common cause of female infertility and ectopic pregnancy

d. Most but not all cases of PID are STDs.
e. Causes of PID
  (1) Most often due to *N. gonorrhoeae* or *C. trachomatis*
    • Coexisting infection in 45% of cases
  (2) Other pathogens (*not* STD)
    • *B. fragilis*, streptococci, *Clostridium perfringens*, *Mycobacteria tuberculosis*, cytomegalovirus (CMV)
2. Gross findings
  a. Fallopian tubes are filled with pus (Fig. 21-23).
  b. Most common cause of hydrosalpinx
    • Pus resorbs, leaving a clear fluid distending the tube.
3. Clinical findings
  a. Fever usually >38.3°C (101°F)
  b. Lower abdominal pain
  c. Cervical motion, adnexal, uterine tenderness on pelvic examination
  d. Abnormal uterine bleeding; vaginal discharge
  e. Mucopurulent discharge in cervical os
  f. Right upper quadrant pain (5%)
    • Perihepatitis (Fitz-Hughes–Curtis syndrome; see Table 21-1)
4. Diagnosis
  a. Finding of cervical motion tenderness and adnexal tenderness
  b. Culture of cervical discharge
  c. Laparoscopy
  d. Transvaginal ultrasound; MRI (best sensitivity and specificity)
5. Treatment
  a. Empiric treatment with uterine, adnexal, and cervical motion tenderness
  b. Ceftriaxone + doxycycline (covers both *N. gonorrhoeae* and *C. trachomatis*)

C. Salpingitis isthmica nodosa (SIN)
1. Invagination of the mucosa into the muscle ("tubal diverticulosis")
  a. Produces nodules in the tube that narrow the lumen
  b. Probably a postinfectious reaction (e.g., previous *C. trachomatis* infection)
2. Complications
  • Infertility, ectopic pregnancy
3. Diagnose with hysterosalpingography
  • Beading appearance in areas of constriction

D. Ectopic pregnancy (EP)
1. Epidemiology and pathogenesis
  a. Implantation of a fetus outside the normal uterine location
  b. Occurs in 1% to 2% of pregnancies
  c. Accounts for 13% of maternal deaths
  d. Risk factors
    (1) Scarring from previous PID (most common cause)
    (2) Endometriosis
    (3) Altered tubal motility, SIN
    (4) Progestin-only pill; previous tubal ligation

PID: most common cause is N. gonorrhoeae and C. trachomatis; both present in 45% of cases

PID: cervical motion, adnexal, uterine tenderness highly predictive of PID

Rx PID: ceftriaxone (for N. gonorrhoeae) + doxycycline (for C. trachomatis)

SIN: tubal diverticulosis

EP: most common cause is previous PID

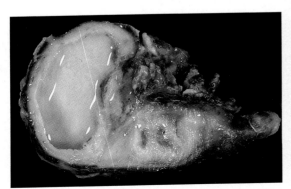

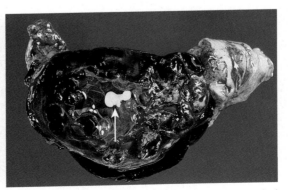

21-23: Pelvic inflammatory disease. Note the pus filling the lumen of the fallopian tube. (*From Rosai J, Ackerman LV: Surgical Pathology, 9th ed. St. Louis, Mosby, 2004, p 1638, Fig. 19-192B.*)

21-24: Ruptured ectopic tubal pregnancy showing marked hemorrhage (hematosalpinx) and an embryo (*arrow*) in the center of the clot material. (*From Rosai J, Ackerman LV: Surgical Pathology, 9th ed. St. Louis, Mosby, 2004, p 1639, Fig. 19-198.*)

e. Sites of implantation
  (1) Majority occur within the tubes (Fig. 21-24)
      • Most are in the broad ampullary portion below the fimbriae.
  (2) Ovaries, abdominal cavity

2. Clinical findings

  a. Sudden onset of lower abdominal pain and tenderness (95%)
      • Usually ~6 weeks after a previous normal menstrual period
  b. Adnexal tenderness (87–99%)
  c. Peritoneal signs (rebound tenderness; >70%)
  d. Abnormal uterine bleeding (75%)
  e. Hypovolemic shock (intraperitoneal bleeding; 2–17%)

3. Complications

  a. Rupture with intra-abdominal bleed
      • Most common cause of death in early pregnancy
  b. Most common cause of hematosalpinx
      • Blood in the tube

4. Diagnosis
  a. β-hCG is the best screening test.
      (1) Urine screen is usually sensitive enough.
      (2) Serum test is used if the urine screen is negative.
      (3) Positive test does *not* prove that an ectopic pregnancy is present.
  b. Vaginal ultrasound is the confirmatory test.
      • Check for an amniotic sac.
  c. Laparoscopy is used in equivocal cases.

5. Treatment
  a. Methotrexate if stable and no hemorrhage
  b. Conservative surgery; salpingectomy

VIII. Ovarian Disorders

A. Follicular cyst

1. Most common ovarian mass
2. Non-neoplastic cyst
   • Accumulation of fluid in a follicle or previously ruptured follicle
3. Rupture produces sterile peritonitis with pain.
4. Most regress spontaneously.
5. Ultrasound is the best screening test.
6. Surgical removal if symptomatic

B. Corpus luteum cyst

1. Most common ovarian mass in pregnancy
2. Non-neoplastic cyst
   a. Accumulation of fluid in the corpus luteum during pregnancy
   b. May be confused with an amniotic sac
   c. Most regress spontaneously.
3. Surgical removal if symptomatic

C. Oophoritis

   • May be a complication of mumps or pelvic inflammatory disease

D. Stromal hyperthecosis

1. Epidemiology
   a. Occurs primarily in obese postmenopausal women
      • Causes bilateral ovarian enlargement
   b. Hypercellular ovarian stroma
      (1) Vacuolated (luteinized) stromal hilar cells are present
          • Synthesize excess androgens
      (2) May cause hirsutism or virilization

2. Clinical findings
   a. Hirsutism or virilization
   b. Association with acanthosis nigricans and insulin resistance
   c. Hypertension
3. Treatment is oophorectomy.

E. Ovarian tumors

1. Epidemiology and pathogenesis
   a. Tumors are more likely benign in women < 45 years of age.

(1) Risk increases with age.
(2) Median age of presentation is 61 years of age.
(3) Peaks in the late 70s
(4) Approximately 60% present with advanced disease.

b. Risk factors
  (1) Nulliparity
    (a) Increased number of ovulatory cycles increases risk.
    (b) Increased risk for surface-derived ovarian tumors
  (2) Genetic factors
    (a) Mutations of *BRCA1* and *BRCA2* suppressor genes
    (b) Lynch syndrome (refer to Chapter 8)
    (c) Turner's syndrome (refer to Chapter 5)
      • Increased risk for dysgerminoma
    (d) Peutz-Jeghers syndrome (refer to Chapter 17)
      • Increased incidence of sex cord tumors with annular tubules
  (3) History of breast cancer
  (4) Postmenopausal estrogen therapy; obesity (increased estrogen)
  (5) OCPs/pregnancy decrease risk for surface-derived ovarian cancers.
    • Decreased number of ovulatory cycles

2. Classification of ovarian tumors (Table 21-4 and Fig. 21-25)
  a. Surface-derived tumors
    (1) Account for 65% to 70% of ovarian tumors
    (2) Derive from coelomic epithelium
    (3) Account for the greatest number of malignant ovarian tumors
    (4) Malignant tumors commonly seed the omentum (refer to Chapter 8).
  b. Germ cell tumors
    (1) Account for 15% to 20% of ovarian tumors
    (2) Cancers are similar to those seen in the testicle (refer to Chapter 20).
    (3) A relatively small number of tumors are malignant.
  c. Sex cord stromal tumors
    (1) Account for 3% to 5% of ovarian tumors
    (2) Derive from stromal cells
    (3) May be hormone-producing
    (4) Majority of tumors are benign.
  d. Metastasis
    (1) Accounts for 5% of ovarian tumors
    (2) Common primary cancers metastasizing to ovaries
      • Breast, stomach (e.g., Krukenberg tumors)

3. Clinical findings
  a. Abdominal enlargement due to fluid (most common sign)
    (1) Malignant ascites most often due to seeding
    (2) Signs of malignant ascites due to seeding
      (a) Induration in the rectal pouch on digital rectal examination
      (b) Intestinal obstruction with colicky pain
  b. Palpable ovarian mass in a postmenopausal woman
    • Ovaries should *not* be palpable in menopausal women.
  c. Malignant pleural effusion
    • Common site for ovarian cancer metastasis
  d. Cystic teratomas undergo torsion leading to infarction.
    • Radiographs show calcification from bone or teeth (see Fig. 8-3).
  e. Signs of hyperestrinism from estrogen-secreting tumors
    (1) Bleeding from endometrial hyperplasia/cancer
    (2) 100% superficial squamous cells in a cervical Pap smear
  f. Hirsutism or virilization from androgen-secreting tumors

4. Tumor markers
  a. Increased serum cancer antigen 125 (CA125)
  b. Only increased in surface-derived malignant tumors

5. Treatment
  • Surgery, chemotherapy, occasionally radiation

6. Prognosis
  a. Better prognosis if <65 years old
  b. Overall 1- and 5-year relative survival rates for ovarian cancer are 75% and 45%, respectively.

Margin notes:

Ovarian cancer: risk increases with age

Ovarian cancer: genetic factors; excess estrogen exposure

OCPs/pregnancy: ↓ risk for surface-derived ovarian cancers

Surface-derived tumors: most common group of ovarian tumors

Serous cystadenocarcinoma: most common ovarian cancer; bilaterality; psammoma bodies

Malignant surface-derived cancers: commonly seed the abdominal cavity

Germ cell tumors: teratoma and dysgerminoma most common benign and malignant, respectively

Sex cord stromal tumors: hormone producing tumors; most are benign

Ovarian cancer: abdominal enlargement due to fluid most common sign

Ovarian cancer: palpable ovaries in postmenopausal women is cancer until proved otherwise

Sex cord stromal tumors: ↑ estrogen/androgens

Surface-derived tumors: ↑ CA125

TABLE 21-4. **CLASSIFICATION OF OVARIAN TUMORS**

TUMOR	CHARACTERISTICS
Surface-Derived Tumors	
Serous tumors	Most common group of primary benign and malignant tumors Most common group of tumors that can be bilateral Cysts are lined by ciliated cells (similar to fallopian tube) Serous cystadenoma (benign; most common benign ovarian tumor); serous cystadenocarcinoma has psammoma bodies (dystrophically calcified tumor cells); most common malignant tumor that is bilateral
Mucinous tumors	Cysts lined by mucus-secreting cells (similar to endocervix) Large, multiloculated tumors Seeding produces pseudomyxoma peritonei Mucinous cystadenoma (benign); may be associated with Brenner tumors; mucinous cystadenocarcinoma
Endometrioid	Malignant tumors associated with endometrial carcinoma (15–30% of cases); tumor resembles endometrial carcinoma Commonly bilateral
Brenner tumor	Usually benign Contain Walthard's rests (transitional-like epithelium)
Germ Cell Tumors	
Cystic teratoma	Usually benign; less than 1% become malignant (usually squamous cancer) Most common benign germ cell tumor Ectodermal differentiation (hair, sebaceous glands, teeth) most prominent Most of these derivatives are found in a nipple-like structure in the cyst wall called Rokitansky tubercle Immature malignant types contain mature and immature components (e.g., muscle, neuroepithelium) Struma ovarii type has functioning thyroid tissue
Dysgerminoma	Most common malignant germ cell tumor; characteristic increase in serum LDH; same histologic picture as seminoma of testis Associated with streak gonads of Turner syndrome
Yolk sac tumor	Malignant tumor; most common ovarian cancer in girls < 4 years old Contain Schiller-Duval bodies (resemble yolk sac) Increased α-fetoprotein
Sex-Cord Stromal Tumors	
Thecoma-fibroma	Benign tumor associated with Meigs' syndrome (ascites, right-sided pleural effusion); regression of effusions follows removal of tumor Commonly calcify
Granulosa-theca cell tumor	Low-grade malignant tumor Feminizing tumor (produces estrogen) that contains Call-Exner bodies
Sertoli-Leydig cell	Benign masculinizing tumor (produces androgens) Pure Leydig cell tumors contain cells with crystals of Reinke
Gonadoblastoma	Malignant tumor with mixture of germ cell tumor (dysgerminoma) and sex-cord stromal tumor; associated with abnormal sexual development in 80% of cases Commonly calcify
Tumors Metastatic to Ovary	
Krukenberg tumor	May affect both ovaries; contains signet-ring cells from hematogenous spread of a gastric cancer

LDH, lactate dehydrogenase.

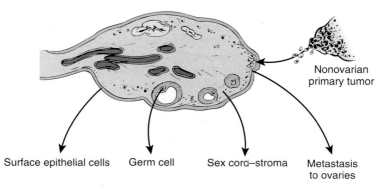

21-25: Schematic showing the derivation of primary ovarian tumors. *(From Kumar V, Abbas AK, Fausto N, Mitchell RN: Robbins Basic Pathology, 8th ed. Philadelphia, Saunders Elsevier, 2007, p 729, Fig. 19-16.)*

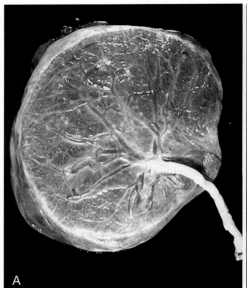

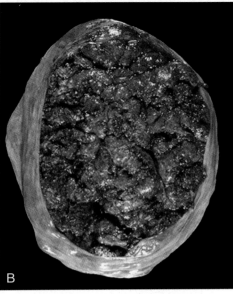

21-26: Normal placenta, showing the fetal side (**A**) and the maternal side (**B**). See text for discussion. *(From Klatt E: Robbins and Cotran's Atlas of Pathology. Philadelphia, WB Saunders, 2006, p 326, Fig. 13-108.)*

IX.   Gestational Disorders
A. Placental anatomy
1. Fetal surface (Fig. 21-26A)
   a. Entirely covered by the chorionic plate
   b. Chorionic villi vessels converge with the umbilical cord.
   c. Chorion is covered by the amnion.
2. Maternal surface (Fig. 21-26B)
   • Contains cotyledons covered by a layer of decidua basalis
3. Chorionic villus/umbilical cord
   a. Chorionic villi project in the intervillous space (Fig. 21-27).
      (1) Space contains maternal blood from which oxygen is extracted.
      (2) Spiral arteries from the uterus empty into the space.
   b. Chorionic villi are lined by trophoblastic tissue.
      (1) Outside layer is composed of syncytiotrophoblast.
         (a) Synthesizes hCG (see earlier discussion)
         (b) Synthesizes human placental lactogen (HPL)
            • Directly correlates with placental mass and has anti-insulin activity
      (2) Inside layer is composed of cytotrophoblast.
   c. Chorionic villus vessels coalesce to form the umbilical vein.
   d. Umbilical cord
      (1) Contains one umbilical vein and two umbilical arteries
         • Umbilical vein contains oxygenated blood.
      (2) Single umbilical artery

Fetal surface: chorionic plate

Maternal surface: cotyledons

Chorionic villi: extract O_2 from maternal blood

Trophoblast: lines villi; syncytiotrophoblast (synthesizes hCG, HPL) and cytotrophoblast

HPL: directly correlates with placental mass, anti-insulin activity

Umbilical cord: 2 arteries, 1 vein; umbilical vein has most O_2

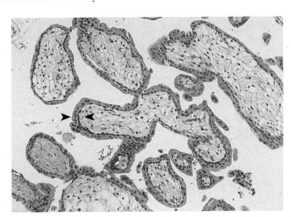

21-27: Chorionic villi. The outer layer of the villus is covered by two layers of cells called the trophoblast (*arrowheads*). The outer layer of the trophoblast is lined by syncytiotrophoblast, while the inner layer is lined by cytotrophoblast. *(From Klatt E: Robbins and Cotran's Atlas of Pathology. Philadelphia, WB Saunders, 2006, p 326, Fig. 13-109.)*

(a) Increased incidence of congenital anomalies (20% of cases)
(b) Defects—cardiovascular; trisomy 18; esophageal atresia

B. Placental infections

1. Epidemiology
   a. Most are due to ascending bacterial infections
      (1) Complication of premature rupture of membranes
         - If culture is negative for group B streptococcus, treat prophylactically with IV ampicillin + IV erythromycin followed by amoxicillin + erythromycin by mouth
      (2) Group B streptococcus is common pathogen.
         - If culture is positive during labor, treat with penicillin G or ampicillin IV.
      (3) Other pathogens—*B. fragilis*, *Prevotella bivius*, group A streptococcus
   b. Congenital infections (e.g., cytomegalovirus, syphilis)
2. Funisitis and placentitis
   - Infection of the umbilical cord and placenta, respectively
3. Chorioamnionitis
   a. Infection of the fetal membranes
   b. Danger of neonatal sepsis and meningitis
   c. Treatment
      - Cefoxitin; ticarcillin-clavulanate

C. Selected placental abnormalities

1. Placenta previa (Fig. 21-28)
   a. Epidemiology
      (1) Implantation over cervical os
      (2) Previous cesarean section is a risk factor (approaches 10%).
   b. Clinical findings
      (1) Presents with painless vaginal bleeding
         - Usually in second or third trimester
      (2) Uterus soft and nontender
      (3) Fetal distress usually not present.
   c. Diagnosis
      (1) Pelvic examination should *not* be performed.
      (2) Transabdominal ultrasound localizes placenta.
      (3) Transvaginal ultrasound confirms placenta previa.
   d. Treatment
      (1) Careful observation of fetus and mother
      (2) Delivery by cesarean section
2. Abruptio placentae (Fig. 21-29)
   a. Epidemiology

Margin notes:

Placenta infections: group B streptococcus most common

Chorioamnionitis: infection fetal membranes; danger neonatal sepsis/meningitis

Placenta previa: implantation over cervical os; previous C-section risk factor

Placenta previa: painless vaginal bleeding

Placenta previa: do not perform pelvic exam; diagnose by ultrasound

Abruptio placentae: retroplacental clot

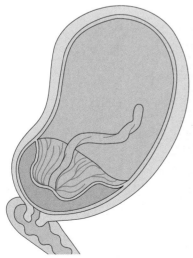

21-28: Schematic of placenta praevia. Note how the placenta is implanted over the cervical os. *(From Greer I, Cameron IT, Kitchener HC, Prentice A: Mosby's Color Atlas and Text of Obstetrics and Gynecology. St. Louis, Mosby, 2000, p 184, Fig. 7-28.)*

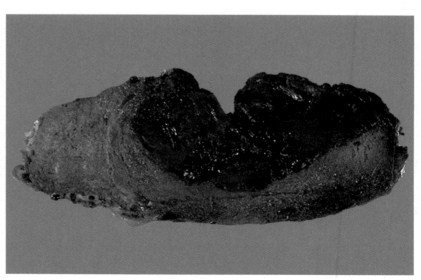

21-29: Abruptio placentae. Note the retroplacental blood clot that separated the placenta from its implantation site. *(From Klatt E: Robbins and Cotran's Atlas of Pathology. Philadelphia, WB Saunders, 2006, p 327, Fig. 13-112.)*

        (1) Premature separation of placenta due to formation of a retroplacental clot
           (a) Separates the placenta from the implantation site
           (b) Most common cause of late pregnancy bleeding
           (c) Occurs in 1:830 pregnancies
        (2) Fetal mortality rate is 20% to 40%.
        (3) Risk factors
           (a) Hypertension (greatest risk factor; 40–50% of cases)
           (b) Smoking cigarettes
           (c) Cocaine addiction; advanced maternal age
           (d) Trauma; chorioamnionitis
           (e) Premature rupture of membranes
           (f) Previous abruptio placentae
    b. Clinical findings
        (1) Painful uterine bleeding
          • Concealed (20%) or vaginal bleeding (80%)
        (2) Forceful uterine contractions (~15%) or signs of preterm labor
        (3) Evidence of fetal distress is usually present.
    c. Diagnosis
        (1) Pelvic examination should *not* be done.
        (2) Ultrasound
    d. Treatment
        (1) Fetal heart monitoring
        (2) Monitor maternal hemodynamic status
        (3) Deliver baby
  3. Placenta accreta
    a. Direct implantation into muscle *without* intervening decidua
      • Occurs in 1:2500 pregnancies
    b. Great risk for hemorrhage during delivery
    c. Commonly requires surgery to control bleeding
      • Hysterectomy is often necessary.
  4. Velamentous insertion
    a. Umbilical cord inserts away from the placental edge.
      • Vessels pass to the placenta through the membranes between the amnion and the chorion.
    b. Increased risk for hemorrhage if vessels are torn
    c. Can be diagnosed by ultrasound
    d. Often delivered by cesarean section to avoid vessel tear
  5. Accessory lobes
    • Increased risk for hemorrhage if they are detached
  6. Enlarged placenta
    a. Diabetes mellitus
    b. Rh hemolytic disease of newborn (HDN)
    c. Congenital syphilis
  7. Twin placentas (Fig. 21-30)
    a. Monochorionic types are associated with identical twins.
        (1) Identical twins derive from a single fertilized egg.
        (2) Monoamniotic with a single amniotic sac (Fig. 21-30A)
          • Type for Siamese twins or tangling of umbilical cords
        (3) Diamniotic with separate amniotic sacs (Fig. 21-30B)
        (4) Fetal-to-fetal transfusion can occur in either type.
    b. Dichorionic placentas
        (1) Can be identical or fraternal twins
          • Fraternal twins occur when separate eggs are fertilized.
        (2) Placentas can be diamniotic (Fig. 21-30C) or separated (Fig. 21-30D).

D. Preeclampsia/eclampsia
  • Toxemia of pregnancy
  1. Epidemiology
    a. Usually occurs in the third trimester (24th to 25th weeks)
    b. Occurs in ~6% of primigravidas and ~7% of multigravidas
    c. Risk factors
        (1) More common in women < 20 years of age and >35 years of age
        (2) History of previous preeclampsia

Margin notes:

Abruptio placentae: most common cause of late pregnancy bleeding

Abruptio placentae: hypertension greatest risk factor

Abruptio placentae triad: painful vaginal bleeding, tetanic contractions, fetal compromise

Placenta accreta: implantation into muscle; danger of hemorrhage at delivery

Velamentous insertion: cord inserts away from placental edge; danger of tearing vessels

Accessory lobe: increased risk for hemorrhage if detached

Enlarged placenta: Rh HDN, congenital syphilis, diabetes mellitus

Monochorionic twin placentas: identical twins, single fertilized egg

Dichorionic twin placentas: identical or fraternal (separate fertilized eggs)

Preeclampsia: usually occurs during third trimester

21-30: Twin placentas. See text for description. *(Redrawn from Goljan EF: Star Series: Pathology. Philadelphia, WB Saunders, 1998, Fig. 18-2.)*

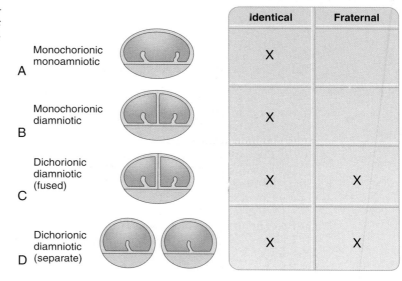

	Identical	Fraternal
A Monochorionic monoamniotic	X	
B Monochorionic diamniotic	X	
C Dichorionic diamniotic (fused)	X	X
D Dichorionic diamniotic (separate)	X	X

(3) Positive family history
(4) Multiple gestations
(5) Blacks
(6) Thrombocytosis; obesity
   d. May be associated with hydatidiform moles (see later discussion)
     (1) Complete mole, 2%
     (2) Partial mole, 5%
 2. Pathogenesis
   a. Abnormal placentation
     (1) Causes mechanical or functional obstruction of the spiral arteries
     (2) Abnormal trophoblastic tissue invades the spiral arteries.
   b. Imbalance favoring vasoconstrictors over vasodilators
     (1) Normal vasodilators are decreased.
      • Examples—PGE_2, nitric oxide
     (2) Vasoconstrictors are increased.
      (a) Examples—thromboxane A_2, angiotensin II
      (b) Increased sensitivity to the effect of angiotensin II
     (3) Increase in various growth factors (e.g., vascular growth factor)
   c. Net effect is placental hypoperfusion.
 3. Pathologic findings
   a. Premature aging of the placenta
   b. Multiple placental infarctions
   c. Spiral arteries show intimal atherosclerosis.
 4. Clinical and laboratory findings
   a. Hypertension (increased vasoconstrictors)
     • Ranges from just below 140/90 mm Hg to >160/110 mm Hg
   b. Proteinuria in nephrotic range (>3.5 g/24 hours)
     • Usually >5 g/24 hour urine collection
   c. Dependent pitting edema
     • Due to loss of albumin in the urine
   d. Weight gain > 4 pounds/week
     • Due to retention of sodium
   e. Generalized seizures
     (1) Preeclampsia + seizures is called eclampsia.
     (2) Magnesium sulfate is used for treatment.
   f. Renal disease
     (1) Swollen endothelial cells in the glomerular capillaries
     (2) Produces oliguria
   g. Liver disease
     (1) Right upper quadrant pain and hepatomegaly
     (2) Periportal necrosis with increased transaminases

Preeclampsia: placental hypoperfusion; vasoconstriction overrides vasodilation

Preeclampsia: premature aging of placenta; placental infarctions

Preeclampsia: hypertension, proteinuria, pitting edema

h. HELLP syndrome (refer to Chapter 18)
   • Hemolytic anemia and disseminated intravascular coagulation
5. Treatment
   a. Delivery is the treatment of choice and the only cure for the disease.
   b. Magnesium sulfate is given for seizures.

E. Gestational trophoblastic neoplasms
1. Hydatidiform moles
   a. Benign tumors of the chorionic villus
      • Complete and partial moles
   b. More common at the extremes of age
   c. Occurs in 1:1200 pregnancies in the United States
      • Occurs in 1:200 pregnancies in Indonesia
   d. Complete mole is the most common type.
      (1) The entire placenta is neoplastic.
      (2) Dilated, swollen villi without fetal blood vessels (Fig. 21-31)
      (3) *No* embryo is present.
      (4) 46,XX (90% of cases)
         (a) Both chromosomes are of male origin.
         (b) Egg is fertilized by two haploid spermatozoa with X chromosomes.
      (5) Increased risk for developing choriocarcinoma (20% chance)
      (6) Clinical findings
         (a) Painless vaginal bleeding in fourth or fifth month of pregnancy
         (b) Severe vomiting
         (c) Preeclampsia is present in 2% of patients.
         (d) Uterus is too large for gestational age.
         (e) Increased hCG for the gestational age
         (f) "Snowstorm appearance" with ultrasound (Fig. 21-32)
      (7) Treatment
         (a) Dilation and curettage
            • Must remove all material
         (b) Follow patient with hCG levels
            • Should go down to zero
   e. Partial mole
      (1) Not all villi are neoplastic or dilated.
      (2) Normal embryo is present (no chromosome abnormality).
         (a) Triploid (69,XY)
         (b) Egg with 23,X is fertilized by a 23,X and a 23,Y sperm.

Rx preeclampsia: delivery is treatment of choice; magnesium sulfate for seizures

Hydatidiform mole: benign tumor of chorionic villus

Complete mole: whole placenta is neoplastic; no embryo; 46,XX (both male Xs)

Complete mole: ultrasound with "snowstorm" appearance; too large for gastrointestinal age

Partial mole: part of placenta neoplastic; embryo present; 69 chromosomes

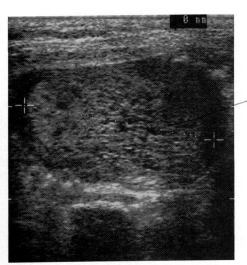

21-32: Ultrasound of a complete hydatidiform mole showing the classic "snowstorm" appearance. No fetus is present. *(From Greer I, Cameron IT, Kitchener HC, Prentice A: Mosby's Color Atlas and Text of Obstetrics and Gynecology. St. Louis, Mosby, 2000, p 94, Fig. 4-22.)*

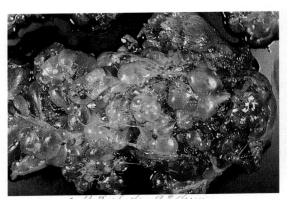

21-31: Complete hydatidiform mole. The enlarged and edematous villi are interconnected by thin cord-like structures. No fetus is present. *(From Damjanov I, Linder J: Pathology: A Color Atlas. St. Louis, Mosby, 2000, p 290, Fig. 13-111A.)*

(3) Preeclampsia in 5% of patients

(4) Low risk (2–3%) risk for developing a choriocarcinoma

2. Choriocarcinoma

   a. Malignant tumor composed of syncytiotrophoblast and cytotrophoblast

     • Chorionic villi are *not* present.

   b. Risk factors

     (1) Complete mole (50% of cases)

     (2) Spontaneous abortion (25% of cases)

     (3) Normal pregnancy (25% of cases)

   c. Common sites of metastasis

     (1) Lungs and vagina

     (2) Lesions are hemorrhagic.

   d. Excellent response to chemotherapy (methotrexate); low mortality rate

     • Good response does *not* apply to non–gestationally derived cancer.

F. Amniotic fluid

1. Composition

   a. Predominantly fetal urine

   b. High salt content causes ferning when dried on a slide.

     • Excellent sign of premature rupture of the amniotic sac

   c. Swallowed and recycled by the fetus

   d. Polyhydramnios

     (1) Excessive amniotic fluid

     (2) Causes

       (a) Tracheoesophageal (TE) fistula (refer to Chapter 17)

       (b) Duodenal atresia (refer to Chapter 17)

       (c) Maternal diabetes (20%)

         • Maternal hyperglycemia → fetal hyperglycemia → fetal polyuria

   e. Oligohydramnios

     (1) Decreased amount of amniotic fluid

     (2) Causes

       (a) Juvenile polycystic kidney disease (refer to Chapter 19)

       (b) Fetal genitourinary obstruction

       (c) Uteroplacental insufficiency

       (d) Premature rupture of membranes

2. α-Fetoprotein (AFP) in pregnancy

   a. Increased maternal AFP

     (1) Open neural tube defect

     (2) Related to folate deficiency

     (3) Folate stores should be adequate *before* pregnancy.

       • Neural tube is already developed by the end of the first month of gestation.

   b. Decreased maternal AFP

     • Down syndrome

3. Lecithin/sphingomyelin (L:S) ratio

   a. Lecithin

     (1) Synthesized by type II pneumocytes

     (2) Decreases alveolar surface tension to prevent atelectasis

   b. L:S ratio greater than 2 in amniotic fluid indicates adequate surfactant.

   c. Cortisol and thyroxine increase surfactant synthesis.

     • Maternal administration of glucocorticoids increases surfactant synthesis if babies must be delivered before term.

   d. Insulin inhibits surfactant synthesis.

G. Urine estriol in pregnancy

1. Derived from the fetal adrenal gland, placenta, and maternal liver

   a. Fetal zone of the adrenal cortex

     (1) Converts pregnenolone synthesized in the placenta to DHEA-sulfate

     (2) Fetal zone is absent in anencephaly (absent brain).

   b. Fetal liver

     • DHEA-sulfate is 16-hydroxylated to 16-OH-DHEA-sulfate.

   c. Maternal placenta

     (1) Placental sulfatase cleaves off the sulfate from 16-OH-DHEA-sulfate.

     (2) 16-OH-DHEA is converted by aromatase to free unbound estriol.

Marginal notes (left column):

Choriocarcinoma: malignancy of trophoblastic tissue; no chorionic villi

Choriocarcinoma: complete mole (50%); spontaneous abortion (25%); normal pregnancy (25%)

Amniotic fluid: high salt content causing ferning when dried on glass slide

Polyhydramnios: TE fistula, duodenal atresia, maternal diabetes (fetal polyuria)

Oligohydramnios: juvenile polycystic kidney disease

Increased AFP in pregnancy: open neural tube defect

L:S ratio > 2: adequate surfactant

Estriol: derived from fetal adrenal gland, placenta, maternal liver

d. Maternal liver
(1) Free estriol is conjugated to estriol sulfate and estriol glucosiduronate.
(2) Both compounds are excreted in maternal urine and bile.
2. Decreased levels of estriol
- Sign of fetal-maternal-placental dysfunction
3. Down syndrome triad
a. Decreased urine estriol
b. Decreased serum AFP
c. Increased serum β-hCG

X. **Breast Disorders**
A. Clinical anatomy
1. High-density locations of breast tissue
a. Upper outer quadrant
- Underscores why cancer is most commonly located in this quadrant
b. Beneath the nipple
2. Hormone effects during menstrual cycle
a. Estrogen
- Stimulates ductal and alveolar growth
b. Progesterone
- Stimulates alveolar differentiation
3. Hormone effects in lactation
a. Prolactin
- Stimulates and maintains lactogenesis
b. Oxytocin
(1) Released by suckling reflex
(2) Expulsion of milk into ducts
4. Lymph nodes
a. Outer quadrant cancers
- Drain to the axillary lymph nodes
b. Inner quadrant cancers
- Drain to the internal mammary nodes
B. Locations for breast lesions (Fig. 21-33)
C. Nipple discharges
1. Galactorrhea; causes other than lactation:
a. Mechanical stimulation of the nipple
(1) Prolonged sucking of nipple
(2) Sexual intercourse
(3) Most common physiologic cause of galactorrhea
b. Prolactinoma (refer to Chapter 22)
- Most common pathologic cause of galactorrhea (Fig. 21-34)
c. Primary hypothyroidism (refer to Chapter 22)
(1) Most common nonpituitary endocrine disease causing galactorrhea
(2) Decreased serum thyroxine increases thyrotropin-releasing factor (TRF).
- TRF stimulates prolactin.
d. Drugs
- Examples—OCPs, phenothiazines, methyldopa, H_2-receptor blockers, anxiolytics

Margin notes:

Decreased estriol: fetal-maternal-placental dysfunction

Down syndrome triad: ↓ urine estriol, serum AFP; ↑ serum hCG

Upper outer quadrant: most common location for cancer

Outer quadrant cancer: axillary node involvement

Inner quadrant cancer: internal mammary node involvement

Galactorrhea: mechanical stimulation of nipple most common physiologic cause

Prolactinoma: most common pathologic cause of galactorrhea

Galactorrhea: primary hypothyroidism; ↑ TRH stimulates prolactin release

Galactorrhea: drugs very common cause

Nipple/areola complex	Lactiferous sinus	Major duct	Terminal duct	Lobule	Stroma
Paget's disease Breast abscess	Intraductal papilloma Breast abscess Plasma cell mastitis	Fibrocystic change Ductal cancer	Tubular carcinoma	Lobular carcinoma Sclerosing adenosis	Fibroadenoma Phyllodes tumor

21-33: Locations for breast lesions. See text for discussion. *(Redrawn from Goljan EF: Star Series: Pathology. Philadelphia, WB Saunders, 1998, Fig. 18-3.)*

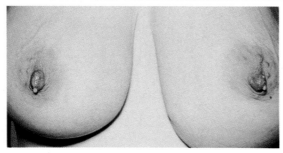

21-34: Galactorrhea in a patient with a prolactinoma. *(From Mansel R, Bundred N: Color Atlas of Breast Disease. St. Louis, Mosby, 1995.)*

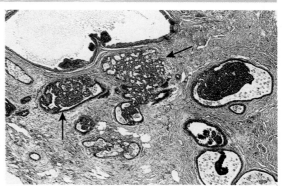

21-35: Fibrocystic change. The microscopic section shows cystic spaces surrounded by a dense fibrous stroma. The large cyst at the top has eosinophilic staining cells exhibiting apocrine metaplasia. The smaller cysts *(arrows)* show extensive ductal hyperplasia with a sieve-like pattern. *(From Rosai J, Ackerman LV: Surgical Pathology, 9th ed. St. Louis, Mosby, 2004, p 1780, Fig. 20-30.)*

2. Bloody nipple discharge
   - Intraductal papilloma, ductal cancer
3. Purulent nipple discharge
   a. Acute mastitis due to *Staphylococcus aureus*
   b. Usually occurs during lactation or breast-feeding
   c. Treatment
      (1) If not methicillin resistant, dicloxacillin or cephalexin
      (2) If methicillin resistant, trimethoprim-sulfamethoxazole
4. Greenish brown nipple discharge
   - Mammary duct ectasia (plasma cell mastitis)

D. Breast pain
   1. Most common cause is fibrocystic change
   2. Mondor's disease
      a. Superficial thrombophlebitis of veins overlying the breast
      b. Presents as a palpable, painful cord

E. Fibrocystic change (FCC)
   1. Epidemiology and pathogenesis
      a. Most common painful breast mass in women < 50 years old
      b. Occurs in >50% of women in the reproductive period of life
      c. Distortion of normal cyclic breast changes
   2. Small and large cysts (Fig. 21-35)
      a. Some cysts have hemorrhage into the cyst fluid.
         - Called "blue-domed" cysts
      b. Vary in size with the menstrual cycle
      c. *No* malignant potential
      d. May have to surgically remove if recurrent
   3. Fibrosis
      - *No* malignant potential
   4. Sclerosing adenosis
      a. Proliferation of small ductules/acini in the lobule
         - Pattern is often confused with infiltrating ductal cancer.
      b. Often contain microcalcifications
   5. Ductal hyperplasia
      a. Ducts are estrogen-sensitive.
      b. Pathologic findings
         (1) Papillary proliferation is called papillomatosis.
         (2) Apocrine metaplasia refers to the presence of large, pink-staining cells.
         (3) Atypical ductal hyperplasia
            - Increased risk for developing cancer, because it is due to excess estrogen stimulation

F. Inflammation
   1. Acute mastitis (see earlier discussion)

Margin notes:

Bloody discharge: intraductal papilloma; ductal cancer

Purulent discharge: acute mastitis during breast feeding

Breast pain: most common cause is fibrocystic change

FCC: most common breast mass in women < 50 years old

Cysts and fibrosis: "lumpy bumpy" feeling on breast examination

Sclerosing adenosis: often contain microcalcifications seen on mammogram

Atypical ductal hyperplasia: increased risk for breast cancer

2. Mammary duct ectasia (plasma cell mastitis)
   a. Epidemiology
      (1) Affects 25% of women in menopause
      (2) Main ducts fill up with debris.
         (a) Causes dilation, rupture, and inflammation
         (b) Greenish brown nipple discharge
      (3) May produce skin and nipple retraction simulating cancer
      (4) *No* increased risk for breast cancer
   b. Treatment
      (1) Antibiotics if infection is present
      (2) Surgical removal of blocked duct
3. Traumatic fat necrosis
   a. Trauma to breast tissue
   b. Microscopic findings
      (1) Lipid-laden macrophages with foreign body giant cells
      (2) Fibrosis, dystrophic calcification
   c. Painless, indurated mass
      • Painful in acute stage
   d. May produce skin retraction simulating cancer
4. Silicone breast implant
   a. Polymer of silica, oxygen, and hydrogen
   b. Silicone gel can leak or the implant can rupture
      (1) Produces foreign body giant cells and chronic inflammation
      (2) Association with autoimmune disease is *not* proved.

G. Benign breast tumors
1. Fibroadenoma
   a. Epidemiology
      (1) Most common breast tumor in women < 35 years old
      (2) Most commonly diagnosed breast tumor
      (3) Develop in 50% of women who receive cyclosporine after renal transplantation
      (4) Discrete movable, painless or painful mass (Fig. 21-36).
         • Multiple lesions may be present (10–15%).
      (5) Benign tumor derived from the stroma
         (a) Stroma proliferates and compresses the ducts (Fig. 21-37).
         (b) Duct epithelium is *not* neoplastic.
      (6) Increases in size during pregnancy
         • Estrogen-sensitive
      (7) May spontaneously disappear or involute during menopause
      (8) Do *not* progress into cancer; however, breast cancer may secondarily develop within duct epithelial cells as a separate event (3%)
   b. Diagnosis
      • Fine needle or core needle biopsy

Mammary duct ectasia: common in menopause; greenish brown nipple discharge

Traumatic fat necrosis: usually painless indurated mass; associated with trauma to breast tissue

Silicone breast implant rupture: foreign body giant cell reaction

Fibroadenoma: most common breast tumor women < 40 years old

Fibroadenoma: commonly develop in women taking cyclosporine

Fibroadenoma: benign tumor derived from stroma

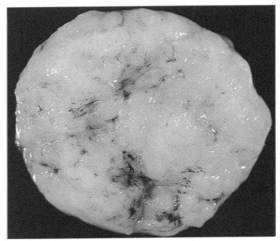

21-36: Fibroadenoma. Note the bulging gray-white surface of this benign stromal tumor. *(From Damjanov I, Linder J: Pathology: A Color Atlas. St. Louis, Mosby, 2000, p. 298, Fig. 14-3.)*

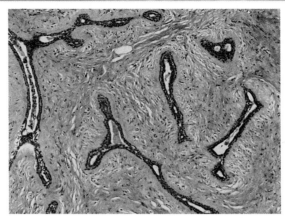

21-37: Fibroadenoma: A microscopic section shows compressed, elongated ducts surrounded by neoplastic stromal tissue. *(From Damjanov I: Pathology for the Health-Related Professions, 2nd ed. Philadelphia, WB Saunders, 2000, p 405, Fig. 16-5B.)*

c. Treatment
   (1) Surgical removal
   (2) Cryoablation
2. Phyllodes tumor
   a. Bulky tumor derived from stromal cells
   b. Most often benign but can be malignant in some cases
      • Hypercellular stroma with mitoses are signs of malignancy.
   c. Lobulated tumor with cystic spaces containing leaf-like extensions
      • Often reach massive size
   d. Treat by wide excision.
3. Intraductal papilloma
   a. Most common cause of bloody nipple discharge in women < 50 years old
   b. Develop in the lactiferous ducts or sinuses
   c. No increased risk for cancer
   d. Surgically remove the duct or sinus.
H. Breast cancer
   1. Epidemiology
      a. Most common cancer in adult women (1:8 lifetime risk)
         (1) Mean age is 64 years old.
         (2) Risk increases with age.
      b. Most common breast mass in women > 50 years old
      c. Slightly decreasing in incidence due to early detection and treatment
      d. Second most common cancer-producing death in women
         • It is also the second most common cancer producing death in adults (includes men and women as a group).
   2. Risk factors
      a. Common denominators for increased risk of cancer
         (1) Prolonged estrogen stimulation
         (2) Genetically susceptible background
      b. Family history and genetics
         (1) Increased risk if breast cancer involves first-generation relatives
            • Mother, sister
         (2) Genetic basis is involved in <10% of cases (refer to Chapter 8).
            (a) Autosomal dominant *BRCA1* and *BRCA2* association
               • Breasts or ovaries are frequently prophylactically removed.
            (b) Li-Fraumeni multicancer syndrome
               • Inactivation of *TP53* suppressor gene
            (3) Other gene relationships
               • *RAS* oncogene, *ERBB2*, *RB* suppressor gene
      c. Prolonged estrogen stimulation
         (1) Early menarche/late menopause
         (2) Nulliparity

Phyllodes tumor: benign, borderline, or malignant; depends on stromal cellularity

Intraductal papilloma: most common cause of bloody nipple discharge in women < 50 years old

Breast cancer: most common cancer in women

Breast cancer risk: prolonged estrogen stimulation, genetically susceptible background

Genetic basis: <10%

(3) Postmenopausal obesity
  - Aromatization of androstenedione to estrone
(4) Hormone replacement therapy
d. Atypical ductal hyperplasia
e. Endometrial cancer, ionizing radiation, smoking cigarettes
f. High breast density (determined by mammogram)
g. Recent use of OCPs; obesity after menopause
h. Use of postmenopausal hormone therapy (estrogen and progestin therapy)
3. Factors that decrease the risk for breast cancer
  a. Breast-feeding
  b. Moderate or vigorous physical training
  c. Healthy body weight
4. Clinical findings
  a. Painless mass in the breast
    - Usually in the upper outer quadrant
  b. Skin or nipple retraction
  c. Painless axillary lymphadenopathy
  d. Hepatomegaly; bone pain if metastasis has occurred
5. Mammography
  a. Primarily a screening test
    - Detects nonpalpable breast masses (detects 80–90%)
  b. Does *not* distinguish benign from malignant lesions
  c. Screening usually starts annually at age 40; earlier if patient is high risk
  d. Identifies microcalcifications (Fig. 21-38) and spiculated masses with or without microcalcifications (30–50%)
    (1) Most often occur in ductal carcinoma in situ (DCIS) and sclerosing adenosis
    (2) Microcalcification pattern suggesting malignancy
      - Five or more tightly clustered microcalcifications that are punctate, microlinear, or branching
6. Types of breast cancer (Table 21-5 and Fig. 21-39)
7. Natural history, treatment, and prognosis
  a. Spread first by lymphatics and then hematogenously
    (1) Outer quadrant cancer spreads to axillary nodes.
    (2) Inner quadrant cancers spread to internal mammary nodes.
  b. Extranodal metastasis
    (1) Common sites of metastasis
      - Lungs, bone, liver, brain, ovaries
    (2) May metastasize 10 to 15 years after treatment
    (3) Pain in bone metastasis is relieved with radiation.

Risk factors: unopposed estrogen; recent use of OCPs

Factors reducing risk: breast-feeding; exercise; healthy body weight

Clinical: painless mass; skin/nipple retraction

Mammography: detect nonpalpable masses

Initial management of breast mass: fine needle aspiration

Microcalcifications: DCIS, sclerosing adenosis

Breast cancer: most common cancer metastatic to lungs and bone

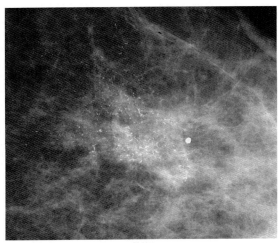

21-38: Mammogram with microcalcifications. The biopsy in this patient shows breast cancer. *(From Pretorius ES, Solomon JA: Radiology Secrets, 2nd ed. St. Louis, Mosby, 2006, p 43, Fig. 6-5.)*

TABLE 21-5. **TYPES OF BREAST CANCER**

TYPE	COMMENTS
Noninvasive	
Ductal carcinoma in situ (DCIS) (see Fig. 21-39A)	Nonpalpable Patterns: cribriform (sieve-like), comedo (necrotic center) Commonly contain microcalcifications; cannot be detected by mammogram unless microcalcifications are present One third eventually invade Treated with "lumpectomy"
Lobular carcinoma in situ (see Fig. 21-39B)	Nonpalpable; virtually always an incidental finding in a breast biopsy for other reasons; cannot be identified by mammography Lobules distended with bland neoplastic cells; one third eventually invade; usually estrogen and progesterone receptor positive Increased incidence of cancer in the opposite breast (50–75%); does *not* have to be a lobular cancer
Invasive	
Infiltrating ductal carcinoma (see Fig. 21-39C and D)	Stellate morphology, indurated, gray-white tumor One third have amplification of *ERBB2* oncogene Gritty on cut section Induration caused by reactive fibroplasia (desmoplasia)
Paget's disease of nipple (see Fig. 21-39E)	Extension of DCIS into lactiferous ducts and skin of nipple producing a rash with or without nipple retraction Paget's cells are present Palpable mass present in 50–60%
Medullary carcinoma	Associated with *BRCA1* mutations Bulky, soft tumor with large cells and lymphoid infiltrate Majority are estrogen and progesterone receptor negative
Inflammatory carcinoma (see Fig. 21-39F)	Erythematous breast with dimpling like an orange (peau d'orange) due to fixed opening of the sweat glands, which cannot expand with lymphedema Plugs of tumor blocking lumen of dermal lymphatics cause localized lymphedema Very poor prognosis Combination chemotherapy followed by surgery and irradiation
Invasive lobular carcinoma	Neoplastic cells arranged in linear fashion or form concentric circles (bull's-eye appearance)
Tubular carcinoma	Develops in terminal ductules Increased incidence of cancer in opposite breast (10–40%)
Colloid (mucinous) carcinoma	Usually occurs in elderly women Neoplastic cells are surrounded by extracellular mucin

c. Staging
  (1) Extranodal metastasis has greater significance than nodal metastasis (refer to Chapter 9)
  (2) Sentinel node biopsy
    (a) Sampling of the initial node that drains the tumor
    (b) If negative for metastasis, the other nodes in that group are usually negative.
    (c) If positive for metastasis, there is a one-third chance that other nodes in that group have metastases.
d. Estrogen and progesterone receptor assays (ERA and PRA, respectively)
  (1) Most often positive in postmenopausal women
  (2) Clinical significance
    (a) Confers an overall better prognosis
    (b) Candidate for antiestrogen therapy with tamoxifen or raloxifene
e. Other tests performed on tissue
  (1) S phase fraction
    • Above 5% is poor prognosis.
  (2) DNA ploidy
    • Diploid tumor is better than an aneuploid tumor.
  (3) *ERBB2* oncogene status
    • Poor prognosis if amplification (multiple copies) is present (refer to Chapter 8).
f. Treatment for high-risk patients *without* breast cancer
  • Treatment with tamoxifen or raloxifene reduces risk.

Breast cancer: extranodal spread has greater significance than nodal metastasis alone

Sentinel node: initial node draining the tumor

ERA-PRA receptor assays: positive assay confers better prognosis

ERBB2 oncogene: if positive in breast tissue, poor prognosis

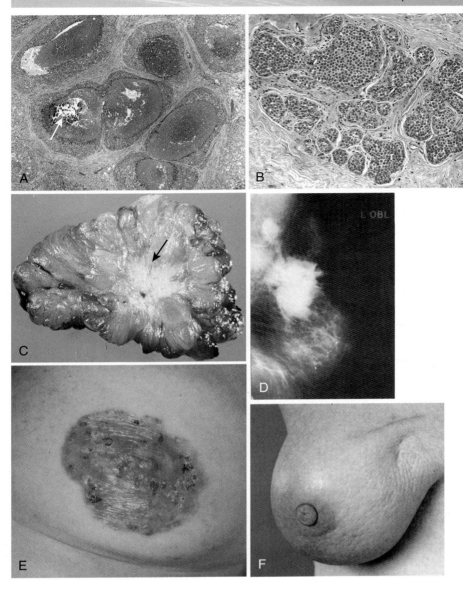

21-39: A, Ductal carcinoma in situ (DCIS) showing dilated ducts lined by layers of neoplastic cells. Central areas of necrosis (comedo pattern) are present, some of which contain microcalcifications (*arrow*). **B,** Lobular carcinoma in situ showing complete replacement and expansion of a lobule by a monomorphic population of cells. **C,** Infiltrating ductal carcinoma showing a stellate-shaped scar (*arrow*) in the fat tissue of the breast. **D,** Mammogram showing a large irregular spicular mass lesion, which on biopsy showed an infiltrating ductal carcinoma. **E,** Paget's disease of the breast showing an erythematous rash around the nipple. **F,** Inflammatory carcinoma of the right breast. Note the dimpled appearance of the breast (peau d'orange) and retraction of the skin. (*A and B from Kumar V, Fausto N, Abbas A: Robbins and Cotran's Pathologic Basis of Disease, 7th ed. Philadelphia, WB Saunders, 2004, pp 1139, 1142, Figs. 23-16B, 23-20, respectively; C from Damjanov I, Linder J: Pathology: A Color Atlas. St. Louis, Mosby, 2000, p 304, Fig. 14-14A; D and F from Grieg JD: Color Atlas of Surgical Diagnosis. London, Mosby-Wolfe, 1996, p 33, Figs. 6-22, 6-23, respectively; E from Swartz MH: Textbook of Physical Diagnosis, 5th ed. Philadelphia, Saunders Elsevier, 2006, p 468, Fig. 16-13.*)

g. Surgical procedures
   (1) Modified radical mastectomy; includes:
       (a) Nipple/areolar complex
       (b) All breast tissue
       (c) Pectoralis minor
       (d) Level I and II axillary lymph nodes in continuity
           • Level I nodes are inferior to the pectoralis minor muscle; level II nodes are beneath the pectoralis minor.
       (e) Level III nodes if level I and II nodes are grossly involved
           • Level III nodes are medial and superior to the pectoralis minor.

A **winged scapula** may occur due to damage of the long thoracic nerve. There is also a danger for developing lymphedema.

Winged scapula: damage to long thoracic nerve

   (2) Breast conservation therapy
       (a) Lumpectomy with microscopically free margins
       (b) Sentinel node biopsy (preferable) or removal of level I and II axillary nodes
       (c) Breast irradiation

Breast conservation therapy has similar survival rate as modified radical mastectomy

h. Prognosis
(1) The 5-year relative survival rate for localized breast cancer (no node involvement) is 98%.
(2) The 5-year relative survival rate for breast cancer with nodal involvement is 84%.
(3) The 5-year relative survival rate for breast cancer with distant spread is 27%.
(4) Survival rate at 5 years for all stages combined is 89%.
(5) Survival rate at 10 years for all stages combined is 80%.

I. Gynecomastia

Gynecomastia: benign glandular proliferation of male breast tissue

1. Benign glandular proliferation in the male breast due to estrogen
   a. Subareolar mass (see Fig. 18-9)
   b. More often unilateral than bilateral
   c. Due to increased estrogen stimulation
      (1) Increase in estrogen
      (2) Decrease in androgens (leaves estrogen unopposed)
      (3) Defect in androgen receptors (leaves estrogen unopposed)

Estrogen sources: peripheral aromatization of androgens; Leydig cells in testis

   d. Source of estrogen
      (1) Peripheral aromatization (85%)
         (a) Testosterone to estradiol
         (b) Androstenedione to estrone
      (2) Leydig cells (15%)

Gynecomastia: normal in newborn, adolescence, elderly

2. Physiologic gynecomastia
   a. Normal in the following:
      (1) Newborn (60–90%)
      (2) Puberty (peaks at ages 13–14 years)
      (3) Elderly (occurs between 50–80 years of age)
   b. In general, surgery is *not* indicated.
3. Pathologic gynecomastia

Gynecomastia: most common pathologic cause is cirrhosis (hyperestrinism)

   a. Cirrhosis
      (1) Inability to metabolize estrogen
      (2) Inability to metabolize 17-ketosteroids
         • Peripherally aromatized to estrone

Genetic causes: Klinefelter's syndrome, testicular feminization

   b. Genetic diseases
      (1) Klinefelter's syndrome (refer to Chapter 5)
         • Increased aromatization of androgens to estrogens in Leydig cells
      (2) Testicular feminization (refer to Chapter 5)
         • Decreased androgen receptor synthesis

Drug causes: spironolactone, ketoconazole, DES, digoxin, flutamide, leuprolide

   c. Drugs
      (1) Drug displacement of estrogen from SHBG
         • Spironolactone, ketoconazole
      (2) Drugs with estrogen activity
         • Diethylstilbestrol, digoxin (activates estrogen receptors)
      (3) Drugs that block androgen receptors
         • Spironolactone, flutamide
      (4) Drugs that decrease androgen production
         • Leuprolide

Cancer causes: choriocarcinoma

   d. Cancer
      • Choriocarcinoma of testis producing hCG (LH analogue)
   e. Disorders with decreased androgen production
      (1) Primary hypogonadism
         • Leydig cell dysfunction (refer to Chapter 20)
      (2) Secondary hypogonadism
         • Pituitary/hypothalamic dysfunction (refer to Chapter 22)

J. Breast cancer in men

Breast cancer in men: Klinefelter's; inactivation of *BRCA2* suppressor gene

1. Risk factors
   a. Inactivation of *BRCA2* suppressor gene
   b. Klinefelter's syndrome
2. Usually have a poor prognosis

CHAPTER 22
ENDOCRINE DISORDERS

I. **Overview of Endocrine Disease**
  A. **Negative feedback loops**
    1. Control an increase or decrease in hormone production
    2. Example—increased calcium decreases parathyroid hormone (PTH).
  B. **Stimulation tests**
    1. Evaluate hypofunctioning disorders
      • Example—adrenocorticotropic hormone (ACTH) stimulation test is used in the workup of hypocortisolism.
    2. Causes of hypofunction
      a. Autoimmune destruction
        • Examples—Addison's disease, Hashimoto's thyroiditis
      b. Infarction
        • Example—Sheehan's postpartum necrosis, Waterhouse-Friderichsen syndrome
      c. Decreased hormone stimulation
        • Example—decreased thyroid-stimulating hormone in hypopituitarism
      d. Enzyme deficiency, infection, neoplasia, congenital disorder
  C. **Suppression tests**
    1. Evaluate hyperfunctioning disorders
      • Example—dexamethasone suppression test evaluates hypercortisolism.
    2. Most hyperfunctioning disorders *cannot* be suppressed.
      • Notable *exceptions* are prolactinoma and pituitary Cushing syndrome.
    3. Causes of hyperfunction
      • Adenoma, acute inflammation, hyperplasia, cancer
II. **Hypothalamus Disorders**
  A. **Tumors altering hypothalamic function**
    1. Pituitary adenoma (see section IV)
      • Most common tumor affecting the hypothalamus
    2. Craniopharyngioma (see section IV)
    3. Midline hamartoma
      • *Not* a neoplasm
    4. Langerhans histiocytosis (refer to Chapter 13)
  B. **Inflammatory disorders altering hypothalamic function**
    1. Sarcoidosis (refer to Chapter 16)
      • Produces granulomatous inflammation
    2. Meningitis (refer to Chapter 25)
  C. **Clinical findings of hypothalamic dysfunction**
    1. Secondary hypopituitarism
      • *No* releasing hormones to stimulate the anterior pituitary
    2. Central diabetes insipidus (CDI)
      • Antidiuretic hormone (ADH) is synthesized in the hypothalamus.
    3. Hyperprolactinemia
      • Loss of dopamine inhibition causes galactorrhea.
    4. Precocious puberty
      • Most common cause in boys is a midline hamartoma.

Margin notes:

Negative feedback: ↑ calcium, ↓ PTH; ↓ calcium, ↑ PTH

Endocrine gland hypofunction: use stimulation tests

Endocrine gland hypofunction: most common cause is autoimmune disease

Endocrine gland hyperfunction: use suppression tests

Endocrine gland hyperfunction: pituitary Cushing syndrome and prolactinoma can suppress

Endocrine gland hyperfunction: most common cause is a benign adenoma

Hypothalamic dysfunction: secondary hypopituitarism, CDI, ↑ prolactin; precocious puberty, visual field defects, mass effects (hydrocephalus)

Precocious puberty: true if CNS origin, pseudo if peripheral cause

"True" precocious puberty implies a central nervous system (CNS) origin for the disorder, but pseudo-precocious puberty implies a peripheral cause (e.g., adrenogenital syndrome). True precocious puberty in boys is the onset of puberty *before* 9 years of age. The most common cause is a midline hamartoma in the hypothalamus. True precocious puberty in girls is the onset of puberty *before* 8 years of age. In most cases, it is idiopathic and less likely to be caused by a midline hamartoma.

5. Visual field disturbances
   - Usually bitemporal hemianopia
6. Mass effects
   - Produces obstructive hydrocephalus (refer to Chapter 25)
7. Growth disorders
   - Dwarfism in children
8. Kallmann's syndrome (refer to Chapter 20)

III. **Pineal Gland Disorders**
   A. **Clinical anatomy**

Pineal gland: midline above quadrigeminal plate

   1. Midline location above the quadrigeminal plate
   2. Site for melatonin production
      a. Superior cervical sympathetic ganglia stimulates receptors on pinealocytes.
         - Causes release of melatonin into spinal fluid and blood

Melatonin: chemical messenger of darkness

      b. Melatonin functions
         (1) Important in sleep/moods and circadian rhythms
            - Released at night
         (2) Used in the treatment of sleep and mood disorders
   B. **Disorders**

Pineal gland: commonly undergoes dystrophic calcification

   1. Dystrophic calcification of the pineal gland begins in childhood.
      a. Useful in showing shifts due to mass lesions in the brain
      b. Approximately 80% are calcified between 70 and 80 years old.

Pineal gland: majority are germ cell tumors

   2. Pineal tumors
      a. Majority are germ cell tumors resembling seminomas.
      b. Minority of tumors are teratomas.
   C. **Clinical findings**

Pineal gland tumors: paralysis of upward gaze ("setting sun" sign)

   1. Visual disturbances
      - Paralysis of upward conjugate gaze (Parinaud's syndrome; see Fig. 25-5)
   2. Obstructive hydrocephalus
      - Due to compression of the aqueduct of Sylvius in the third ventricle

IV. **Pituitary Gland Disorders**
   A. **Anterior pituitary hypofunction**
   1. Epidemiology
      a. Partial or complete loss of secretion of one or more hormones
         - Infarctions of the pituitary invariably lead to panhypopituitarism
      b. Increased incidence of vascular or cerebrovascular disease

Pituitary infarction: invariably produces panhypopituitarism

      c. Types of pituitary dysfunction
         (1) Primary hypopituitarism (pituitary dysfunction)
            - Approximately 75% of the gland must be destroyed.
         (2) Secondary hypopituitarism (hypothalamic dysfunction)
            - Decreased hypothalamic releasing factors
   2. Causes of hypopituitarism

Hypopituitarism in adults: most common cause is nonfunctioning adenoma

      a. Nonfunctioning (null) pituitary adenoma (Fig. 22-1)
         (1) Most common cause
         (2) Microadenoma < 10 mm; macroadenoma > 10 mm

MEN I: pituitary adenoma, hyperparathyroidism, pancreatic tumor

         (3) Association with multiple endocrine neoplasia (MEN) I syndrome
         (4) MEN I syndrome findings include pituitary adenoma, hyperparathyroidism, pancreatic tumor (Zollinger-Ellison syndrome or insulinoma).

Hypopituitarism in children: most common cause is craniopharyngioma

      b. Craniopharyngioma
         (1) Most common cause of hypopituitarism in children
         (2) Benign pituitary tumor derived from Rathke's pouch remnants

Rathke's pouch is an ectodermal derivative derived from the oral cavity. It develops into the anterior lobe of the pituitary gland.

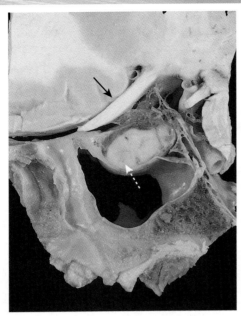

22-1: Pituitary adenoma. The *interrupted arrow* shows a well-circumscribed mass that has almost completely replaced the pituitary gland. A thin rim of sella turcica is present at the base of the tumor. The *solid arrow* shows the optic nerve and its proximity to the sella turcica. *(From Burger PC, Scheithauer BW, Vogel KS: Surgical Pathology of the Nervous System, 4th ed. London, Churchill Livingstone, 2002, p 444, Fig. 9-20.)*

    (3) Located *above* the sella turcica
       • Extends into sella turcica and destroys the gland
    (4) Cystic tumor with hemorrhage and calcification
    (5) Commonly causes bitemporal hemianopia
    (6) May produce central diabetes insipidus
  c. Sheehan's postpartum necrosis
    (1) Hypovolemic shock (e.g., blood loss) causes infarction.
    (2) Sudden cessation of lactation due to loss of prolactin
       • Eventual development of hypopituitarism

Rathke's pouch: develops anterior pituitary

Sheehan's postpartum necrosis: sudden cessation of lactation; pituitary infarction secondary to shock

> The **pituitary gland** doubles in size during pregnancy due to synthesis of prolactin. Prolactin release is inhibited by estrogen and progesterone during pregnancy.

  d. Pituitary apoplexy
    (1) Term "apoplexy" refers to a sudden onset of neurologic dysfunction
    (2) Most often due to hemorrhage/infarction of preexisting pituitary adenoma
    (3) Predisposing factors
       • Trauma, pregnancy (Sheehan's postpartum necrosis, a nontumorous cause), treatment of a prolactinoma with bromocriptine
    (4) Clinical findings; sudden onset of
      (a) Headache, mental status dysfunction, visual disturbances
      (b) Hormone dysfunction
  e. Sickle cell anemia
    • Pituitary infarction from vascular occlusion by irreversibly sickled cells
  f. Lymphocytic hypophysitis
    (1) Female dominant autoimmune destruction of the pituitary gland
    (2) Occurs during or after pregnancy
  g. Empty sella syndrome
    (1) Epidemiology
      (a) Radiologic studies show an empty sella turcica.
      (b) Primary and secondary types
    (2) Primary type
      (a) Anatomic defect above pituitary
      (b) Subarachnoid space extends into sella turcica and fills up with cerebrospinal fluid (CSF).

Pituitary apoplexy: hemorrhage into preexisting adenoma

Lymphocytic hypophysitis: autoimmune destruction; occurs during or after pregnancy

Empty sella syndrome: subarachnoid space extends into sella; ↑ CSF pressure compresses gland

Empty sella syndrome: obese with hypertension

(c) Increase in pressure on the pituitary gland causes it to flatten out.
(d) Often associated with women who are obese and have high blood pressure
(3) Secondary type
• Regression in size due to radiation, trauma, surgery
h. Hypothalamic dysfunction (see section II)
3. Clinical and laboratory findings of pituitary hypofunction (Table 22-1 and Fig. 22-2)
4. Diagnosis
a. CT scan or MRI (better test) of sella turcica
b. Stimulation tests for the various deficiencies
5. Treatment
a. Surgery for tumors (usually transsphenoidal)
b. Hormone replacement for deficiencies

TABLE 22-1. **CLINICAL FINDINGS IN HYPOPITUITARISM**

TROPHIC HORMONE DEFICIENCY	DISCUSSION
Gonadotropins (FSH, LH) (see Fig. 22-2A and B)	Children have delayed puberty Adult females have secondary amenorrhea; produces osteoporosis, hot flashes (lack of estrogen), decreased libido Males have impotence, due to decreased libido from decreased testosterone (refer to Chapter 20) GnRH stimulation test: *No* significant increase of FSH/LH in hypopituitarism Eventual increase of FSH/LH in hypothalamic disease Metyrapone test: stimulation test of pituitary ACTH reserve; metyrapone inhibits adrenal 11-hydroxylase, which causes a decrease in cortisol and a corresponding increase in plasma ACTH (pituitary) and 11-deoxycortisol (adrenal), which is proximal to the enzyme block; in hypopituitarism, neither ACTH or 11-deoxycortisol are increased
Growth hormone (GH)	Decreased GH decreases synthesis and release of IGF-1 Children have growth delay: delayed fusion of epiphyses; bone growth does *not* match the age of the child Adults have hypoglycemia: decreased gluconeogenesis; loss of muscle mass; increased adipose around waist Arginine and sleep stimulation tests: *no* increase in GH or IGF-1; normally, GH and IGF-1 are released at 5 AM
Thyroid-stimulating hormone (TSH)	Secondary hypothyroidism: decreased serum T_4 and TSH Cold intolerance, constipation, weakness *No* increase in TSH after TRF stimulation
Adrenocorticotropic hormone (ACTH)	Secondary hypocortisolism: decreased ACTH and cortisol Hypoglycemia: decreased gluconeogenesis Hyponatremia: mild SIADH (loss of inhibitory effect of cortisol on ADH) Weakness, fatigue Short ACTH stimulation test: *no* increase in serum cortisol over decreased baseline levels Prolonged ACTH stimulation test: eventual increase in cortisol over the decreased baseline value once the adrenal gland is restimulated Metyrapone test: no increase in ACTH or 11-deoxycorticosterone (see above gonadotropin discussion)

ADH, antidiuretic hormone; FSH, follicle-stimulating hormone; GnRH, gonadotropin-releasing hormone; IGF, insulin growth factor; LH, luteinizing hormone; SIADH, syndrome of inappropriate antidiuretic hormone; T_4, thyroxine; TRF, thyrotropin-releasing factor.

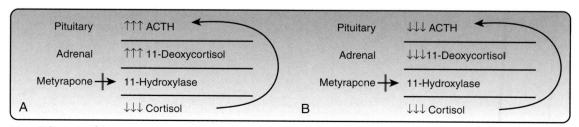

22-2: Schematic of the metyrapone test: a normal response (**A**) and the response expected in hypopituitarism (**B**). See text for discussion. ACTH, adrenocorticotropic hormone.

B. Posterior pituitary hypofunction
1. Normal function of posterior pituitary
    a. Stores ADH
        (1) Controls total body water
        (2) Presence of ADH produces concentration of urine.
        (3) Absence of ADH produces dilution of urine.
    b. Releases oxytocin
        • Produces milk ejection and uterine contractions
2. Refer to Chapter 4 for discussion of diabetes insipidus
C. Pituitary hyperfunction disorders
1. Prolactinoma
    a. Epidemiology
        (1) Benign adenoma
        (2) Overall most common pituitary tumor (35%)
        (3) Secrete growth hormone as well in 7% of cases
    b. Clinical and laboratory findings
        (1) Women
            (a) Secondary amenorrhea
                • Prolactin inhibits gonadotropin-releasing hormone (GnRH).
            (b) Galactorrhea (see Fig. 21-34)
        (2) Men
            (a) Impotence
                • Loss of libido due to decrease in testosterone
            (b) Headache
                • Tumors tend to be larger than in women.
            (c) *Not* enough estrogen-dependent breast tissue to produce galactorrhea
        (3) Serum prolactin level is usually >200 ng/mL.
        (4) Decreased follicle-stimulating hormone (FSH) and luteinizing hormone (LH)
            • Due to decreased GnRH
    c. Other causes of galactorrhea (refer to Chapter 21)
    d. Treatment
        (1) Dopamine analogues (e.g., cabergoline)
            (a) Tumor does respond to suppression.
                • Shrinks in <50% of cases
            (b) Restores gonadal function in 70% to 90% of cases
        (2) Surgery if macroadenomas
2. Growth hormone (GH) adenoma
    a. Epidemiology
        (1) Accounts for 20% of all pituitary adenomas
        (2) Functions of GH
            (a) Stimulates liver synthesis/release of insulin growth factor (IGF)-1
            (b) Stimulates gluconeogenesis and amino acid uptake in muscle
            (c) Negative feedback relationship with glucose and IGF-1
            (d) Antinatriuretic action (retains sodium)
        (3) Functions of IGF-1
            • Stimulates growth of bone (linear and lateral), cartilage, soft tissue
    b. Clinical and laboratory findings
        (1) Children develop gigantism.
            (a) Due to increased linear bone growth (epiphyses have not fused)
            (b) Lateral bone growth also increased
        (2) Adults develop acromegaly (Fig. 22-3)
            (a) Increased lateral bone growth (e.g., hands, feet, jaw)
                • *No* linear growth because epiphyses are fused
            (b) Prominent jaw
                • Spacing between the teeth
            (c) Frontal bossing
                • Enlarged frontal sinus increases the hat size.
            (d) Macroglossia, cardiomyopathy (cause of death)
        (3) Increased GH and IGF-1 (more sensitive test than GH)
            • Hormones are *not* suppressed by glucose administration.
        (4) Hyperglycemia
            • Due to increase in gluconeogenesis

Posterior pituitary: storage of ADH and release of oxytocin

Prolactinoma: most common pituitary tumor

Prolactinoma: secondary amenorrhea + galactorrhea

Prolactinoma in men: impotence due to loss of libido; headache

Rx prolactinoma: dopamine analogues; surgery

GH: gluconeogenesis; ↑ amino acid uptake in muscle; stimulate IGF-1 in liver

IGF-1: stimulates bone, cartilage, soft tissue growth

Gigantism: ↑ linear/ lateral bone growth in children; epiphyses *not* fused

Acromegaly: ↑ lateral bone growth only (epiphyses not fused), organomegaly, hyperglycemia

Acromegaly: comparing old versus new photograph is valuable diagnostic tool

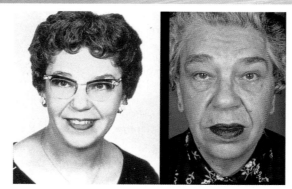

22-3: Acromegaly showing the patient before development of the tumor (*left*) and after development of the tumor (*right*). Note the coarse facial features and enlargement of the jaw and lips. *(From Damjanov I: Pathology for the Health-Related Professions, 2nd ed. Philadelphia, WB Saunders, 2000, p 407.)*

Acromegaly: heart failure from cardiomyopathy is a common cause of death

(5) Hypertension
- Sodium retention related to increased GH and insulin (hyperglycemia increases its release)

(6) Visceral organomegaly with dysfunction
- Heart, liver, kidneys, thyroid

(7) Muscle weakness (myopathy); cardiomyopathy

(8) Headache and visual field defects
- Enlarged sella turcica

c. Diagnosis
(1) Imaging with CT scan, MRI (best study)
(2) Suppression tests

d. Treatment
(1) Transsphenoidal surgery
(2) If surgery does not correct
- Somatostatin and dopamine analogues; GH receptor antagonists

3. Syndrome of inappropriate ADH (SIADH)
- Refer to Chapter 4 for complete discussion of SIADH

V. **Thyroid Gland Disorders**

A. **Steps in thyroid hormone synthesis**
1. Trapping of iodide is thyroid-stimulating hormone (TSH)–mediated.
2. Oxidation of iodides to iodine is peroxidase-mediated.
3. Organification
   a. Iodine is incorporated into tyrosine to form MIT (monoiodotyrosine) and DIT (diiodotyrosine).
   b. It is TSH-mediated.
4. Coupling of MIT with DIT produces triiodothyronine (T_3).
5. Coupling of DIT with DIT produces thyroxine (T_4).
6. Hormones are stored as colloid.
7. Proteolysis of colloid by lysosomal proteases is TSH-mediated.
8. T_4 and T_3 bind to thyroid-binding globulin (TBG).
   - One third of TBG binding sites are normally occupied.
9. Free T_4 (FT_4) is peripherally converted to free T_3 (FT_3) by an outer ring deiodinase.
   a. FT_3 is a metabolically active hormone.
   b. FT_4 is considered a prohormone.
   c. FT_4 and FT_3 have a negative feedback relationship with TSH.
      (1) An increase in FT_4/FT_3 should produce a decrease in TSH.
      (2) A decrease in FT_4/FT_3 should produce an increase in TSH.

B. **Functions of thyroid hormone**
1. Control of total energy expenditure
2. Growth and maturation of tissue
3. Turnover of hormones and vitamins
4. Cell regeneration

C. **Thyroid function tests**
1. Total serum T_4 (Fig. 22-4A)

Thyroid hormone: iodide attached to tyrosine

TSH: mediates trapping, organification, and proteolysis

FT_4: prohormone; rendered metabolically active by outer ring deiodinase (FT_3)

FT_4/FT_3: negative feedback with TSH

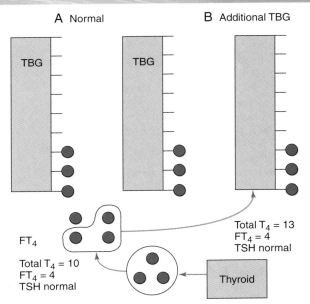

A Normal

B Additional TBG

TBG

TBG

TBG

FT$_4$

Total T$_4$ = 10
FT$_4$ = 4
TSH normal

Total T$_4$ = 13
FT$_4$ = 4
TSH normal

Thyroid

22-4: Schematic of total serum thyroxine (T$_4$) in a normal individual (**A**) and an individual with an increase in thyroid-binding globulin (TBG) (**B**). The actual numbers do not represent the true concentration of T$_4$ and free T$_4$ (FT$_4$). The bars represent TBG and the circles are T$_4$ bound to TBG and T$_4$ that is free (FT$_4$). FT$_4$ normally has a negative feedback with thyroid-stimulating hormone (TSH). Refer to the text for a complete discussion. *(From Goljan EF: Star Series: Pathology. Philadelphia, WB Saunders, 1998, Fig. 19-1.)*

a. Represents T$_4$ bound to TBG and free (unbound) T$_4$ (FT$_4$)
  • Note: the values used in the schematic do *not* represent true values for each of the components.
  (1) Figure 22-2A shows one third of TBG binding sites on two TBGs occupied by T$_4$.
    • Total of 6 T$_4$ bound to TBG
  (2) There are 4 FT$_4$.
  (3) The total serum T$_4$ is 10.
  (4) TSH is normal, because FT$_4$ is normal.
b. Increase in TBG synthesis increases total serum T$_4$ (Fig. 22-4B).
  (1) Estrogen increases the synthesis of TBG.
    • Pregnancy, oral contraceptive pill, hormone replacement
  (2) Extra TBG automatically has one third of its binding sites occupied by T$_4$.
    • Total of 9 T$_4$ bound to TBG
  (3) The 3 T$_4$ used to bind to the extra TBG are replaced by 3 T$_4$ released from the thyroid gland.
  (4) FT$_4$ remains normal (4).
  (5) Total serum T$_4$ is increased (9 + 4 = 13).
  (6) TSH is normal, because FT$_4$ is normal.
  (7) *No* signs of thyrotoxicosis are present.
c. Decrease in TBG synthesis decreases total serum T$_4$.
  (1) Causes of a decreased TBG
    • Anabolic steroids, nephrotic syndrome (urinary loss)
  (2) Total serum T$_4$ is decreased.
  (3) FT$_4$ and TSH remain normal.
  (4) *No* signs of hypothyroidism
d. Normal TBG with increase or decrease in total serum T$_4$
  (1) Increase or decrease in FT$_4$ must be present.
  (2) Increased FT$_4$—Graves' disease, thyroiditis
  (3) Decreased FT$_4$—hypothyroidism
2. Serum TSH
  a. Best overall screening test for thyroid dysfunction
  b. Increased TSH
    • Primary hypothyroidism

Total serum T$_4$: T$_4$ bound to TBG + FT$_4$

Estrogen: ↑ TBG which ↑ total serum T$_4$ but *not* FT$_4$

↓ TBG: ↓ total serum T$_4$ but *not* FT$_4$

Alterations in TBG: alter total serum T$_4$; no effect on FT$_4$ and TSH

Serum TSH: best screening test for thyroid dysfunction

c. Decreased TSH
  (1) Thyrotoxicosis (e.g., Graves' disease)
  (2) Hypopituitarism/hypothalamic dysfunction
     • Causes secondary/tertiary hypothyroidism, respectively
3. ^{131}I radioactive uptake
  a. Evaluates synthetic activity of the thyroid gland
     • Iodide is used to synthesize thyroid hormone.
  b. Increased uptake indicates increased synthesis of T$_4$.
     • Examples—Graves' disease, toxic nodular goiter
  c. Decreased uptake of ^{131}I
    (1) Inactivity of the gland
       • Example—patient taking thyroid hormone
    (2) Inflammation of the gland
       • Example—acute/subacute/chronic thyroiditis
  d. Evaluates functional status of thyroid nodules
    (1) Decreased uptake in a nodule
       • "Cold" nodule—cyst, adenoma, cancer (Fig. 22-5)
    (2) Increased uptake in a nodule
       • "Hot" nodule—toxic nodular goiter
4. Thyroglobulin
   • Marker for thyroid cancer
D. Lingual thyroid
  1. Failed descent of thyroid anlage from the base of the tongue
     • Usually represents all of the thyroid tissue
  2. Clinical findings
    a. Dysphagia for solids
    b. Mass lesion
  3. ^{131}I scan locates the lesion
     • Also identifies any other thyroid tissue that is present
  4. Treatment
    a. Suppression with thyroxine
       • Lingual thyroids are usually hypofunctional.
    b. Ablation with radioactive iodine
    c. Surgery if obstructive
E. Thyroglossal duct cyst
  1. Cystic midline mass that is close to or within the hyoid bone (Fig. 22-6)
  2. Surgery with removal of the proximal duct and hyoid bone
F. Thyroiditis
  1. Acute thyroiditis
    a. Bacterial infection (e.g., *Staphylococcus aureus*)

Margin notes (left column):

^{131}I uptake: evaluates synthetic activity of thyroid gland

↑ ^{131}I uptake: increased synthesis of thyroid hormone; Graves' disease

↓ ^{131}I uptake: thyroiditis; patient taking excess thyroid hormone

Cold nodule: ↓ ^{131}I uptake

Hot nodule: ↑ ^{131}I uptake

Mass at base of the tongue: lingual thyroid

Thyroglossal duct cyst: cystic midline mass

Branchial cleft cyst: located in the anterolateral neck

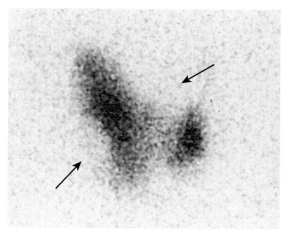

22-5: Nuclear scan of thyroid showing "cold" nodules (lack of uptake or radioactive iodine) in both lobes of the thyroid (*arrows*). (*From Katz D, Math K, Groskin S: Radiology Secrets. Philadelphia, Hanley & Belfus, 1998, p 531, Fig. 2.*)

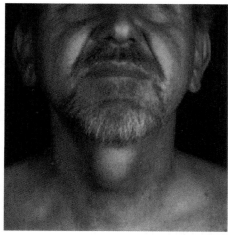

22-6: Patient with a midline thyroglossal duct cyst. (*From Bouloux P: Self-Assessment Picture Tests: Medicine, Vol. 1. London, Mosby-Wolfe, 1997, p 52, Fig. 103.*)

b. Clinical findings
(1) Fever
(2) Tender gland with painful cervical adenopathy
(3) Initial thyrotoxicosis from gland destruction
   • Increased serum T_4, decreased serum TSH
(4) Permanent hypothyroidism is uncommon.
c. Decreased ^{131}I uptake
d. Treatment
   • Penicillin or ampicillin
2. Subacute granulomatous thyroiditis
a. Viral infection (e.g., coxsackievirus, mumps)
b. Occurs most often in women 40 to 50 years old
c. Granulomatous inflammation with multinucleated giant cells
d. Clinical findings
(1) Most common cause of a painful thyroid gland
(2) Often preceded by an upper respiratory infection
(3) Cervical adenopathy is *not* prominent.
(4) Initial thyrotoxicosis from gland destruction
   • Increased serum T_4, decreased serum TSH
(5) Permanent hypothyroidism is uncommon.
e. Decreased ^{131}I uptake
f. Self-limited; does *not* require treatment
3. Hashimoto's thyroiditis
a. Epidemiology
(1) Autoimmune thyroiditis
(2) Incidence increases with age
(3) More common in women than men
(4) Human leukocyte antigen (HLA)-Dr3 and -Dr5 associations
(5) Increased incidence in:
   • Turner's syndrome, Down syndrome, Klinefelter's syndrome
(6) Increased incidence of other autoimmune diseases (e.g., pernicious anemia)
b. Pathogenesis
(1) Cytotoxic T cells destroy parenchyma (type IV hypersensitivity).
   • Initial thyrotoxicosis, eventual hypothyroidism
(2) Blocking IgG autoantibodies against the TSH receptor
   • Decrease hormone synthesis; type II hypersensitivity
(3) Antimicrosomal and thyroglobulin antibodies
   • Develop as a *result* of gland injury; no causal role
c. Gross and microscopic
(1) Enlarged, gray gland
(2) Lymphocytic infiltrate with prominent germinal follicles (Fig. 22-7)
d. Clinical findings
(1) Most common cause of primary hypothyroidism
(2) Initial thyrotoxicosis from gland destruction
   • Known as *hashitoxicosis*
(3) Signs of hypothyroidism (see later discussion)
(4) Risk factor for primary B-cell malignant lymphoma of the thyroid
4. Reidel's thyroiditis
a. Fibrous tissue replacement of the gland
b. Extension of fibrosis into surrounding tissue
   • Can produce tracheal obstruction
c. Associated with other sclerosing conditions
   • Example—sclerosing mediastinitis
d. Hypothyroidism may occur.
e. Treatment
(1) Initial treatment with corticosteroids
(2) Tamoxifen
   • First-line therapy or if corticosteroids are unsuccessful
(3) Surgery
5. Subacute painless lymphocytic thyroiditis
a. Autoimmune disease that develops post partum

Acute thyroiditis: thyrotoxicosis; ↓ ^{131}I uptake

Subacute granulomatous thyroiditis: most common cause of painful thyroid; virus induced; no adenopathy

Hashimoto's thyroiditis: autoimmune thyroiditis

Hashimoto's thyroiditis: type IV (mainly) and type II hypersensitivity

Hashimoto's thyroiditis: most common cause of hypothyroidism

Reidel's thyroiditis: fibrous tissue replacement of gland and surrounding tissue

Subacute painless lymphocytic thyroiditis: develops post partum; progression to hypothyroidism

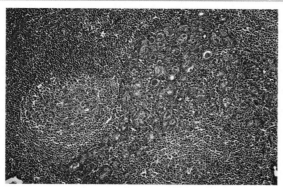

22-7: Microscopic section of Hashimoto's thyroiditis. Note the prominent germinal follicle and heavy infiltrate of lymphocytes throughout the gland with destruction of the thyroid follicles. *(From Rosai J, Ackerman LV: Surgical Pathology, 9th ed. St. Louis, Mosby, 2004, p 522, Fig. 9-10.)*

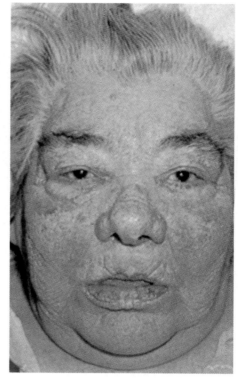

22-8: Primary hypothyroidism in a patient with Hashimoto's thyroiditis. The patient has a puffy face, particularly around the eyes, and coarse hair. *(From Forbes C, Jackson W: Color Atlas and Text of Clinical Medicine, 2nd ed. St. Louis, Mosby, 2003, p 325, Fig. 7-72.)*

  b. Gland lacks germinal follicles.
  c. Clinical findings
   (1) Abrupt onset of thyrotoxicosis due to gland destruction
   (2) Gland is slightly enlarged and painless.
   (3) Progresses to primary hypothyroidism in 40% to 50% of cases
   (4) Antimicrosomal antibodies (50–80%)
  d. Treatment
   • Levothyroxine in the hypothyroid stage
 G. Hypothyroidism
  1. Reduced secretion of thyroid hormone
   a. Patients are hypometabolic.
   b. Decrease in the basal metabolic rate
  2. Causes
   a. Hashimoto's thyroiditis (90% of cases)
   b. Subacute painless lymphocytic thyroiditis
   c. Hypopituitarism, iodine deficiency, enzyme deficiency
   d. Drugs
    • Amiodarone, lithium, sulfonamides, phenylbutazone
   e. Hypothalamic dysfunction/hypopituitarism (see sections II and IV, respectively)
   f. Congenital (see later discussion)
  3. Cretinism
   a. Hypothyroidism in infancy or early childhood
   b. Brain requires thyroxine for its maturation.
   c. Causes
    (1) Maternal hypothyroidism
     • *Before* the fetal thyroid is developed
    (2) Enzyme or iodine deficiency
   d. Clinical findings
    (1) Severe mental retardation

Hypothyroidism: hypometabolic

Brain: requires thyroxine for maturation

Cretinism: most often caused by maternal hypothyroidism before fetal thyroid is developed

      (2) Increased weight and short stature
        • Pituitary dwarfism—decreased weight and short stature
   e. Treatment is thyroid hormone replacement.
 4. Clinical findings in adult hypothyroidism
   a. Proximal muscle myopathy
      (1) Very common finding
      (2) Increased serum creatine kinase
   b. Weight gain
      • Due to hypometabolic state with retention of water and salt
   c. Dry and brittle hair; loss of outer one-third of eyebrow
   d. Bradycardia (slow heart rate)
   e. Coarse yellow skin
      • Yellow skin due to less conversion of β-carotenes into retinoic acid
   f. Periorbital puffiness, hoarse voice
      (1) Both of these are due to myxedema (Fig. 22-8)
      (2) Increased hyaluronic acid and chondroitin sulfate in interstitial tissue
      (3) Nonpitting edema
   g. Fatigue, cold intolerance, constipation
   h. Menstrual irregularities
      • Most often menorrhagia
   i. Diastolic hypertension
      • Due to retention of sodium and water
   j. Congestive (dilated) cardiomyopathy with biventricular heart failure
   k. Atherosclerotic coronary artery disease
   l. Delayed recovery of Achilles reflex, mental slowness, dementia
 5. Laboratory findings
   a. Decreased serum T_4, increased serum TSH
   b. Antimicrosomal, antiperoxidase, and antithyroglobulin antibodies
      • Present in Hashimoto's thyroiditis
   c. Hypercholesterolemia
      • Due to decreased synthesis of low-density lipoprotein (LDL) receptors
 6. Treatment
   a. Levothyroxine in small increments every 6–8 weeks
   b. Bring serum TSH into the normal range (euthyroid state)
 7. Myxedema coma
   a. Causes
      (1) Idiopathic; cold exposure
      (2) Use of sedatives/opiates
      (3) Acute illness
   b. Clinical findings
      (1) Progressive stupor
      (2) Hypothermia
      (3) Bradycardia; hypoventilation
      (4) Hypoglycemia, hypocortisolism, SIADH
   c. Treatment
      (1) Ventilatory support
      (2) Treat hypothermia
      (3) IV levothyroxine
      (4) High doses of corticosteroids
   d. Mortality rate is 20% to 50%.
H. Thyroid hormone excess
 1. Classification
   a. Thyrotoxicosis
      • Describes hormone excess regardless of cause
   b. Hyperthyroidism
      (1) Describes hormone excess due to increased synthesis
      (2) Examples—Graves' disease, toxic nodular goiter
 2. Patients are hypermetabolic.
   • Increase in the basal metabolic rate
 3. Graves' disease
   a. Epidemiology
      (1) Most common cause of hyperthyroidism and thyrotoxicosis

Cretinism: severe mental retardation

Hashimoto's thyroiditis: muscle weakness common complaint; weight gain; dry, brittle hair

Hashimoto's thyroiditis: periorbital puffiness, hoarse voice; signs of myxedema

Hashimoto's thyroiditis: cold intolerance, constipation

Hashimoto's thyroiditis: hypertension from sodium retention; delayed reflexes

Primary hypothyroidism: ↓ serum T_4/FT_4; ↑ serum TSH, cholesterol

Myxedema coma: stupor, hypothermia, hypoventilation; IV levothyroxine, corticosteroids

Thyrotoxicosis: hormone excess from any cause

Hyperthyroidism: thyrotoxicosis due to excess synthesis of thyroid hormone

Graves' disease: most common cause of hyperthyroidism and thyrotoxicosis

(2) Female dominant autoimmune disease

(3) HLA-B8 and HLA-Dr3 association

b. Pathogenesis

(1) T cells induce specific B cells to produce IgG antibodies against the TSH-receptor

(a) Stimulating type of antibody as opposed to a blocking antibody

(b) Type II hypersensitivity reaction

(2) Antimicrosomal and thyroglobulin antibodies are present.

(3) Inciting events that may initiate onset of the disease

- Infection, withdrawal of steroids, iodide excess, post partum

c. Symmetrical, nontender thyromegaly

(1) Scant colloid

(2) Papillary infolding of the glands

d. Clinical features unique to Graves' disease

(1) Infiltrative ophthalmopathy (exophthalmos; 50%)

(a) Proptosis and muscle weakness of the eye (Figs. 22-9 and 22-10)

Graves' disease: anti-TSH receptor antibody, type II hypersensitivity

Unique to Graves': exophthalmos, pretibial myxedema, thyroid acropachy

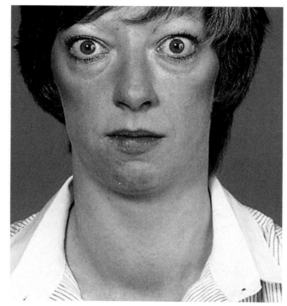

22-9: Graves' disease. The patient has exophthalmos and a diffuse enlargement of the thyroid gland (goiter). *(From Forbes C, Jackson W: Color Atlas and Text of Clinical Medicine, 2nd ed. St. Louis, Mosby, 2003, p 323, Fig. 7-61.)*

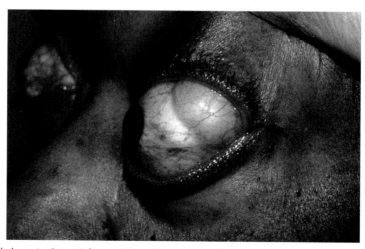

22-10: Severe exophthalmos in Graves' disease. Note the proptosis of the eye, increased vascularity of the conjunctiva, and the enlarged lacrimal gland. *(From Swartz MH: Textbook of Physical Diagnosis, 5th ed. Philadelphia, Saunders Elsevier, 2006, p 232, Fig. 10-35.)*

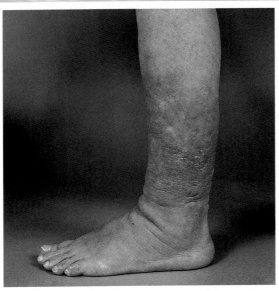

22-11: Pretibial myxedema in Graves' disease. Note the thickened area of erythema involving the pretibial area and dorsum of the foot. *(Courtesy of R.A. Marsden, MD, St. George's Hospital, Lodon.)*

      (b) Due to adipose and glycosaminoglycans deposited in orbital tissue
      (c) IgG-TSH receptor antibodies can cross placenta and produce transient hyperthyroidism in fetus

    (2) Pretibial myxedema (1–2%; Fig. 22-11)
      • Due to excess glycosaminoglycans in the dermis

    (3) Thyroid acropachy
      (a) Digital swelling and clubbing of fingers
      (b) Nails separate from nail bed (lifted up)
      (c) Exophthalmos and pretibial myxedema usually present

4. Graves' disease in the elderly (apathetic hyperthyroidism)
  a. Cardiac abnormalities
    • Atrial fibrillation, congestive heart failure
  b. Muscle weakness, apathy
  c. Thyromegaly

5. Toxic multinodular goiter (Plummer's disease)
  a. One or more nodules in a multinodular goiter become TSH-independent.
  b. See "hot" nodules with ^{131}I scan
  c. Distinctions from Graves' disease
    • *Lack* exophthalmos and pretibial myxedema
  d. Treatment is surgery.

6. Clinical findings in all causes of thyrotoxicosis
  a. Constitutional signs
    (1) Weight loss (good appetite)
    (2) Fine tremor of the hands
    (3) Heat intolerance, diarrhea, anxiety
    (4) Menstrual irregularities
      • Usually oligomenorrhea
    (5) Lid stare
      • Due to increased sympathetic stimulation of eyelid muscles
  b. Cardiac findings
    (1) Sinus tachycardia (>90 beats/min)
    (2) Increased risk for atrial fibrillation
    (3) Systolic hypertension, high-output heart failure
      (a) Thyroid hormone increases β-receptor synthesis in the heart.
      (b) Excess hormone increases inotropic and chronotropic effect on the heart.
  c. Brisk reflexes, osteoporosis (increased bone turnover)

Transient hyperthyroidism in fetus

Thyroid acropachy: digital swelling and clubbing

Graves' disease in elderly: cardiac and muscle findings predominate; apathetic appearing

Toxic multinodular goiter: one or more nodules in a multinodular goiter becomes TSH-independent

Thyrotoxicosis: weight loss with a good appetite; heat intolerance; diarrhea

Thyrotoxicosis: oligomenorrhea; lid stare; sinus tachycardia; systolic hypertension; brisk reflexes

Atrial fibrillation: always order a TSH test to rule out hyperthyroidism

Graves' hyperthyroidism: ↑ serum T_4/ FT_4, ↑ ^{131}I uptake, ↓ serum TSH

Thyrotoxicosis: ↑ glucose, calcium, lymphocytes; ↓ cholesterol

Treatment for Graves' disease: β-blockers, thionamides

Thyroid storm: tachyarrhythmias, hyperpyrexia, coma, shock

ESS: serum T_3 and T_4 abnormalities; normal gland function

ESS: block in outer ring deiodinase conversion of T_4 to T_3; T_4 converted to inactive reverse T_3

ESS: ↓ serum T_3 and ↑ reverse T_3

Goiter: thyroid enlargement

7. Laboratory findings
  a. Increased serum T_4, decreased serum TSH
  b. Increased ^{131}I uptake
    • Graves' disease and toxic multinodular goiter
  c. Decreased ^{131}I uptake
    • Thyroiditis, patient taking excess thyroid hormone
  d. Hyperglycemia
    • Increased glycogenolysis
  e. Hypocholesterolemia
    • Increased LDL receptor synthesis
  f. Hypercalcemia
    • Increased bone turnover
  g. Absolute lymphocytosis
8. Treatment of Graves' disease
  a. β-Blockers decrease adrenergic effects.
  b. Thionamides decrease hormone synthesis.
  c. Ablative ^{131}I therapy in 1 year if above regimen does not work
9. Thyroid storm
  a. Causes
    (1) Inadequately treated patients with Graves' disease undergo surgery.
    (2) Infection; trauma
    (3) Iodine; pregnancy
  b. Clinical findings
    (1) Tachyarrhythmias
    (2) Hyperpyrexia
    (3) Shock
      • Volume depletion from vomiting
    (4) Coma
  c. Treatment
    (1) Inhibit hormone synthesis
      (a) Propylthiouracil
      (b) Iodide
    (2) Sympathetic blockade with β-blockers
    (3) Hydrocortisone
    (4) Cooling blanket
10. Euthyroid sick syndrome (ESS)
  a. Epidemiology
    (1) Abnormalities in serum T_3 and T_4 but gland function appears normal
    (2) Associated with:
      • Malignancy, heart failure, chronic renal failure, sepsis, myocardial infarction
    (3) Laboratory test alterations usually return to normal with resolution of the illness.
  b. Pathogenesis
    (1) Normally, a peripheral tissue outer ring deiodinase converts T_4 into metabolically active T_3.
    (2) In ESS, outer ring deiodinase is blocked and inner ring deiodinase converts T_4 into inactive reverse T_3.
      • There are also abnormalities in thyroid-binding globulin.
    (3) Most common variant of ESS
      (a) Normal/decreased serum T_4
      (b) Decreased serum T_3
      (c) Normal/decreased serum TSH
      (d) Increased serum reverse T_3
  c. Treatment
    • Varies from no treatment to levothyroxine during the time of the illness
  I. Summary of laboratory findings in thyroid disorders (Table 22-2)
  J. Nontoxic goiter
    1. Thyroid enlargement from excess colloid (Fig. 22-12)
    2. Types of goiter
      a. Endemic type
        • Due to iodide deficiency (most common)
      b. Sporadic type; causes include:
        • Goitrogens (e.g., cabbage), enzyme deficiency, puberty, pregnancy

TABLE 22-2. **LABORATORY FINDINGS IN THYROID DISEASE**

DISORDER	SERUM T$_4$	FREE T$_4$	SERUM TSH	^{131}I UPTAKE
Graves' disease	↑	↑	↓	↑
Patient taking excess hormone	↑	↑	↓	↓
Initial phase of thyroiditis	↑	↑	↓	↓
Primary hypothyroidism	↓	↓	↑	↔
Secondary hypothyroidism (hypopituitarism)	↓	↓	↓	↔
Increased TBG (e.g., excess estrogen)	↑	N	N	↔
Decreased TBG (e.g., anabolic steroids)	↓	N	N	↔

N, normal; T$_4$, thyroxine; TBG, thyroid-binding globulin; TSH, thyroid-stimulating hormone; ↔, not indicated.

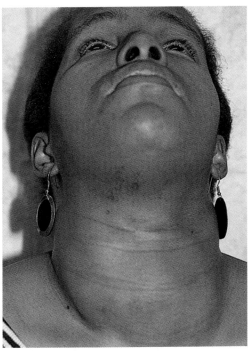

22-12: Patient with a multinodular goiter. Note the diffuse enlargement of the lower anterior neck. *(From Swartz MH: Textbook of Physical Diagnosis, 5th ed. Philadelphia, Saunders Elsevier, 2006, p 199, Fig. 9-7.)*

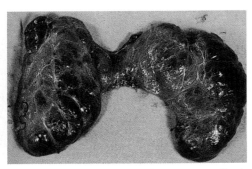

22-13: Gross of multinodular goiter. Note the diffusely enlarged gland with numerous cystic nodules filled with excess colloid. Hemorrhage has occurred into many of the cysts. *(From Grieg JD: Color Atlas of Surgical Diagnosis. London, Mosby-Wolfe, 1996, p 268, Fig. 33-3.)*

3. Pathogenesis
   a. Absolute or relative deficiency of thyroid hormone
   b. Hyperplasia/hypertrophy
      • Attempt to increase hormone synthesis
   c. Hyperplasia/hypertrophy is followed by gland involution.
      • Failure of gland to sustain synthesis
   d. Initial diffuse thyromegaly is followed by multinodular goiter (Fig. 22-13)
4. Complications
   a. Hemorrhage into cyst
      • Produces sudden, painful, gland enlargement
   b. Compression of jugular vein causing neck congestion
      • Called Pemberton's sign
   c. Primary hypothyroidism
   d. Toxic nodular goiter
      • One or more nodules become TSH-independent; "hot" nodule.
   e. Hoarseness (compresses laryngeal nerve)
   f. Dyspnea (compresses trachea)

Nontoxic goiter: absolute or relative deficiency of thyroid hormone

Nontoxic goiter: hyperplasia/hypertrophy followed by involution; initially diffuse then nodular

Toxic nodular goiter: one or more nodules become TSH-independent

5. Treatment
   a. Levothyroxine reduces gland size and achieves the euthyroid state.
   b. Surgery if compressive symptoms persist

K. Solitary thyroid nodule

1. Epidemiology
   a. Majority are cold nodules (95%).
   b. Causes in adult women
      (1) Majority are cysts in a goiter (60%) or a follicular adenoma (25%).
      (2) Approximately 15% are malignant.
      (3) Approximately 85% to 90% of solitary nodules are euthyroid.
   c. Causes in adult men and children
      • Similar to women, but there is a greater chance of malignancy
   d. Prior history of radiation to head and neck
      • Nodule is more likely to be malignant (40% of cases).
2. Diagnosis
   a. Fine needle aspiration (FNA) most important initial step
   b. Thyroid hormone studies
3. Treatment
   a. Depends on the FNA result
   b. If malignant, surgical removal
   c. If benign and asymptomatic, periodic follow-up

L. Benign and malignant tumors

1. Follicular adenoma
   a. Most common benign tumor
      • Surrounded by a complete capsule
   b. Presents as a solitary "cold" nodule (see Fig. 22-5)
   c. Approximately 10% progress into a follicular carcinoma.
2. Papillary adenocarcinoma
   a. Epidemiology
      (1) Most common endocrine cancer
      (2) Papillary adenocarcinoma most common thyroid cancer (>75%)
      (3) More common in women than men (3:1)
         • Usually occur in second and third decades
      (4) Associated with radiation exposure
   b. Gross and microscopic findings
      (1) Usually multifocal
      (2) Papillary fronds intermixed with follicles
      (3) Psammoma bodies (35–45% of cases)
         • Dystrophically calcified cancer cells (Fig. 22-14)
      (4) Empty-appearing nuclei
         • Called Orphan Annie nuclei
      (5) Lymphatic invasion
   c. Metastasize to cervical nodes, lung
   d. Diagnose with FNA

Solitary nodule in a woman: majority are benign; 15% malignant

Solitary nodule in man/ child: more likely to be malignant

Solitary nodule with history of radiation exposure: more likely to be malignant (40%)

First step in management of solitary thyroid nodule: fine needle aspiration

Follicular adenoma: most common benign thyroid tumor

Papillary carcinoma: most common endocrine cancer

Papillary carcinoma: most common thyroid cancer; psammoma bodies

Papillary carcinoma: lymphatic invasion

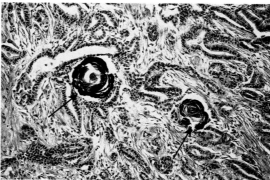

22-14: Papillary carcinoma of thyroid showing branching papillae and blue concretions (*arrows*) representing psammoma bodies. (*From Rosai J, Ackerman LV: Surgical Pathology, 9th ed. St. Louis, Mosby, 2004, p 534, Fig. 9-37A.*)

e. Treatment
(1) Usually subtotal or near total thyroidectomy with sampling of cervical nodes
(2) Followed in a few weeks by radiotherapy with ^{131}I
(3) Suppressive therapy with thyroid hormone
- Tumor is TSH dependent.
f. Five-year survival rate > 95%

3. Follicular carcinoma
a. Epidemiology
(1) Most common thyroid cancer presenting as a solitary cold nodule
(2) Female dominant cancer
b. Gross and microscopic findings
(1) Encapsulated or invasive
(2) Neoplastic follicles invade blood vessels.
(3) Lymph node metastasis is uncommon.
c. Metastasize to lung and bone
d. Treatment
- Similar to papillary cancer
e. Five-year survival rate ~80%.

4. Medullary carcinoma
a. Epidemiology
(1) Types
(a) Sporadic (80% of cases)
(b) Familial (20% of cases)
(2) Familial type
(a) Associated with autosomal dominant MEN IIa/IIb
(b) MEN IIa syndrome
- Medullary carcinoma, hyperparathyroidism (HPTH), pheochromocytoma
(c) MEN IIb (III) syndrome
- Medullary carcinoma, mucosal neuromas (lips/tongue), pheochromocytoma
(3) Familial type has a better prognosis than sporadic type.
(4) Ectopic hormones
- ACTH, which can produce Cushing syndrome
b. Pathogenesis
(1) Tumors derive from parafollicular C cells.
(2) C cells synthesize calcitonin.
(a) Tumor marker
(b) May produce hypocalcemia
(c) Converted into amyloid
(3) C-cell hyperplasia is a precursor lesion.
- Calcitonin levels increase with infusion of pentagastrin.
c. Diagnosis
(1) FNA
(2) Serum calcitonin
d. Treatment
(1) Total thyroidectomy
(2) Genetic screening for familial cases
(a) Detection of mutation of *RET* proto-oncogene
(b) Thyroidectomy is performed if patient is a gene carrier.

5. Primary B-cell malignant lymphoma
- Most often develop from Hashimoto's thyroiditis

6. Anaplastic thyroid cancer
a. Most often occurs in elderly women
b. Risk factors
- Multinodular goiter, history of follicular cancer
c. Rapidly aggressive and uniformly fatal
d. Treatment
(1) Palliative surgery; often compresses trachea
(2) Irradiation or chemotherapy
e. Five-year survival rate is 5%.

Side notes:

Follicular carcinoma: most common thyroid cancer presenting as a solitary cold nodule

Follicular carcinoma: hematogenous rather than lymphatic spread

MEN IIa: medullary carcinoma, HPTH, pheochromocytoma

MEN IIb (III): medullary carcinoma, mucosal neuromas lips/tongue, pheochromocytoma

Medullary carcinoma: derives from C cells; calcitonin is tumor marker

Medullary carcinoma: calcitonin converted into amyloid

Primary B-cell lymphoma: most often derives from Hashimoto's thyroiditis

Anaplastic thyroid cancer: rapidly aggressive; uniformly fatal

VI. **Parathyroid Gland Disorders**
   A. **Clinical anatomy and physiology**

1. Superior and inferior parathyroid glands
   • Derive from fourth pharyngeal pouch and third pharyngeal pouch, respectively
2. PTH
   a. Increases calcium reabsorption in the early distal tubule
   b. Decreases bicarbonate reclamation in the proximal tubule
   c. Decreases phosphorus reabsorption in the proximal tubule
   d. Maintains ionized calcium level in blood
      • Increases bone resorption and renal reabsorption of calcium
   e. Increases synthesis of 1-α-hydroxylase in proximal renal tubule
      (1) Increases synthesis of 1, 25-(OH)$_2$D (dihydroxycholecalciferol; calcitriol)
      (2) Inhibits 24-hydroxylase in proximal tubule, which normally converts 25-hydroxycholecalciferol synthesized in the liver to inactive 24,25-(OH)$_2$D.
   f. Stimulated by hypocalcemia and hyperphosphatemia
   g. Suppressed by hypercalcemia and hypophosphatemia

3. Role of vitamin D in calcium metabolism (see Fig. 7-3)
   a. Preformed vitamin D in the diet consists of cholecalciferol (fish) and ergocalciferol (plants).
   b. Endogenous synthesis of vitamin D in the skin occurs by photoconversion of 7-dehydrocholesterol via sunlight to vitamin D$_3$ (cholecalciferol).
   c. Reabsorption of vitamin D occurs in the small intestine.
   d. Liver hydroxylation of precursor vitamin D to 25-hydroxyvitamin D (25-(OH)D; calcidiol)
      • Occurs in the cytochrome P-450 system.
   e. 25-(OH)D is secreted into the blood and bound to a protein for delivery to the proximal tubules of the kidneys.
   f. Kidney hydroxylation of 25-(OH)D by 1α-hydroxylase produces 1,25-(OH)$_2$-D (active form of vitamin D; calcitriol).
      • If PTH is decreased, 1α-hydroxylase is decreased, and 24-hydroxylase in the proximal tubule converts 25-(OH)D to metabolically inactive 24,25-(OH)$_2$D.
   g. Calcitriol attaches to nuclear receptors in target tissues.
   h. Functions of calcitriol
      (1) Increased calcium reabsorption in duodenum
      (2) Increased phosphorus reabsorption in jejunum and ileum
      (3) Increases bone resorption
         • Induces monocytic stem cells to become osteoclasts
   i. Feedback control of calcitriol is calcium-mediated.
      (1) Decreased serum calcium: ↑ PTH → ↑ synthesis of 1α-hydroxylase → ↑ synthesis 1,25-(OH)$_2$-D and via inhibition of 24-hydroxylase → ↓ synthesis of metabolically inactive 24,25-(OH)$_2$D.
      (2) Increased serum calcium: ↓ PTH → ↓ synthesis of 1α-hydroxylase → ↓ synthesis 1,25-(OH)$_2$-D and via activation of 24-hydroxylase → ↑ synthesis of metabolically inactive 24,25-(OH)$_2$D.

4. Total serum calcium
   a. Components of the total serum calcium (Fig. 22-15A)
      (1) Calcium bound to albumin (40%) and phosphorus and citrate (13%)
         (a) Albumin has the most acidic amino acids.
         (b) At a normal pH of 7.4, ~40% of the acidic groups are COO$^-$ and can bind to positively charged calcium.
      (2) Free, ionized calcium (47%)
         • Metabolically active fraction has a negative feedback with PTH.
   b. Hypoalbuminemia (Fig. 22-15B)
      (1) Decreased total serum calcium
         • Due to a decrease in calcium bound to albumin
      (2) Normal free ionized level, normal PTH
      (3) *No* evidence of tetany
   c. Effect of respiratory or metabolic alkalosis (Fig. 22-15C)
      (1) Increases negative charges on albumin
         (a) Due to fewer hydrogen ions on the COOH groups of acidic amino acids
            • Change of COOH groups to COO$^-$

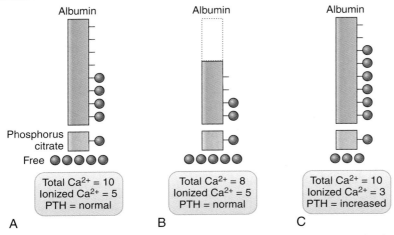

22-15: Total serum calcium in a normal individual (**A**), individual with hypoalbuminemia (**B**), and individual with alkalosis (**C**). Refer to the text for discussion. PTH, parathyroid hormone.

        (b) Extra negative charges bind some of the ionized calcium (arrows in schematic).
    (2) Total serum calcium remains normal.
    (3) Decreased ionized calcium, increased PTH
    (4) Patient develops tetany.
        • Although serum PTH is in equilibrium with ionized calcium, it cannot keep pace with the binding of ionized calcium to the negative charges on albumin; hence, tetany occurs.
  d. Tetany is due to a decreased ionized calcium level.
    (1) Causes partial depolarization of nerves and muscle
        (a) Lowers the threshold potential (E_t)
            • Comes closer to the resting membrane potential (E_m)
        (b) A smaller stimulus is required to initiate an action potential.
    (2) Clinical findings of tetany
        (a) Carpopedal spasm
            • Thumb flexes into the palm.
        (b) Chvostek's sign
            • Facial twitch after tapping the facial nerve

B. Hypoparathyroidism
  • Hypofunction of the parathyroid glands leads to hypocalcemia.
  1. Causes
    a. Autoimmune hypoparathyroidism (most common cause)
    b. Previous thyroid surgery
      • *Not* common in current day surgery
    c. DiGeorge syndrome
      (1) Failure of descent of third and fourth pharyngeal pouches
        • Absence of parathyroid glands
      (2) Absent thymus (pure T-cell deficiency)
    d. Hypomagnesemia
      (1) Magnesium is a cofactor for adenylate cyclase.
        • Cyclic adenosine monophosphate (cAMP) is required for PTH activation.
      (2) Causes of hypomagnesemia
        • Diarrhea, aminoglycosides, diuretics, alcoholism
  2. Clinical findings
    a. Tetany
    b. Calcification of basal ganglia
      (1) Due to metastatic calcification
      (2) Increased phosphorus drives calcium into the brain tissue.
    c. Cataracts, *Candida* infections (? cause)
  3. Laboratory findings
    • Hypocalcemia, hyperphosphatemia, decreased PTH

Alkalosis: normal total serum calcium; decreased ionized calcium, increased PTH; tetany

Tetany: E_t comes close to E_m; initiates action potential

Tetany: thumb adduct into palm; facial twitching after tapping facial nerve

Hypoparathyroidism: autoimmune hypoparathyroidism most common cause

DiGeorge syndrome: failure of descent of 3rd/4th pharyngeal pouches; absent parathyroids and thymus

Hypomagnesemia: most common pathologic cause of hypocalcemia in the hospital

Hypomagnesemia: diarrhea, aminoglycosides, diuretics, alcohol

Hypoparathyroidism: ↓ serum calcium, PTH; ↑ serum phosphorus

4. Other causes of hypocalcemia (Table 22-3 and Fig. 22-16)
5. Treatment
   a. Calcium and vitamin D_3 (calcitriol)
   b. Teriparatide (recombinant PTH) may be used in near future.

C. Primary hyperparathyroidism (HPTH)
1. Epidemiology
   a. Most common nonmalignant cause of hypercalcemia
   b. Occurs most frequently in postmenopausal women
   c. Asymptomatic in >50% of patients
   d. Association with MEN I and MEN IIa
   e. Causes
     (1) Adenoma (~80% of cases; Fig. 22-17)
       (a) Usually a single adenoma
       (b) Sheets of chief cells with *no* intervening adipose
       (c) Remainder of the gland plus all other glands show atrophy.
         • Hypercalcemia suppresses PTH produced from normal tissue.
       (d) Right inferior parathyroid gland is most often involved.

Chronic renal failure: most common cause of hypocalcemia; causes hypovitaminosis D

Primary HPTH: MEN I, IIa association

Most common cause of primary HPTH: benign adenoma

TABLE 22-3. OTHER CAUSES OF HYPOCALCEMIA

DISORDER	COMMENTS
Acute pancreatitis	Calcium is bound to fatty acids in enzymatic fat necrosis Poor prognostic sign
Hypovitaminosis D	Lack of sunlight: decreased photoconversion of cholesterol to (nonrenal) vitamin D_3 (cholecalciferol) in the skin Malabsorption (e.g., celiac disease): ↓ reabsorption of fat-soluble vitamin D; ↓ synthesis of 25-(OH)D; ↓ serum calcium causes ↑ serum PTH, which ↑ synthesis of 1,25-(OH)$_2$D even though there is a ↓ 25-(OH)D (more enzyme than normal for the conversion); serum phosphorus is usually normal because of the opposing effects of an ↑ serum PTH (phosphaturic effect) and ↑ 1,25-(OH)$_2$D, increases bowel reabsorption of phosphorus Cirrhosis: decreased synthesis of 25-(OH)D; similar findings to malabsorption regarding calcium, phosphorus, PTH, and 1,25-(OH)$_2$D Drugs enhancing cytochrome system (e.g., alcohol, phenytoin): increased metabolism of 25-(OH)D into an inactive metabolite; hence, ↓ 25-(OH)D → ↓ 1,25-(OH)$_2$D Chronic renal failure: ↓ synthesis of 1,25-(OH)$_2$D (↓ 1α-hydroxylation); 25-(OH)D normal or slightly ↓; ↓ serum calcium, ↑ serum phosphorus, ↑ serum PTH
Vitamin D–dependent rickets	*Autosomal recessive type I:* absent 1α-hydroxylase, so ↓ 1,25-(OH)$_2$D; normal 25-(OH)D, ↓ serum calcium, normal to ↓ serum phosphorus, ↑ serum PTH Treatment: calcitriol *Autosomal recessive type II:* absent receptors for calcitriol, so calcitriol cannot function properly; ↑ 1,25-(OH)$_2$D, normal 25-(OH)D, ↓ serum calcium, normal to ↓ serum phosphorus, ↑ serum PTH
Pseudohypoparathyroidism (see Fig. 22-16)	Autosomal dominant disease End-organ resistance to PTH (includes its ability to synthesize 1α-hydroxylase in the proximal tubule) Mental retardation, basal ganglia calcification, short fourth and fifth metacarpals ("knuckle-knuckle-dimple-dimple" sign) Hypocalcemia, normal to ↑ PTH; normal 25-(OH)D, ↓ 1,25-(OH)$_2$D

25-(OH)D, calcidiol; 1,25-(OH)$_2$D, calcitriol; PTH, parathyroid hormone.

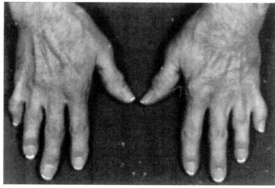

22-16: Pseudohypoparathyroidism. Note the short fourth and fifth digits, producing the classic "knuckle-knuckle-dimple-dimple" sign. *(From Bouloux P: Self-Assessment Picture Tests: Medicine, Vol. 3. London, Mosby-Wolfe, 1997, p 14, Fig. 27.)*

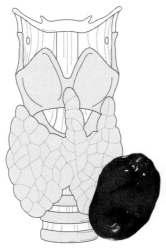

22-17: Parathyroid adenoma in primary hyperparathyroidism. *(From Rosai J, Ackerman LV: Surgical Pathology, 9th ed. St. Louis, Mosby, 2004, p 597, Fig. 10-2.)*

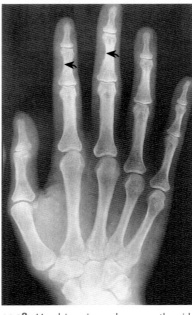

22-18: Hand in primary hyperparathyroidism. The radiograph shows a concavity at the radial aspect of the middle phalanges of the index and middle fingers *(arrows)*. *(From Katz D, Math K, Groskin S: Radiology Secrets. Philadelphia, Hanley & Belfus, 1998, p 309, Fig. 3.)*

    (2) Primary hyperplasia (~20% of cases)
        (a) All four glands are involved.
        (b) Usually a chief cell hyperplasia
        (c) Clear cell hyperplasia (wasserhelle cell hyperplasia)
          • Associated with markedly increased serum calcium levels
    (3) Carcinoma (uncommon)
2. Clinical findings
  a. Renal
    (1) Calcium stones
      • Most common presentation.
    (2) Nephrocalcinosis (refer to Chapters 1 and 19)
      • Causes polyuria and renal failure
  b. Gastrointestinal
    (1) Peptic ulcer disease (PUD)
      • Calcium stimulates gastrin, which increases gastric acid.
    (2) Acute pancreatitis
      • Calcium activates phospholipase.
    (3) Constipation
  c. Bone and joints
    (1) Osteitis fibrosa cystica
        (a) Cystic and hemorrhagic bone lesion
          • Caused by increased osteoclastic activity
        (b) Commonly involves the jaw
    (2) Radiographic findings
        (a) Subperiosteal bone resorption of phalanges (Fig. 22-18) and tooth sockets
        (b) "Salt and pepper" appearance of the skull
    (3) Osteoporosis
    (4) Chondrocalcinosis (pseudogout)
  d. Diastolic hypertension
    • Due to hypercalcemia

Marginal notes:

Primary hyperplasia: all 4 glands involved

Primary HPTH: renal stones most common presentation

Primary HPTH: PUD; acute pancreatitis

Primary HPTH: osteitis fibrosa cystica; subperiosteal bone resorption; osteoporosis; pseudogout

Primary HPTH: diastolic hypertension

e. Eyes
  (1) Band keratopathy in the limbus of the eye
  (2) Due to metastatic calcification
f. Central nervous system
  • Myriad of different findings—psychosis, confusion, anxiety, coma
3. Laboratory findings
  a. Increased serum PTH, increased calcium, decreased phosphorus
    (1) Intact serum PTH is best initial screening test
    (2) Distinguishes it from hypercalcemia related to malignancy
  b. Normal anion gap metabolic acidosis
    (1) Due to decreased proximal tubule reclamation of bicarbonate
    (2) Type II renal tubular acidosis (refer to Chapter 4)
  c. Chloride:phosphorus ratio > 33
    • Ratio < 29:1 *excludes* primary HPTH.
  d. Increased serum 1,25-$(OH)_2$D
    • PTH increases synthesis of 1α-hydroxylase in proximal renal tubule
  e. Electrocardiogram shows shortening of QT interval.
4. Localization of adenoma
  • Technetium-99m-sestamibi radionuclide scan
5. Treatment
  a. Surgical removal of the adenoma
  b. Treatment of hypercalcemia
    (1) IV hydration with normal saline followed by IV furosemide
      • Most common therapy
    (2) Bisphosphonates
    (3) Cinacalcet directly lowers PTH levels
      • Increases the calcium-sensing receptor to extracellular calcium
6. Other causes of hypercalcemia (Table 22-4)
  a. Primary HPTH and the hypercalcemia of malignancy (refer to Chapter 8) account for ~80% of all cases of hypercalcemia.
  b. The primary differentiating feature between the above two diagnoses is serum PTH.
    (1) Serum PTH is increased in primary HPTH.
    (2) Serum PTH is decreased in hypercalcemia of malignancy.
  c. Hypercalcemia in pregnancy can produce hypocalcemia in fetus.
    • Suppression of PTH in the fetus

TABLE 22-4. OTHER CAUSES OF HYPERCALCEMIA

DISORDER	COMMENTS
Hypervitaminosis D	Increased calcium reabsorption in the jejunum and kidneys
Malignancy-induced	Mechanisms: Bone metastasis with local activation of osteoclasts (most common): produces lytic lesions in bone; ↓ serum PTH; normal 25-(OH)D, ↓ 1,25-$(OH)_2$D (↓ PTH, therefore no 1α-hydroxylase) Ectopic secretion of a PTH-related protein (squamous cell carcinoma of lung, renal cell carcinoma): generalized activation of osteoclasts *without* producing lytic lesions in bone; uses the same receptor site as PTH to perform its functions; ↓ serum PTH; normal 25-(OH)D, ↓ 1,25-$(OH)_2$D (no 1α-hydroxylase) Multiple myeloma: localized increased secretion of osteoclast-activating factor (IL-1) by malignant plasma cells; produces lytic lesions in bone; ↓ serum PTH; normal 25-(OH)D, ↓ 1,25-$(OH)_2$D (no 1α-hydroxylase)
Familial hypocalciuric hypercalcemia	Autosomal dominant with 100% penetrance Mutation causing altered set-point for calcium-sensing receptor on renal tubule and parathyroid gland; normal to slightly increased serum PTH but very low urinary calcium levels (increased in primary hyperparathyroidism)
Sarcoidosis	Mechanism: macrophages in granulomas synthesize 1α-hydroxylase, causing hypervitaminosis D
Thiazides	Mechanism: volume depletion increases renal tubule reabsorption of calcium; always consider a possible underlying parathyroid adenoma (order serum intact PTH)

IL, interleukin; 25-(OH)D, calcidiol; 1,25-$(OH)_2$D, calcitriol; PTH, parathyroid hormone.

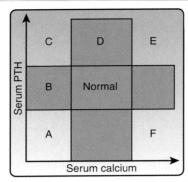

22-19: Schematic showing serum calcium and serum PTH in different disorders. The center square with the shaded areas represent the normal serum calcium and PTH. Area A describes primary hypoparathyroidism (↓ serum calcium, ↓ serum PTH); area B represents hypoalbuminemia (↓ serum calcium, normal serum PTH); area C represents secondary hyperparathyroidism (↓ serum calcium, ↑ serum PTH); D represents respiratory alkalosis (normal serum calcium, ↑ serum PTH); E represents primary hyperparathyroidism (↑ serum calcium, ↑ serum PTH); and F represents hypercalcemia associated with malignancy (↑ serum calcium, ↓ serum PTH). PTH, parathyroid hormone.

D. Secondary hyperparathyroidism
1. Hyperplasia of all four parathyroid glands
    a. Compensation for hypocalcemia
    b. Example—hypovitaminosis D due to renal failure and malabsorption
2. Decreased calcium, increased PTH
3. May develop tertiary hyperparathyroidism
    a. Glands become autonomous regardless of calcium level.
    b. May bring serum calcium into a normal or increased range

E. Schematic summarizing serum PTH and calcium relationships (Fig. 22-19)

F. Phosphorus disorders
1. Causes of hypophosphatemia (Table 22-5)
2. Clinical findings in hypophosphatemia
    a. Muscle weakness
        (1) Decreased synthesis of adenosine triphosphate (ATP) causes muscle weakness.
        (2) Muscle paralysis and rhabdomyolysis may occur.
    b. RBC hemolysis
        • RBCs require ATP to maintain pumps and membrane integrity.
    c. Osteomalacia (soft bones)
        • Phosphorus is required to mineralize bone (refer to Chapter 7).
3. Causes of hyperphosphatemia (Table 22-6)
4. Clinical findings in hyperphosphatemia
    a. Metastatic calcification
        • Excess phosphorus drives calcium into normal tissue
    b. Hypovitaminosis D
        • Hyperphosphatemia inhibits the synthesis of 1α-hydroxylase.

Secondary HPTH: compensation for hypocalcemia

Insulin therapy: danger of developing hypophosphatemia

Hypophosphatemia: alkalosis most common cause

Hyperphosphatemia: most common cause is renal failure

TABLE 22-5. CAUSES OF HYPOPHOSPHATEMIA

DISORDER	COMMENTS
Hypovitaminosis D (extrarenal causes)	Decreased reabsorption of phosphorus from the small intestine and kidneys
Insulin Rx in DKA	Increased uptake of glucose into cells requires phosphorus for phosphorylation (traps glucose in the cell)
Primary HPTH	Increased PTH decreases phosphorus reabsorption in the proximal tubules
PTH-related peptide	Uses same receptor as PTH; decreases phosphorus reabsorption in the proximal tubules
Respiratory/metabolic alkalosis	Alkalosis activates phosphofructokinase, the rate-limiting reaction of glycolysis, causing increased phosphorylation of glucose; most common cause of hypophosphatemia in the hospital
Vitamin D–resistant rickets	X-linked dominant disorder Defect in renal and gastrointestinal reabsorption of phosphorus

DKA, diabetic ketoacidosis; HPTH, hyperparathyroidism; PTH, parathyroid hormone; Rx, treatment.

TABLE 22-6. CAUSES OF HYPERPHOSPHATEMIA

DISORDER/CONDITION	COMMENTS
Chronic renal failure (most common cause)	Decreased excretion of phosphorus as titratable acid
Normal child	Children require increased serum phosphorus to drive calcium into bone for mineralization
Primary hypoparathyroidism	Decreased excretion of phosphorus as titratable acid
Pseudohypoparathyroidism	Autosomal dominant disease (see Table 22-3) End-organ resistance to PTH (includes its ability to synthesize 1α-hydroxylase in the proximal tubule)

PTH, parathyroid hormone.

G. **Summary table integrating calcium, phosphorus, 25-(OH)D, 1,25-(OH)D, and PTH in calcium and phosphorus disorders** (Table 22-7)

VII. **Adrenal Gland Disorders**

A. **Adrenal cortex hormones** (Fig. 22-20)

1. Zona glomerulosa produces mineralocorticoids (e.g., aldosterone).
   - Angiotensin II activates 18-hydroxylase, which converts corticosterone to aldosterone.
2. Zona fasciculata produces glucocorticoids.
   - 11-Deoxycortisol and cortisol are 17-hydroxycorticoids (17-OH).
3. Zona reticularis produces sex hormones.
   a. 17-Ketosteroids (17-KS)
      - Dehydroepiandrosterone (DHEA) and androstenedione
   b. Testosterone
      - Converted to dihydrotestosterone (DHT) by 5α-reductase in peripheral tissue sites

B. **Adrenal medulla**

1. Neural crest origin
2. Produces catecholamines
   - Epinephrine (EPI) and norepinephrine (NOR)
3. Metabolic products of EPI and NOR
   - Metanephrine and vanillylmandelic acid (VMA)
4. Metabolic product of dopamine is homovanillic acid (HVA).

C. **Adrenocortical hypofunction (primary hypocortisolism)**

1. Acute adrenocortical insufficiency
   a. Causes
      (1) Abrupt withdrawal of corticosteroids
      (2) Waterhouse-Friderichsen syndrome (see later discussion)
      (3) Anticoagulation therapy
   b. Waterhouse-Friderichsen syndrome
      (1) Usually associated with septicemia from *Neisseria meningitidis*

Margin notes:

Adrenal cortex: glomerulosa → mineralocorticoids, fasciculata → glucocorticoids, reticularis → sex hormones

Peripheral tissue sites: skin, testis, prostate, seminal vesicles, epididymis, liver

Adrenal medulla: produce catecholamines

Metabolic end-products of EPI/NOR: metanephrines, VMA

Abrupt withdrawal of corticosteroids: most common cause of acute adrenocortical insufficiency

TABLE 22-7. SUMMARY OF CALCIUM AND PHOSPHORUS DISORDERS

DISORDER	SERUM CALCIUM	SERUM PHOSPHORUS	SERUM PTH	SERUM 25-(OH)D	SERUM 1,25-(OH)$_2$D
Primary hypoparathyroidism	↓	↑	↓	N	↓
Vitamin D deficiency (renal)	↓	↑	↑	N to ↓	↓
Vitamin D deficiency (nonrenal)	↓	N*	↑	↓	↑*
Vitamin D–dependent rickets (type I)	↓	N to ↓	↑	N	↓
Vitamin D–dependent rickets (type II)	↓	N to ↓	↑	N	↑
Primary HPTH	↑	↓	↑	N	↑
Malignancy-induced hypercalcemia (lytic)	↑	N	↓	N	↓
Malignancy-induced hypercalcemia (PTHr)	↑	↓†	↓	N	↓

*See comments in Table 22-4 concerning why 1,25-(OH)$_2$D is increased when 25-(OH)D is decreased, and why serum phosphorus is normal.
†PTHr uses same receptor as for PTH.
HPTH, hyperparathyroidism; N, normal; 25-(OH)D, calcidiol; 1,25-(OH)$_2$D, calcitriol; PTH, parathyroid hormone; PTHr, PTH-related peptide.

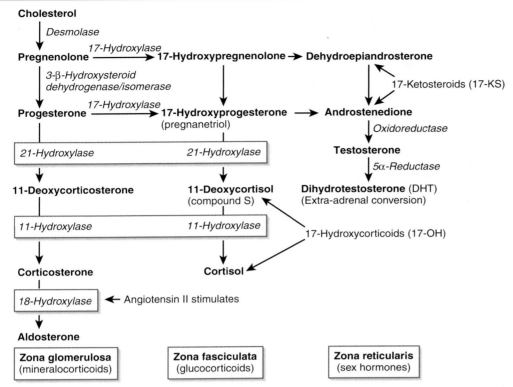

22-20: Adrenocortical hormone synthesis. The zona glomerulosa produces mineralocorticoids (e.g., aldosterone), the zona fasciculata produces glucocorticoids (e.g., cortisol), and the zona reticularis produces sex hormones (e.g., testosterone). The 17-hydroxycorticoids (17-OH) are 11-deoxycortisol and cortisol. The 17-ketosteroids (17-KS, weak androgens) are dehydroepiandrosterone and androstenedione. Testosterone is converted to dihydrotestosterone (DHT) by 5α-reductase in extra-adrenal tissue.

    (2) Patients develop endotoxic shock.
- Release of tissue thromboplastin causes disseminated intravascular coagulation (DIC).

    (3) Bilateral adrenal hemorrhage
- Fibrin clots in vessels cause hemorrhagic infarction.

2. Chronic adrenal insufficiency (Addison's disease)
  a. Epidemiology
    (1) Causes
      (a) Autoimmune destruction
- Most common cause (80% of cases)

      (b) Miliary tuberculosis (15% of cases/histoplasmosis)
      (c) Adrenogenital syndrome (see later discussion)
      (d) Metastasis
- Most often from a primary lung cancer

      (e) AIDS (30% of patients)
  b. Clinical findings
    (1) Weakness and hypotension
- Due to sodium loss from mineralocorticoid and glucocorticoid deficiency

    (2) Diffuse hyperpigmentation (Fig. 22-21)
      (a) Increased plasma ACTH stimulates melanocytes.
      (b) Buccal mucosa, skin, skin creases
  c. Laboratory findings
    (1) Short and prolonged ACTH stimulation test
- *No* increase in cortisol or 17-OH

    (2) Metyrapone test (Fig. 22-22)
- Increased ACTH but *no* increase in 11-deoxycortisol

    (3) Increased plasma ACTH
    (4) Electrolyte findings (refer to Chapter 4)
- Hyponatremia, hyperkalemia, and metabolic acidosis

Waterhouse-Friderichsen syndrome: *N. meningitidis* sepsis → DIC → bilateral adrenal hemorrhage

Autoimmune disease: most common cause of Addison's disease in U.S.

Miliary TB: most common cause of Addison's disease in developing countries

Most common cause of Addison's disease in children: adrenogenital syndrome

Addison's disease: diffuse hyperpigmentation; hypotension, weakness

Metyrapone test: ↓ cortisol → ↑ ACTH → ↓ 11-deoxycortisol

Addison's disease: ↓ serum sodium, cortisol, bicarbonate; ↑ serum potassium, ACTH

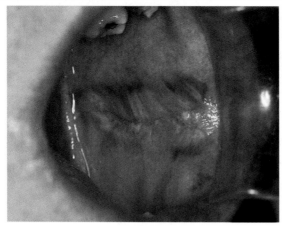

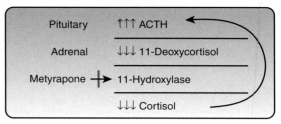

22-22: Schematic of the metyrapone test in Addison's disease. Metyrapone blocks 11-hydroxylase in the adrenal gland. This further decreases cortisol leading to a marked increase in adrenocorticotropic hormone (ACTH) due to a loss of negative feedback. However, the increase in ACTH does *not* increase the synthesis of 11-deoxycortisol in the adrenal cortex, which is destroyed in Addison's disease.

22-21: Addison's disease. Note the increased melanin pigmentation of the buccal mucosa. *(From Savin JAA, Hunter JAA, Hepburn NC: Diagnosis in Color: Skin Signs in Clinical Medicine. London, Mosby-Wolfe, 1997, p 1105, Fig. 4.44.)*

Aldosterone enhances the exchange of sodium for potassium in the kidneys. Hence, its deficiency leads to a hypertonic loss of sodium in the urine (hyponatremia) and retention of potassium (hyperkalemia). Aldosterone also enhances the proton pump. Deficiency leads to retention of protons and metabolic acidosis (normal anion gap type).

Addison's disease: hypoglycemia, eosinophilia, lymphocytosis, neutropenia

↑ 17-KS, testosterone, DHT: ambiguous genitalia females; precocious puberty males and females

Newborn with ambiguous genitalia: first step is to determine genetic sex with chromosome analysis

    (5) Fasting hypoglycemia
        • Due to decrease in cortisol (cortisol is gluconeogenic)
    (6) Eosinophilia, lymphocytosis, and neutropenia
        • Due to decrease in cortisol (refer to Chapter 12)
  d. Treatment
    • Glucocorticoid and mineralocorticoid replacement
3. Adrenogenital syndrome (congenital adrenal hyperplasia)
  a. Autosomal recessive disorders
    • Use Figure 22-20 to understand changes in steroid synthesis
  b. Enzyme deficiency causes hypocortisolism and corresponding increase in ACTH.
    (1) Increase in ACTH
        • Causes adrenocortical hyperplasia and diffuse skin pigmentation
    (2) Increase in 17-KS, testosterone, and DHT; causes:
      (a) Ambiguous genitalia in females (Fig. 22-23)
        • Primarily due to DHT; first step is to check the genetic sex of the newborn with a chromosome analysis

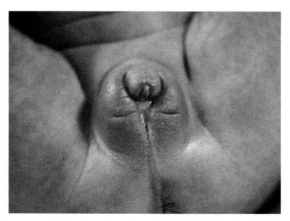

22-23: Newborn girl with ambiguous genitalia. Note the enlarged clitoris and the partially fused labia majora suggesting the presence of a scrotum. *(Courtesy of Patrick C. Walsh, MD, Johns Hopkins School of Medicine.)*

(b) Precocious puberty may develop in males and females.
- In girls, excess androgens are aromatized in peripheral tissue to estrogen.

(c) Girls experience irregular menses and infertility as adults.

(d) Both sexes have rapid growth in childhood, but early fusion of epiphyses.
- Majority have short stature as adults.

(3) Decrease in 17-KS, testosterone, and DHT causes hypogonadism in both sexes.

   (a) Females have delay in menarche and development of secondary sex characteristics; recall that female hormones come from androgens.

   (b) Males develop pseudohermaphroditism.
- Male external genitalia development requires DHT (refer to Chapter 5).

(4) Increase in mineralocorticoids
- Causes sodium retention leading to hypertension

(5) Decrease in mineralocorticoids; causes:

   (a) Sodium loss (hyponatremia), hyperkalemia

   (b) Hypotension and possible hypovolemic shock

c. Substrates proximal to the enzyme block increase

d. Substrates distal to the enzyme block decrease

e. Classic 21-hydroxylase (OHase) deficiency

  (1) Most common enzyme deficiency (90–95% of cases)

  (2) Increase in 17-KS, testosterone, and DHT

  (3) Decrease in mineralocorticoids (salt losers)

  (4) Decrease in 17-OH

  (5) Increase in 17-hydroxyprogesterone

f. Nonclassic 21-hydroxylase deficiency

  (1) Impaired cortisol production but normal mineralocorticoid production (not sodium wasting)

  (2) Ambiguous genitalia in females and virilization; precocious puberty in boys

g. 11-Hydroxylase deficiency

  (1) Increase in 17-KS, testosterone, and DHT

  (2) Increase in mineralocorticoids (11-deoxycorticosterone); salt retainers

  (3) Increase in 17-OH (11-deoxycortisol is proximal to the block)

  (4) Increase in 17-hydroxyprogesterone

h. 17-Hydroxylase deficiency

  (1) Decrease in 17-KS, 17-OH, 17-hydroxyprogesterone, testosterone, and DHT

  (2) Increase in mineralocorticoids (salt retainers)

i. Diagnosis of adrenogenital syndrome

  (1) Serum 17-OH progesterone is an excellent screening test

    (a) Increased in 21- and 11-OHase deficiency

    (b) Decreased in 17-OHase deficiency

    (c) Can measure prenatally with chorionic villous sampling

    (d) Screening test in most but not all states on newborns

  (2) Urine for 17-hydroxycorticoids and 17-ketosteroids

j. Treatment

  (1) Glucocorticoids

  (2) Mineralocorticoids (21-OHase deficiency)

  (3) Estrogen or testosterone at time of puberty

k. Summary of adrenogenital syndrome (Table 22-8)

D. Adrenocortical hyperfunction

  1. Cushing syndrome

    a. Causes

Margin notes:

↓ 17-KS, testosterone, DHT: delayed menarche and secondary sex characteristics; males develop pseudohermaphroditism

↑ Mineralocorticoids: sodium retention with hypertension

↓ Mineralocorticoids: sodium losers with hypotension

Classic 21-OHase deficiency: most common cause of adrenogenital syndrome

Classic 21-OHase deficiency: impaired cortisol and mineralocorticoid production (salt loser); ↑ androgens

Nonclassic 21-OHase deficiency: impaired cortisol synthesis only; virilization

11-OHase deficiency: impaired cortisol + mineralocorticoid excess (salt retainer); ↑ androgens

17-OHase deficiency: impaired cortisol and androgens; ↑ mineralocorticoid production

17-OH progesterone: excellent screening test; ↑ 21- and 11-OHase deficiency; ↓ 17-OHase deficiency

---

TABLE 22-8. SUMMARY OF ADRENOGENITAL SYNDROMES

LABORATORY MEASUREMENT	21-OHASE DEFICIENCY	11-OHASE DEFICIENCY	17-OHASE DEFICIENCY
17-Ketosteroids	↑	↑	↓
17-Hydroxyprogesterone	↑	↑	↓
17-Hydroxycorticoids	↓	↑	↓
Mineralocorticoids	↓	↑	↑

OHase, hydroxylase.

Cushing syndrome: most common cause is corticosteroid therapy (iatrogenic)

Cushing syndrome: pituitary Cushing most common pathologic cause

Pituitary Cushing: ↑ ACTH, ↑ cortisol

Adrenal Cushing: ↓ ACTH, ↑ cortisol

Ectopic Cushing: ↑ ↑ ACTH, ↑ cortisol

(1) Prolonged corticosteroid therapy
  • Most common cause
(2) Pituitary Cushing syndrome (Cushing disease)
  (a) 60% of cases
  (b) Due to a pituitary adenoma
  (c) Increased ACTH and cortisol
(3) Adrenal Cushing syndrome
  (a) 25% of cases
  (b) Most often due to an adenoma
  (c) Markedly decreased ACTH and increased cortisol
(4) Ectopic Cushing syndrome
  (a) 15% of cases
  (b) Usually small cell carcinoma of lung; less commonly thymus, thyroid
    • Ectopic ACTH production
  (c) Markedly increased ACTH and cortisol
b. Clinical findings
  (1) Weight gain
    (a) Due to hyperinsulinism from hyperglycemia
      • Insulin increases storage of fat (triglyceride) in adipose; also has mineralocorticoid effects and retains sodium

Cushing syndrome: truncal obesity, thin extremities, purple stria

    (b) Fat deposition in face ("moon facies"), upper back ("buffalo hump"), and trunk (truncal obesity) (Fig. 22-24)
  (2) Muscle weakness
    (a) Cortisol breaks down muscles in the extremities (thin extremities).
    (b) Muscles supply amino acids (e.g., alanine) for gluconeogenesis.
  (3) Diastolic hypertension

Hypercortisolism: thin extremities, purple stria

Hyperinsulinemia: truncal obesity

    (a) Due to increase in weak mineralocorticoids and glucocorticoids
    (b) Aldosterone is *not* increased (requires angiotensin II)
  (4) Hirsutism
    • Due to increased androgens
  (5) Purple abdominal stria

Cushing: hypertension; hirsutism

    • Cortisol weakens collagen, causing rupture of blood vessels in stretch marks.

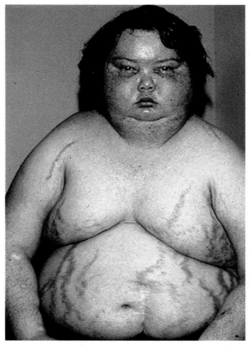

22-24: Patient with Cushing syndrome, showing "moon facies," truncal obesity, and purple abdominal striae. *(From Damjanov I: Pathology for the Health-Related Professions, 2nd ed. Philadelphia, WB Saunders, 2000, p 426.)*

(6) Osteoporosis
  • Hypercortisolism causes increased breakdown of bone.
c. Laboratory findings
  (1) Increased urine for free cortisol
    • Very high positive and negative predictive value
  (2) Low-dose dexamethasone (cortisol analogue) suppression test
    • *Cannot* suppress cortisol in all types
  (3) High-dose dexamethasone suppression test
    • Can suppress cortisol in pituitary Cushing syndrome but *not* the other types
  (4) Hyperglycemia
    (a) Cortisol enhances gluconeogenesis.
    (b) Stimulates the release of insulin
  (5) Hypokalemic metabolic alkalosis
    • Due to increased weak mineralocorticoids
d. Nelson's syndrome
  (1) Bilateral adrenalectomy causes enlargement of a preexisting pituitary adenoma.
    • Sudden drop in cortisol causes an increase in synthesis of ACTH.
  (2) Clinical findings of headache and diffuse hyperpigmentation
e. Summary of Cushing syndrome (Table 22-9)
2. Hyperaldosteronism
a. Primary aldosteronism (Conn's syndrome; refer to Chapter 4 for full discussion)
  (1) Most often due to a benign adenoma in the zona glomerulosa
  (2) Clinical findings
    (a) Diastolic hypertension
    (b) Muscle weakness, tetany (from metabolic alkalosis)
  (3) Laboratory findings (refer to Chapter 4; see Fig. 4-8)
    (a) Hypernatremia, hypokalemia, metabolic alkalosis
    (b) Decreased plasma renin activity

In **primary hyperaldosteronism**, there is increased exchange of sodium (hypernatremia) for potassium (hypokalemia). Sodium exchanges with hydrogen ions when potassium is depleted, causing a loss of hydrogen ions in the urine and a corresponding increase in bicarbonate reabsorption (metabolic alkalosis). Hypernatremia increases plasma volume, which increases renal blood flow and inhibits plasma renin activity. Chronic retention of sodium produces hypertension. Hypokalemia produces muscle weakness.

b. Secondary aldosteronism
  (1) Compensatory reaction related to a decrease in cardiac output
  (2) Decreased renal blood flow activates the renin-angiotensin-aldosterone (RAA) system.
  (3) Plasma renin activity is increased.
E. **Adrenal medulla hyperfunction**
  • Increased production of catecholamines causes hypertension.
  1. Pheochromocytoma
    a. Epidemiology
      (1) Unilateral (~90% of cases)
      (2) Benign adenoma (~90% of cases)

Marginal notes:
Screening tests: ↑ urine free cortisol; no suppression of cortisol with low dose of dexamethasone

Pituitary Cushing syndrome: suppression of cortisol by high-dose dexamethasone

Cushing: hyperglycemia; hypokalemia; metabolic alkalosis

Nelson's syndrome: bilateral adrenalectomy causes enlargement of preexisting pituitary adenoma

Primary hyperaldosteronism: hypertension, hypernatremia, hypokalemia, metabolic alkalosis

Secondary aldosteronism: compensation for ↓ cardiac output; activation of RAA system

TABLE 22-9   SUMMARY OF PITUITARY, ADRENAL, AND ECTOPIC CUSHING SYNDROME (CS)

LABORATORY TEST	PITUITARY CS	ADRENAL CS	ECTOPIC CS
Serum cortisol	↑	↑	↑
Urine free cortisol	↑	↑	↑
Low-dose dexamethasone	Cortisol *not* suppressed	Cortisol *not* suppressed	Cortisol *not* suppressed
High-dose dexamethasone	Cortisol suppressed	Cortisol *not* suppressed	Cortisol *not* suppressed
Plasma adrenocorticotropic hormone (ACTH)	"Normal"* to ↑	↓	Markedly ↑

*"Normal": a plasma ACTH in the normal range is *not* normal in the presence of an increase in serum cortisol.

Pheochromocytoma: majority benign, unilateral, arise in adrenal medulla

Associations: neurofibromatosis; MEN IIa/IIb; von Hippel–Lindau disease

Unique findings: palpitations, paroxysmal hypertension, anxiety, drenching sweats, headache

Pheochromocytoma: orthostatic hypotension, chest pain, ileus

(3) Arises in the adrenal medulla (~90% of cases)
  • Other sites—bladder, organ of Zuckerkandl near the bifurcation of the aorta, posterior mediastinum
(4) *N*-methyltransferase converts NOR to EPI (Fig. 22-25).
  (a) Adrenal medulla and the organ of Zuckerkandl contain the enzyme.
    • Pheochromocytoma produces NOR and EPI.
  (b) Other sites lack the enzyme.
    • Pheochromocytoma produces only NOR.
(5) Associations
  (a) Neurofibromatosis (5% in type 1; refer to Chapter 25)
  (b) MEN IIa and IIb (MEN III)
    • Mutation in RET protooncogene
  (c) Von Hippel–Lindau disease (often bilateral tumors)
    • Mutation in VHL gene
b. Tumor characteristics
  • Brown, hemorrhagic, and often necrotic
c. Clinical findings
  (1) Diastolic hypertension
    (a) Sustained (55%)
    (b) Paroxysmal bursts (45%)
      • *N*ot present in essential hypertension
  (2) Pounding headache (80%)
  (3) Palpitations (70%)
    (a) With or without tachycardia
    (b) Palpitations are *not* present in essential hypertension.
  (4) Drenching sweats (hyperhidrosis; 70%)
    (a) Correlates with paroxysms of hypertension
    (b) Hyperhidrosis is *not* present in essential hypertension.
  (5) Anxiety
    (a) Correlates with paroxysms of hypertension
    (b) Anxiety is *not* present in essential hypertension.
  (6) Chest pain from subendocardial ischemia
  (7) Orthostatic hypotension
    • Plasma volume is reduced owing to vasoconstriction of arterioles/venules

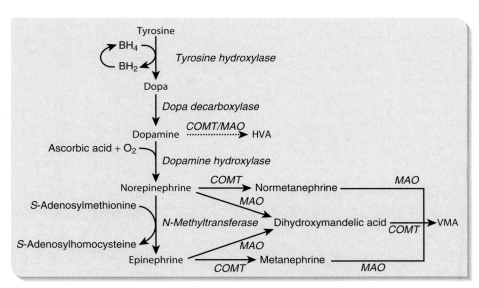

22-25: Schematic of catecholamine synthesis and degradation. Note the role of tyrosine in the synthesis of catecholamines. Catecholamines are important neurotransmitters and are involved in cardiac contraction, vasoconstriction, and gastrointestinal motility. BH₂, dihydrobiopterin; BH₄, tetrahydrobiopterin; COMT, catechol-*O*-methyltransferase; HVA, homovanillic acid; MAO, monoamine oxidase; VMA, vanillylmandelic acid. *(From Pelley J, Goljan E: Rapid Review Biochemistry, 2nd ed. St. Louis, Mosby, 2007, p 144, Fig. 8-6.)*

(8) Ileus
  - Catecholamines inhibit peristalsis.
  d. Laboratory findings
    (1) Increased plasma free metanephrines
      - Best test to screen and confirm pheochromocytoma
    (2) Increased plasma normetanephrine
    (3) Increased 24-hour urine for metanephrine (100% sensitivity)
    (4) Increased 24-hour urine for VMA
    (5) Lack of suppression of plasma norepinephrine with clonidine
    (6) Hyperglycemia
      - Increased glycogenolysis and gluconeogenesis
    (7) Neutrophilic leukocytosis
      - Inhibition of neutrophil adhesion molecules (refer to Chapter 2)
  e. Treatment is surgery.
    (1) Preoperative stabilization
      (a) Phenoxybenzamine
      (b) β-Blocker
      (c) Metyrosine (catecholamine synthesis inhibitor)
      (d) Liberal fluid and salt intake
    (2) Preoperative or intraoperative hypertensive crisis
      - Phentolamine or nitroprusside in concert with a β-adrenergic blocker
2. Neuroblastoma
  a. Malignant tumor
    (1) Neoplasm of postganglionic sympathetic neurons
    (2) Most often occurs in children < 5 years old
      (a) Third most common cancer
      (b) Mean age of onset 18 months
    (3) Primarily located in the adrenal medulla
      - Occasionally located in the posterior mediastinum (paraspinal)
    (4) Amplification of *N-MYC* oncogene (nuclear transcriber)
    (5) Opsoclonus-myoclonus syndrome
      (a) Paraneoplastic syndrome
      (b) Myoclonic jerks of extremities
      (c) Chaotic eye movements in all directions
      (d) Associated with neuroblastoma in 20% to 50% of cases
  b. Commonly metastasize to skin and bones
    - Approximately 70% have metastases at the time of diagnosis.
  c. Prognosis depends on age.
    - Children < 1 year old have a good prognosis.
  d. "Small cell" tumor
    (1) Composed of malignant neuroblasts
    (2) Presence of Homer-Wright rosettes
      - Neuroblasts are located around a central space.
    (3) Electron microscopy shows neurosecretory granules.
  e. Clinical and laboratory findings
    (1) Palpable abdominal mass
    (2) Diastolic hypertension
    (3) Increased urine VMA and HVA (90–95% sensitivity)
  f. Diagnosis
    (1) Urine collections for VMA and HVA
    (2) Imaging studies
      (a) Body scan with ^{131}I-MIBG (metaiodobenzylguanidine)
        - Malignant cells pick up the radioactive material.
      (b) Bone scans to detect lytic lesions
  g. Treatment
    (1) Depends on age, stage of disease
    (2) Surgery; irradiation; multiagent chemotherapy
  h. Prognosis
    (1) Overall survival is 40%.
    (2) Children < 1 year old have 90% cure rate.

VIII. Islet Cell Tumors (Table 22-10)

Margin notes:

Diagnosis: plasma free metanephrines best screen

Urine tests: 24-hour collection for metanephrine (best test), VMA

Pheochromocytoma: hyperglycemia, neutrophilic leukocytosis

Neuroblastoma: malignant tumor postganglionic sympathetic neurons

Neuroblastoma: childhood tumor and cause of hypertension

Opsoclonus-myoclonus syndrome: paraneoplastic syndrome; myoclonic jerk; chaotic eye movements

Neuroblastoma: "small cell" tumor; neurosecretory granules

Neuroblastoma: child with abdominal mass + hypertension

Insulinoma: ↑ serum insulin; ↑ C-peptide

Patient injecting excess insulin: ↑ serum insulin; ↓ C-peptide

TABLE 22-10. **SUMMARY OF ISLET CELL TUMORS**

TUMOR	DESCRIPTION
Glucagonoma	Malignant tumor of α-islet cells Clinical: hyperglycemia, rash (necrolytic migratory erythema) *Treatment*: surgery; octreotide (somatostatin analogue)
Insulinoma	Benign tumor of β-islet cells; most common islet cell tumor; approximately 80% have MEN I syndrome Clinical: fasting hypoglycemia causing mental status abnormalities Laboratory: fasting hypoglycemia; increase in serum insulin and C-peptide, which is an endogenous marker of insulin produced in β-islet cells *Treatment*: surgery is the treatment of choice; streptozotocin Surreptitious injection of insulin: fasting hypoglycemia, increased insulin, *decreased* C-peptide
Somatostatinoma	Malignant tumor of α-islet cells; somatostatin is an inhibitory hormone Inhibition of gastrin causes achlorhydria Inhibition of cholecystokinin causes cholelithiasis and steatorrhea Inhibition of gastric inhibitory peptide causes diabetes mellitus Inhibition of secretin causes steatorrhea *Treatment*: surgery; streptozotocin
VIPoma (pancreatic cholera)	Malignant tumor with excessive secretion of vasoactive intestinal peptide (VIP) Clinical: secretory diarrhea, achlorhydria Laboratory: hypokalemia, normal anion gap metabolic acidosis (loss of bicarbonate in stool) *Treatment*: surgery; octreotide (somatostatin analogue)
Zollinger-Ellison (refer to Chapter 17)	Malignant islet cell tumor that secretes gastrin producing hyperacidity; MEN I association (20–30% of cases) Clinical: peptic ulceration, diarrhea, maldigestion of food Laboratory: serum gastrin >1000 pg/mL *Treatment*: proton inhibitors; surgery; octreotide (somatostatin analogue)

MEN, multiple endocrine neoplasia.

IX. **Diabetes Mellitus (DM)**

A. **Epidemiology**

1. Affects 5% to 7% of population in the United States
   - Increased in Native Americans (35% of Pima Indians)
2. Leading cause in the United States for
   a. Legal blindness
   b. Peripheral neuropathy
   c. Chronic renal failure
   d. Below-the-knee amputation
3. Incidence increases with age.

B. **Classification**

1. Type 1 and type 2 diabetes mellitus (Table 22-11)
2. Secondary causes
   a. Pancreatic disease
      - Examples—cystic fibrosis, chronic pancreatitis
   b. Drugs
      - Examples—glucocorticoids, pentamidine, thiazides, α-interferon
   c. Endocrine disease
      - Examples—pheochromocytoma, glucagonoma, Cushing syndrome
   d. Genetic disease
      - Examples—hemochromatosis, syndrome X (metabolic syndrome), maturity onset diabetes of the young (MODY)
   e. Insulin-receptor deficiency
      - Acanthosis nigricans is a phenotypic marker.
   f. Infections
      - Examples—mumps, cytomegalovirus (AIDS patients)
3. Impaired glucose tolerance (IGT)
4. Gestational diabetes mellitus (GDM)
5. Maturity onset diabetes of the young (MODY)
   a. Autosomal dominant (AD) inheritance
      (1) Various subtypes
      (2) Mutations of transcription factor genes (e.g., glucokinase gene)
   b. Patients < 25 years old and are *not* obese.
   c. Mild to severe hyperglycemia
      - Impaired glucose-induced secretion of insulin release

DM most common cause of blindness, peripheral neuropathy, chronic renal failure, below-knee amputation

MODY: AD inheritance; not obese; impaired glucose-induced secretion of insulin

TABLE 22-11. COMPARISON BETWEEN TYPE 1 AND TYPE 2 DIABETES MELLITUS

CHARACTERISTIC	TYPE 1	TYPE 2
Prevalence	5–10%	90–95%
Age at onset	<30 years	>40 years
Speed of onset	Rapid	Insidious
Body habitus	Usually thin	Usually obese (80% of cases)
Genetics	Family history uncommon Environmental factors required for expression HLA-DR3 and HLA-DR4	Family history common No HLA association Increased in Native Americans and in blacks
Associations	Other autoimmune diseases: Graves' disease, Hashimoto's thyroiditis, pernicious anemia, Addison's disease	No autoimmune associations
Pathogenesis	Lack of insulin Pancreas devoid of β-islet cells Insulitis: T-cell cytokine destruction (type IV HSR) and autoantibodies against β-islet cells and insulin (type II HSR) Triggers for destruction—e.g., viruses Autoantibodies to islet cells (>80%) and insulin (>50%)	Relative deficiency of insulin; early stages have hyperinsulinemia Insulin resistance related to receptor and postreceptor problems Decreased insulin receptors: downregulation by increased adipose Postreceptor defects: most important factor; examples—tyrosine kinase defects, GLUT-4 abnormalities Fibrotic β-islet cells contain amyloid No autoantibodies
Clinical findings	Polyuria, polydipsia, polyphagia, weight loss Ketoacidosis (hyperglycemia, coma; production of ketone bodies); lactic acidosis from shock	Insidious onset of symptoms Recurrent blurry vision: alteration in lens refraction from sorbitol Recurrent infections: bacterial, *Candida* Target organ disease: nephropathy, retinopathy, neuropathy, coronary artery disease Reactive hypoglycemia: too much insulin is released for a glucose load (early finding) Increased risk for Alzheimer's disease (refer to Chapter 25) HNKC: enough insulin to prevent ketoacidosis but *not* enough to prevent hyperglycemia Lactic acidosis may occur due to shock
Treatment	Insulin	Weight loss: upregulates insulin receptor synthesis Oral hypoglycemic agents; may require insulin

GLUT, glucose transport unit; HLA, human leukocyte antigen; HNKC, hyperosmolar nonketotic coma; HSR, hypersensitivity reaction.

    d. Resistance to ketosis

    e. May progress into type 2 diabetes mellitus

    f. Treatment varies with regard to oral hypoglycemic agents or insulin.

  6. Metabolic syndrome

    a. May affect as high as 25% of the U.S. population

    b. Insulin resistance syndrome

      (1) Genetic defect causes insulin resistance that is exacerbated by obesity.

      (2) Commonly associated with polycystic ovary syndrome in women

      (3) May be associated with acanthosis nigricans (refer to Chapter 24)

      (4) Increased risk for developing Alzheimer's disease (refer to Chapter 25)

    c. Clinical and laboratory findings

      (1) Hyperinsulinemia; leads to

        (a) Increased synthesis of very low-density lipoprotein (VLDL; hypertriglyceridemia)

          • Serum triglyceride ≥ 150 mg/dL

        (b) Hypertension (≥130/85 mm Hg)

          • Increased insulin increases sodium retention by the renal tubules.

        (c) Coronary artery disease (CAD)

          • Increased insulin damages endothelial cells.

      (2) Obesity exacerbates insulin resistance.

        • Increased adipose downregulates insulin receptor synthesis.

      (3) Definition for obesity in metabolic syndrome

        (a) Abdominal waistline girth in men > 40 inches (102 cm)

        (b) Abdominal waistline girth in women > 35 inches (88 cm)

      (4) Serum high-density lipoprotein cholesterol (HDL-CH) < 40 mg/dL in men and <50 mg/dL in women

      (5) Fasting serum glucose ≥ 110 mg/dL

Metabolic syndrome: insulin resistance exacerbated by obesity

Associations: acanthosis nigricans; Alzheimer's disease

Hyperinsulinemia: ↑ VLDL, hypertension, CAD; ↓HDL-CH

d. Treatment
  (1) Statin drugs to lower lipids
  (2) Treat hypertension
    • Angiotensin-converting enzyme (ACE) inhibitors or diuretics
  (3) Correct insulin resistance with weight loss.
  (4) Correct insulin resistance with drugs.
    • ? Metformin, thiazolidinediones
C. Pathologic processes and complications in diabetes mellitus (Table 22-12)
  1. Poor glycemic control
    a. Hyperglycemia is the key factor that produces organ damage.
    b. Glucose control reduces onset and severity of complications.
      • Complications are related to retinopathy, neuropathy, and nephropathy in descending order.
  2. Nonenzymatic glycosylation (NEG)
    a. Glucose combines with amino groups in proteins.
    b. Produces advanced glycosylation products
      (1) Increased vessel permeability to protein
      (2) Increased atherogenesis
    c. Role in diabetes
      (1) Production of glycosylated Hb_{A1c}
      (2) Hyaline arteriolosclerosis (refer to Chapter 9)

Good glycemic control prevents complications of diabetes.

NEG: Hb_{A1c}, hyaline arteriolosclerosis, glomerulopathy

TABLE 22-12. COMPLICATIONS OF DIABETES MELLITUS

COMPLICATION CATEGORY	DISCUSSION
Atherosclerotic disease	Increased incidence of strokes, CAD, and peripheral vascular disease Acute MI is the most common cause of death Gangrene of the lower extremities; diabetes is the most common cause of nontraumatic amputation of the lower extremity
Renal disorders (see Fig. 19-7J)	Renal failure due to nodular glomerulosclerosis (refer to Chapter 19) Renal papillary necrosis

Ocular disorders (see Fig. 22-27)	Increased risk for cataracts and glaucoma
	Retinopathy (15%):
	    Nonproliferative: microaneurysm formation; flame hemorrhages; exudates
	    Proliferative: formation of new vessels (neovascularization); increased risk for retinal detachment and blindness; annual ophthalmologic examination is mandatory (photocoagulate microaneurysms)

Peripheral nerve disorders (see Fig. 22-26)	Diabetes mellitus is the most common cause of peripheral neuropathy in the United States; occurs in 70–80% Sensory: paresthesias; patients complain of burning feet; ↓ pinprick sensation; ↓ proprioception (ataxia) Motor dysfunction: muscle weakness; ↓ deep tendon reflexes Neuropathy is the most important risk factor for pressure ulcers on the bottom of the feet (patient cannot feel pain) *Treatment* for neuropathy: duloxetine (selective serotonin and norepinephrine reuptake inhibitor); topical capsaicin; amitriptyline
Autonomic nervous system disorders	Autonomic neuropathy: gastroparesis (delayed emptying of stomach); impotence; neurogenic bladder; orthostatic hypotension *Treatment* for gastroparesis: prokinetic agents (e.g., metoclopramide)
Cranial nerve (CN) disorders	Diabetes is the most common cause of multiple cranial nerve palsies Cranial nerves most often involved: CN III, IV, and V
Infectious disorders	Urinary tract infections *Candida* infections: e.g., vulvovaginitis Malignant external otitis due to *Pseudomonas aeruginosa* Rhinocerebral mucormycosis: *Mucor* extends from the frontal sinuses to the frontal lobes, producing infarction (vessel invader) and abscesses Cutaneous infections: usually *Staphylococcus aureus* abscesses
Skin disorders	Necrobiosis lipoidica diabeticorum: well-demarcated yellow plaques over the anterior surface of the legs/dorsum of ankles Lipoatrophy: atrophy at insulin injection sites due to impure insulin Lipohypertrophy: increased fat synthesis at insulin injection sites
Joint disorders	Neuropathic joint: related to lack of sensation; bone or joint deformity from repeated trauma (refer to Chapter 23)

CAD, coronary artery disease; MI, myocardial infarction.

(3) Diabetic glomerulopathy (refer to Chapter 19)

(4) Ischemic heart disease, strokes, peripheral vascular disease

3. Osmotic damage

   a. Aldose reductase

     (1) Converts glucose to sorbitol

     (2) Sorbitol draws water into tissue causing damage.

   b. Role in diabetes mellitus

     (1) Formation of cataracts

     (2) Peripheral neuropathy

       (a) Osmotic damage of Schwann cells produces demyelination and sensorimotor peripheral neuropathy

       (b) Peripheral neuropathy leads to neuropathic pressure ulcers (Fig. 22-26).

         • Patient cannot feel pain.

     (3) Retinopathy

       • Osmotic damage to pericytes produces microaneurysms of retinal vessels (Fig. 22-27).

4. Diabetic microangiopathy

   a. Increased synthesis of type IV collagen in basement membranes and mesangium

   b. Important in diabetic glomerulopathy (refer to Chapter 19)

D. Clinical findings

1. Insulin-induced hypoglycemia

   a. Most common complication

   b. Produces irreversible brain damage by destroying neurons

   c. Clinical findings

     (1) Sympathetic nervous system signs

       • Sweating, tachycardia, palpitations, and tremulousness

     (2) Parasympathetic nervous system signs

       • Nausea and hunger

     (3) Focal neurologic deficits, mental confusion, coma

2. Diabetic ketoacidosis (DKA; Fig. 22-28)

   a. Complication of type 1 diabetes

   b. Precipitated by medical illness or omission of insulin

   c. Produces severe volume depletion and coma

     • Volume depletion due to loss of sodium and water with osmotic diuresis

Aldose reductase: converts glucose to sorbitol; osmotic damage

Osmotic damage: cataracts, peripheral neuropathy, retinopathy

Microangiopathy: diabetic glomerular disease

Insulin-induced hypoglycemia: most common complication of diabetes

DKA: complication of type 1 DM

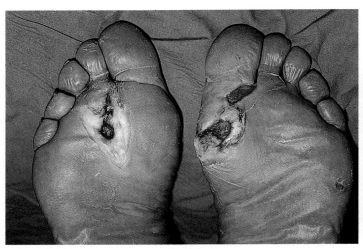

22-26: Neuropathic pressure ulcers. Note the areas of ulcerations over the pressure points on the plantar surfaces of both feet. The patient had no sensation for pain in these areas due to a peripheral neuropathy. This emphasizes the importance for checking pain sensation of the feet in all diabetic patients. *(From Swartz MH: Textbook of Physical Diagnosis, 5th ed. Philadelphia, Saunders Elsevier, 2006, p 641, Fig. 20-72.)*

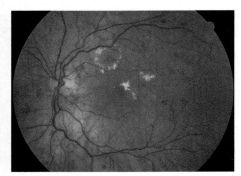

22-27: Diabetic retinopathy. The retina shows tiny dots representing retinal hemorrhages from ruptured microaneurysms and retinal exudates (sharply defined white areas). *(From Goldman L, Ausiello D: Cecil's Textbook of Medicine, 23rd ed. Philadelphia, Saunders Elsevier, 2008, p 2858, Fig. 449-15.)*

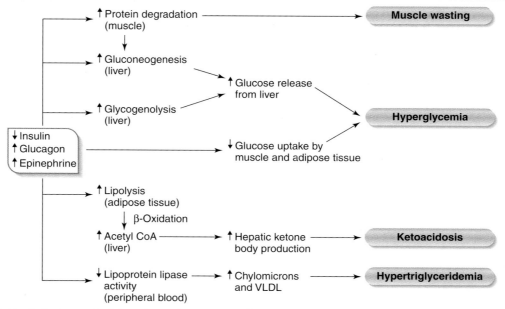

22-28: Metabolic changes in diabetic ketoacidosis (DKA). Refer to the text for discussion. VLDL, very low-density lipoprotein. *(From Pelley J, Goljan EF: Rapid Review: Biochemistry. St. Louis, Mosby, 2004, p 176, Fig. 9-5.)*

Gluconeogenesis: most important mechanism of hyperglycemia in diabetic ketoacidosis

Ketoacids: synthesized from acetyl CoA derived from β-oxidation of fatty acids

Hypertriglyceridemia: ↓ capillary lipoprotein lipase activity; ↓ hydrolysis of chylomicrons and VLDL

DKA electrolytes: ↓ serum sodium, bicarbonate (metabolic acidosis); ↑ serum potassium, anion gap

  d. Mechanisms for hyperglycemia
    (1) Increased gluconeogenesis
      (a) Due to increase in glucagon and epinephrine
      (b) Most important mechanism of hyperglycemia
    (2) Increased glycogenolysis in the liver
  e. Mechanism for ketone bodies
    (1) Increased lipolysis with release of fatty acids
      • *No* inhibition of hormone-sensitive lipase
    (2) Increased β-oxidation of fatty acids increases production of acetyl CoA.
      • *No* malonyl Co-A to inhibit carnitine acyltransferase, the rate-limiting enzyme of β-oxidation
    (3) Acetyl CoA is converted by the liver to ketone bodies.
      • Acetone (fruity odor), acetoacetic and β-hydroxybutyric acid
  f. Mechanism for hypertriglyceridemia
    (1) Lack of insulin decreases capillary lipoprotein lipase activity in peripheral blood.
    (2) Accumulation of chylomicrons and VLDL in the blood
      • Type V hyperlipoproteinemia (refer to Chapter 9)
    (3) May precipitate acute pancreatitis and eruptive xanthomas in the skin
      • Called the hyperchylomicronemia syndrome
  g. Laboratory findings
    (1) Hyperglycemia
      • Glucose ranges from 250 to 1000 mg/dL.
    (2) Increased $Hb_{A1c} \geq 6\%$
    (3) Dilutional hyponatremia (refer to Chapter 4)
      (a) Glucose overrides sodium in controlling the osmotic gradient.
      (b) Water shifts out of the intracellular fluid compartment into the extracellular fluid compartment.
    (4) Hyperkalemia (refer to Chapter 4)
      • Transcellular shift as excess H^+ ions enter cells in exchange of potassium
    (5) Increased anion gap metabolic acidosis (refer to Chapter 4)
      • Due to ketoacidosis and lactic acidosis
    (6) Prerenal azotemia (refer to Chapter 19)
      • Due to volume depletion

h. Mortality rate in DKA is 5% to 10%.
3. Hyperosmolar nonketotic coma (see Table 22-11)
   a. Complication of type 2 diabetes
   b. Increased mortality rate (20–50%)
      • Patients are older and usually have underlying cardiac and renal problems.

Hyperomolar nonketotic coma: complication of type 2 DM

General treatment for type 1 diabetes. Split dose insulin mixtures: split doses of regular insulin + neutral protamine hagedorn (NPH) twice daily (morning [AM] and evening [PM]). **Intensive insulin therapy** involves three injections, including regular insulin + NPH in the AM; regular insulin to cover PM dinner; and NPH at bedtime. **Long-acting insulin** may be used for maintaining a basal level throughout the day plus insulin lispro (peaks at 13 hours) to cover each meal. **Pramlintide** is a synthetic analogue of human amylin, which is a hormone normally secreted along with insulin by β-islet cells. It can be used as adjunctive treatment in type 1 or 2 diabetics who inject insulin at meal time. An **insulin pump** allows continuous infusion of insulin throughout the day at preset levels. It is also possible to program doses of insulin as needed at meal times. In patients on a split dose insulin regimen, a problem may occur in evaluating the cause of an increased early morning glucose level. To sort out the cause of the hyperglycemia, a 3 AM glucose is useful. If both the 3 AM and 7 AM glucose levels are increased, more NPH insulin is required at dinner or bedtime (called the waning effect). If the 3AM glucose is decreased and the 7 AM glucose is increased, then less NPH insulin should be given at dinner or bedtime. This phenomenon (called Somogyi effect) is caused by the rebound release of counterregulatory hormones (e.g., glucagon, catecholamines) in response to the hypoglycemia at 3 AM. If the 3 AM glucose is normal but the 7 AM glucose is increased, this is called the dawn effect. It is caused by the release of growth hormone at 5 AM. Growth hormone is gluconeogenic; hence, it has an anti-insulin effect. Dividing the NPH dose between dinner and bedtime usually corrects this problem. If the lunch time glucose is high, then more regular insulin should be given in the AM. If the glucose is increased at dinner time, then more NPH should be given at breakfast.

General principles in treatment of DKA. Volume replacement is the most important initial step in management of DKA because of the tremendous loss of water and sodium in the urine by osmotic diuresis. Patients are frequently in hypovolemic shock. Volume replacement with crystalloids is best accomplished with 0.9% normal saline until the volume deficit is corrected and the patient is stabile with regard to blood pressure and mental status. At this point, the infusion is switched to 5% dextrose in 0.45% saline and insulin therapy is initiated. Serum glucose, electrolytes, arterial blood gases, and serum ketones should all be closely monitored throughout treatment. Particular concerns related to treatment with insulin include hypophosphatemia (phosphate goes along with glucose into the cell) and hypokalemia (lost in the urine by osmotic diuresis). It should be understood that the hyperkalemia that one initially sees in DKA is most often related to a transcellular shift of potassium moving out of the cell as hydrogen ions move in for buffering (refer to Chapter 4). Total body potassium is in fact decreased in DKA, because it is lost along with sodium in the urine by osmotic diuresis. Hence, when the pH is restored to normal and there is no transcellular shift, the physician often finds a very low serum potassium. Severe hypokalemia or hypophosphatemia can cause respiratory paralysis; hence, monitoring potassium and phosphorus levels is very important once insulin therapy is initiated.

General principles in treatment of type 2 diabetes mellitus. Oral hypoglycemic agents are most often used in treatment, because most patients are *not* insulin deficient. The primary mechanism of action (MOA) of **metformin** is to decrease hepatic output of glucose. Because metformin, a biguanide, does *not* produce hypoglycemia, it is a preferred drug for most patients. Side effects include diarrhea and lactic acidosis. **Sulfonylureas** (e.g., glyburide, glipizide) increase pancreatic secretion of insulin. They are a common cause of hypoglycemia in a type 2 diabetic. **Acarbose** and **miglitol** inhibit α-glucosidase. In this regard, they work by competitively inhibiting pancreatic amylase and small intestinal glucosidases from breaking down glucose in the bowel, hence decreasing glucose reabsorption after eating. Side effects include flatulence and diarrhea. **Pioglitazone** and **rosiglitazone** (thiazolidinediones) increase insulin sensitivity. They accomplish this by decreasing peripheral insulin resistance, increasing glucose disposal, and decreasing hepatic glucose production. Side effects include hepatotoxicity with an increase in serum transaminases. **Repaglinide** and **nateglinide** (meglitinides) acutely increase pancreatic insulin secretion as their MOA. Hypoglycemia may occur as a side effect. **Exenatide** is a synthetic peptide that stimulates release of insulin from pancreatic β-islet cells. Combinations of oral hypoglycemic drugs are commonly used if one drug does *not* produce adequate glycemic control. If oral hypoglycemic agents alone or in combination are still ineffective in glycemic control, then insulin is utilized.

E. Laboratory diagnosis
   1. Criteria
      a. Random plasma glucose ≥ 200 mg/dL plus classic symptoms
      b. Fasting plasma glucose ≥ 126 mg/dL
         • Set for high sensitivity
      c. Two-hour glucose level after 75-g glucose challenge is ≥200 mg/dL.
      d. One of the preceding three criteria must be present on a subsequent day to confirm the diagnosis of diabetes.

HbA1c: marker of long-term glycemic control

   2. Glycosylated hemoglobin (Hb$_{A1c}$)
      a. Evaluates long-term glycemic control
      b. Represents the mean glucose value for the preceding 8 to 12 weeks
      c. Test is currently *not* used to diagnose diabetes.
      d. Goal in therapy is <7% (some use 6.5%).
   3. Fructosamine
      • Reflects glycemic control for the preceding 2 weeks

F. Impaired glucose tolerance (IGT)
   1. Patient has hyperglycemia that is nondiagnostic of diabetes.
      a. Fasting glucose > 110 mg/dL, but <126 mg/dL
      b. Two-hour glucose > 140 mg/dL, but <200 mg/dL after 75-g oral glucose tolerance test

IGT: prediabetic state; insulin resistance

   2. Pathogenesis
      • Prediabetic state with insulin resistance
   3. Increased risk for macrovascular disease and neuropathy
   4. Approximately 30% develop type 2 diabetes within 10 years.
   5. Treatment is to exercise regularly and to reduce sugar intake.

G. Gestational diabetes (GDM)
   1. Glucose intolerance develops during pregnancy.
      a. Anti-insulin effect of human placental lactogen (HPL), cortisol, and progesterone
      b. Increased risk for GDM in future pregnancies

GDM: anti-insulin effect of HPL, cortisol, progesterone

   2. Screening
      a. All pregnant women are screened between 24 and 28 weeks' gestation.
      b. 50-g glucose challenge followed by 1-hour glucose level
         • Above 140 mg/dL is a positive screen.
      c. Positive screen is confirmed with a 3-hour oral glucose tolerance test.
   3. Newborn risks
      a. Macrosomia

Macrosomia: ↑ insulin causes ↑ in adipose and muscle

         (1) Hyperglycemia in the fetus causes release of insulin.
         (2) Insulin increases fat stored in adipose tissue.
         (3) Insulin increases muscle mass by increasing amino acid uptake in muscle.
      b. Respiratory distress syndrome (RDS)
         • Insulin inhibits fetal surfactant production.

RDS: ↑ insulin inhibits fetal surfactant production

      c. Increased risk for open neural tube defects
      d. Neonatal hypoglycemia
         • High insulin levels at birth drives glucose into the hypoglycemic range (give newborn glucose after birth).

Neonatal hypoglycemia: ↑ insulin drives glucose into hypoglycemic range; give newborn glucose at birth

   4. Maternal risk
      • Diabetes may develop at a later date (>50% of cases).
   5. If patients cannot keep their blood glucose in control by diet alone, then insulin is recommended.

X. Polyglandular deficiency syndromes
A. Type I polyglandular syndrome
   1. Autosomal recessive
   2. Mean age of onset is 12 years old.
   3. No HLA relationship
   4. Clinical findings
      a. Addison's disease
      b. Primary hypoparathyroidism
      c. Mucocutaneous candidiasis

Type I: Addison's disease, primary hypoparathyroidism, mucocutaneous candidiasis

B. Type II polyglandular syndrome
   1. Autosomal dominant

2. Mean age of onset is 24 years old.
3. HLA-DR3 and -DR4
4. Clinical findings
    a. Addison's disease
    b. Hashimoto's thyroiditis
    c. Type 1 diabetes mellitus

XI. **Hypoglycemia**
A. **Definition**
    1. Difficult to arrive at a consensus for a cut-off point
    2. Ranges have been anywhere from 40 to 70 mg/dL (normal fasting 70–110 mg/dL)
    3. Reasonable cut-off point is <50 mg/dL.
B. **Fed state hypoglycemia**
    1. Reactive type of hypoglycemia
    2. Causes
        a. Insulin treatment in type 1 diabetes
            (1) Most common cause
            (2) Sulfonylurea-related hypoglycemia is less common.
        b. IGT or type 2 diabetes
            • Excessive amount of insulin is released for the glucose absorbed.
    3. Develop adrenergic symptoms ~1 to 5 hours after eating:
        a. Sweating, trembling, anxiety
        b. Palpitations, tachycardia, mydriasis
        c. Numbness and tingling
    4. Treatment
        a. Carbohydrate intake (grape juice, candy)
        b. Glucagon IM injection

Idiopathic postprandial syndrome (IPS): This syndrome is characterized by the presence of adrenergic symptoms *without* demonstrable evidence of hypoglycemia. Patients also complain of lack of energy, mental dullness, and inability to concentrate. Symptoms usually disappear if mixed carbohydrate-protein meals are eaten at frequent intervals.

C. **Fasting type of hypoglycemia**
    1. Fasting state hypoglycemia
    2. Causes
        a. Alcohol (see Chapter 6)
            (1) Increased nicotinamide adenine dinucleotide (NADH) converts pyruvate to lactate.
                • Less pyruvate for gluconeogenesis
            (2) Decreased glycogen stores in severe liver disease
        b. Renal failure
            • Kidney is a site of gluconeogenesis.
        c. Malnutrition
        d. Chronic liver disease
            • Decreased gluconeogenesis, glycogen depletion
        e. Insulinoma, hypopituitarism (decreased GH and cortisol)
        f. Ketotic hypoglycemia in childhood
            (1) Most common cause of hypoglycemia from 18 months to mid-childhood
            (2) Multiple etiologies
                (a) Maple syrup urine disease, galactosemia, hereditary fructose intolerance, von Gierke's glycogen storage disease (refer to Chapter 5)
                (b) Carnitine deficiency

Carnitine is required for the synthesis of carnitine acyltransferase (CAT). CAT is the rate-limiting reaction of β-oxidation of fatty acids, which are an important source of energy in the fasting and starvation states for muscle tissue. Any excess of acetyl CoA, the end-product of β-oxidation, is used by the liver to synthesize ketone bodies. Ketone bodies are used for energy by muscle in the fasting state and by the brain in starvation. Therefore, in carnitine deficiency, a decrease in CAT significantly reduces the amount of fatty acids and ketone bodies as sources of energy. This leaves glucose as the only fuel available for all tissues to use for energy, which results in hypoglycemia.

Type II: Addison's disease, Hashimoto's thyroiditis, type 1 diabetes mellitus

Hypoglycemia: subdivided into fed state and fasting state

Reactive hypoglycemia: excess insulin most common cause; adrenergic symptoms

Fasting hypoglycemia: alcohol excess; insulinoma; cirrhosis

Alcohol excess: ↓ glycogen stores; ↓ gluconeogenesis (pyruvate converted to lactate)

Fasting hypoglycemia children: look for inborn errors of metabolism

Neuroglycopenia: dizziness, mental status changes, motor disturbances

Diagnosis: prolonged fast; satisfy Whipple's triad

3. Neuroglycopenic symptoms
   a. Dizziness, confusion, headache, inability to concentrate
   b. Motor disturbances, seizures, visual disturbances, coma
4. Diagnosis
   a. Prolonged fast
   b. Must satisfy Whipple's triad:
      (1) Symptoms occur.
      (2) Hypoglycemia is demonstrated.
      (3) Symptoms are relieved by glucose.

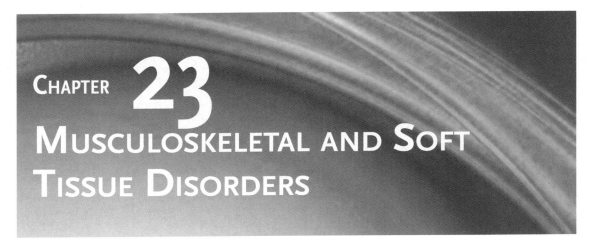

CHAPTER 23

MUSCULOSKELETAL AND SOFT TISSUE DISORDERS

I. **Bone Disorders**
   A. **Osteogenesis imperfecta ("brittle bone" disease)**
      1. Autosomal dominant (AD)
      2. Defective synthesis of type I collagen
      3. Clinical findings
         a. Pathologic fractures at birth
         b. Blue sclera (Fig. 23-1)
         c. Deafness in some patients
      4. Treatment
         • Bisphosphonates to increase bone mineralization
   B. **Achondroplasia**
      1. Autosomal dominant
      2. Pathogenesis
         a. Mutation in fibroblast growth factor receptor gene
            • Gene mutations increase with paternal age
         b. Impaired proliferation of cartilage at the growth plate
      3. Clinical findings
         a. Normal-sized head and vertebral column
         b. Shortened arms and legs
         c. Normal growth hormone and insulin growth factor-1 levels
      4. No treatment
   C. **Osteopetrosis ("marble bone" disease)**
      1. Autosomal recessive (severe)
         • Autosomal dominant (less severe)
      2. Pathogenesis
         a. Deficiency osteoclasts
         b. Normal balance of osteoblasts making bone and osteoclasts breaking down bone is disrupted favoring increased bone formation.
         c. Overgrowth and sclerosis of cortical bone ("too much bone")
      3. Clinical findings
         a. Pathologic fractures
         b. Anemia
            • Replacement of marrow cavity
         c. Cranial nerve compression
            • Visual and hearing loss
      4. No treatment
   D. **Osteomyelitis**
      1. Osteomyelitis in children and adults
         a. Most commonly due to sepsis with subsequent spread to bone
         b. Metaphysis is the most common site.
            • Favors the tibia and fibula in children
         c. Most often due to *Staphylococcus aureus* (90% of cases)
            • Other pathogens: *Streptococcus pyogenes, Haemophilus influenzae*

Osteogenesis imperfecta: AD; defect in synthesis type 1 collagen

Blue sclera: reflection of underlying choroidal veins

Achondroplasia: AD; mutation in fibroblast growth factor receptor gene

Achondroplasia: normal head/axial skeleton; short arms/legs

Osteopetrosis: deficiency of osteoclasts; "too much bone"

Osteopetrosis: pathologic fractures; visual/hearing loss

Osteomyelitis: usually hematogenous spread to bone; metaphysis most common site

Staphylococcus aureus: most common pathogen causing osteomyelitis

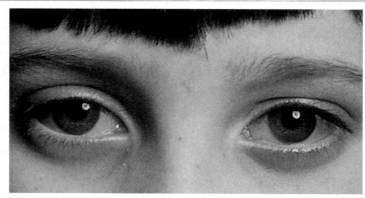

23-1: Osteogenesis imperfecta. Note the faint blue tint of the sclera representing the reflection of the underlying choroidal veins. *(From Mir MA: Atlas of Clinical Diagnosis. London, Saunders, 1995.)*

Salmonella paratyphi: osteomyelitis in sickle cell disease

Tuberculous osteomyelitis: commonly involves vertebral column (Pott's disease)

P. aeruginosa osteomyelitis: puncture of foot through rubber footwear

Sequestra: devitalized bone

Involucrum: reactive bone formation in periosteum

Draining sinuses: danger of squamous cancer

2. Osteomyelitis in sickle cell disease (refer to Chapter 11)
   • Most often due to *Salmonella paratyphi*
3. Tuberculous osteomyelitis
   a. Hematogenous spread from a primary lung focus
   b. Targets vertebral column (Pott's disease)
4. *Pseudomonas aeruginosa* osteomyelitis
   • Most often due to puncture of foot through rubber footwear
5. Neutrophils enzymatically destroy bone (Fig. 23-2).
   a. Devitalized bone is called sequestra.
   b. Chronic disease produces reactive bone formation in periosteum.
      • Called involucrum
   c. Draining sinus tracts to the skin surface often occur.
      • Danger of squamous cell carcinoma developing at orifice of sinus tract
6. Clinical findings
   • Fever, bone pain
7. Diagnosis
   a. Bone biopsy for culture
   b. Imaging studies: CT scan or MRI
8. Treatment
   a. Surgical débridement
   b. *Staphylococcus aureus*: vancomycin + ceftazidime
   c. *Salmonella paratyphi* (sickle cell): ciprofloxacin

Osteoporosis: most common metabolic abnormality of bone

E. Osteoporosis
   1. Epidemiology
      a. Most common metabolic abnormality of bone

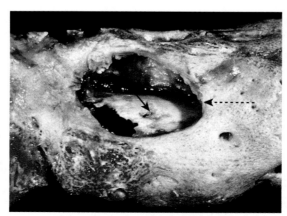

23-2: Chronic osteomyelitis. The *solid arrow* points to necrotic bone in the center of a draining abscess (sequestrum). The *interrupted arrow* is a rim of new bone formation (involucrum). *(From Kumar V, Abbas AK, Fausto N, Mitchell RN: Robbins Basic Pathology, 8th ed. Philadelphia, Saunders Elsevier, 2007, p 810, Fig. 21-7.)*

b. Loss of both organic bone matrix and minerals
  (1) Decreased bone mass and density
    • Radiograph shows osteopenia (washed out appearance).
  (2) Decreased thickness of cortical and trabecular bone
c. More common in women than men
  • Men have greater bone mass to begin with; takes longer to develop osteoporosis
d. Osteoporosis-related fractures: 50% in women > 65 years old
e. Osteoporosis-related fractures: 20% in men > 65 years old
f. Classification
  (1) Primary
    (a) Most common type (80% women, 60% men)
    (b) Idiopathic type in children and young adults
    (c) Postmenopausal type (most common)
    (d) Senile type in men and women
  (2) Secondary
    (a) Underlying disease (e.g., hypercortisolism)
    (b) Drugs (e.g., heparin)
    (c) Hypogonadism (e.g., hypopituitarism)
    (d) Malnutrition (e.g., anorexia nervosa)
    (e) Space travel
      • Lack of gravity reduces bone stress.
2. Postmenopausal osteoporosis
  a. Due to estrogen deficiency
    (1) Increased resorption of bone by osteoclasts
    (2) Decreased formation of bone by osteoblasts
  b. Clinical findings
    (1) Compression fractures of vertebral bodies (Fig. 23-3)
      • Most common fracture
    (2) Colles' fracture of distal radius
    (3) Dowager's hump (Fig. 23-4)

Osteoporosis: loss of mineralized bone + organic bone matrix (osteoid)

Osteoporosis: more common in women than men

Secondary causes: ↑ cortisol, heparin, hypogonadism, malnutrition, space travel

Estrogen: inhibits production of osteoclasts; enhances osteoblasts

↓ Estrogen: ↑ osteoclastic activity, ↓ osteoblastic activity

Postmenopausal osteoporosis: compression vertebral fractures most common

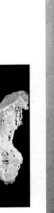

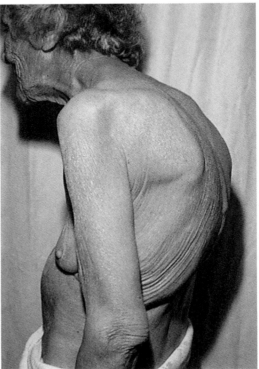

23-3: Osteoporosis of vertebral column. The vertebral body on the right shows decreased bone mass caused by compression fractures when compared with a normal vertebral body on the left. *(From Kumar V, Fausto N, Abbas A: Robbins and Cotran's Pathologic Basis of Disease, 7th ed. Philadelphia, WB Saunders, 2004, p 1284, Fig. 26-12.)*

23-4: Elderly woman with osteoporosis showing the classic Dowager's hump. *(From Seidel HM, Ball JW, Danis JE, Benedict GW: Mosby's Guide to Physical Examination, 6th ed. St. Louis, Mosby Elsevier, 2006, p 756, Fig. 21-78.)*

c. Dual-photon absorptiometry
   • Noninvasive test that evaluates bone density
d. Prevention
   (1) Role of estrogen replacement is being reevaluated.
   (2) Calcium and vitamin D supplements
   (3) Stop smoking (inhibits osteoblast activity)
   (4) Weight-bearing exercise
      (a) Weight lifting; vigorous walking
      (b) Excludes swimming, which decreases bone stress
e. Treatment
   (1) Bisphosphonates inhibit bone resorption.
      • First-line treatment
   (2) Calcitonin inhibits osteoclasts.
3. Senile osteoporosis
   • Decreased ability of osteoblasts to divide and produce osteoid

F. Aseptic (avascular) necrosis of bone
1. Disruption of microcirculation causes bone infarctions.
   a. The term "avascular" is sometimes used because the problem involves the blood supply to the bone.
   b. Causes
      (1) Corticosteroids (35%)
      (2) Alcohol (22%)
      (3) Other causes (43%)
         (a) Idiopathic
         (b) Fractures
   c. Sites of aseptic necrosis
      (1) Femoral head and condyle
      (2) Humeral head
      (3) Scaphoid (navicular) and lunate bones in wrist
      (4) Talus bone
         • Located between the calcaneus and the tibia and fibula
   d. Femoral head aseptic necrosis
      (1) Fracture in elderly persons
         (a) Pertrochanteric fracture (Fig. 23-5A) is extracapsular and does *not* compromise blood supply to the femoral head; hence, no aseptic necrosis.
         (b) Subcapsular fracture (Fig. 23-5B) disrupts blood supply (retinacular arteries from medial circumflex femoral artery); hence, aseptic necrosis occurs.
      (2) Sickle cell disease (due to vasoocclusive disease; refer to Chapter 11)
      (3) Long-term use of corticosteroids
   e. Scaphoid bone
      (1) Located on the thumb side of the wrist
      (2) Most common bone in the wrist that is fractured
      (3) Normally has a poor blood supply
   f. Digits
      • Dactylitis in sickle cell anemia (refer to Chapter 11)
2. Clinical findings
   a. Asymptomatic
   b. Localized pain exacerbated by movement
   c. Functional limitation of activity
3. Bone shows increased density on radiographs (Fig. 23-6).
   a. Magnetic resonance imaging
      (1) Early finding—margin of low signal and inner border of high signal produce a "double line sign."
      (2) Most sensitive test (75–100%) for early detection of aseptic necrosis
   b. CT scan
      • Shows central necrosis and area of collapse before regular x-ray
   c. Bone scan
      (1) Early—shows no uptake (cold area; sensitivity 70%)
      (2) Later—increased uptake (result of bone remodeling)
   d. X-ray study
      (1) Most insensitive test in early phases

Marginal notes (left column):

Diagnosis osteoporosis: dual photon absorptiometry

Prevention: weight-bearing exercises; calcium, vitamin D; stop smoking

Rx for osteoporosis: bisphosphonates first-line drug

Aseptic necrosis: disruption of microcirculation causes bone infarctions

Aseptic necrosis: most common metabolic abnormality of bone

Aseptic necrosis: femoral head most common site

Aseptic necrosis: corticosteroids most common cause

Aseptic necrosis: subcapsular fracture disrupts blood supply

Scaphoid bone: most common wrist bone fractured; susceptible to aseptic necrosis

Aseptic necrosis: localized pain

Aseptic necrosis: MRI most sensitive early test for aseptic necrosis

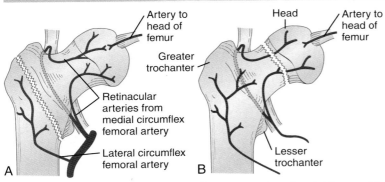

23-5: Schematic showing a pertrochanteric fracture (**A**) and a subcapital fracture (**B**). See text for discussion. *(From Moore NA, Roy WA: Rapid Review Gross and Developmental Anatomy, 2nd ed. St. Louis, Mosby Elsevier, 2007, p 147, Fig. 5-4.)*

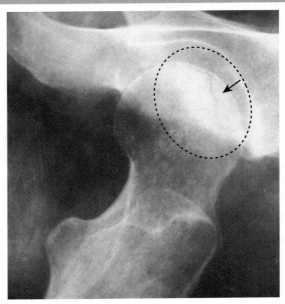

23-6: Radiograph showing avascular necrosis of the femoral head. The *interrupted circle* highlights an area of increased bone density within which is a fracture site *(arrow)*. *(From Rosai J, Ackerman LV: Surgical Pathology, 9th ed. St. Louis, Mosby, 2004, p 2144, Fig. 24-8A.)*

      (2) Early—may show osteopenia (radiolucency)
      (3) Later—flattening, collapsed bone
   e. Treatment
     • Core decompression; bone graft; joint replacement
  4. Osteochondrosis
   a. Aseptic necrosis of ossification centers in children
   b. Legg-Calvé-Perthes disease
      (1) Aseptic necrosis involving the femoral head ossification center
      (2) Occurs most often in boys 3 to 10 years of age
      (3) Presents with pain in the knee or a limp
      (4) Secondary osteoarthritis is common.

G. Osteochondritis dissecans
  1. Variant of osteochondrosis limited to the articular epiphysis
   a. Articular epiphyses fail as a result of compression.
   b. Trauma is the primary insult.
   c. Ischemia is a secondary injury.
   d. Portion of cartilage and underlying subchondral bone separates.
  2. Occurs between 10 and 50 years of age
  3. No sex predilection
  4. Most common joint is knee.
   a. Lateral surface of the medial femoral condyle is the most frequent site.
   b. Cartilage may become detached.
  5. Other sites
   a. Capitellum of humerus
   b. Dome of talus bone in foot
   c. Shoulder, hip, elbow
  6. Clinical findings
   a. Localized pain, stiffness, swelling
   b. Locking of joint by loose body
   c. Tenderness at site of lesion
  7. Complication
   • Osteoarthritis
  8. Diagnosis
   a. Imaging studies used depend on the site involved.
   b. X-ray; spiral (helical CT); MRI

Osteochondrosis: aseptic necrosis of ossification centers

Legg-Calvé-Perthes disease: aseptic necrosis of femoral head ossification center

Osteochondritis dissecans: variant of osteochondrosis limited to articular epiphysis

Osteochondritis dissecans: trauma primary insult; ischemia secondary injury

Osteochondritis dissecans: distal femur most common site

Osteochondritis dissecans: osteoarthritis late complication

9. Treatment
    a. Ice after exercise
    b. NSAIDs for pain
    c. Immobilization
    d. Arthroscopic surgery

H. Osgood-Schlatter disease
1. Affects physically active boys 11 to 15 years of age
2. Painful swelling of tibial tuberosity
    • Inflammation of proximal tibial apophysis at insertion of patellar tendon
3. Clinical findings
    a. Pain aggravated by
        (1) Squatting
        (2) Walking upstairs
        (3) Extending knee with resistance
    b. Permanent knobby-appearing knees
4. *No* effect on bone growth
5. Treatment
    a. Ice after exercise
    b. NSAIDs for pain
    c. Knee splint 2 to 4 weeks in resistant cases

I. Paget's disease of bone (osteitis deformans)
1. Epidemiology
    a. Primarily occurs in men > 50 years of age
    b. Cause unknown (? virus—slow virus, respiratory syncytial virus)
    c. Targets the pelvis, skull (enlarged), and femur
2. Pathogenesis
    a. Early phase of osteoclastic resorption of bone
        • Causes shaggy-appearing lytic lesions
    b. Late phase of increased osteoblastic bone formation
        (1) Markedly increased serum alkaline phosphatase
        (2) Production of thick, weak bone (mosaic bone; Fig. 23-7)
3. Clinical findings
    a. Bone pain is the most common complaint.
    b. Headaches, hearing loss if it affects skull
    c. Increased hat size with skull involvement

Osgood-Schlatter disease: painful swelling tibial tuberosity in boys

Osgood-Schlatter disease: permanent knobby-appearing knees

Paget's disease: primarily occurs in men > 50 years old; ? viral etiology

Paget's disease: osteoclastic phase followed by an osteoblastic phase

Paget's disease: ↑ alkaline phosphatase in osteoblastic phase

Paget's disease: weak, thick, vascular bone

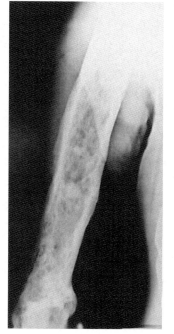

23-7: Radiograph of the humerus in Paget's disease. Note the cortical thickening of the bone and the ragged appearing lytic areas throughout the bone matrix. *(From Katz D, Math K, Groskin S: Radiology Secrets. Philadelphia, Hanley & Belfus, 1998, p 311, Fig. 1.)*

4. Complications
   a. Pathologic fractures
   b. Risk for developing osteogenic sarcomas
   c. Risk for developing high-output heart failure (refer to Chapter 10)
      • Due to arteriovenous connections in vascular bone

Complications: fractures, osteogenic sarcoma, high-output heart failure

5. Diagnosis
   a. Radiographs show thickened bone with shaggy areas of radiolucency.
   b. Markedly increased serum alkaline phosphatase with normal serum calcium and phosphorus
6. Treatment
   a. Bisphosphonates
   b. Calcitonin

J. Fibrous dysplasia
1. Skeletal developmental anomaly
   a. Defect in bone-forming mesenchyme with replacement of medullary bone by fibrous tissue
      • Defect in osteoblastic differentiation and maturation
   b. Cysts may develop in the fibrous tissue matrix that manifests as a defect in osteoblastic differentiation and maturation.

Fibrous dysplasia: defect in osteoblastic differentiation and maturation

Fibrous dysplasia: medullary bone replaced by fibrous tissue with cyst formation

2. May involve single (monostotic; 70–80%) or multiple bones (polyostotic)
3. No sex predilection
4. Occurs between 10 and 30 years of age
5. Most common locations
   a. Ribs (28%)
   b. Femur (23%)
   c. Tibia or craniofacial bones (10–25%)
      • In craniofacial bone, it produces cherubism
   d. Humerus, vertebra

Fibrous dysplasia: ribs most common site

6. Polyostotic bone involvement is associated with Albright's syndrome.
   a. Café au lait spots on skin
   b. Precocious sexual development

Albright's syndrome: polyostotic bone involvement; café au lait spots; precocious puberty

7. Clinical findings
   a. Pain overlying the bone
   b. Swelling of bone
8. Complications
   a. Risk for a pathologic fracture
   b. Malignant degeneration in <1%
      (1) Osteogenic sarcoma
      (2) Fibrosarcoma

Complications: pathologic fracture, osteogenic sarcoma, fibrosarcoma

9. Diagnose with imaging studies.
10. Treatment is surgery.

K. Neoplastic disorders of bone
1. Metastasis is the most common malignancy of bone (see Figs. 8-7A to D).
   • Breast cancer is the most common primary site.

Metastasis: most common bone malignancy

2. Primary malignant tumors of bone, in descending order of frequency
   • Multiple myeloma, osteogenic sarcoma, chondrosarcoma, Ewing's sarcoma
3. Treatment for primary bone tumors is surgery.
4. Summary of bone tumors (Table 23-1; see Fig. 8-1F)

Osteochondroma: most common benign bone tumor

II. Joint Disorders
A. Synovial fluid (SF) analysis
1. Routine studies
   • WBC count and differential, crystal analysis, mucin clot, culture, Gram stain

Giant cell tumor: epiphysis distal femur, proximal tibia

2. Crystal identification
   a. Monosodium urate (MSU)
      (1) Needle-shaped (monoclinic) crystal
      (2) Special polarization shows negative birefringence.
         • Crystal is yellow when parallel to the slow ray (Fig. 23-8).

MSU crystals: negative birefringence (yellow when parallel to slow ray)

   b. Calcium pyrophosphate
      (1) Monoclinic-like or triclinic (rhomboid) crystals
      (2) Special polarization shows positive birefringence.
         • Crystal is blue when parallel to the slow ray.

Calcium pyrophosphate: positive birefringence (blue when parallel to slow ray)

TABLE 23-1. **TUMORS OF BONE**

TUMOR TYPE	EPIDEMIOLOGY	PRIMARY LOCATION	CHARACTERISTICS
Benign			
Osteochondroma	Males, 10–30yr Solitary or multiple	Metaphysis of distal femur	Outgrowth of bone (exostosis) capped by benign cartilage Most common benign tumor
Enchondroma	Equal distribution, 20–50yr Solitary or multiple	Medullary location Small tubular bones in hands and feet	Multiple enchondromas Risk for chondrosarcoma
Osteoma	Males, any age	Facial bones	Associated with Gardner's polyposis syndrome
Osteoid osteoma	Males, 10–20yr	Cortex of proximal femur	Radiographic finding: radiolucent focus surrounded by sclerotic bone Nocturnal pain relieved by aspirin
Osteoblastoma	Males, 10–20yr	Vertebra	Similar to osteoid osteoma
Giant cell tumor	Females, 20–40yr	Epiphysis of distal femur or proximal tibia	Reactive multinucleated giant cells resemble osteoclasts Neoplastic mononuclear cells
Malignant			
Chondrosarcoma	Males, 30–60yr	Pelvic bones, proximal femur	Grade determines biologic behavior Metastasizes to lungs
Osteogenic sarcoma (see Fig. 8-1F)	Males, 10–25yr Risk factors: Paget's disease, familial retinoblastoma, irradiation, fibrous dysplasia	Metaphysis of distal femur, proximal tibia Most common primary bone cancer (some authors say multiple myeloma)	Malignant osteoid Radiographic findings: "sunburst" appearance (spiculated pattern from calcified malignant osteoid) "Codman's triangle" (tumor lifting the periosteum) Metastasizes to lungs
Ewing's sarcoma	Males, 10–20yr	Pelvic girdle, diaphysis and metaphysis of proximal femur or rib	Small, round cell tumor Radiographic finding: "onionskin" appearance around bone (periosteal reaction) Possible fever and anemia

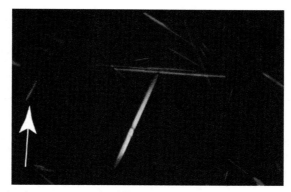

23-8: Synovial fluid with special polarization. Special red filter causes the background to be red. Crystals are aligned parallel to the slow ray (axis) of the compensator (*arrow*). If the crystal is yellow when parallel to the slow ray, as in this figure, the crystal demonstrates negative birefringence. If the crystal is blue when parallel to the slow ray, the crystal demonstrates positive birefringence. *(From Henry JB: Clinical Diagnosis and Management by Laboratory Methods, 20th ed. Philadelphia, WB Saunders, 2001, Plate 19-7.)*

    c. Mucin clot
       (1) Evaluates joint viscosity
       (2) Acid added to synovial clots hyaluronic acid
         • Hyaluronic acid is the normal joint lubricant
       (3) Poor clot formation reflects decreased hyaluronic acid
         • Sign of joint inflammation

B. Classification of joint disorders
1. Group I
   a. Noninflammatory
   b. Examples—osteoarthritis, neuropathic joint
2. Group II
   a. Inflammatory
   b. Examples—rheumatoid arthritis, gout
3. Group III
   a. Septic
   b. Examples—Lyme disease, disseminated gonococcemia
4. Group IV
   a. Hemorrhagic
   b. Examples—trauma, hemophilia A and B

C. Signs and symptoms of joint disease
1. Arthralgia is a general term for joint pain.
2. Arthritis connotes pain associated with joint swelling, tenderness, warmth
3. Morning stiffness
   a. Pain in the joints that lasts >30 minutes
   b. Characteristic finding in
      (1) Rheumatoid arthritis (RA)
      (2) Polymyalgia rheumatica
      (3) Systemic lupus erythematosus (SLE)
4. Abnormal joint mobility
   a. Due to damage to ligaments/joint capsule
   b. Example—tear of anterior cruciate ligament
5. Swelling of the joint (effusion)
   a. Due to due increased joint fluid
   b. Examples—exudate, blood
6. Redness and warmth of the joint
   a. Sign of acute inflammation
   b. Example—septic arthritis
7. Joint crepitus with motion
   a. Crackling feeling when moving a joint
   b. Example—osteoarthritis

D. Osteoarthritis (OA)
1. Epidemiology
   a. Noninflammatory joint disease
   b. No sex predilection
   c. Almost universal >65 years of age
   d. Secondary causes
      (1) Legg-Calvé-Perthes disease
      (2) Osteochondritis dissecans
      (3) Obesity, trauma, neuropathic joint
      (4) Meniscus injuries, hemochromatosis

Ochronosis (alkaptonuria) is an autosomal recessive (AR) disease caused by deficiency of homogentisic acid oxidase and accumulation of homogentisic acid (urine turns black when oxidized). Homogentisic acid deposits in the intervertebral disks, causing osteoarthritis and other systemic findings.

   e. Common sites
      (1) Femoral head, knee
      (2) Cervical and lumbar vertebrae
      (3) Hands (usually genetic)
   f. Less common sites
      (1) Shoulder
      (2) Elbow
      (3) Feet with exception of first metatarsophalangeal joint
         • Site for bunion formation
2. Progressive degeneration of articular cartilage
   a. Primarily targets weight-bearing joints

Margin notes:

Group I: noninflammatory; osteoarthritis, neuropathic joint

Group II: inflammatory; rheumatoid arthritis, gout

Group III: septic; Lyme disease, disseminated gonococcemia

Group IV: hemorrhage; trauma, hemophilia

Morning stiffness: RA, SLE, polymyalgia rheumatica

Joint effusion: blood, exudate

Hot joint: acute inflammation; septic arthritis

Joint crepitus: crackling feeling; osteoarthritis

Osteoarthritis: most common disabling joint disease

Alkaptonuria: homogentistic acid deposits in intervertebral disks; black color

OA: femoral head, knee, cervical/lumbar vertebrae, hands

Ochronosis: AR; deficiency homogentisic acid; osteoarthritis

Articular cartilage: proteoglycans, type II collagen

OA: wearing down of articular cartilage; bone rubs on bone

OA: osteophytes at joint margins

OA: clefts, subchondral cysts

OA: no fusion of the joint

OA: pain most common complaint

OA: joint stiffness after inactivity

OA fingers: Heberden's nodes; DIP joint enlargement/pain

OA fingers: Bouchard's nodes; PIP joint enlargement/pain

OA vertebral column: cervical/lumbar; degenerative disk disease, compressive neuropathies

    b. Components of articular cartilage
      (1) Proteoglycans that provide elasticity
      (2) Type II collagen that provides tensile strength
    c. Cytokines activate metalloproteinases
      • Causes degradation of proteoglycans and collagen
    d. Joint findings (Fig. 23-9)
      (1) Erosion and clefts in articular cartilage
      (2) Reactive bone formation at joint margins (osteophytes)
        • Causes a slight increase in serum alkaline phosphatase
      (3) Subchondral cysts
      (4) Bone eventually rubs on bone.
        • Produces dense, sclerotic bone
      (5) *No* ankylosis (fusion) of the joint
      (6) Joint mice
        • Fragments of articular cartilage that break free into the joint space
  3. Clinical findings
    a. Pain is the most common complaint
      (1) Osteophytes irritating synovial lining; bone rubbing on bone
      (2) Hip OA may refer pain to the groin
    b. Joint stiffness after inactivity
      (1) Waking up in morning
      (2) After sitting
      (3) Aggravated by activity
    c. Hand involvement (Fig. 23-10)
      (1) Enlargement of distal interphalangeal joints (DIPs)
        • Called Heberden's nodes (osteophytes)
      (2) Enlargement of proximal interphalangeal joints (PIPs)
        • Called Bouchard's nodes (osteophytes)
    d. Pain with passive motion of the joint
      • Due to secondary synovitis
    e. Vertebral findings
      • Degenerative disk disease and compressive neuropathies
  4. Diagnosis
    • Imaging studies
  5. Treatment
    a. Heat; decrease weight bearing; range of motion exercises
    b. Use of a cane
    c. Analgesics (NSAIDs, acetaminophen)
    d. Viscosupplementation
      • Oral chondroitin sulfate, glucosamine
    e. Joint replacement

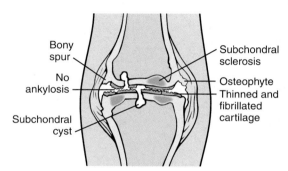

23-9: Schematic of osteoarthritis in a joint. See text for description. *(From Kumar V, Abbas AK, Fausto N, Mitchell RN: Robbins Basic Pathology, 8th ed. Philadelphia, Saunders Elsevier, 2007, p 820, Fig. 7-18 on the right.)*

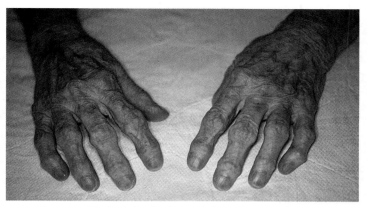

23-10: Osteoarthritis. Both the distal interphalangeal (DIP) and proximal interphalangeal (PIP) joints in both hands show protuberances along their lateral margins representing osteophyte formation in the joints. The DIP protuberances are called Heberden's nodes and the PIP protuberances are called Bouchard's nodes. *(From Swartz MH: Textbook of Physical Diagnosis, 5th ed. Philadelphia, Saunders Elsevier, 2006, p 636, Fig. 20-59.)*

E. Neuropathic arthropathy (Charcot's joint)
 1. Noninflammatory joint disease
 2. Secondary to a neurologic disease
    • Loss of proprioception and deep sensation leading to recurrent trauma
 3. Causes
    a. Diabetes mellitus (15%)
       • Primarily affects the tarsometatarsal joint
    b. Syringomyelia (20–25%)
       • Primarily affects the shoulder, elbow, wrist joints
    c. Tabes dorsalis (10–20%)
       • Primarily affects the hip, knee, ankle joints
 4. Treatment
    a. Immobilization
    b. Pneumatic walking braces

F. Rheumatoid arthritis (RA)
 1. Epidemiology
    a. Occurs more often in women 30 to 50 years of age
    b. HLA-DR4 association
    c. ? Initial inciting agents
       • Epstein-Barr virus, parvovirus, human herpesvirus 6, *Mycoplasma*
 2. Pathogenesis of joint disease is unclear; key points:
    a. B and T cells are activated leading to damage of synovial cells
    b. Synovial cells express an antigen that triggers B cells to produce rheumatoid factor (RF).
    c. RF is an IgM autoantibody that has specificity for the Fc portion of IgG.
    d. RF and IgG join together to form immunocomplexes (type III hypersensitivity).
    e. Immunocomplexes activate the complement system to produce C5a, a chemotactic agent for neutrophils and other leukocytes to enter the joint space.
    f. Chronic synovitis and pannus formation eventually occur (Fig. 23-11).
    g. Pannus is granulation tissue that is formed within the synovial tissue by fibroblasts and inflammatory cells (refer to Chapter 2).
    h. Pannus proliferates and releases cytokines that eventually destroy the articular cartilage leading to fusion of the joint by scar tissue (called ankylosis).
 3. Clinical findings
    a. Symmetric involvement of second/third metacarpophalangeal (MCP) and PIP joints
       (1) Produces ulnar deviation, morning stiffness (Fig. 23-12)
       (2) Swan neck deformity
          (a) Flexion of DIP joint
          (b) Extension of PIP joint
       (3) Boutonnière deformity

Neuropathic joint: loss of proprioception, deep sensation leading to recurrent trauma

Common causes: diabetes, syringomyelia, tabes dorsalis

RA: B cells produce RF, an IgM antibody with specificity against Fc portion of IgG

RA: RF combines with IgG to produce immunocomplexes that activate the complement system

Pannus (granulation tissue): releases cytokines that destroy articular cartilage

Repair by fibrosis causes fusion of the joint (ankylosis)

RA hand: involves MCP and PIP joints; bilateral ulnar deviation

---

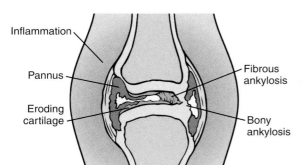

23-11: Schematic of rheumatoid arthritis in a joint. See text for description. *(From Kumar V, Abbas AK, Fausto N, Mitchell RN: Robbins Basic Pathology, 8th ed. Philadelphia, Saunders Elsevier, 2007, p 820, Fig. 7-18 on the left.)*

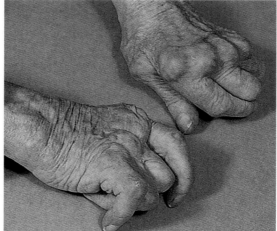

23-12: Patient with rheumatoid arthritis showing bilateral ulnar deviation of the hands and prominent swelling of the second and third metacarpophalangeal joints. *(From Forbes C, Jackson W: Color Atlas and Text of Clinical Medicine, 2nd ed. St. Louis, Mosby, 2003, p 121, Fig. 3-3.)*

(a) Extension of DIP joint
(b) Flexion of PIP joint
(4) Other joints commonly involved
(a) Knees, cervical spine, hips
(b) Shoulders, elbows
b. Lung disease
• Chronic pleuritis with effusions, interstitial fibrosis
c. Hematologic disease
(1) Anemia of chronic disease (ACD)
(2) Felty's syndrome
• Autoimmune neutropenia and splenomegaly
(3) Autoimmune hemolytic anemia (AIHA)
d. Carpal tunnel syndrome (see section V)
• Entrapment of median nerve under transverse carpal ligament
e. Cervical spine
(1) Entire cervical spine is frequently involved
(2) Subluxation of atlantoaxial joint particularly dangerous
(a) Possible compression of spinal cord
(b) Possible compression of vertebral artery causing stroke
f. Rheumatoid nodules
(1) Extensor surface of the forearm, lungs
(2) Fibrinoid necrosis present in center of nodule (refer to Chapter 1)
(3) Correlates with very high titers of RF
g. Cardiovascular disease
(1) Fibrinous pericarditis
(2) Aortitis
(3) Immunocomplex vasculitis
(a) Located around the ankles
(b) Correlates with high RF titers
h. Popliteal (Baker's) cyst behind the knee joint
(1) Outpouching of synovial sack into the posterior joint space due to increased intra-articular pressure
(2) Sometimes ruptures and dissects into the calf
• Frequently misdiagnosed as deep venous thrombosis (DVT)
(3) Sometimes confused with popliteal artery aneurysm
• Ultrasound easily makes the distinction.
4. Laboratory findings in RA
a. Positive serum antinuclear antibody (ANA) test (30%)
b. Positive serum RF (70–90%)
c. Normal to increased serum C3
d. Decreased synovial C3
e. Increased serum total protein
(1) Due to increase in γ-globulins (IgG) in chronic inflammation
(2) Polyclonal gammopathy on serum protein electrophoresis (refer to Chapter 2)
5. Diagnosis
• Laboratory tests are listed in previous section.
6. Treatment
a. Physical therapy emphasizing movement of joints
• Swimming pool exercises are very useful.
b. Initial treatment with NSAIDS
c. Early treatment with disease-modifying drugs
(1) Minimizes long-term joint damage
(2) Methotrexate (most commonly used agent)
(3) Cyclosporine; corticosteroids; hydroxychloroquine; gold compounds
(4) Tumor necrosis factor (TNF)-α blockers effective if disease-modifying drugs ineffective

G. Sjögren's syndrome (SS)
1. Female dominant autoimmune disease
2. Pathogenesis
• Autoimmune destruction of minor salivary glands and lacrimal glands
3. Clinical findings
a. Rheumatoid arthritis

RA lung: interstitial fibrosis, effusions

RA blood: ACD, AIHA, Felty's syndrome (autoimmune neutropenia, splenomegaly)

RA cervical spine: subluxation atlantoaxial joint; cord/vertebral artery compression

Caplan syndrome: rheumatoid nodules in lung plus pneumoconiosis

RA cardiovascular: pericarditis, aortitis, vasculitis

Baker's cyst: outpouching of posterior joint space in knee

RA lab: + serum RF, ANA

Sjögren's syndrome: destruction minor salivary glands and lacrimal glands

b. Keratoconjunctivitis sicca
  (1) Dry eyes described as "sand in my eyes"
  (2) Due to autoimmune destruction of lacrimal glands
c. Xerostomia or dry mouth
  (1) Autoimmune destruction of minor salivary glands
    • "Doctor, I can't swallow dry crackers."
  (2) Dental caries
4. Laboratory findings
  a. Positive serum ANA in most cases
  b. Positive serum RF (90%)
  c. Anti-SS-A antibodies (Ro; 70–95%)
  d. Anti-SS-B antibodies (La; 60–90%)
5. Confirm with lip biopsy
  • Must demonstrate lymphoid destruction of minor salivary glands
6. Treatment
  a. Artificial tears
  b. Pilocarpine or cyclosporine eye drops
  c. Cevimeline (cholinergic agent with muscarinic agonist activity
    • Used for dry mouth

H. Juvenile rheumatoid arthritis (JRA)
  1. Epidemiology
    a. Occurs in children < 16 years of age
    b. More common in girls
    c. RF is usually absent.
  2. Still's disease (20% of cases)
    a. Commonly presents as an "infectious disease"
    b. Fever, rash, polyarthritis
    c. Generalized lymphadenopathy
    d. Neutrophilic leukocytosis
  3. Polyarticular JRA (40% of cases)
    • Disabling arthritis predominates.
  4. Pauciarticular JRA (40% of cases)
    a. Arthritis limited to a few joints.
    b. Uveitis with the potential for blindness
I. Gouty arthritis
  1. Epidemiology
    a. Occurs more often in men > 30 years of age (95%)
    b. Uncommon in women before menopause (5%)
    c. Primary gout arises from inborn errors of metabolism involving purine metabolism.
      • Example—deficiency of hypoxanthine-guanine phosphoryltransferase (HGPRT) in Lesch-Nyhan syndrome (refer to Chapter 5)
    d. Secondary causes are more common causes of gout.
      (1) Underexcretion of uric acid in kidneys (80–90%)
        • Examples—lead poisoning; alcoholism; diets rich in red meat, seafood, beer
      (2) Overproduction of uric acid (increased nucleated cell turnover; 10–20%)
        • Examples—treating leukemia; psoriasis
    e. Clinical conditions commonly associated with gout
      (1) Urate nephropathy, renal stones (refer to Chapter 19)
      (2) Hypertension, coronary artery disease
      (3) Lead poisoning
        • Produces interstitial nephritis, which interferes with uric acid excretion
  2. Recurrent acute attacks of gout are the rule.
    a. Most commonly involve the first metatarsophalangeal joint (called podagra)
    b. Often precipitated by dietary indiscretions, illness, exercise, emotional stress
    c. Free uric acid crystals in the synovial fluid are proinflammatory.
      (1) Activate synovial cells, leukocytes, and the complement cascade, the latter releasing C5a, which attracts neutrophils into the joint producing acute inflammation
        • Neutrophils also phagocytose uric acid crystals.
      (2) Another common site for acute gout is the extensor tenosynovium on the dorsum of the midfoot

---

Sjögren's syndrome: dry eyes; dry mouth

Lab: + serum ANA, RF, anti-SS-A/anti-SS-B; lip biopsy confirms

JRA: RF is usually negative

JRA, Still's disease: fever, rash, polyarthritis

JRA, polyarticular: disabling arthritis predominates

JRA, pauciarticular: limited arthritis; uveitis and potential for blindness

Gout: male dominant disease

Gout: most cases due to underexcretion of uric acid

Gout associations: urate nephropathy, renal stones, hypertension, artery disease, Pb poisoning

Acute gout: 1st metatarsophalangeal joint most often involved

Acute gout: free uric acid crystals responsible for initiating the attack

d. Clinical findings acute gout
  (1) Sudden onset of severe pain in the big toe
  (2) Joint is hot, red, and swollen (Fig. 23-13).
  (3) Fever, tachycardia, and other constitutional signs
e. Laboratory findings
  (1) Hyperuricemia
    (a) Increased serum uric acid > 7 mg/dL in men
    (b) Increased serum uric acid > 6 mg/dL in women
  (2) Absolute neutrophilic leukocytosis
  (3) Joint aspiration is confirmatory.
    • Negatively birefringent MSU crystals
3. Chronic gout
  a. Chronic gout is likely to occur if gout is poorly controlled.
  b. Uric acid crystals accumulate in the joint and produce a tophus.
    (1) Due to MSU crystals leaking into the soft tissue around the joint
      (Fig. 23-14)
    (2) MSU excites a brisk granulomatous reaction in the periarticular tissue.
      • Microscopic sections reveal numerous multinucleated giant cells within which
        are MSU crystals that polarize.
  c. Tophi destroy subjacent bone causing erosive arthritis.
4. Treatment
  a. Modify diet to eliminate diets high in purine.
  b. Moderation in alcohol intake (refer to Chapter 6)
  c. Drugs
    (1) Treatment for acute gouty arthritis
      (a) NSAIDs or colchicine
      (b) Corticosteroids if intolerant to above drugs
    (2) Chronic treatment to prevent acute gout
      (a) Goal is to normalize serum uric acid.
      (b) Uricosuric agents for underexcretors (e.g., probenecid)
        • If 24-hour urine collection of uric acid < 700 mg
      (c) Allopurinol (xanthine oxidase inhibitor) for overproducers
        • If 24-hour urine collection of uric acid > 900 mg
J. Calcium pyrophosphate dihydrate deposition (CPPD) disease
  1. Epidemiology
    a. Deposition of calcium pyrophosphate in tissues
      (1) Deposition in cartilage (called chondrocalcinosis)

Margin notes:

Acute gout: must confirm with joint aspiration; hyperuricemia does *not* define gout

Tophus: MSU deposits in soft tissue around the joint

Nonpharmacologic Rx of gout: eliminate high-purine diet; moderation in alcohol intake

Pharmacologic Rx of acute gout: NSAIDs or colchicine

Drugs to prevent gout: uricosuric agents for underexcretors; allopurinol for overproducers

CPPD disease: deposition of calcium pyrophosphate in tissues

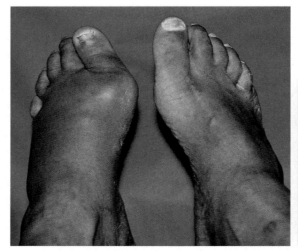

23-13: Acute gouty arthritis involving the left big toe. Note the erythema and swelling of the joint. *(From Swartz MH: Textbook of Physical Diagnosis, 5th ed. Philadelphia, Saunders Elsevier, 2006, p 634, Fig. 20-55.)*

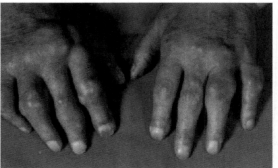

23-14: Tophi involving the soft tissue around the joints in both hands. The white material represents crystals of monosodium urate. *(From Bouloux P: Self-Assessment Picture Tests: Medicine, Vol. 1. London, Mosby-Wolfe, 1997, p 55, Fig. 109.)*

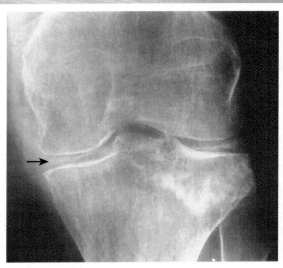

23-15: Chondrocalcinosis (pseudogout). The radiograph shows linear calcifications in the fibrocartilage in the knee joint (*arrow*) in a patient with the osteoarthritis variant of calcium pyrophosphate deposition. *(From Katz D, Math K, Groskin S: Radiology Secrets. Philadelphia, Hanley & Belfus, 1998, p 278, Fig. 10.)*

  (2) Less commonly in tendons, ligaments, synovial tissue, bursa
 b. Incidence of CPPD increases in the presence of:
  (1) Hemochromatosis, hemosiderosis
   (a) Pyrophosphate inhibitor is increased in these diseases.
   (b) Causes an increase in inorganic pyrophosphate concentration
  (2) Primary hyperparathyroidism (HPTH)
   • Increase in calcium is responsible.
 c. Four variants are associated with the disease.
 d. Most common variant is osteoarthritis (OA).
  (1) Most common in elderly population
   • Present in 50% of patients who are 85 years old
  (2) Degenerative arthritis with symptoms similar to OA
  (3) Most common joint involved is the knee.
  (4) Calcium pyrophosphate crystals deposit in articular cartilage (usually knee).
   (a) Crystals produce linear deposits in articular cartilage (Fig. 23-15).
   (b) Called chondrocalcinosis when it deposits in articular cartilage
  (5) Crystals phagocytosed by neutrophils show positive birefringence.
  (6) Treatment
   • NSAIDs; colchicine; arthroscopic surgery

K. Seronegative spondyloarthropathies (spondyloarthritis)
 1. Characteristics
  a. Rheumatoid factor (RF) negative (meaning of seronegative)
  b. Involve the axial skeleton (spondylitis)
  c. Individuals HLA-B27 positive
  d. Male dominant
  e. Sacroiliitis with or without peripheral arthritis
 2. Types of spondyloarthropathy
  a. Ankylosing spondylitis
  b. Reiter's syndrome
  c. Psoriasis
  d. Enteropathic
   • Associated with ulcerative colitis, shigellosis
 3. Ankylosing spondylitis (AS)
  a. Initially targets sacroiliac joint in young men
   • Bilateral sacroiliitis with morning stiffness

Margin notes:

CPPD disease: ↑ with hemochromatosis, hemosiderosis, primary HPTH

CPPD OA variant: knee most common joint; chondrocalcinosis present

Chondrocalcinosis: linear deposits of calcium pyrophosphate in articular cartilage

Seronegative: RF negative arthritis

Key points: – RF; + HLA-B27; male; sacroiliitis; spondylitis

AS: begins with sacroiliitis

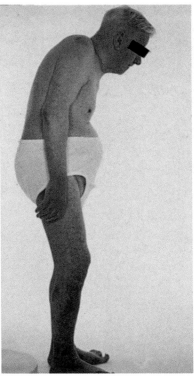

23-16: Man with ankylosing spondylitis. The patient cannot bend forward owing to fusion of the vertebra. *(From Forbes C, Jackson W: Color Atlas and Text of Clinical Medicine, 2nd ed. St. Louis, Mosby, 2003, Fig. 3-48.)*

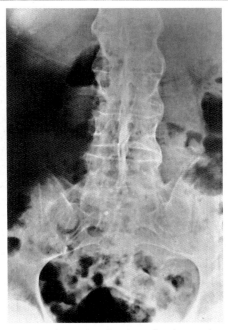

23-17: Radiograph showing fused vertebra ("bamboo" spine) in ankylosing spondylitis. *(From Katz D, Math K, Groskin S: Radiology Secrets. Philadelphia, Hanley & Belfus, 1998, p 277, Fig. 7.)*

b. Eventually involves the vertebral column (Fig. 23-16)
  (1) Fusion of vertebrae ("bamboo spine") causes forward curvature (kyphosis; Fig. 23-17).
  (2) Kyphosis interferes with chest wall movement.
    (a) Nonpulmonary restrictive lung disease
    (b) Schober test evaluates degree of restriction to forward bending.
c. Aortitis with aortic regurgitation
d. Anterior uveitis (20%)
  (1) Blurry vision
  (2) Potential for blindness
e. Treatment
  (1) NSAIDs
  (2) Disease-modifying agents
    • Methotrexate, cyclosporine, corticosteroids
  (3) TNF-α inhibitors
    • Extremely effective in slowing down progression of the disease
4. Reiter's syndrome
  a. Urethritis due to *Chlamydia trachomatis*
  b. Arthritis and Achilles tendon periostitis
    • Achilles tendon periostitis is a confirmatory radiologic sign.
  c. Conjunctivitis (noninfectious)
5. Psoriatic arthritis
  a. Sausage-shaped DIP joints (finger or toe)
  b. Radiographs show erosive joint disease.
    • "Pencil-in-cup" deformity (Fig. 23-18)
  c. Extensive nail pitting

L. Septic arthritis
1. *Staphylococcus aureus*
  a. Most common nongonococcal cause of septic arthritis

AS: over time develop fusion of vertebrae ("bamboo spine")

AS: aortitis; uveitis with potential for blindness

Reiter's syndrome: *C. trachomatis* urethritis, arthritis, conjunctivitis

Reiter's syndrome: Achilles tendon periostitis is diagnostic sign

Psoriatic arthritis: sausage-shaped DIP joints; "pencil-in-cup" deformity

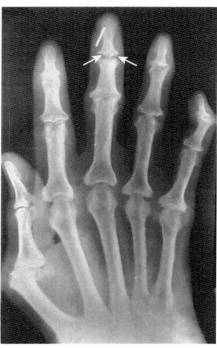

23-18: Radiograph of the hand in psoriatic arthritis. The distal interphalangeal joint of the middle finger shows the classic "pencil-in-cup" deformity *(arrows)*. The metallic foreign body in the soft tissue was an incidental finding. *(From Katz D, Math K, Groskin S: Radiology Secrets. Philadelphia, Hanley & Belfus, 1998, p 276, Fig. 6.)*

    b. Treatment
      • Nafcillin + cephalosporin (third generation)
  2. *Neisseria gonorrhoeae*
    a. Most common cause of septic arthritis in urban populations
    b. May produce disseminated gonococcemia
      (1) More common in young women
        • Deficiency of C6–C9 predisposes to dissemination
      (2) Septic arthritis (knee)
      (3) Tenosynovitis (wrists and ankles)
      (4) Dermatitis (pustules on wrists or ankles)
      (5) Treatment is ceftriaxone.
  3. Lyme disease
    a. Epidemiology
      (1) Transmitted by bite of *Ixodes* tick; *Borrelia burgdorferi* (spirochete)
      (2) White-tailed deer is a reservoir for the organism.
    b. Early disease
      (1) Erythema chronicum migrans develops at tick bite site (Fig. 23-19).
      (2) Red, expanding lesion with concentric circles ("bull's-eye" lesion)
      (3) Pathognomonic lesion of Lyme disease
    c. Late disease
      (1) Disabling arthritis (usually involves the knee)
      (2) Bilateral Bell's palsy
        • Highly predictive of Lyme disease
      (3) Myocarditis and pericarditis
    d. Diagnosis
      (1) ELISA (enzyme-linked immunosorbent assay) testing first as screen (highly sensitive
      (2) Western blot assay for equivocal or positive ELISA test
        • High specificity (94–96%)
      (3) PCR (polymerase chain reaction) test is also available
    e. Treatment
      (1) Adults—doxycycline or amoxicillin or erythromycin or ceftriaxone
      (2) Child—amoxicillin

Neisseria gonorrhoeae: most common cause of septic arthritis in urban populations

Disseminated gonococcemia: septic arthritis, tenosynovitis, dermatitis

Borrelia burgdorferi: gram-negative spirochete; cause of Lyme disease

Lyme disease: vector *Ixodes* tick; reservoir white-tailed deer

Erythema chronicum migrans: pathognomonic of Lyme disease

Lyme disease: disabling arthritis, Bell's palsy, myocarditis

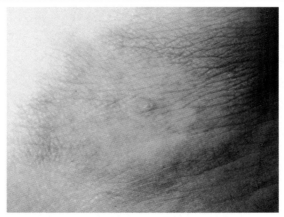

23-19: Erythema chronicum migrans in a patient with Lyme disease. Raised central area is the site of the tick bite. Concentric area of erythema surrounds the bite site. *(From Lookingbill D, Marks J: Principles of Dermatology, 3rd ed. Philadelphia, WB Saunders, 2000, p 269, Fig. 17-5A.)*

Babesiosis: tick-transmitted hemolytic anemia

    f. Babesiosis
       (1) Intraerythrocytic protozoal disease due to *Babesia microti*
       (2) Secondary infection transmitted by *Ixodes*
         • Often presents concurrently with Lyme disease
       (3) Fever, headache, hemolytic anemia
       (4) Diagnosis
         (a) Wright- or Giemsa-stained peripheral smear to look for organisms
         (b) Serologic testing
       (5) Treatment
         • Atovaquone + azithromycin

Pasteurella multocida: septic arthritis/tendinitis due to cat/dog bite

   4. Septic arthritis and tendinitis due to cat/dog bite
     a. Causal agent is *Pasteurella multocida*.
     b. Most common infection secondary to animal injury
     c. Types of infection
       (1) Cellulitis (most common)
       (2) Septic arthritis/tendinitis
       (3) Osteomyelitis
       (4) Endocarditis, meningitis
     d. Rapid onset of infection at the bite site (usually within 24 hours)
     e. Treatment
       • Amoxicillin-clavulanate

III. Muscle Disorders
  A. Muscle fibers
    1. Innervation of the muscle determines fiber type.
    2. Type I fibers

Type I: slow-twitch (red); rich in mitochondria, oxidative enzymes, poor in ATPase enzymes

     a. Slow-twitch (red) fibers
       (1) Slow contraction but repetitive
       (2) Do *not* fatigue easily
       (3) Example—long muscles in the back
     b. Rich in mitochondria, myoglobin, and oxidative enzymes
     c. Weak in ATPase enzymes
    3. Type II fibers

Type II: fast-twitch (white); poor in mitochondria, oxidative enzymes; rich in ATPase enzymes

     a. Fast-twitch (white) fibers
       (1) Fast contraction, but fatigue easily
       (2) Specialized for fine, skilled movement
       (3) Examples—extraocular muscles, some muscles in the hand
     b. Poor in mitochondria, myoglobin, oxidative enzymes
     c. Rich in ATPase enzymes

  B. Muscle disorders

Muscle weakness: motor neuron, neuromuscular synapse, muscle dysfunction

    1. Pathogenesis of muscle weakness
     a. Abnormality in the motor neuron pathways
       • Example—poliomyelitis

b. Abnormality in the neuromuscular synapse
  • Example—myasthenia gravis
c. Abnormality in muscle
  • Example—muscular dystrophy
2. Neurogenic atrophy
  a. Motor neuron or its axon degenerates.
  b. Produces atrophy of type I and II fibers
3. *Trichinella spiralis* infection
  a. Epidemiology
    (1) Causative agent *Trichinella spiralis* (nematode)
    (2) Transmission
      (a) Eating raw or poorly cooked pork containing the encysted larvae in muscle
      (b) Common on pig farms where pigs are fed uncooked garbage
      (c) Bear and seal meat are other sources
      (d) Larva excyst and develop into adult worms within small intestine mucosa.
      (e) Eggs hatch within the adult female worm.
      (f) Larvae are released into the blood stream.
      (g) Larvae encyst in striated muscle.
        • Commonly undergo dystrophic calcification; visible on x-ray
      (h) Larvae die if deposited in other sites.
  b. Trichinosis
    (1) Muscle pain
    (2) Periorbital edema (larva)
    (3) Splinter hemorrhages in nails
    (4) Complications
      • Myocarditis, encephalitis
    (5) Diagnosis
      • Pronounced eosinophilia; muscle biopsy
    (6) Treatment is albendazole.
4. Invasive infections due to group A streptococcus
  a. Types of invasive infections
    (1) Necrotizing fasciitis
    (2) Myositis
    (3) Streptococcal toxic shock syndrome (STSS)
  b. Related to various toxins produced by the streptococcus
    (1) Pyrogenic exotoxin A
      • Superantigen associated with STSS
    (2) Exotoxin B
      • Protease that destroys tissue associated with necrotizing fasciitis
  c. Treatment
    (1) Intravenous penicillin G + clindamycin
    (2) Intravenous immunoglobulin
  d. Death rates range from 20% to 100%.
5. Duchenne's muscular dystrophy (DMD)
  a. Epidemiology
    (1) X-linked recessive (XR)
    (2) Incidence 1:3500 male births
  b. Pathogenesis
    (1) Absence of dystrophin
      (a) Dystrophin normally anchors actin to membrane glycoprotein.
      (b) Becker's type has deficiency/defective dystrophin.
    (2) Most common childhood muscular dystrophy
    (3) Progressive degeneration of type I and II fibers
    (4) Fibrosis and infiltration of muscle tissue by fatty tissue
      • Produces pseudohypertrophy of calf muscles (Fig. 23-20A)
  c. Clinical findings
    (1) Symptoms occur between 2 and 5 years of age.
    (2) Weakness and wasting of pelvic muscles
      (a) Child places hands on the knees for help in standing (Gower's maneuver; Fig. 23-20B).
      (b) Waddling gait (duck-like)

Neurogenic atrophy: motor neuron or axon degenerates

Trichinosis: *Trichinella spiralis* (nematode); from eating encysted larvae in pig muscle

Trichinosis: calcified larvae visible on x-ray

Trichinosis: muscle pain, periorbital edema, splinter hemorrhages

Trichinosis: pronounced eosinophilia

Invasive group A streptococcus: necrotizing fasciitis, myositis, STSS

Invasive group A streptococcus: exotoxin A (superantigen), exotoxin B (protease)

DMD: XR; absence of dystrophin

DMD: pseudohypertrophy of calf muscles

DMD: waddling gait due to weakness of pelvic muscles

23-20: Duchenne's muscular dystrophy (DMD). **A,** Pseudohypertrophy of the calf. **B,** A child with DMD performing the Gower's maneuver. *(From Perkin GD: Mosby's Color Atlas and Text of Neurology. St. Louis, Mosby, 2002, p 269, Figs. 14-10 and 14-12.)*

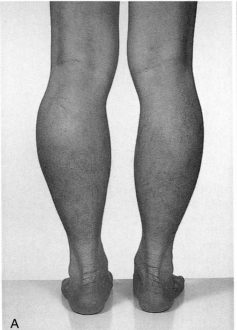
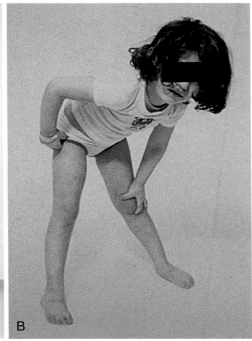

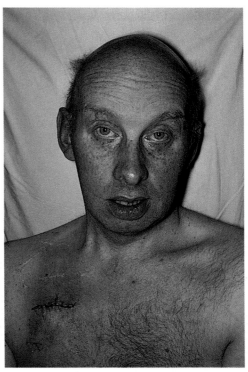

23-21: Myotonic dystrophy. The patient shows frontal balding, drooping of the eyelids, sagging of the facial muscles, and atrophy of the sternocleidomastoid muscles. *(From Perkin GD: Mosby's Color Atlas and Text of Neurology. St. Louis, Mosby, 2002, p 272, Fig. 14-16.)*

(3) Cardiac involvement may be present.

(4) Death usually occurs by 20 years of age.

d. Laboratory findings

    (1) Serum creatine kinase (CK) is increased at birth.

       • Progressively declines as muscle degenerates

    (2) Female carriers have increased levels of serum CK.

e. Diagnosis

    (1) Muscle biopsy

    (2) DNA testing available (Western blot)

       • Diagnosed prenatally via chorionic villous sampling

f. Treatment

    • Corticosteroids improve muscle strength and function.

6. Myotonic dystrophy (MD)

  a. Epidemiology and pathogenesis

    (1) Autosomal dominant

    (2) Most common adult muscular dystrophy

    (3) Trinucleotide repeat (CTG) disorder (refer to Chapter 5)

    (4) Selective atrophy of type I fibers

  b. Clinical findings (Fig. 23-21)

    (1) Facial muscle weakness

       • Sagging face; problem in closing the mouth

    (2) Percussion and grip myotonia

       • Inability to relax muscles (sustained grip)

    (3) Frontal balding; cataracts

    (4) Testicular atrophy; glucose intolerance

    (5) Cardiac involvement (conduction defects)

  c. Increased serum CK

  d. No specific treatment

7. Myasthenia gravis (MG)

  a. Epidemiology

    (1) Afflicts men in sixth and seventh decades of life

    (2) Afflicts women in second and third decades of life

  b. Pathogenesis

    (1) Autonomic disorder of postsynaptic neuromuscular transmission

    (2) Autoantibody against acetylcholine receptors

       (a) Type II hypersensitivity reaction

       (b) Antibodies inhibit or destroy the receptors.

       (c) Decrease in functional ACh receptors

    (3) Antibody is synthesized in the thymus.

       • Thymic hyperplasia with germinal follicles (85% of cases)

  c. Clinical findings

    (1) Fluctuating muscle weakness

       • Worsened with exercise, improved with rest

    (2) Ptosis is the most common initial finding (Fig. 23-22).

       • Diplopia is due to eye muscle weakness.

> DMD: ↑ serum CK at birth; ↓ as muscles degenerate

> MD: most common adult muscular dystrophy; CTG trinucleotide repeat

> Myotonia: inability to relax muscles

> MD: sagging face; frontal balding; cataracts; testicular atrophy; cardiac involvement

> MG: autoantibodies against ACh receptors; synthesized in thymus

> MG: ptosis, diplopia common initial finding

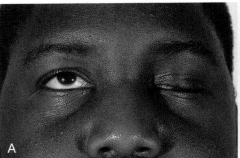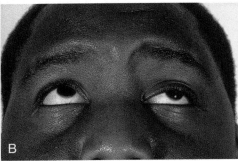

23-22: Patient with myasthenia gravis showing ptosis of the left eye (**A**) followed by opening of the eye (**B**) after intravenous injection of Tensilon. *(From Perkin GD: Mosby's Color Atlas and Text of Neurology. St. Louis, Mosby, 2002, p 263, Fig. 14-5A and B.)*

MG: oropharyngeal
dysphagia for solids/
liquids

(3) Weakness in proximal muscles, diaphragm, neck extension (85%)
(4) Dysphagia for solids and liquids
  • Occurs in the upper esophagus (striated muscle)
(5) Normal reflexes, sensation, and coordination
(6) Increased risk for developing a thymoma (15%)
  d. Diagnosis

Tensilon: inhibits
acetylcholinesterase

(1) Tensilon (edrophonium) test
  (a) Inhibits acetylcholinesterase
  (b) Increase in acetylcholine reverses muscle weakness
(2) Single-fiber electromyography (abnormal in 95% of MG)
  e. Treatment
(1) Avoid certain medications
  • β-Blockers; aminoglycosides; quinolone antibiotics; class 1
    antiarrhythmics
(2) Pyridostigmine (acetylcholinesterase inhibitor)
(3) Immunosuppressive drugs
  • Corticosteroids; azathioprine; mycophenolate mofetil;
    cyclosporine
(4) Plasmapheresis (short-term treatment; removes antibodies)
(5) Thymectomy (removes site for antibody production)

IV. Soft Tissue Disorders
  A. Fibromatosis
  1. Non-neoplastic, proliferative connective tissue disorder
  2. Fibrous tissue infiltrates tissue (usually muscle).

Dupuytren's contracture:
fibromatosis palmar
fascia

  3. Dupuytren's contracture (Fig. 23-23)
    a. Fibromatosis involving palmar fascia
    b. Causes contraction of single or multiple fingers
    c. Associated with alcoholism
  4. Desmoid tumor
    a. Fibromatosis of the anterior abdominal wall in women

Liposarcoma: most
common adult sarcoma

Unhappy triad: damage to
medial meniscus, medial
collateral ligament,
anterior cruciate ligament

    b. Associated with previous trauma
    c. Associated with Gardner's polyposis syndrome
  B. Selected soft tissue tumors (Table 23-2; see also Figs. 8-1B
    and 21-4)
V. Selected Orthopedic Disorders (Table 23-3 and Fig. 23-24A to D)

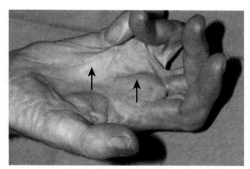

23-23: Dupuytren's contractures in the hand. The *arrows* show thickening of the palmar fascia producing cords that cause the fingers to have a hook-like deformity. *(From Grieg JD: Color Atlas of Surgical Diagnosis. London, Mosby-Wolfe, 1996, p 40, Fig. 7-4.)*

TABLE 23-2. **SOFT TISSUE TUMORS**

TUMOR TYPE	LOCATION	COMMENT
Lipoma (see Fig. 8-1B)	Trunk, neck, proximal extremities	Most common benign soft tissue tumor Arises in subcutaneous tissue *No* clinical significance
Liposarcoma	Thigh, retroperitoneum	Most common adult sarcoma Lipoblasts identified with fat stains
Fibrosarcoma	Thigh, upper limb	May arise after irradiation
Dermatofibroma	Lower extremities	Benign, nonencapsulated proliferation of spindle cells confined to the dermis Red nodule that umbilicates (has a central dimple) when squeezed
Malignant fibrous histiocytoma	Retroperitoneum, thigh	Associated with radiation therapy and scarring
Rhabdomyoma	Heart, also tongue and vagina	Benign heart tumor associated with tuberous sclerosis
Embryonal rhabdomyosarcoma (see Fig. 21-4)	Penis and vagina	Most common sarcoma in children Grape-like, necrotic mass protrudes from penis or vagina
Leiomyoma	Uterus, stomach	Most commonly located in uterus Most common benign tumor in gastrointestinal tract
Leiomyosarcoma	Gastrointestinal tract, uterus	Most common sarcoma of gastrointestinal tract and uterus
Neurofibrosarcoma	Major nerve trunks	Associated with neurofibromatosis
Synovial sarcoma	Around joints	Does not arise from synovial cells in joints but from mesenchymal cells around joints Biphasic pattern: epithelial cells forming glands + intervening spindle cells

TABLE 23-3. **SELECTED ORTHOPEDIC DISORDERS**

DISORDER	DISCUSSION
Colles' fracture (see Fig. 23-24A)	Common fracture when falling on outstretched hand Fracture of distal radius with or without fracture of ulnar styloid
Rotator cuff tear	Components: tendon insertions of supraspinatus, infraspinatus, teres minor, subscapularis muscles Pain/weakness with active shoulder abduction Diagnosis: arthrography; MRI *Treatment*: physical therapy; arthroscopic surgery
Tennis elbow	Causes: racquet sports, repetitive use of a hammer or screwdriver Pain where extensor muscle tendons insert near the lateral epicondyle (lateral epicondylitis); pain when gripping something *Treatment*: NSAIDs; rest; local injection with corticosteroids; localized pressure
Golfer's elbow	Pain where the flexor muscle tendons insert near the medial epicondyle (medial epicondylitis) Pain duplicated by flexing hand muscles and supinating the arm (arm wrestling movement) *Treatment*: NSAIDs; rest; local injection with corticosteroids; localized pressure
DeQuervain's tenosynovitis	Chronic stenosing tenosynovitis of the first dorsal compartment of the wrist; overuse of the hands and wrist; first dorsal compartment has abductor pollicis longus and extensor pollicis brevis Excessive friction thickens tendon sheath causing stenosis of the osseofibrous tunnel Pain on the ulnar aspect of the wrist aggravated by moving the thumb Finkelstein's test: patient puts thumb in the palm, closes fist, tilt hand toward little finger (ulnar deviation); pain occurs in first dorsal compartment *Treatment*: corticosteroid injection; spica splint

Continued

TABLE 23-3. **SELECTED ORTHOPEDIC DISORDERS—cont'd**

DISORDER	DISCUSSION
Ganglion (synovial) cyst (see Fig. 23-24B)	Bulge on the dorsum of the wrist when the wrist is flexed More common in women than in men Cyst communicates with synovial sheaths on the dorsum of the wrist *Treatment*: aspiration; excision by arthroscopy
Compartment syndrome	Increase of pressure in a confined space (fascial compartment); pressure reduces perfusion, which may cause ischemic contractures of the muscle(s) Most common locations anterior and posterior compartments in the leg; forearm muscle compartment 5 Ps: *pain, paresthesias, pallor, paralysis, pulselessness* Risk factors: fractures, injuries to arteries/soft tissue; excessive use of the muscles (cyclists; arm wrestlers) Volkmann's ischemic contracture: displaced supracondylar fracture of distal humerus causing compression of brachial artery and median nerve; forearm muscles (superficial and deep flexor muscles) may undergo contracture; although most of the muscles are innervated by the median nerve, the flexor carpi ulnaris is innervated by the ulnar nerve Diagnosis: measure pressures *Treatment*: fasciotomy if pressure cannot be relieved with supportive therapy (ice packs)
Carpal tunnel syndrome	Entrapment syndrome of the median nerve in the transverse carpal ligament of the wrist Causes: rheumatoid arthritis and pregnancy most common causes; obesity, excessive use of hands, acromegaly Pain, numbness, or paresthesias in the thumb, index finger, 2nd finger, 3rd finger, and the radial side of 4th finger; thenar atrophy produces "ape hand" appearance Diagnosis: nerve conduction; electromyography *Phalen's maneuver*: gently flexing of the wrist as far as possible and holding this position reproduces the findings within 1 minute *Tinel's sign*: light tapping over the transverse carpal ligament produces numbness and tingling in the median nerve *Treatment*: wrist splint at night; corticosteroid injection; surgery
Intervertebral disk disease	Degeneration of fibrocartilage/nucleus pulposus; ruptured disk material may herniate posteriorly and compress the nerve root and/or spinal cord Radicular pain; leg pain aggravated by straight leg raising Herniation of L3–L4 disk: loss of knee jerk (femoral nerve L2–L4) Herniation of L4–L5 disk: no loss of reflexes (ankle and knee reflexes intact) Herniation of L5–S1 disk: loss of ankle reflex (tibial nerve L4–S3) *Treatment*: physical therapy; traction; surgery
Knee joint injuries (see Fig. 23-24C)	Valgus injury: angulation away from the midline Laterally originating force is applied to the knee (e.g., clipping injury in football) Varus injury: angulation toward the midline Medially originating force is applied to the knee McMurray test: meniscus injuries Anterior and posterior draw test: cruciate injuries "Unhappy triad": most common internal derangement of knee joint Valgus injury; damage to medial meniscus, medial collateral ligament, anterior cruciate ligament *Treatment*: physical therapy; arthroscopic surgery
Scoliosis (see Fig. 23-24D)	Lateral curvature of the spine (S- or C-shaped on x-ray) Congenital, idiopathic, related to another disease (e.g., cerebral palsy) Idiopathic type: usually affects adolescent girls between 10 and 16 years of age; usually a right thoracic curve; forward bending causes a paraspinous prominence on the right from a hump in the ribs due to a rotational component of the vertebra *Treatment*: bracing; surgery

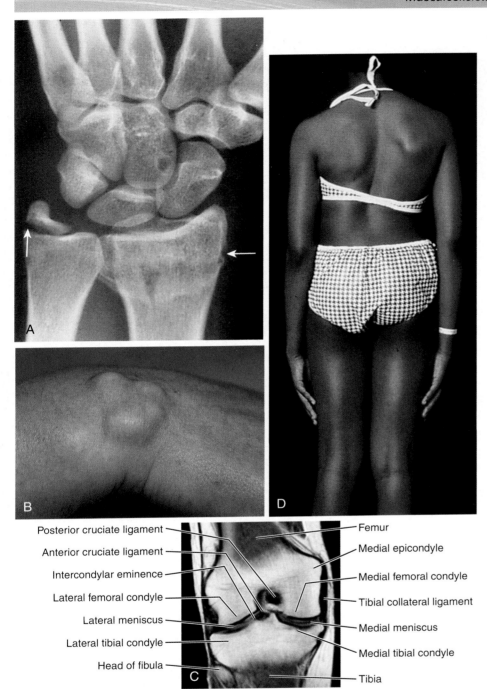

23-24: **A,** Radiograph showing a Colles fracture. Note the fracture lines (*arrows*) in the distal radius and the styloid process of the ulna. **B,** Ganglion cyst on the dorsum of the wrist. **C,** Magnetic resonance image of a normal knee joint and its structures. **D,** Patient with scoliosis. The patient has lateral curvature of the spine with increased convexity to the right. There is obvious scapular asymmetry in the upright position. (*A from Katz D, Math K, Groskin S: Radiology Secrets. Philadelphia, Hanley & Belfus, 1998, p 440, Fig. 9;* ***B*** *from Swartz MH: Textbook of Physical Diagnosis, 5th ed. Philadelphia, Saunders Elsevier, 2006, p 171, Fig. 8-74;* ***C*** *from Moore NA, Roy WA: Rapid Review Gross and Developmental Anatomy, 2nd ed. St. Louis, Mosby Elsevier, 2007, p 148, Fig. 5-6;* ***D*** *from Zitelli B: Atlas of Pediatric Physical Diagnosis, 3rd ed. St. Louis, Mosby, 1997.*)

Posterior cruciate ligament

Anterior cruciate ligament

Intercondylar eminence

Lateral femoral condyle

Lateral meniscus

Lateral tibial condyle

Head of fibula

Femur

Medial epicondyle

Medial femoral condyle

Tibial collateral ligament

Medial meniscus

Medial tibial condyle

Tibia

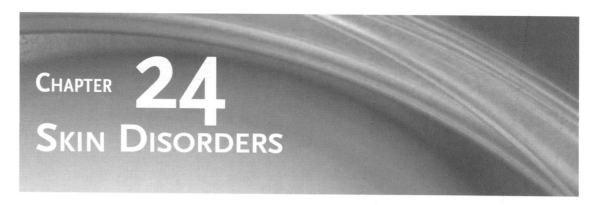

CHAPTER **24**
SKIN DISORDERS

I. Skin Histology and Terminology
   A. Normal skin histology
     1. Epidermis

> Stratum basalis: stem cells for division

       a. Stratum basalis
         (1) Actively dividing stem cells along the basement membrane
         (2) Mitoses should be limited to this area.
       b. Stratum spinosum
         • Contains prominent desmosome attachments
       c. Stratum granulosum
         • Granular layer with keratohyaline granules
       d. Stratum corneum

> Stratum corneum: site for superficial dermatophyte infections

         (1) Anucleate cells with keratin
         (2) Site for superficial dermatophyte infections
     2. Dermis
       a. Papillary
         • Loose connective tissue beneath the epidermis
       b. Reticular
         • Dense dermal collagen
     3. Melanocytes

> Melanocytes: neural crest origin

       a. Derived from neural crest cells
       b. Located in stratum basalis
         • Dendritic processes extend between keratinocytes.

> Melanin: synthesized from tyrosine; synthesized in melanosomes

       c. Melanin is synthesized in membrane-bound melanosomes.
         (1) Tyrosinase converts tyrosine to 3,4-dihydroxyphenylalanine (DOPA).
         (2) DOPA is converted to melanin.

> Melanosomes: transferred by dendritic processes to keratinocytes

         (3) Melanosomes are transferred by dendritic processes to keratinocytes.
       d. Skin color
         (1) Number of melanocytes is essentially the *same* in all races.
         (2) Melanin is degraded more rapidly in whites than in blacks.
         (3) In whites, melanosomes are concentrated in the basal layer.

> Blacks: melanosomes in all layers; melanocytes larger/more dendritic processes

         (4) In blacks, melanosomes are present throughout all layers.
          • Melanocytes are larger and have more dendritic processes.
       e. Sunlight and adrenocorticotropic hormone stimulate melanin synthesis.
   B. Common terms used in dermatology (Table 24-1)
II. Selected Viral Disorders
   A. Common warts

> Common wart: HPV

     1. Caused by human papillomavirus (HPV; DNA virus)
     2. Common sites are the fingers and soles.
     3. Verrucous papular lesions covered by scales (Fig. 24-1A)
     4. Treatment
       a. Physical therapy—e.g., cryotherapy with liquid nitrogen
       b. Chemotherapy—e.g., salicylic acid, trichloroacetic acid
       c. Biologic therapeutic agent—imiquimod (induces cytokines)
   B. Molluscum contagiosum

> Molluscum contagiosum: poxvirus; umbilicated lesions with viral particles

     1. Caused by a poxvirus (DNA virus)
     2. Bowl-shaped lesions with central depression filled with keratin (Fig. 24-1B)
       • Depression contains viral particles called molluscum bodies.

TABLE 24-1. **COMMON TERMS IN DERMATOLOGY**

TERM	DEFINITION	EXAMPLE
Macroscopic		
Macule	Pigmented or erythematous flat lesion on epidermis	Tinea versicolor
Papule	Peaked or dome-shaped surface elevation < 5 mm in diameter	Acne vulgaris
Nodule	Elevated, dome-shaped lesion > 5 mm in diameter	Basal cell carcinoma
Plaque	Flattened, elevated area on epidermis > 5 mm in diameter	Psoriasis
Vesicle	Fluid-filled blister < 5 mm in diameter	Varicella (chickenpox)
Bulla	Fluid-filled blister > 5 mm in diameter	Bullous pemphigoid
Pustule	Fluid-filled blister with inflammatory cells	Impetigo
Wheal (hive)	Edematous, transient papule or plaque caused by infiltration of dermis by fluid	Urticaria
Scales	Excessive number of dead keratinocytes produced by abnormal keratinization	Seborrheic dermatitis
Microscopic		
Hyperkeratosis	Increased thickness of stratum corneum produces scaly appearance of skin	Psoriasis
Parakeratosis	Persistence of nuclei in stratum corneum layer	Psoriasis
Papillomatosis	Spire-like projections from surface of skin or downward into papillary dermis	Verruca vulgaris
Acantholysis	Loss of cohesion between keratinocytes	Pemphigus vulgaris

3. Transmission
   a. Can be sexually transmitted in adults (common in AIDS)
   b. Self-inoculation by scratching the infective viral particles out of the crater

Molluscum contagiosum: common in AIDS

4. Treatment
   a. Spontaneous remission occurs in 6 to 9 months if immunocompetent.
      • Cell-mediated immunity
   b. Cryotherapy

C. Rubeola (measles)
  1. RNA paramyxovirus
  2. Vaccination has reduced the incidence of rubeola.
  3. Prodrome
    • Fever, cough, coryza (runny nose), conjunctivitis
  4. Koplik spots develop on the buccal mucosa.
    • Koplik spots are white spots overlying an erythematous base (Fig. 24-1C).
  5. Maculopapular rash develops *after* Koplik spots disappear (Fig. 24-1D).
   a. Cytotoxic T cell damage of endothelial cells containing the virus
   b. Typically begins on the head and then to the trunk and extremities
   c. Tends to become confluent on face and trunk but discrete on extremities
  6. Complications
   a. Giant cell pneumonia
    • Warthin-Finkeldey multinucleated giant cells
   b. Acute appendicitis in children
   c. Otitis media
   d. Encephalitis
    • Before immunization, encephalitis was a common cause of death in measles.
   e. *Not* teratogenic
  7. Prevented through vaccinations

Rubeola: regular measles

Prodrome 3 Cs: cough, coryza, conjunctivitis

Rubeola: rash after Koplik spots disappear

Rubeola: giant cell pneumonia; acute appendicitis (children); otitis media

D. Rubella (German measles)
  1. RNA togavirus
    • Produces "3-day measles"
  2. Vaccination has reduced the incidence of rubella.
  3. Forchheimer's spots (see Fig. 21-1E)
   a. Dusky red spots that develop on posterior soft/hard palate
   b. Develop at beginning of the rash.
  4. Maculopapular rash lasts 3 days (see Fig. 21-1F).
   a. Pinkish, red maculopapular eruption
   b. Begins first at hairline and rapidly spreads cephalocaudally
   c. Unlike rubeola, the macules and papules are discrete and do *not* become confluent.
   d. Fades in 3 days

Rubella: maculopapular rash with discrete lesion; not confluent; fades in 3 days

24-1: Viral infections. **A,** Verruca vulgaris (common wart) on the fingers, showing scaling, verrucous papules with interrupted skin lines. **B,** Molluscum contagiosum, showing small bowl-shaped lesions with central areas of depression (umbilication). **C,** Rubeola (regular measles). Note the Koplik spots on the buccal mucosa. **D,** Rubeola. A macular rash begins on the face and neck and then becomes maculopapular (this patient) and spreads to the trunk and extremities in irregular confluent patches. **E,** Rubella. Note the red Forchheimer spots on the soft and hard palate. **F,** Rubella. Note the fine pinkish red maculopapular rash. The lesions remain discrete and do not become confluent as they do in rubeola. **G,** Erythema infectiosum. Note the "slapped face" appearance. **H,** Roseola infantum. Note the maculopapular rash, which normally blanches with pressure. There are subtle peripheral halos due to vasoconstriction around some of the lesions. **I,** Varicella. Note the vesicles and pustules surrounded by an erythematous base. The lesions are at different stages of development. **J,** Herpes zoster (shingles). Note the erythematous vesicular rash with the characteristic "band" distribution, which starts from the midline and extends to the lateral trunk. (**A** from Lookingbill D, Marks J: Principles of Dermatology, 3rd ed. Philadelphia, WB Saunders, 2000, p 68, Fig. 6-1A; **B** and **G** from Savin JA, Hunter JAA, Hepburn NC: Diagnosis in Color: Skin Signs in Clinical Medicine. London, Mosby-Wolfe, 1997, pp 79 and 6, Figs. 2-47 and 1-10, respectively; **C** from Centers for Disease Control and Prevention Web site—Public Health Image Library. Image #4500. Available at http://phil.cdc.gov/phil/details.asp; **D** from Zitelli B: Atlas of Pediatric Physical Diagnosis, 3rd ed. St. Louis, Mosby, 1997; **E** from Eisen D, Lynch DP: The Mouth: Diagnosis and Treatment. St. Louis, Mosby, 1998; **F** courtesy of Dr. Michael Sherlock; **H** from Paller AS, Mancinin AJ [eds]: Hurwitz Clinical Pediatric Dermatology, 3rd ed. Philadelphia, Elsevier, 2006, p 434; **I** courtesy of The Honickman Collection of Medical Images in memory of Elaine Garfinkel and The Jefferson Clinical Images Collection [through the generosity of JMB, AKR, LKB and DA]; **J** from Forbes C, Jackson W: Color Atlas and Text of Clinical Medicine, 2nd ed. St. Louis, Mosby, 2003, p 29, Fig. 1-85.)

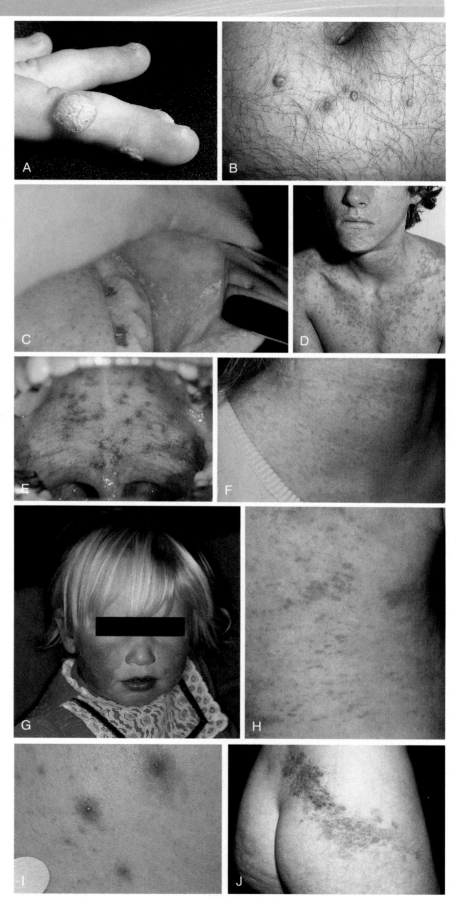

5. Painful <u>postauricular lymphadenopathy</u> (characteristic) *of rubella*
6. Polyarthritis is common in adults.
7. Infection during <u>first</u> trimester may produce <u>congenital anomalies</u>
   (refer to Chapter 5).
8. Prevent through <u>vaccination</u>

E. **Erythema infectiosum (fifth disease)**
1. Caused by <u>parvovirus B19</u> (DNA virus)
2. Most often occurs in school age children
   • Often occurs in epidemics
3. <u>Confluent net-like erythema</u> type of rash
   a. Begins on the cheeks ("<u>slapped face</u>" appearance; Fig. 24-1G)
   b. Extends to the trunk and <u>proximal</u> extremities
4. <u>Polyarthritis</u> is common in adults.

> Other disorders caused by parvovirus B19 include pure red blood cell aplasia and aplastic anemia in chronic hemolytic diseases (e.g., hereditary spherocytosis) and chronic arthritis. Pregnant mothers exposed to a child with the infection may abort the fetus.

F. **Roseola infantum**
1. Caused by <u>human herpesvirus 6</u> (DNA virus)
2. <u>Most common viral exanthem</u> in children < 2 years old
3. Erythematous macules develop on <u>soft palate 48 hours *before*</u> rash.
4. <u>Maculopapular rash</u> occurs abruptly after 3 to 7 days of high fever (Fig. 24-1H).
5. High fever may <u>precipitate</u> a febrile convulsion. *Fever → Rash*

G. **Disorders caused by varicella-zoster virus**
1. DNA herpesvirus
   • Remains latent in cranial and thoracic sensory ganglia
2. Varicella (chickenpox)
   a. Predominantly a childhood disease
      (1) Approximately 90% of cases occur in those <10 years of age.
      (2) Peaks in spring months
   b. Incubation 2 to 3 weeks
   c. Patient is infectious <u>1 week *before*</u> the rash appears.
      • Infectious an additional 4 to 5 days until vesicles become crusted
   d. Pruritic rash progresses <u>from macules, to vesicles, to pustules</u> (Fig. 24-1I).
      (1) All stages of development are <u>simultaneously present</u>.
      (2) Lesions are most prominent on the trunk.
         (a) Also involves extremities (including palms and soles), mucous membranes in mouth, conjunctiva
         (b) Vesicles are often <u>umbilicated</u> (depressed center) and hemorrhagic.
   e. Positive Tzanck test similar to herpes simplex virus (refer to Chapter 21)
   f. Complications
      (1) Association with Reye syndrome
      (2) Pneumonia, self-limited cerebellitis
      (3) In adults—hepatitis, pneumonia, encephalitis
         • Treated with acyclovir
   g. Treatment
      (1) Prevention with immunization
      (2) Antihistamine; oatmeal bath; calamine lotion
3. Herpes zoster (shingles)
   a. Occurs in 10% to 20% of people in their lifetime.
   b. Incidence increases with age.
   c. Incidence increased in patients with cancer and AIDS
   d. Prodrome of radicular pain and itching *before* rash occurs
   e. Eruption characterized by groups of vesicles on an erythematous base
      (1) Rash follows sensory dermatomes in the distribution of cranial nerves or spinal nerves (Fig. 24-1J).
      (2) Like varicella, pustules form that rupture, causing crusting and weeping.
   f. Treatment
      (1) Prevention with previous immunization for varicella

Margin notes:

Rubella: painful postauricular lymphadenopathy

Rubella: teratogenic

Erythema infectiosum: parvovirus; slapped face appearance

Polyarthritis in adults: rubella and parvovirus

Roseola: HHV-6; most common viral exanthem children < 2 years old

Roseola: common cause of febrile convulsions

Varicella: predominantly a childhood disease

Infectious: week before rash; week after rash until vesicles become crusted

Varicella: macules, vesicles, pustules

Complications: children—Reye syndrome, cerebellitis; adult—pneumonia, encephalitis, hepatitis

Herpes zoster: incidence increases with age; cancer; immunocompromised state

Herpes zoster: painful vesicles/pustules follow sensory dermatomes

(2) Prevention with zoster vaccine
  • Greater than 50% reduction in infection
(3) Analgesics commensurate with amount of pain
(4) Immunocompromised patients are often treated with acyclovir, valacyclovir, or famiciclovir.
  • Best started *before* the rash has erupted

III. **Selected Bacterial Disorders**
    A. ***Staphylococcus aureus* skin infections**

S. aureus: gram-positive coccus in clumps

TSST: produces desquamating sunburn-like rash

      1. Gram-positive coccus (Fig. 24-2A)
      2. Toxic shock syndrome
        a. Production of toxic shock syndrome toxin (TSST)
          • Superantigen that stimulates release of cytokines
        b. Usually occurs in tampon-using menstruating women
        c. Clinical findings
          (1) Fever, hypotension
          (2) Desquamating, sunburn-like rash
      3. Other infections
        a. Skin abscess (see Fig. 2-6)
          • Treatment: trimethoprim-sulfamethoxazole (TMP-SMX; community acquired)

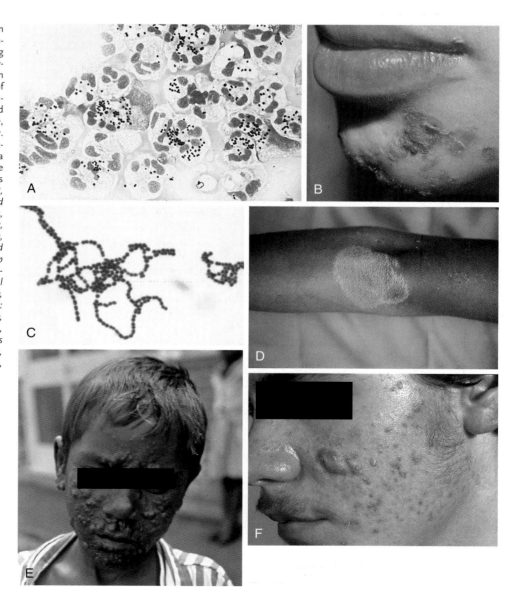

24-2: Bacterial infections. **A,** Gram stain of *Staphylococcus aureus*. Note the gram-positive cocci, some of which are forming clusters. **B,** Impetigo of the face showing "honey-colored" crusts overlying an erythematous base. **C,** Gram stain of *Streptococcus pyogenes*. Note the gram-positive cocci in chains. **D,** Tuberculoid leprosy. Note the hypopigmented macule, an early finding in tuberculoid leprosy. **E,** Lepromatous leprosy. Note the nodular lesions on the face giving the patient a leonine facies. **F,** Acne vulgaris. Note the severe facial acne with inflamed papules and cystic lesions. (*A from McPherson R, Pincus M: Henry's Clinical Diagnosis and Management by Laboratory Methods, 21st ed. Philadelphia, WB Saunders, 2007, p 1018, Fig. 56-2; **B** from Lookingbill D, Marks J: Principles of Dermatology, 3rd ed. Philadelphia, WB Saunders, 2000, pp 217 and 213, Figs. 13-9 and 13-4A, respectively; **C** from Murray PR, Shea YR: Medical Microbiology, 2nd ed. St. Louis, Mosby, 2002, p 238, Fig. 23-1; **D** from Cohen J: Infectious Disease, 2nd ed. St. Louis, Mosby, 2003; **E** and **F** from Savin JA, Hunter JAA, Hepburn NC: Diagnosis in Color: Skin Signs in Clinical Medicine. London, Mosby-Wolfe, 1997, pp 23 and 135, Figs. 1-48 and 5-20, respectively.*)

b. Hidradenitis suppurativa
(1) Chronic condition characterized by:
(a) Swollen, painful, inflamed apocrine glands usually in the axillae and groin
(b) Infection can also involve adjacent subcutaneous tissue and fascia.
(c) Hallmark is the presence of sinus tracts.
(2) Must aspirate and culture pus
(3) Difficult to treat; may require surgery
c. Postsurgical wound infection (most common pathogen)
(1) If not septic, treat with TMP-SMX double strength.
(2) If septic, treat with IV vancomycin.
d. Impetigo
(1) Most often caused by *Staphylococcus aureus*
• *Streptococcus pyogenes* second most common cause
(2) Rash usually begins on the face (Fig. 24-2B).
• Vesicles and pustules rupture to form honey-colored, crusted lesions.
(3) Bullae commonly occur.
(4) Treatment
• Mupirocin ointment + dicloxacillin (or oxacillin, amoxicillin-clavulanate, azithromycin)

B. *Streptococcus pyogenes* skin infections
1. Gram-positive coccus (Fig. 24-2C)
2. Scarlet fever
a. Particular strains of *S. pyogenes* produce an erythrogenic toxin.
b. Patients are febrile and have a sore throat due to streptococcal pharyngitis.
c. An erythematous rash develops that involves the skin and tongue.
(1) It initially occurs on the face and neck before spreading to other parts of the body.
(2) It spares the mouth producing conspicuous circumoral pallor.
(3) It has a sandpapery feeling.
(4) The tongue is covered by a white exudate studded with prominent red papillae.
(5) The rash begins to fade after 6 days and desquamation (peeling) begins, which may last up to 10 days.
(6) The white exudate on the tongue disappears; tongue is beefy red, hence the term "strawberry tongue."
d. Increased risk for developing poststreptococcal glomerulonephritis (refer to Chapter 19) and rheumatic fever (refer to Chapter 10)
e. Treatment is penicillin V.
3. Erysipelas
a. Type of cellulitis
(1) Border is raised and surface appears like an orange peel (see Fig. 2-1).
(2) Skin surface is hot and bright red (rubor of acute inflammation).
b. Commonly occurs on the face and lower extremities
c. Patient feels ill and is febrile.
d. Treatment is IV penicillin G if on extremities; vancomycin if on the face

C. Leprosy
1. Caused by *Mycobacterium leprae*
• Grows in footpads of mice and armadillos; *cannot* be cultured
2. Tuberculoid type
a. Granulomas present
• Very few acid-fast bacteria are present in the granulomas.
b. Positive lepromin skin test
• Indicates intact cellular immunity
c. Localized skin lesions with nerve involvement
(1) Autoamputation of digits
(2) Anesthetic macules with hypopigmentation (Fig. 24-2D)
d. Treatment
• Dapsone + rifampin
3. Lepromatous type
a. Absence of granulomas
(1) Numerous bacteria are present in foamy macrophages.
(2) Macrophages are located under a subepidermal zone free of organisms.
• Called the Grenz zone

S. aureus infections: abscess, postsurgical wound infection; hidradenitis; impetigo

S. pyogenes: gram-positive coccus in chains

Scarlet fever: erythrogenic toxin; erythematous sandpapery rash that desquamates

Scarlet fever: ↑ risk poststreptococcal glomerulonephritis, rheumatic fever

Erysipelas: cellulitis with raised borders

Tuberculoid: granuloma; intact cellular immunity; + lepromin skin test

Tuberculoid: digital autoamputation; hypopigmented skin

Lepromatous: organisms present; impaired cellular immunity; – lepromin skin test

Lepromatous: leonine facies

      b. Negative lepromin skin test
- Indicates a lack of cellular immunity

      c. Nodular lesions produce the classic leonine facies (Fig. 24-2E).

      d. Treatment
- Dapsone + rifampin + clofazimine

D. Acne vulgaris

Acne vulgaris: chronic inflammation of pilosebaceous unit

1. Chronic inflammation of the pilosebaceous unit
2. Most common disease seen by dermatologists
3. Begins at an early age (9–11 years old)
4. Increases in severity in teenage years
5. Clinical lesions
- Inflammatory papules, pustules, nodules, cysts
6. Noninflamed comedones

Comedones: open ("blackhead"), closed ("whitehead")

      a. Plugging of the outlet of a hair follicle by keratin debris

      b. Open comedone is called a "blackhead."

      c. Closed comedone is called a "whitehead."

7. Inflammatory type

Acne vulgaris: androgen receptors located on sebaceous glands

      a. Abnormal keratinization of the follicular epithelium

      b. Increased sebum production (androgen-dependent)

Acne vulgaris: *Propionibacterium acnes* produces lipase

      c. Bacterial lipase *(Propionibacterium acnes)* produces irritating fatty acids.
- Produces the inflammatory reaction (Fig. 24-2F)

8. Treatment

      a. Topical agents—e.g., topical retinoid + benzoyl peroxide

      b. Systemic antibiotics—e.g., tetracycline (first choice); erythromycin

      c. Systemic retinoids—isotretinoin (decreases follicular keratinization, sebum production, bacterial count)

      d. Hormonal therapy—oral contraceptives (women; reduce free testosterone levels); antiandrogens (spironolactone)

IV.   Selected Fungal Disorders

A. Superficial mycoses (dermatophytoses)

1. Fungi confined to the stratum corneum or its adnexal structures

Superficial dermatophytes: live in stratum corneum

      a. Incidence increases in warm, humid climates.

      b. Most infections present with a scaling rash.

      c. Tinea actually means "worm" in Latin, but is applied to describe superficial fungal infections.

        (1) Tinea is followed by a word that qualifies its location (e.g., capitis, pedis, corporis)

        (2) Most common infections in decreasing order—tinea pedis (foot), tinea unguim (nail), tinea versicolor (describes color variation rather than location), tinea cruris (groin)

Wood's lamp: detects fluorescent fungal metabolites

Wood's lamp and potassium hydroxide (KOH)–treated skin scrapings from lesions are commonly used for diagnosis of the dermatophytoses. Wood's lamp (ultraviolet A light) detects fluorescent metabolites produced by organisms (e.g., fungi, some bacteria). KOH preparations identify yeasts and hyphae in the stratum corneum or hair shafts (Fig. 24-3A).

2. Tinea capitis

      a. Superficial fungal infection of scalp

      b. Pathogens

T. tonsurans: most common cause in blacks; – Wood's lamp

        (1) Most often caused by *Trichophyton tonsurans*
          (a) Infects the inner hair shaft
          (b) Negative Wood's lamp
          (c) Predominant type present in blacks

M. canis/audouinii: most common cause in whites; + Wood's lamp

        (2) *Microsporum canis* and *Microsporum audouinii*
          (a) Former type is associated with exposure to dogs.
          (b) Both infect the outer hair shaft.
          (c) Positive Wood's lamp
          (d) Predominant pathogens in whites

Tinea capitis: oral terbinafine; topical imidazoles do not work

      c. Circular or ring-shaped patches of hair loss (alopecia)
- Black dot is present where hair breaks off (Fig. 24-3B).

      d. Treatment is oral terbinafine.

T. rubrum: most common cause of all other tineas (except versicolor)

3. Other infections are most often caused by *Trichophyton rubrum*.

      a. Tinea corporis (body surface) (Fig. 24-3C)

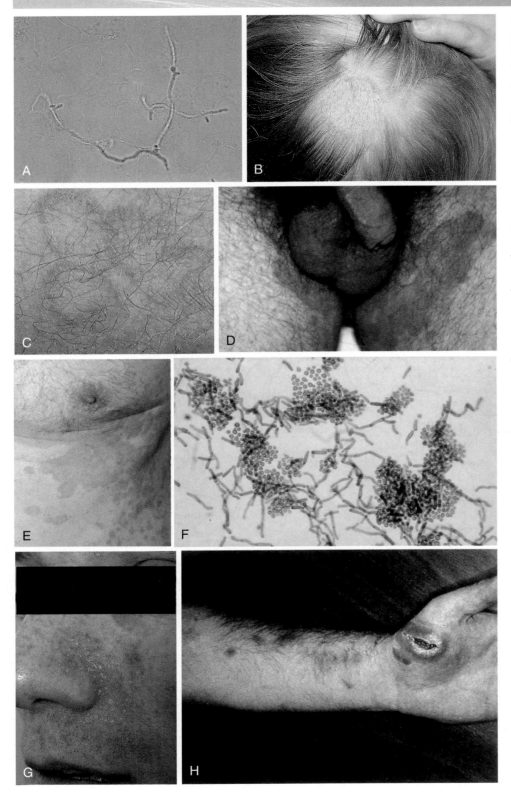

24-3: A, Potassium hydroxide (KOH) preparation of skin scrapings showing hyphae and yeasts. **B,** Tinea capitis due to *Trichophyton tonsurans*. Note the area of alopecia (hair loss) with black dots representing broken off hairs and scaling of the skin. **C,** Tinea corporis showing annular lesions with erythematous margins and clear centers. **D,** Tinea cruris. Note the scaly, erythematous rash in the groin. **E,** Tinea versicolor showing skin with pink-tan patches (hyperpigmentation) intermixed with normal skin. The hyperpigmented lesions should be scraped for a KOH preparation. **F,** *Malassezia furfur.* Note the classic spaghetti (hyphae) and meatball (yeasts) morphologic appearance. **G,** Seborrheic dermatitis. Note the erythematous, greasy scaling rash in the nasolabial fold. It is caused by *M. furfur.* **H,** Lymphocutaneous sporotrichosis showing a linear array of suppurating subcutaneous nodules. *(A and B from Goldstein BG: Practical Dermatology, 2nd ed. St. Louis, Mosby, 1997, pp 24, 97, Fig. 3-2 and Fig. 10-1, respectively; C from Forbes C, Jackson W: Color Atlas and Text of Clinical Medicine, 2nd ed. St. Louis, Mosby, 2003, p 97, Fig. 2-57; D and G from Savin JA, Hunter JAA, Hepburn NC: Diagnosis in Color: Skin Signs in Clinical Medicine. London, Mosby-Wolfe, 1997, pp 123 and 9, Figs. 4.78 and 1.17, respectively; E from Lookingbill D, Marks J: Principles of Dermatology, 3rd ed. Philadelphia, WB Saunders, 2000, p 227, Fig. 14-2; F from Midgley G, Clayton Y, Hay RJ: Diagnosis in Color: Medical Mycology. London, Mosby-Wolfe, 1997, p 73, Fig. 93; H from Murray PR, Shea YR: Medical Microbiology, 2nd ed. St. Louis, Mosby, 2002, p 163, Fig. 43-14.)*

(1) Sometimes called "ringworm"
(2) May have history of exposure to cat or dog
(3) One or more lesions may be present.
(4) Typically are annular with an elevated red, scaly border
   • Tendency for central clearing

Tinea corporis: annular; outer border raised/scaly; central clearing

(5) Treatment uses topical agents (e.g., miconazole, clotrimazole).
   • Can use oral terbinafine as an alternative
b. Tinea pedis ("athlete's foot")

   (1) Most common site for infection
   (2) Most common in patient with sweaty feet
   (3) Macerated scaling rash between the toes
   (4) Elderly people have diffuse plantar scaling
      • "Moccasin" appearance
   (5) Treatment is with topical agents (e.g., miconazole, clotrimazole).
      • Can use oral terbinafine as an alternative
c. Tinea cruris (groin; "jock itch") (Fig. 24-3D)

   (1) Frequently also have tinea pedis
   (2) Both are areas for excessive sweating.
   (3) Rash is *not* annular but has elevated, scaly borders.
   (4) Scrotum is involved.
   (5) Treatment uses topical agents (e.g., miconazole, clotrimazole).
      • Can use oral terbinafine as an alternative
d. Tinea unguium (nail; onychomycosis)
   (1) Second most common superficial dermatophyte infection

   (2) *T. rubrum* (most common) and *T. mentagrophytes* most common dermatophytes
   (3) Nail is raised and nail plate is white, thick, and crumbly.
   (4) Nail is frequently discolored.
   (5) Treatment
      (a) Topical agents do not work.
      (b) Oral therapy with terbinafine (best) or itraconazole
4. Tinea versicolor
   a. Tinea with alteration with skin pigmentation

      (1) Hypopigmented type is due to decrease in melanin synthesis.
      (2) Hyperpigmented type is due to an enlargement of melanosomes.
   b. Wood's lamp accentuates the color variation in skin.
   c. Caused by *Malassezia furfur*
      (1) In hypopigmented type, fungus-derived acids inhibit tyrosinase in melanocytes from synthesizing melanin.
      (2) In hyperpigmented type, fungus induces enlargement of melanosomes in melanocytes along the basal cell layer.

   d. Affected skin does *not* tan ("white spots"); normal skin does (Fig. 24-3E).
      • Lesions become hyperpigmented and scaly in winter months.
   e. KOH findings (Fig. 24-3F)
      (1) Hypopigmented/hyperpigmented areas have the organism.
      (2) Short hyphae have the appearance of "spaghetti."
      (3) Yeasts have the appearance of "meatballs."
   f. Treatment
      (1) Topical selenium sulfide
      (2) Oral ketoconazole (best treatment)
5. Infections caused by *Candida albicans*
   a. Intertrigo
      (1) Erythematous rash in body folds
         • KOH shows pseudohyphae and yeast (see Fig. 21-1A).

      (2) Examples—rash under pendulous breasts, diaper rash
      (3) Treatment is topical agents (e.g., miconazole, clotrimazole)
   b. Onychomycosis
      (1) Nail infection
      (2) Treatment
         (a) Topical—amphotericin B, clotrimazole, econazole
         (b) Oral ketoconazole
6. Seborrheic dermatitis (dandruff)
   a. Affects 3% to 5% of population
   b. Caused by *M. furfur*
   c. Common associations

      (1) Parkinson's disease
      (2) AIDS and AIDS-related complex
   d. Scaly, yellowish, greasy dermatitis (Fig. 24-3G)
   e. Locations

(1) Scalp (dandruff), eyebrows, and nasal creases

(2) Called cradle cap in newborns

 f. Treatment

  • Shampoo—selenium sulfide, zinc pyrithione; may need higher prescription doses of these over-the-counter shampoos

B. Sporotrichosis

 1. Caused by *Sporothrix schenckii*

  a. Subcutaneous mycotic infection

  b. Dimorphic fungus

   • Mold in soil, yeast in tissue

 2. Traumatic implantation of fungus

  a. Rose gardening

  b. Sphagnum peat moss for packing material

  c. Splinters from carpentry work

  d. Landscapers; berry-pickers

 3. Lymphocutaneous disease

  • Chain of suppurating lymphocutaneous nodules (Fig. 24-3H)

 4. Treatment

  a. Oral itraconazole

  b. Saturated solution of potassium iodide (SSKI)

   • Poorly tolerated; not the treatment of choice

V. Selected Parasitic and Arthropod Disorders

A. Cutaneous larva migrans

 1. Caused by *Ancyclostoma braziliense* (dog and cat hookworm; nematode)

  a. Transmission

   (1) Dogs and cats are the definitive host.

    • Sexually mature host that can mate and lay eggs

   (2) Larvae evolve in sand/soil from eggs passed in the feces.

   (3) Larvae penetrate the skin in children/adults (intermediate hosts).

  b. Cutaneous larva migrans (creeping eruption)

   (1) Larvae penetrate the skin.

    (a) Commonly contracted while playing in sand

    (b) Cover sandboxes so dogs/cat do not use them as litter boxes.

   (2) Produce serpiginous tunnels in the skin (Fig. 24-4A)

    • Causes intense pruritus and scratching and eosinophilia

   (3) Treatment is ivermectin.

B. Arthropod disorders: mites

 1. Chiggers

  a. Small, red to orange-colored mite

  b. Produces a pruritic dermatitis

   (1) Bright red papular, urticarial, or vesicular rash

   (2) Favor the legs and areas of tight-fitting clothing

  c. Treatment

   • Topical antipruritic agents (crotamiton and calamine lotion)

 2. Human itch mite (*Sarcoptes scabiei* var. *hominis*)

  a. Adult females bore into the stratum corneum.

   (1) Burrows are visible as dark lines between the fingers, at the wrists, on the nipples, or on the scrotum.

   (2) Females lay eggs at the end of the tunnel.

    • Eggs are responsible for the intensely pruritic lesion.

  b. Adults

   (1) Disease limited to the webs between the fingers (Fig. 24-4B), intertriginous areas

   (2) Spares the soles, palms, face and head

  c. Infants

   (1) *No* burrows are present.

   (2) Pruritic rash occurs on the palms, soles, face or head.

  d. Treatment is permethrin cream.

C. Arthropod disorders: lice

 1. *Pediculus humanis capitis* (head louse)

  a. Adults lay eggs ("nits") on hair shafts (Fig. 24-4C).

  b. Itching of the scalp

24-4: A, Cutaneous larva migrans. Note irregular, erythematous tracts beneath the skin surface. **B,** Scabies. Note the erythematous area in the web between the fingers. The *arrows* show raised burrows. **C,** Pediculus capitis. Note the white nits (eggs) attached to the hair shafts. **D,** Pediculus corporis. Note the numerous erythematous papules over the back of this homeless person. **E,** Phthirus pubis. Note the crab-like appearance of the louse. (*A and B courtesy of R.A. Marsden, MD, St. George's Hospital, London;* **C** *from Kliegman RM, Jenson HB, Behrman RE, Stanton BF: Nelson's Textbook of Pediatrics, 18th ed. Philadelphia, Saunders Elsevier, 2007, p 2758, Fig. 667-6;* **D** *from Savin JA, Hunter JAA, Hepburn NC: Diagnosis in Color: Skin Signs in Clinical Medicine. London, Mosby-Wolfe, 1997, p 214, Fig. 9.3;* **E** *from Klatt E: Robbins and Cotran's Atlas of Pathology. Philadelphia, WB Saunders, 2006, p 399, Fig. 16-90 right.*)

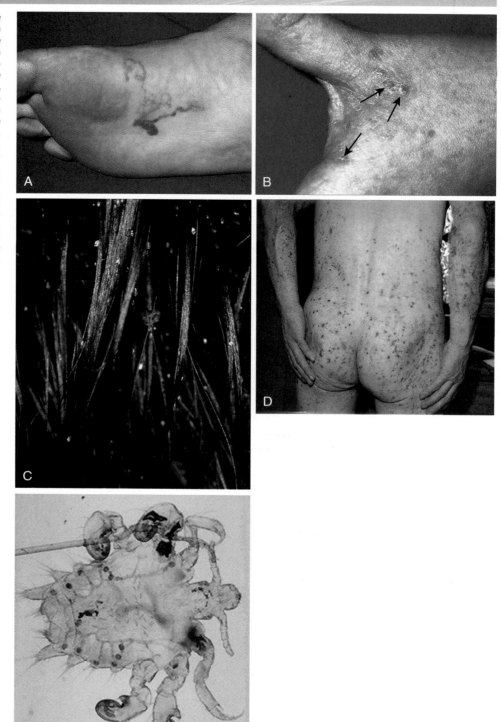

Body louse: *Pediculus hominis corporis;* adults live on skin and breed in clothing

Body louse: treat clothing *not* the patient

c. Treatment
   (1) Permethrin (kills newly hatched lice)
   (2) Followed by lindane (Kwell), if the initial treatment is unsuccessful
2. *Pediculus humanis corporis* (body louse)
   a. Adults live on the surface of the skin and breed in the clothing.
   b. Skin lesions are papular and produce intense itching (Fig. 24-4D).
   c. Treat the clothing, *not* the patient.
      • Treat clothing with malathion or DDT powder or discard clothes

3. *Phthirus pubis* (pubic louse, crabs)
   a. Adults live in the pubic hairs
      • Looks like a crab
   b. Treatment is permethrin or malathion.
D. **Arthropod disorders: bedbug**
   1. Common bedbug is *Cimex lectularius*
   2. Commonly completely infest dwellings (houses, motels)
   3. Feed on human blood
      a. Active just before dawn
      b. Attracted by warmth and CO_2
   4. Skin lesions
      a. Intensely pruritic red papules/wheals
      b. Allergic reaction to anesthetic in saliva
   5. Treatment
      • Exterminators use permethrin.

VI. **Melanocytic Disorders**
A. **Solar lentigo**
   1. Common finding in elderly individuals
   2. Brown, macules located on sun-exposed areas ("liver spots") (Fig. 24-5A)
      a. Increased number of melanocytes
      b. In contradistinction, freckles have a normal number of melanocytes but an increase in melanosomes.
   3. *Not* precancerous
   4. No treatment
B. **Vitiligo**
   1. Common in blacks
   2. Autoimmune destruction of melanocytes
      a. Causes localized to extensive areas of skin depigmentation (Fig. 24-5B).
      b. In contradistinction, albinism is due to a deficiency of tyrosinase leading to absence of melanin in melanocytes.
   3. Often associated with other autoimmune conditions
      • Examples—Hashimoto's thyroiditis, hypoparathyroidism
C. **Melasma**
   1. Macular, hyperpigmented lesions on the forehead and cheeks (Fig. 24-5C)
   2. Female predominance; exacerbated (melanocytes produce more melanin) by:
      a. Oral contraceptives (OCP)
      b. Pregnancy ("pregnancy mask")
      c. Sunlight
   3. Treatment
      • Application of hydroquinone (bleaching agent) to skin
D. **Nevocellular nevus (mole)**
   1. Neoplastic melanocytic disorder
   2. Whites have an average of 15 to 40 nevi on their skin.
   3. Frequently contain hair
   4. Benign tumor of neural crest–derived nevus cells
      • Nevus cells are modified melanocytes.
   5. Begins in early childhood as junctional nevus (Fig. 24-5D)
      a. Pigmented macular (flat) lesion
      b. Nests of nevus cells occur along the basal cell layer.
   6. Junctional nevus develops into a compound nevus.
      a. Usually occurs in children and adolescents
      b. Nevus cells extend into the superficial dermis.
         • Junctional and intradermal components are present.
      c. Pigmented lesion with a papillomatous surface (Fig. 24-5E)
   7. Intradermal nevus
      • Develop when a compound nevus loses its junctional component (Fig. 24-5F)
   8. Dysplastic nevus (atypical mole)
      a. May arise sporadically
         (1) Controversial on whether they may develop into a malignant melanoma
         (2) Usually >6mm; variegated in color with an erythematous background; irregular borders
      b. May be associated with the dysplastic nevus syndrome (Fig. 24-5G)
         (1) Autosomal dominant syndrome with >100 nevi on the skin

---

Phthirus pubis: louse; pubic hairs

Bedbug: *Cimex lectularius*; commonly infest dwellings; feed on human blood

Solar lentigo: common in elderly; "liver spots"; ↑ melanocytes

Freckles: normal number of melanocytes with increase in melanosomes

Vitiligo: autoimmune destruction of melanocytes

Albinism: deficiency of tyrosinase; absent melanin in melanocytes

Melasma: malar hyperpigmentation pregnancy/OCP

Nevus cells: modified melanocytes

Junctional nevus: most common nevus in children

Intradermal nevus: most common nevus in adults

Dysplastic nevus syndrome: majority develop malignant melanoma

24-5: **A,** Solar lentigo. Note the numerous brown macules on the dorsum of the hand. **B,** Vitiligo. Note the patchy depigmentation of the skin. **C,** Melasma. Note the facial hyperpigmentation in this pregnant woman. **D,** Junctional nevus. Note the oval, uniformly pigmented macular lesion. **E,** Compound nevus. Note the pigmented lesion with the slightly papillomatous appearing surface. **F,** Intradermal nevus. Note the raised, pigmented lesion with the papillomatous appearing surface. **G,** Dysplastic nevus syndrome. Note the numerous pigmented lesions over the back and neck. The inset shows a dysplastic nevus that is >6 mm in diameter and shows variable pigmentation. **H,** Superficial spreading malignant melanoma. The lesion on the patient's forearm is black, is multinodular, and has an irregular border with areas of pale gray discoloration. **I,** Lentigo maligna melanoma. Note that the facial lesion shows asymmetry, border irregularity, color variation, and a diameter >6 mm. **J,** Acral lentiginous malignant melanoma. Note the pigmented lesion under the nail that has spread to involve the proximal nail bed. **K,** ABCD changes in malignant melanoma. See text for discussion. *(A and I from Lookingbill D, Marks J: Principles of Dermatology, 3rd ed. Philadelphia, WB Saunders, 2000, p 94, Figs. 7-2 and 7-4B, respectively; B courtesy of The Honickman Collection of Medical Images in memory of Elaine Garfinkel and The Jefferson Clinical Images Collection [through the generosity of JMB, AKR, LKB and DA]; C, D, E, and F from Habif T: Clinical Dermatology, 4th ed. St. Louis, Mosby, 2004; G from Kumar V, Abbas AK, Fausto N, Mitchell RN: Robbins Basic Pathology, 8th ed. Philadelphia, Saunders Elsevier, 2007, p 854, Fig. 22-20C; H from Damjanov I, Linder J: Pathology: A Color Atlas. St. Louis, Mosby, 2000, p 327, Fig. 15-57A; J from Savin JA, Hunter JAA, Hepburn NC: Diagnosis in Color: Skin Signs in Clinical Medicine, London, Mosby-Wolfe, 1997, p 119, Fig. 4.63; K reproduced with permission from American Academy of Dermatology, copyright © 2009, all rights reserved.)*

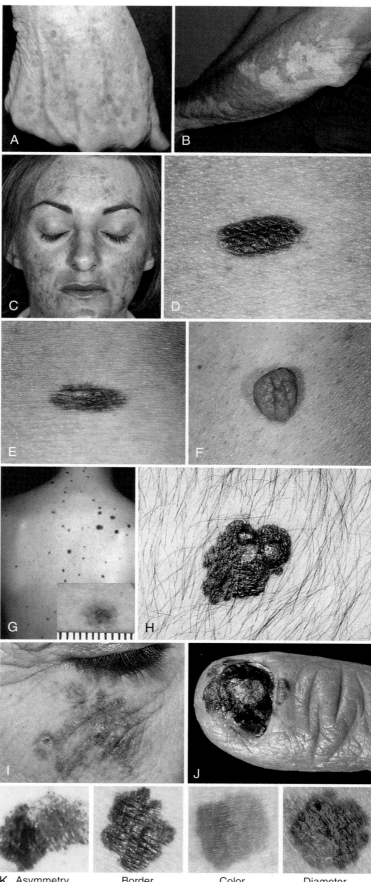

K Asymmetry   Border   Color   Diameter

(2) Dysplastic nevi in this syndrome can develop into malignant melanomas.
- Virtually all members in the family with this syndrome will develop melanomas.

(3) All patients require a yearly dermatologic examination.

E. Malignant melanoma
1. Epidemiology
   a. Malignant tumor of melanocytes
   b. Most rapidly increasing cancer worldwide
      - More common in whites than blacks
2. Leading cause of death due to skin cancer
3. Median age at diagnosis is 53 years.
4. Risk factors
   a. Exposure to excessive sunlight (UVA and UVB) at an early age
      - Single most important risk factor
   b. History of a family member with melanoma
   c. Use of tanning booths
   d. Dysplastic nevus syndrome
   e. History of melanoma in first- or second-degree relative
   f. Xeroderma pigmentosum (refer to Chapter 8)
5. Radial growth phase
   a. Initial phase of invasion
   b. Melanocytes proliferate
      (1) Laterally within the epidermis
      (2) Along the dermoepidermal junction
      (3) Within the papillary dermis
   c. *No* metastatic potential in this phase
6. Vertical growth phase
   a. Final phase of invasion
   b. Malignant cells penetrate the underlying reticular dermis.
   c. Potential for metastasis
7. Types of malignant melanoma
   a. Superficial spreading melanoma (Fig. 24-5H)
      (1) Most common type (70% of cases)
      (2) Develops on lower extremities, arms, and upper back
   b. Lentigo maligna melanoma (4–10% of cases)
      (1) Common in the elderly population
      (2) Extension of lentigo maligna (intraepidermal lesion) into the dermis
      (3) Occurs on parts of the face most exposed to the sun (Fig. 24-5I)
      (4) *Least* likely to have a vertical phase
   c. Nodular melanoma (15–30% of cases)
      (1) *No* radial growth phase
      (2) Can be found in any sun-exposed area
         - Most often the trunk
      (3) No radial phase only vertical phase
      (4) Poor prognosis
   d. Acral lentiginous melanoma (2–8% of cases)
      (1) *Not* related to sun exposure
      (2) Located on the palm, sole, or beneath the nail (Fig. 24-5J)
         - Often confused with a subungual hematoma
      (3) Most often occurs in Asians and blacks
      (4) Poor prognosis
8. Depth of invasion best determines biologic behavior.
9. ABCD criteria for malignancy (Fig. 24-5K)
   a. Asymmetry of shape
   b. Border irregularity
   c. Color variation
   d. Diameter > 6 mm
10. Prevention
   a. Sunscreen > 15 SPF (controversial)
      - Prevention for UVA and UVB light
   b. Protective clothing

Melanoma: leading cause of death due to skin cancer

Melanoma: most rapidly increasing cancer worldwide

Malignant melanoma: exposure to excessive sunlight at early age most significant risk factor

Radial growth phase: initial phase of invasion; spread laterally in papillary dermis; no metastatic potential

Vertical growth phase: final phase of invasion; penetrate reticular dermis; metastatic potential

ABCD signs of melanoma: *a*symmetry; *b*orders irregular; *c*olor changes; *d*iameter increased

Superficial spreading melanoma: most common type of malignant melanoma

Lentigo maligna melanoma: elderly; occurs on face; least likely to have vertical phase

Nodular melanoma: no radial phase only vertical phase

Acral lentiginous melanoma: not UV related; palms/soles; Asians and blacks

Prognosis in malignant melanoma: depth of invasion most important

Melanoma prevention: sunscreen > 15 SPF

11. Treatment
    a. Excision of entire lesion and surrounding normal tissue
       • Sentinel lymph node biopsy to determine stage
    b. More extensive disease
       • Immunotherapy; irradiation

VII. Benign Epithelial Tumors

A. Seborrheic keratosis

1. Epidemiology
   a. Most common benign tumor in older people
   b. Occurs in individuals > 50 years of age
2. Benign pigmented epidermal tumor (Fig. 24-6A)
   a. Coin-like, macular to raised verrucoid lesion with "stuck-on" appearance
   b. Extremities and shoulders most common sites
   c. Occur commonly on the face in elderly patients
3. Leser-Trélat sign (refer to Chapter 8)
   a. Rapid increase in number of keratoses
   b. Phenotypic marker for stomach adenocarcinoma
4. Treatment
   a. Cryotherapy
   b. Curettage
   c. Shave biopsy/excision

B. Acanthosis nigricans (AN)

1. Velvety, pigmented skin lesion
2. Commonly located in the axilla (Fig. 24-6B)
   a. Other sites—neck, axilla, groin, under breasts
3. Pathogenesis
   • Excess insulin noted in many cases
4. Associations
   a. Metabolic syndrome (refer to Chapter 22)
      • Obesity association important because of insulin resistance (down-regulation of insulin receptors)
   b. Insulin receptor deficiency
   c. Polycystic ovary syndrome (POS; refer to Chapter 21)
   d. Phenotypic marker for gastric cancer (refer to Chapters 8 and 17)
   e. Multiple endocrine neoplasia syndrome IIb
5. Treatment
   a. Treating underlying condition causes some regression
   b. Topical tretinoin

C. Keratoacanthoma (KA)

1. Male predominance
2. Rapidly growing, benign crateriform tumor with a central keratin plug (Fig. 24-6C)
   a. Grows within 4 to 6 weeks
   b. Develops in sun-exposed areas
   c. Mimics a well-differentiated squamous cell carcinoma
3. Regresses spontaneously with scarring usually within 6 months
4. Excision is recommended.

D. Benign epidermal cysts

1. Epidermal inclusion cysts (follicular cyst)
   a. Derived from the epidermis of the hair follicle (Fig. 24-6D)
   b. Locations
      • Face, base of ears, and trunk
   c. Cyst wall composed of normal epidermis that produces keratin
      • Keratin intermixed with lipid-rich debris
   d. Spontaneous inflammation and rupture may occur.
   e. Treatment
      • None required; surgical excision if necessary
2. Pilar cyst (wen)
   a. Derived from hair root sheaths
   b. Located on the scalp and face (Fig. 24-6E)
   c. Cyst wall lacks stratum granulosum.
      • Keratin has a laminated appearance.

Seborrheic keratosis: most common benign tumor in older people

Leser-Trélat sign: phenotypic marker for stomach adenocarcinoma

AN: velvety pigmented lesion; common in axilla

AN associations: metabolic syndrome; insulin receptor deficiency; POS; stomach cancer

KA: benign tumor that histologically mimics squamous cancer

KA: appears within 4–6 weeks; disappears within 6 months

Epidermal inclusion cyst: derives from epidermis of hair follicle

Locations: face, base of ears, trunk

Pilar cyst: derives from hair root sheaths

Pilar cyst: located on scalp and face

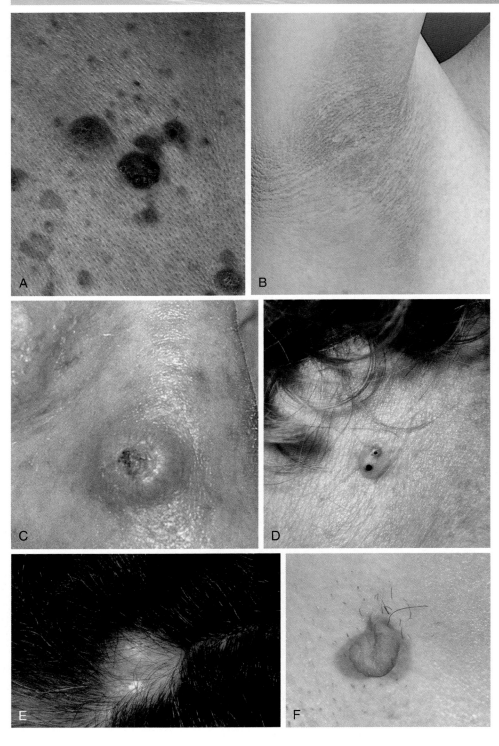

24-6: **A,** Seborrheic keratosis. Note the numerous raised, pigmented lesions with a verrucoid surface. These lesions appeared suddenly (Leser-Trélat sign) in this patient indicating a possible underlying gastric adenocarcinoma. In most cases, they are a common lesion in the elderly population where they frequently occur on the face and axilla. **B,** Acanthosis nigricans. Note the pigmented verrucoid lesion in the axilla. Like the Leser-Trélat sign, these lesions may be associated with an underlying gastric adenocarcinoma or other disorders. **C,** Keratoacanthoma. Note the crateriform tumor with a central keratin plug. This looks very similar to a basal cell carcinoma; however, it appears rapidly and spontaneously resolves, unlike a basal cell carcinoma. A biopsy settles the issue. **D,** Epidermoid cyst. Note the dome-shaped lesion near the hairline on the neck. It has two openings on the surface. **E,** Pilar cyst. Note the dome-shaped swelling on the scalp. **F,** Fibroepithelial tag. Note the flesh-colored pedunculated lesion attached to the body by a narrow stalk. These are common lesions in the elderly. (*A from Kumar V, Cotran RS, Robbins SL: Robbins Basic Pathology, 7th ed. Philadelphia, Saunders, 2003, p 799, Fig. 22-13A; **B** and **C** from Lookingbill D, Marks J: Principles of Dermatology, 3rd ed. Philadelphia, WB Saunders, 2000, pp 350 and 83, Figs. 25-5 and 6-12, respectively; **D** courtesy of R.A. Marsden, MD, St. George's Hospital, London; **E** courtesy of A. du Vivier, MD, King's College Hospital, London; **F** from Habif T: Clinical Dermatology, 4th ed. St. Louis, Mosby, 2004.)*

    d. Spontaneous inflammation and rupture may occur.
    e. Treatment
       • Usually none required; surgical excision if necessary
E. Fibroepithelial polyp (tag)
    1. Flesh-colored soft tag of skin attached to the body by a narrow stalk (Fig. 24-6F)
    2. Common finding in the elderly
    3. Locations
       • Neck, upper chest, upper back
    4. Treatment
       • None required; excise if necessary

Fibroepithelial tag: flesh-colored tag of skin with a stalk; common in elderly

VIII. Premalignant and Malignant Epithelial Tumors
A. Actinic (solar) keratosis (refer to Chapter 8)

Actinic (solar) keratosis: squamous dysplasia; precursor for squamous cancer

1. Associated with prolonged ultraviolet light exposure
2. Precursor (squamous dysplasia) of squamous cell carcinoma
   • Squamous cancer occurs in 2% to 5% of cases.
3. Hyperkeratotic, pearly gray-white appearance

Actinic (solar) keratosis: lesions recur after being scraped off.

   a. Occurs on face, back of neck, dorsum of hands/forearms (Fig. 24-7A)
   b. Commonly recurs when scraped off
4. Treatment
   a. Protection of skin with sunscreen
   b. Topical therapy—5-fluorouracil
   c. Cryotherapy

B. Basal cell carcinoma (BCC)

BCC: most common malignant skin tumor

1. Caused by chronic exposure to ultraviolet light
2. Raised papule or nodule with a central crater (Fig. 24-7B)
   • Sides of the crater are surfaced by telangiectatic vessels.
3. Occurs in sun-exposed areas

BCC: invade but do not metastasize

   a. Inner canthus of the eye, upper lip
   b. Very general rule of thumb is that BCCs favor upper lip and higher.
4. Locally aggressive, infiltrating cancer that does *not* metastasize
   a. Tumor is stromal dependent, hence precluding metastasis.
   b. Arises from the basal cell layer of the epidermis
   c. Multifocal in origin

BCC: arise from basal cell layer

     • This makes it difficult to get free margins after surgery
   d. Cords of basophilic-staining basal cells infiltrate the underlying dermis (Fig. 24-7C).
5. Diagnosis
   • Punch biopsy or shave biopsy
6. Treatment
   a. Varies with location and size of the cancer

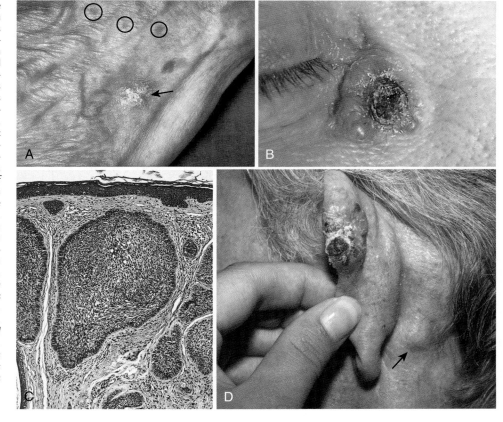

24-7: A, Actinic (solar) keratosis. Note the pearly gray-white hyperkeratotic lesion *(arrow)* on the hand. The other lesions *(circles)* are good examples of solar lentigo. Both of these lesions are common in the elderly population and are located in sun-exposed areas. **B,** Basal cell carcinoma. Note the ulcerated nodular mass on the inner aspect of the nose. This is a particularly common site for this cancer that invades but does *not* metastasize. **C,** Basal cell carcinoma. This microscopic section shows multifocal nests of basophilic staining cells with peripheral palisading. This section does not show a connection with the basal cell layer of skin; however, these tumors arise from multifocal locations and extend into the dermis. **D,** Squamous cell carcinoma. Note the nodular, hyperkeratotic lesion occurring on the ear. This is a common site for this cancer in the elderly population. *Arrow* shows metastasis to a lymph node. (**A** courtesy of R.A. Marsden, MD, St. George's Hospital, London; **B** from Savin JA, Hunter JAA, Hepburn NC: Diagnosis in Color: Skin Signs in Clinical Medicine. London, Mosby-Wolfe, 1997, p 104, Fig. 4-27; **C** from Rosai J, Ackerman LV: Surgical Pathology, 9th ed. St. Louis, Mosby, 2004, p 137, Fig. 4-60; **D** from Kumar V, Abbas AK, Fausto N, Mitchell RN: Robbins Basic Pathology, 8th ed. Philadelphia, Saunders Elsevier, 2007, p 851, Fig. 22-17.)

b. Options include topical 5-fluorouracil, cryotherapy, curettage and electrodesiccation, surgical excision, radiation (usually in elderly).

C. Squamous cell carcinoma (SCC)

1. Risk factors
   a. Excessive exposure to ultraviolet light (most common)
   b. Actinic (solar) keratosis
   c. Arsenic exposure
   d. Scar tissue in a third-degree burn
   e. Orifice of chronically draining sinus tract
   f. Immunosuppressive therapy
2. Scaly to nodular lesions
   a. Nodules are often ulcerated.
   b. Majority occur in sun-exposed areas of the body.
      (1) Examples—ears (Fig. 24-7D), lower lip (see Fig. 17-7), dorsum of the hands
      (2) Very general rule of thumb is that SCCs favor lower lip.
   c. Usually well differentiated
      • Minimal risk for metastasis
3. Treatment
   a. Varies with location and size of the cancer
   b. Options include topical 5-fluorouracil, cryotherapy, curettage and electrodesiccation, surgical excision, radiation (usually in elderly).

IX. Selected Skin Disorders

A. Ichthyosis vulgaris

1. Autosomal dominant
   • Most common inherited skin disorder
2. Defect in keratinization
   a. Causes increased thickness of the stratum corneum
   b. Absent stratum granulosum
3. Hyperkeratotic, dry skin
   • Involves palms, soles, and extensor areas

B. Xerosis

1. Most common cause of dry skin and pruritus in the elderly
   • Due to a decrease in skin lipids
2. Other age-related changes in elderly
   a. Decreased number of hair follicles, sweat glands
   b. Decrease in thickness of epidermis
   c. Decreased dermal collagen/elastic tissue
   d. Decreased subcutaneous fat
      • Example—over dorsum of hands
   e. Increased cross-linking of collagen and elastic tissue

C. Polymorphous light eruption (PLE)

1. Most common photodermatitis
2. Affects ~10% of population
3. Positive family history
   • Very common in Native Americans
4. More common in women than men
5. More common in blacks than whites
6. Rash has a rapid onset after sun exposure (Fig. 24-8A).
   a. Erythematous macules, papules, plaques, or vesicles/bullae
   b. Rash is pruritic and sometimes painful.
   c. *Not* related to drugs
7. Treatment
   a. Broad-spectrum high-potency sunscreen against UVA and UVB
      • Often vitamin E is added to the mixture or given as oral supplement.
   b. Topical corticosteroids

D. Eczema

1. Group of inflammatory dermatoses
   • Characterized by pruritus
2. Acute eczema
   • Weeping, erythematous rash with vesicles
3. Chronic eczema
   • Dry, thickened skin (hyperkeratosis) caused by continual scratching

---

SCC: excessive exposure to UV light; actinic keratosis; scar tissue

SCC: most common cancer complicating immunosuppressive therapy

SCCs favor lower lip; BCCs favor upper lip

Ichthyosis vulgaris: most common inherited skin disorder; ↑ stratum corneum

Xerosis: most common cause of dried skin and pruritus in elderly

Skin changes elderly: ↓ hair follicles, sweat glands, skin thickness

Skin changes in elderly: ↓ dermal collagen/elastic tissue but ↑ cross-linking

PLE: most common photodermatitis

PLE: common in Native Americans

PLE: rash occurs abruptly after sun exposure

PLE: rash begins with sun exposure

Eczema: group of inflammatory dermatoses

Eczema: acute weep; chronic dry

24-8: A, Polymorphous light eruption. Note the erythematous papules and vesicles on the sun-exposed skin. **B,** Atopic dermatitis. Note the erythematous, scaling rash on the cheeks and chin of this infant. Also note the scaling rash on the scalp, which is cradle cap (seborrheic dermatitis). **C,** Atopic dermatitis. Note the erythematous, scaling rash with thickening of the skin (lichenification) from constant scratching in the elbow flexure. **D,** Poison ivy. Note the acute eczematous rash with vesicle formation. **E,** Schematic of a suprabasal vesicle (e.g., pemphigus vulgaris). See text for discussion. **F,** Schematic of a subepidermal vesicle (e.g., bullous pemphigoid). See text for discussion. **G,** Bullous pemphigoid. Note the tense bullae. **H,** Lichen planus. Note the flat-topped violaceous papules. **I,** Psoriasis: The elbow shows a flat, salmon-colored plaque covered by white to silver-colored scales. **J,** Nail pitting in psoriasis. The nails show pitting and separation of the distal nail plate (onycholysis). **K,** Pityriasis rosea. Note the erythematous, scaly papules and plaques following the lines of cleavage of the skin ("Christmas tree" distribution). The initial herald patch was present in the left supraclavicular region. **L,** Erythema multiforme. The palms show the classic target lesions with three zones of color. **M,** Erythema nodosum. Note the raised, erythematous nodular lesions on the anterior shins. This is commonly associated with coccidioidomycosis. **N,** Granuloma annulare. Note the erythematous, annular plaque on the dorsum of the hands. There is an increased association of this skin lesion with diabetes mellitus. **O,** Urticaria. One of the manifestations of urticaria is dermatographism. In this case, there is swelling with the word HIVE. **P,** Cherry angiomas. Note the red, papular lesions on the chest. These are extremely common in the elderly population. **Q,** Acne rosacea. Note the pustules and papules superimposed on a background of erythema and telangiectasias (dilated vessels). There is also enlargement of the nose due to sebaceous gland hyperplasia (rhinophyma). **R,** Pyoderma gangrenosum. Note the large ulcer with the prominent red border. (***A*** and ***D*** courtesy of The Honickman Collection of Medical Images in memory of Elaine Garfinkel and The Jefferson Clinical Images Collection [through the generosity of JMB, AKR, LKB and DA]; ***B*** from Eichenfield L, Frieden I, Esterly N: Textbook of Neonatal Dermatology, Philadelphia, Saunders, 2001, p 242; ***C*** and ***M*** from Savin JA, Hunter JAA, Hepburn NC: Diagnosis in Color: Skin Signs in Clinical Medicine, London, Mosby-Wolfe, 1997, pp 9 and 8, Figs. 1.16 and 1.14, respectively; ***E*** and ***F*** from Goljan EF: Star Series: Pathology. Philadelphia, WB Saunders, 1998, Fig 21-2BC; ***G*** and ***L*** from Callen JP, Paller AS, Greer KE, Swinyer LJ: Color Atlas of Dermatology, 2nd ed. Philadelphia, W.B. Saunders, 2000; ***H, O,*** and ***Q*** from Lookingbill D, Marks J: Principles of Dermatology, 3rd ed. Philadelphia, WB Saunders, 2000, pp 201, 264, and 213, Figs. 12-7A, 17-2, and 13-4A, respectively; ***I*** from Forbes C, Jackson W: Color Atlas and Text of Clinical Medicine, 2nd ed. St. Louis, Mosby, 2003, p 87, Fig. 2-15; ***J, K, N,*** and ***R*** from Goldstein BG: Practical Dermatology, 2nd ed. St. Louis, Mosby, 1997, pp 180, 177, 312, and 321, Figs. 14-16, 14-13, 23-4, and 23-15, respectively; ***P*** from Habif T: Clinical Dermatology, 4th ed. St. Louis, Mosby, 2004.)

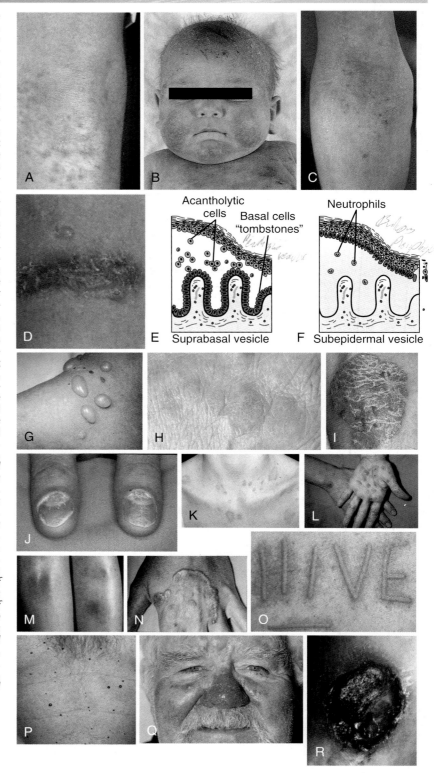

Atopic dermatitis:
type I IgE-mediated
hypersensitivity

4. Atopic dermatitis
   a. Type I IgE-mediated hypersensitivity reaction
   b. Dermatitis in children
      • Dry skin and eczema on cheeks and extensor and flexural surfaces (Fig. 24-8B and C)
   c. Dermatitis in adults
      • Dry skin and eczema on hands, eyelids, elbows, and knees
5. Contact dermatitis

  a. Allergic contact dermatitis
  (1) Type IV hypersensitivity reaction
  (2) Examples—poison ivy (Fig. 24-8D), nickel in jewelry
  b. Irritant contact dermatitis
  • Skin reaction to an irritant (e.g., laundry detergent)
  c. Contact photodermatitis
  (1) Ultraviolet light reacts with drugs that have a photosensitizing effect.
  (2) Example—tetracycline
6. General treatment
  a. Avoid drugs, irritants that produce a rash
  b. Apply moistening agents (emollients) to skin
  c. Topical corticosteroids
  (1) Only low-potency hydrocortisone for the face
  (2) Higher potency corticosteroids for other sites
    (a) High-potency—clobetasol propionate, fluocinonide
    (b) Medium-potency—clobetasone butyrate; triamcinolone

E. Autoimmune skin disorders
1. Chronic cutaneous lupus erythematosus (refer to Chapter 3)
  a. Associated with atrophy of the epidermis
  b. DNA–anti-DNA immunocomplex deposition in the basement membrane
  (1) Degeneration of basal cells and hair shafts (alopecia)
  (2) Positive immunofluorescent (IF) band test
    • IF shows immunocomplexes deposited along the basement membrane.
  c. Clinical findings
  (1) Erythematous maculopapular eruption
    • Usually over malar eminences and bridge of nose ("butterfly" rash) (see Fig. 3-2A)
  (2) Skin lesions are exacerbated by UV light.
  d. Antimalarials remain cornerstone of treatment.
2. Pemphigus vulgaris (PV)
  a. IgG antibodies against intercellular attachment sites (desmosomes) between keratinocytes
    • Type II hypersensitivity reaction
  b. Vesicles and bullae develop on skin and oral mucosa.
  c. Intraepithelial vesicles are located *above* the basal layer (suprabasal; Fig. 24-8E).
  (1) Basal cells resemble a row of tombstones.
  (2) Acantholysis of keratinocytes in the vesicle fluid
  (3) Positive Nikolsky sign
    • Outer epidermis separates from basal layer with minimal pressure
  d. Treatment
    • Corticosteroids and other immunosuppressive agents (e.g., methotrexate, azathioprine)
3. Bullous pemphigoid
  a. IgG antibodies against the basement membrane
    • Type II hypersensitivity reaction
  b. Vesicles are subepidermal (Fig. 24-8F).
  (1) Develop on the skin and oral mucosa (Fig. 24-8G)
  (2) *No* acantholytic cells in vesicle fluid
  (3) Negative Nikolsky sign
  c. Disease usually subsides after months or years.
  d. May requires systemic corticosteroid in resistant cases
4. Dermatitis herpetiformis (DH; see Fig. 17-19)
  a. IgA–anti-IgA complexes deposit at the tips of the dermal papillae.
    • Produces subepidermal vesicles with neutrophils
  b. Strongly correlated with celiac disease
    • Increase in antireticulin and endomysial antibodies
  c. Treatment
  (1) Gluten-free diet
  (2) Dapsone or sulfapyridine

F. Lichen planus (LP)
1. Intensely pruritic, scaly, violaceous, flat-topped papules (Fig. 24-8H)
  a. Fine white reticular pattern on the surface (called Wickham's striae)

Contact dermatitis: type IV hypersensitivity; poison ivy, nickel in earrings

Tetracycline: drug with photosensitizing effect

Lupus skin involvement: immunocomplexes along basement membrane

PV: IgG antibodies against desmosomes between keratinocytes

PV: intraepithelial vesicles; + Nikolsky sign; basal cells resemble tombstones

Bullous pemphigoid: IgG antibodies against basement membrane

Bullous pemphigoid: subepidermal vesicles; – Nikolsky sign

PV and bullous pemphigoid: type II hypersensitivity reactions

DH: associated with celiac disease; subepidermal vesicles with neutrophils

LP: pruritic; violaceous, flat-topped papules

LP: oral mucosa commonly involved; Wickham's striae

LP: associated with hepatitis C

       b. Commonly located on the wrists, ankles
       c. Nails are commonly dystrophic.
       d. Lesions develop in areas of scratching (Koebner's phenomenon)
    2. Women more commonly affected than men
    3. Oral mucosa is often involved (50% of cases).
       a. Produces a fine, white, net-like lesion (Wickham's striae)
       b. Slight risk of developing squamous cell carcinoma
    4. Association with hepatitis C
    5. Treatment
       a. Topical high-potency corticosteroids
       b. Antihistamines (for pruritus)
       c. Systemic corticosteroids
       d. Retinoids
       e. Cyclosporine in resistant cases

G. Psoriasis

Psoriasis: strong HLA relationship

    1. Epidemiology
       a. Afflicts 1% to 3% of the world population
       b. Strong human leukocyte antigen (HLA) relationship
       c. Peak age at onset is bimodal.
         • Adolescents and 60 years of age
       d. No gender difference

Psoriasis: unregulated proliferation of keratinocytes

Psoriasis: commonly preceded by streptococcal pharyngitis

    2. Pathogenesis
       a. Unregulated proliferation (hyperplasia) of keratinocytes
         (1) Genetic factors involved (30% of cases)
         (2) Aggravating factors
           (a) Streptococcal pharyngitis
           (b) HIV
             • Sudden onset of psoriasis is highly suspicious for HIV
           (c) Drugs: lithium, β-blockers, NSAIDs
           (d) Scratching the skin (Koebner's phenomenon)
       b. Microcirculatory changes in superficial papillary dermis

Psoriasis: erythematous plaques with silver scales

Psoriasis: rash in areas of trauma (i.e., elbows); pitting of nails

    3. Well-demarcated, flat, elevated salmon-colored plaques (Fig. 24-8I)
       a. Covered by adherent white to silver-colored scales
         • Pinpoint areas of bleeding occur when scales are scraped off.
       b. Rash commonly develops in areas of trauma (elbows, lower back).
         • Called Koebner's phenomenon
    4. Pitting of the nails (Fig. 24-8J)
    5. Microscopic findings
       a. Hyperkeratosis and parakeratosis
       b. Elongation of rete pegs
         • Downward extensions of basal layer
       c. Extension of the papillary dermis close to the surface epithelium
         • Blood vessels in dermis rupture when scales are picked off (Auspitz sign).

Psoriasis: Munro microabscesses in stratum corneum: Auspitz sign

       d. Neutrophil collections in the stratum corneum
         • Called Munro microabscesses
    6. Treatment modalities
       a. Topical high-potency corticosteroids
       b. Topical calcipotriene (vitamin D analogue)
       c. Ultraviolet light A plus psoralen applied to plaques
       d. Ultraviolet light B plus coal tar applied to plaques
       e. Retinoids
       f. Systemic treatment
         • Methotrexate, cyclosporine

H. Pityriasis rosea

Pityriasis rosea: herald patch (plaque) followed by rash in "Christmas tree" distribution

    1. Initially presents as a single, large, oval, scaly, rose-colored plaque on the trunk
       a. Called the "herald patch"
       b. Frequently misdiagnosed as tinea corporis ("ringworm")
    2. Days or weeks later, a papular eruption develops on the trunk (Fig. 24-8K).
       a. Rash follows the lines of cleavage ("Christmas tree" distribution).
       b. Lesions tend to be pruritic.
       c. Rash remits spontaneously in 2 to 10 weeks.
    3. Antihistamines control pruritus; UV light therapy hastens resolution.

I. Erythema multiforme (EM)

1. Immunologic reaction of skin
2. Triggered by:
   a. Infection
      - *Mycoplasma pneumoniae*, herpes simplex virus (HSV; primary agent if recurrent EM occurs)
   b. Drugs
      - Sulfonamides, penicillin, barbiturates, phenytoin
3. Vesicles and bullae have a "targetoid" appearance (Fig. 24-8L).
   - Located on the palms, soles, and extensor surfaces
4. Stevens-Johnson syndrome
   a. EM that involves the skin and mucous membranes
   b. Can be fatal
5. Treatment
   a. Treat with systemic corticosteroids
   b. Treat triggering infection
   c. Discontinue drug

J. Erythema nodosum (EN)

1. Inflammatory lesion of subcutaneous fat (panniculitis)
2. More common in women than men
3. Raised, erythematous, painful nodules
   - Usually located on the anterior portion of the shins (Fig. 24-8M)
4. Common associations
   a. Coccidioidomycosis, histoplasmosis
   b. Tuberculosis, leprosy
   c. Streptococcal pharyngitis
   d. *Yersinia* enterocolitis
   e. Sarcoidosis, ulcerative colitis
   f. Pregnancy, OCPs
5. Treatment
   a. Identify and treat precipitating causes.
   b. NSAIDs
   c. Systemic corticosteroids if severe

K. Granuloma annulare

1. Chronic inflammatory dermal disorder
   - Unknown etiology
2. Occurs in children and adults
   - Female predominance
3. Begin as erythematous papules
   - Papules evolve into annular plaques (Fig. 24-8N).
4. Occur on the dorsum of the hands and feet
   - Disseminated type may be associated with diabetes mellitus.
5. Spontaneously resolve within 2 years
   - Recurrence in 40% of cases
6. Treatment
   a. High-potency topical corticosteroids
   b. Intralesional injection of corticosteroids

L. Porphyria cutanea tarda (PCT)

1. Genetic or acquired disease involving porphyrin metabolism
2. Deficiency of uroporphyrinogen decarboxylase
   a. Urine is wine-red color on voiding.
   b. Uroporphyrin I is increased in urine.
3. Precipitating factors
   a. Hepatitis C (HCV)
   b. Excessive alcohol intake
   c. OCPs
   d. Iron
4. Clinical findings
   a. Photosensitive bullous skin lesions
      (1) Caused by porphyrin metabolites deposited in the skin
      (2) Patients avoid light.
   b. Hyperpigmentation, fragile skin, hypertrichosis

EM: triggered by infection (*Mycoplasma*, HSV), drugs

EM: rash has targetoid appearance; palmar involvement

EM: Stevens-Johnson syndrome involves skin and mucous membranes

EN: panniculitis involving anterior portion of shins

EN: systemic fungal infections, TB, leprosy, sarcoid, pregnancy, OCPs

Granuloma annulare: association with diabetes mellitus

PCT: deficiency uroporphyrinogen decarboxylase; association with HCV, alcohol abuse

Precipitating factors: HCV, alcohol abuse, OCPs, iron

5. Treatment
   a. Avoid alcohol, OCPs
   b. Phlebotomy (decrease iron)
   c. Chloroquine

M. Urticaria

Urticaria: mast cell release of histamine

1. Pruritic elevations of the skin
   a. Most often due to mast cell release of histamine
   b. Type I IgE-mediated reactions associated with certain exposure:
     (1) Certain foods (e.g., peanuts)
     (2) Insect bites (e.g., fire ant)
     (3) Drugs (e.g., penicillin, morphine, aspirin, laxative)
     (4) Emotional stress
     (5) Hepatitis B (part of serum sickness prodrome)
       • This is a type III hypersensitivity reaction.

Urticaria: may exhibit dermatographism

2. Dermatographism (Fig. 24-8O)
   • Urticaria develops in areas of mechanical pressure on skin.
3. Treatment
   a. Discontinue offending drug.
   b. Avoid aspirin and other NSAIDs.
   c. Antihistamines
   d. Tricyclic drugs (e.g., doxepin)
   e. Systemic steroids

N. Cherry angiomas

Cherry angiomas: bright red papules; invariably present in elderly

1. Tiny, bright red papules (Fig. 24-8P)
   • Turn brown with time
2. Invariably occur in all individuals > 30 years old.
3. No treatment is required.

O. Acne rosacea

Acne rosacea: causal relationship with mite (*Demodex folliculorum*)

1. Inflammatory reaction of the pilosebaceous units of facial skin
   • Causal relationship with a mite (*Demodex folliculorum*)
2. Pustules and flushing of the cheeks (Fig. 24-8Q)
   • Exacerbated by drinking alcohol, stress, eating spicy foods

Acne rosacea: pustules and flushing of cheeks; rhinophyma

3. Sebaceous gland hyperplasia (Fig. 24-8Q)
   • Produces enlargement of the nose (rhinophyma)
4. Treatment
   a. Topical metronidazole gel
   b. Systemic treatment
     (1) Isotretinoin
     (2) Tetracycline

P. Pyoderma gangrenosum

Pyoderma gangrenosum: ulcerative cutaneous disease associated with systemic disease

1. Epidemiology
   a. Ulcerative cutaneous condition often associated with systemic disease (>50%)
   b. Systemic disease associations

Pyoderma gangrenosum: ulcerative colitis/Crohn's disease; MPD; RA

     (1) Ulcerative colitis/Crohn's disease
     (2) Myeloproliferative disease (MPD); monoclonal gammopathy
     (3) Seronegative spondyloarthropathy
     (4) Rheumatoid arthritis (RA)
2. Pathogenesis
   a. Probable dysregulation of immune system
   b. Neutrophil dysfunction often present

Pyoderma gangrenosum: dysregulation of immune system

   c. Trauma may initiate the event (called pathergy).
3. Clinical findings
   a. Small red pustule/papule that ulcerates and enlarges (Fig. 24-8R)
     (1) Reminiscent of a brown recluse spider bite
     (2) Single or multiple ulcers
   b. Violaceous border overhangs ulcer crater.
4. Diagnosis
   a. Culture to rule out secondary infection
   b. Biopsy
5. Treatment
   a. Topical—high-potency corticosteroids
   b. Systemic—corticosteroids; tumor necrosis factor-α inhibitors, cyclosporine

X. Selected Skin Disorders in Newborns

A. Erythema toxicum
1. Self-limited benign eruption of unknown cause
   a. Occurs in 30% to 70% of full-term newborns (*not* premature newborns)
   b. Lasts 2 to 3 weeks
2. Erythematous papules, macules, and pustules (Fig. 24-9A)
3. Locations
   * All sites *except* palms and soles

B. Sebaceous hyperplasia
1. Profuse yellow-white papules
   a. Hyperplastic sebaceous glands
   b. Disappear in first weeks of life
2. Locations
   * Forehead, nose (Fig. 24-9B), upper lip, cheeks

C. Milia
1. Superficial epidermal inclusion cysts
   * Pearly white papules contain laminated keratin material.
2. Location in neonates
   * Face (Fig. 24-9C), gingiva, midline of palate and gingiva (called Epstein's pearls)
3. Exfoliate spontaneously or can be unroofed with fine needle

Margin notes:

Erythema toxicum: 30–70% newborns; self-limited

Sebaceous hyperplasia: yellow-white papules on face; self-limited

Milia: superficial epidermal inclusion cysts; pearly white papules

Milia: called Epstein's pearls when in mouth

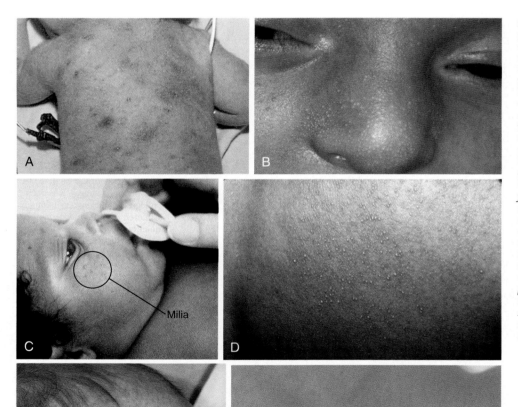

24-9: **A,** Erythema toxicum. Note the yellow-white papules and pustules with a surrounding erythematous flare over the chest and arms of this newborn. **B,** Sebaceous gland hyperplasia. Note the yellow papules on the nose of the newborn. **C,** Milia. Note the white papules on the face of the newborn. **D,** Miliaria crystallina. Note the clear vesicles on the skin of the newborn. **E,** Miliaria rubra. Note the erythematous maculopapular rash on the face of the newborn. **F,** Mongolian spot. Note the area of black discoloration above the crease of the buttocks in the newborn. (*A, B, and D from Kliegman RM, Jenson HB, Behrman RE, Stanton BF: Nelson's Textbook of Pediatrics, 18th ed. Philadelphia, Saunders Elsevier, 2007, pp 2662, 2661, 2725, Figs. 646-3, 646-1, 660-1, respectively; C from Seidel HM, Ball JW, Danis JE, Benedict GW: Mosby's Guide to Physical Examination, 6th ed. St. Louis, Mosby Elsevier, 2006, p 199, Fig. 8-25; E from Habif T: Clinical Dermatology, 4th ed. St. Louis, Mosby, 2004; F from Lemmi FO, Lemmi CAE: Physical Assessment Findings CD-ROM, Philadelphia, WB Saunders, 2000.*)

Miliaria crystallina:
pinpoint clear vesicles;
sweat in occluded sweat
glands

Miliaria rubra: prickly
heat; erythematous
papulovesicles

Both types of miliaria
respond to cooling

Mongolian spot: bluish
black to gray spot; dark-
skinned babies

Mongolian spot:
disappears in preschool
years

Anagen phase: new
hair shaft; hair length
determined

Telogen phase: resting
phase; loss of hair

Estrogen: causes
synchronous hair growth;
risk for massive hair loss

Massive hair loss:
postpartum; OCPs; stress;
radiation/chemotherapy

Alopecia areata: hairs
in areas of hair loss
have appearance of
exclamation marks

D. Miliaria
 1. Miliaria crystallina
    a. Pinpoint clear vesicles on skin
    b. Retention of sweat in occluded eccrine sweat glands
    c. May suddenly erupt in profusion over large areas of the body (Fig. 24-9D)
    d. Often associated in warm, humid conditions or fever
    e. Responds dramatically to cooling the patient and removal of excess clothing
 2. Miliaria rubra ("prickly heat")
    a. Retention of sweat in occluded eccrine glands
    b. Erythematous, minute papulovesicles that impart a prickly sensation (Fig. 24-9E)
    c. Like miliaria crystallina, it responds dramatically to cooling
E. Mongolian spot
 1. Bluish black to slate gray spots
 2. Usually occur in dark-skinned babies
 3. Locations
    a. Buttocks (Fig. 24-9F), back, shoulders, legs
 4. Disappears in the preschool years
XI. Selected Hair and Nail Disorders
A. Phases of hair growth in succession
 1. Anagen phase
    a. Development of new shaft of hair comes from hair bulb.
    b. Hair length is determined in this stage.
    c. Growth stops at end of this phase.
 2. Telogen phase
    a. Resting phase
    b. Matrix portion shrivels and hair within the follicle is shed.
    c. New matrix is formed at the bottom of the follicle.
    d. Cycle repeats itself.
 3. Length of each phase varies in the body.
    • Scalp hair—anagen phase 6 years, telogen phase 4 months
 4. Hair growth is usually asynchronous; for scalp hair:
    a. At any one time, ~80% is in anagen phase; ~10% to 20% is in telogen phase.
    b. Only a small percentage of hair is lost at any point in time.
 5. Estrogen effect on hair growth
    a. Causes synchronous hair growth
    b. All the hairs enter the resting phase at once.
B. Massive hair loss
 1. Post partum
    • Most common cause
 2. Oral contraceptive pills
 3. Stress
 4. Radiation/chemotherapy
    • Inhibition of anagen phase when cells in the hair bulb are dividing
C. Alopecia areata
 1. Affects both sexes equally
 2. Onset most commonly in young adults
 3. Cause is not known.
    a. May have an autoimmune association in some cases
       • Hashimoto's thyroiditis, pernicious anemia
    b. Family history in 20% to 25% of patients
 4. Clinical findings
    a. Well-circumscribed, round to oval patches of hair loss
       • Hair loss may occur on scalp, beard, eyebrows, eyelashes.
    b. Hairs have the appearance of exclamation marks (Fig. 24-10A).
    c. Hair loss occurs over a period of weeks.
    d. Regrowth of hair occurs over several months.
    e. May recur in up to one third of cases
 5. Treatment
    a. Topical—clobetasol
    b. Intralesional triamcinolone
    c. Systemic corticosteroids
    d. Psoralen + UVA, immunotherapy

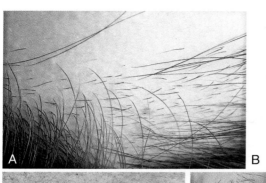

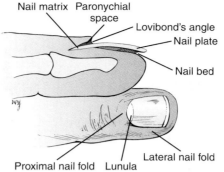

Nail matrix   Paronychial space

Lovibond's angle

Nail plate

Nail bed

Proximal nail fold   Lunula

Lateral nail fold

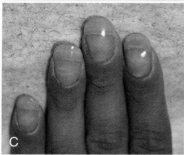

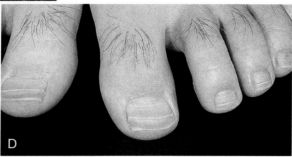

24-10: A, Alopecia areata. Note the area of baldness and the short hairs that have the appearance of exclamation marks. **B,** Nail anatomy. See text for discussion. **C,** Mees bands. Note the transverse white lines in the nail plate that extend proximally until they are pared off. **D,** Beau's lines. Note the transverse grooves or depressions that are oriented parallel to the lunula. (**A** from Savin JA, Hunter JAA, Hepburn NC: Diagnosis in Color: Skin Signs in Clinical Medicine. London, Mosby-Wolfe, 1997, p 96, Fig. 4.5; **B** and **C** from Swartz MH: Textbook of Physical Diagnosis, 5th ed. Philadelphia, Saunders Elsevier, 2006, pp 140 and 146, Figs. 8-3 and 8-7, respectively; **D** from Callen JP, Paller AS, Greer KE, Swinyer LJ: Color Atlas of Dermatology, 2nd ed. Philadelphia, WB Saunders, 2000.)

D. Nail disorders
1. Nail anatomy (Fig. 24-10B)
   a. Lunula
      (1) White half-moon–shaped area proximal to the cuticle
      (2) Underlying nail bed is partially keratinized, which produces the white color.
   b. Nail plate
      • Attached to the nail bed *except* distally where it separates from the hyponychium
   c. Nail matrix
      (1) Underneath the cuticle (eponychium)
      (2) Germinative zone where the nail plate originates
2. Nail disorders
   a. Psoriasis (see Fig. 24-8J)
      • Greater than 80% have nail pitting.
   b. Iron deficiency
      • Koilonychia (spoon nails; see Fig. 11-10)
   c. Subacute infective endocarditis and trichinosis
      • Splinter hemorrhages in nails (see Fig. 10-21)
   d. Mees lines
      (1) Sign of arsenic poisoning and systemic illness of any kind
      (2) Transverse white lines in the nail plate (Fig. 24-10C)
         • Extend proximally until they are pared off
   e. Beau's lines
      (1) Transverse grooves or depressions parallel to lunula (Fig. 24-10D)
      (2) Caused by conditions that cause the nail to grow slowly
         • Examples—infections, nutritional disorders, hypothyroidism
   f. Subungual hematoma
      (1) Blood clot under the nail plate due to trauma
      (2) Often confused with acral lentiginous melanoma

Nail anatomy: lunula, nail plate, nail matrix

Psoriasis: nail pitting

Iron deficiency: koilonychia (spoon nails)

Splinter hemorrhages: subacute infective endocarditis; trichinosis

Mees lines: transverse white lines; arsenic poisoning; systemic illness

Beau's lines: transverse grooves parallel to lunula; infections

Subungual hematoma: blood clot under nail plate; confused with acral lentiginous melanoma

I.   **Cerebral Edema, Pseundotumor Cerebri, Herniations, Hydrocephalus**
A. **Cerebral edema**
1. Subdivided into intracellular and extracellular types (Fig. 25-1)
2. Intracellular edema
a. Water moves into cells.
b. Causes
(1) Dysfunctional Na^+/K^+-ATPase pump (e.g., global hypoxia)
(2) Hyponatremia causing osmotic shift (e.g., syndrome of inappropriate antidiuretic hormone, SIADH)
3. Extracellular edema
a. Due to increased vessel permeability (vasogenic)
b. Causes
(1) Acute inflammation (e.g., meningitis, encephalitis)
(2) Metastasis, trauma, lead poisoning

A patient with **head trauma** is purposely hyperventilated to produce respiratory alkalosis, which causes cerebral vessel constriction. This decreases the risk of increased vessel permeability and cerebral edema. Respiratory acidosis and hypoxemia cause vasodilation of cerebral vessels, which increases cerebral vessel permeability, resulting in cerebral edema. Both conditions cause increased activity of the K^+ channels in smooth muscle cells → produces hyperpolarization → relaxes smooth muscle cells ($\downarrow$ intracellular calcium) producing vasodilation with increased vessel permeability.

4. Produces signs of increased intracranial pressure (intracranial hypertension)
a. Papilledema
• Swelling of the optic disk (Fig. 25-2)
b. Headache, projectile vomiting *without* nausea
c. Sinus bradycardia, hypertension
d. Potential for herniation (see below)
B. **Pseudotumor cerebri**
• Benign intracranial hypertension
1. Epidemiology
a. Increased intracranial pressure
• Papilledema is present
b. Absence of tumor and obstruction to cerebrospinal fluid (CSF) flow
c. *No* mental status alterations as one would see with cerebral edema
d. *No* focal neurologic signs
e. Most commonly seen in obese women of childbearing age
f. Other risk factors
(1) All-trans-retinoic acid used in treating acute promyelocytic leukemia (refer to Chapter 12)
(2) Hypothyroidism; Cushing disease
(3) Isotretinoin in treating acne; tamoxifen

Cerebral edema: intracellular and extracellular types

Intracellular: $\downarrow$ serum Na^+ (SIADH); dysfunctional Na^+/K^+-ATPase pump (global hypoxia)

Extracellular: $\uparrow$ vessel permeability; meningitis, metastasis

Respiratory acidosis, hypoxemia: $\uparrow$ cerebral vessel permeability; enhance cerebral edema

Papilledema: sign of cerebral edema

Intracranial hypertension: papilledema, bradycardia, projectile vomiting, hypertension

Pseudotumor cerebri: $\uparrow$ intracranial pressure *without* evidence of tumor or obstruction

Pseudotumor cerebri: most common in young obese women

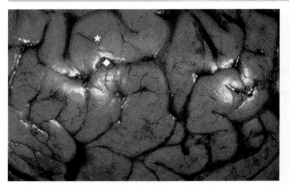

25-1: Cerebral edema. Note the widening and flattening of the gyri and the narrowing of the sulci. *(From Klatt E: Robbins and Cotran's Atlas of Pathology. Philadelphia, WB Saunders, 2006, p 449, Fig. 19-11.)*

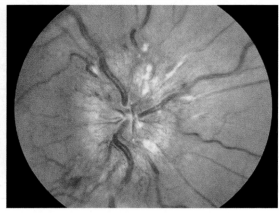

25-2: Optic disk with papilledema showing loss of the disk margin and hard exudates (white streaks). *(From Perkin GD: Mosby's Color Atlas and Text of Neurology. St. Louis, Mosby, 2002, p 160, Fig. 9-4.)*

2. Pathogenesis
   a. Decreased CSF resorption in arachnoid granulations
   b. Eventual equilibration occurs with inflow and outflow.
3. Clinical findings
   a. Headache
   b. Rhythmic sound heard in one or both ears
   c. Diplopia; blurry vision
4. Diagnosis
   a. MRI shows flattening of the posterior globe (100% positive predictive value)
   b. Increased CSF pressure
     • Usually >300 mm H_2O (normal, 70–180 mm H_2O)
   c. Decreased CSF protein
5. Treatment
   a. Medical
     • Carbonic anhydrase inhibitor or systemic corticosteroids if visual disturbances (lowers CSF pressure)
   b. Surgery
     (1) Lumboperitoneal shunt
     (2) Optic nerve sheath fenestration (regresses papilledema in the eye)

C. Cerebral herniation
1. Pathogenesis
   a. Complication of increased intracranial pressure
   b. Portions of the brain become displaced (Fig. 25-3).
     (1) Openings of dural partitions
     (2) Openings of the skull
2. Subfalcine herniation
   a. Cingulate gyrus herniates under the falx cerebri.
   b. Causes compression of the anterior cerebral artery (ACA)
3. Uncal herniation
   a. Medial portion of temporal lobe herniates through the tentorium cerebelli.
   b. Complications
     (1) Compression of the midbrain
       • Produces Duret's hemorrhages
     (2) Compression of oculomotor nerve
       (a) Eye is deviated down and out.
       (b) Pupil is mydriatic (dilated).
         • Compression of parasympathetic postganglionic fibers
     (3) Compression of posterior cerebral artery (PCA)
       • Causes hemorrhagic infarction of occipital lobe
4. Tonsillar herniation
   a. Cerebellar tonsils herniate into the foramen magnum.
   b. Causes "coning" of the cerebellar tonsils (Fig. 25-4)
   c. Produces cardiorespiratory arrest

Margin notes:

Pseudotumor cerebri: ↓ CSF resorption in arachnoid granulations

Pseudotumor cerebri: headache, blurry vision, diplopia

Cerebral herniation: complication of intracranial hypertension

Subfalcine herniation: compression of ACA

Uncal herniation: compression CN III, PCA, parasympathetic fibers

Uncal herniation: eye deviated down and out; mydriasis

Tonsillar herniation: coning of cerebellar tonsils; cardiorespiratory arrest

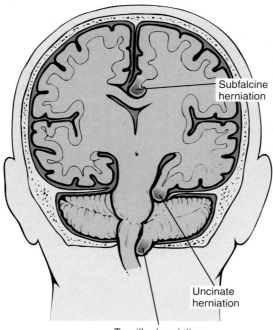

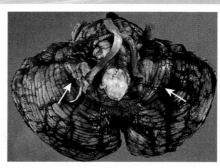

25-4: Cerebellar coning. Note the notching in the cerebellar tonsils (*arrows*) due to downward displacement of the cerebellar tonsils through the foramen magnum. (*From Grieg JD: Color Atlas of Surgical Diagnosis. London, Mosby-Wolfe, 1996, p 312, Fig. 39-2.*)

Subfalcine herniation

Uncinate herniation

Tonsillar herniation

25-3: Brain herniations. See text for discussion. (*Adapted from Fishman RA: Brain edema. N Engl J Med 1975; 293: 706 in Kumar V, Abbas AK, Fausto N, Mitchell RN: Robbins Basic Pathology, 8th ed. Philadelphia, Saunders Elsevier, 2007, p 862, Fig. 23-4.*)

D. Hydrocephalus

Hydrocephalus: enlargement of ventricles

CSF: produced by choroid plexus; reabsorbed by arachnoid granulations

- Increase in the CSF volume causes enlargement of the ventricles.
  1. Production and movement of CSF
     a. Produced by the choroid plexus in the ventricles
     b. Exits fourth ventricle through foramina and enters subarachnoid space
     c. Reabsorbed by the arachnoid granulations into the dural venous sinuses
     d. CSF analysis (Box 25-1)
  2. Communicating (nonobstructive) hydrocephalus
     a. Open communication between ventricles and subarachnoid space

---

BOX 25-1   CEREBROSPINAL FLUID (CSF) ANALYSIS

CSF derives from the choroid plexus in the ventricles and enters the subarachnoid space. It cushions the brain and spinal cord and transmits chemicals to reach other parts of the brain. CSF is reabsorbed by the arachnoid granulations and drained into dural venous sinuses, which eventually drain into the jugular vein.

CSF normally is clear and colorless. **Turbidity** may be caused by an increase in protein, cells, microbial pathogens, or a combination of all three elements. **Bloody CSF** from spinal taps is most commonly iatrogenic but can also represent a pathologic hemorrhage into the subarachnoid space (e.g., ruptured berry aneurysm, intracerebral bleed near the surface of the brain or ventricles). If the bloody tap is iatrogenic, the supranate should be clear after centrifugation, particularly in the last tube collected in the spinal tap. In pathologic bleeds, there are sequential color changes that occur. CSF colors after centrifugation may be pink- or orange-tinged. A pink color is due to oxyhemoglobin (oxyHb) from ruptured red blood cells. It first occurs 2–4 hours post-bleed, peaks in 24–36 hours, and subsides in 4–8 days. A yellow to orange color (xanthochromia) is due to oxyHb breakdown into bilirubin. It first appears 12 hours post-bleed, peaks in 2–4 days, and subsides in 2–4 weeks. **CSF protein** normally is 15–45 mg/dL. CSF prealbumin and albumin derive from plasma; therefore, increased levels of these proteins must be due to increased capillary permeability (e.g., acute inflammation). **CSF gamma (γ) globulins** derive from the synthesis of IgG by plasma cells within the central nervous system (CNS). In a CSF electrophoresis, CSF γ-globulins account for <12% of the total protein. An increase in CSF IgG is due to either increased synthesis of IgG in the CNS (e.g., multiple sclerosis) or an increase in capillary vessel permeability in acute inflammation (e.g., meningitis). It is clinically important to make this distinction. A **CSF IgG index** (calculated with a formula) is useful in distinguishing acute inflammation from demyelinating diseases, the most common CNS disease producing an increase in IgG. An increase in the CSF IgG index correlates with a CNS origin of the IgG, and a decreased index indicates

BOX 25-1   CEREBROSPINAL FLUID (CSF) ANALYSIS—cont'd

acute inflammation. **Routine CSF electrophoresis** quantitates the amount of γ-globulins that are present when CSF protein is increased. **High-resolution CSF electrophoresis**, however, is most useful in detecting demyelinating disease, of which multiple sclerosis is the most common cause. Other demyelinating diseases include neurosyphilis and Guillain-Barré syndrome. High-resolution detects **oligoclonal bands** in the γ-globulin region (see Fig. 25-27D). These are discrete, discontinuous bands originating from single clones of immunocompetent B cells. Another test for demyelinating disease is **myelin basic protein (MBP),** a protein that is normally present in myelin. An increased CSF MBP occurs with active demyelinating disease. CSF MBP is decreased when a demyelinating disease is in remission.

   CSF glucose does *not* have the same concentration as serum glucose. A normal value for CSF glucose is 50–75 mg/dL, but a normal value in serum glucose is 70–110 mg/dL. A rough estimate of what the CSF glucose should be is to multiply a serum sample value obtained 30–90 minutes *before* the lumbar puncture by 0.66. For example, if the serum glucose is 100 mg/dL, then the CSF glucose should be around 66 mg/dL. A decreased CSF glucose (hypoglycorrhachia) is defined as a glucose level < 40 mg/dL. It implies that there has been increased uptake of glucose by cellular elements in the CSF (e.g., neutrophils in acute bacterial meningitis, malignant cells) or a defect in the glucose carrier system (frequently occurs in bacterial/fungal meningitis). CSF glucose is usually normal in viral meningitis, neurosyphilis, demyelinating disease, and a cerebral abscess. Exceptions in which viral infections of the CNS produce a decreased CSF glucose include infections associated with mumps, herpes simplex, and the lymphocytic choriomeningitis virus. **CSF chloride** is usually greater than the serum chloride (limited usefulness). The **CSF white blood cell count** normally is 0–5 mononuclear cells/mm³. Neutrophils are *never* normal in the CSF. An increased CSF WBC count is most often due to meningitis caused by microbial pathogens. Bacterial meningitis usually has a predominance of neutrophils, while viral meningitis initially has a neutrophil response in the first 24 hours that changes to a predominantly lymphocytic response in 2–3 days. Fungal meningitis is characterized by a predominance of lymphocytes and monocytes. A parasitic meningitis usually has a mixed inflammatory infiltrate (eosinophils suggest a helminth infection). A **Gram stain** is useful for detecting bacteria (75–80% sensitivity) in the sediment after ultracentrifugation of the CSF. Other tests include culture, India ink for *Cryptococcus neoformans* (sensitivity is 50%), antigen detection (sensitivity depends on the pathogen; specificity is 96–100%), enzyme immunoassay (96–100% sensitivity/specificity), and polymerase chain reaction studies that detect DNA (sensitivity 94%, specificity 96%).

   b. Causes
      (1) Increased CSF production
         • Example—choroid plexus papilloma
      (2) Obstruction in reabsorption of CSF by arachnoid granulations
         • Examples—postmeningitic scarring, tumor
   3. Noncommunicating (obstructive) hydrocephalus
      a. Obstruction of CSF flow out of the ventricles
      b. Causes
         (1) Stricture of the aqueduct of Sylvius
            (a) Most common cause in newborns
            (b) Paralysis of upward gaze (Parinaud's syndrome; Fig. 25-5)
         (2) Tumor in the fourth ventricle
            • Examples—ependymoma, medulloblastoma
         (3) Scarring at the base of the brain
            • Example—tuberculous meningitis
         (4) Colloid cyst in the third ventricle
         (5) Developmental disorders (see section II)
   4. Clinical findings
      a. Newborns
         • Ventricles dilate and enlarge the head circumference (see Fig. 25-5).
      b. Adults
         • Ventricles enlarged but *no* increase in head circumference
   5. Hydrocephalus ex vacuo
      a. Dilated appearance of the ventricles when the brain mass is decreased
      b. Example—Alzheimer's disease
   6. Normal pressure hydrocephalus
      a. Epidemiology
         (1) Dilated ventricles + symptom complex of:
            (a) Wide-based gait
            (b) Urinary incontinence
            (c) Dementia

Communicating hydrocephalus: ↑ production CSF; ↓ reabsorption CSF

Noncommunicating hydrocephalus: obstruction CSF outflow into ventricles

Blockage aqueduct of Sylvius: most common cause of hydrocephalus in newborns

Hydrocephalus children: ventricles dilate and enlarge head circumference

Hydrocephalus adults: no increase in head size; dementia, gait disturbance, urinary incontinence

Hydrocephalus ex vacuo: dilated ventricles secondary to brain atrophy

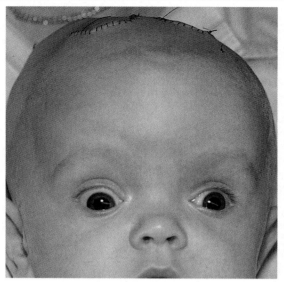

25-5: Hydrocephalus and Parinaud's syndrome. Note the increased head circumference and paralysis of upward gaze in this newborn with stenosis of the aqueduct of Sylvius. *(Courtesy of Dr. Albert Biglan, Children's Hospital of Pittsburgh.)*

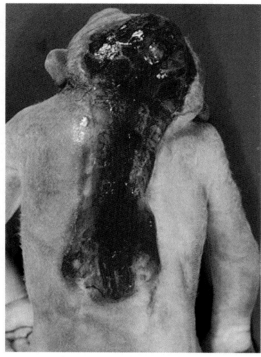

25-6: Anencephaly showing absence of the brain and opening of the spinal canal. *(From Damjanov I: Pathology for the Health-Related Professions, 2nd ed. Philadelphia, WB Saunders, 2000, p 126, Fig. 5-23B.)*

Normal pressure hydrocephalus: dilated ventricles + triad—dementia, urinary incontinence, wide-based gait

Normal pressure hydrocephalus: potentially reversible cause of dementia with shunting

Wide-based gait/urinary incontinence: stretching of sacral motor fibers

Dementia: stretching of the limbic fibers

      (2) Dilated ventricles but normal CSF pressure
      (3) Accounts for 5% of dementia cases
      (4) Potentially reversible cause of dementia
    b. Causes
      (1) Idiopathic (50%)
      (2) Secondary causes
        (a) Prior subarachnoid hemorrhage
        (b) Prior intracranial surgery
        (c) Prior trauma
    c. Pathogenesis
      (1) Increased subarachnoid space volume
      (2) Ventricular dilation is out of proportion to sulcal atrophy ("ventriculomegaly")
      (3) Wide-based gait and urinary incontinence due to stretching of sacral motor fibers near the dilated ventricle
      (4) Dementia due to stretching of limbic fibers near the dilated ventricle
    d. Diagnosis
      (1) MRI documents ventriculomegaly and sulcal atrophy.
      (2) Large volume of CSF is removed at lumbar puncture.
        • Symptoms improve with removal of the fluid.
    e. Treatment
      • Ventriculoperitoneal or ventriculoatrial shunting

II. Developmental Disorders
  A. Neural tube defects
    1. Pathogenesis
      a. Failure of fusion of the lateral folds of the neural plate
      b. Rupture of a previously closed neural tube
    2. Maternal findings
      • Increased maternal α-fetoprotein (AFP) in serum or amniotic fluid
    3. Anencephaly
      a. Complete absence of brain (Fig. 25-6)
      b. Frog-like appearance
      c. Maternal polyhydramnios

Neural tube defects: failure of fusion of lateral folds of neural plate; ↑AFP

Maternal folate level must be adequate *before* pregnancy

Anencephaly: absence of brain; maternal polyhydramnios

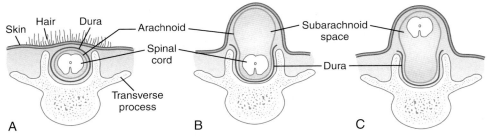

25-7: Types of spina bifida: spina bifida occulta (**A**), meningocele (**B**), meningomyelocele (**C**). *(From Moore NA, Roy WA: Rapid Review Gross and Developmental Anatomy, 2nd ed. St. Louis, Mosby Elsevier, 2007, p 12, Fig. 1-13.)*

    4. Spina bifida occulta (Fig. 25-7A)
       a. Defect in closure of the posterior vertebral arch
       b. Dimple or tuft of hair in the skin overlying L5–S1
    5. Meningocele (Fig. 25-7B)
       a. Spina bifida with cystic mass containing meninges
       b. Most common in lumbosacral region
    6. Meningomyelocele (Fig. 25-7C)
       a. Spina bifida with cystic mass containing meninges and spinal cord
       b. Most common in lumbosacral region

B. Arnold-Chiari malformation
    1. Caudal extension of medulla and cerebellar vermis through foramen magnum
    2. Noncommunicating hydrocephalus
    3. Platybasia (flattening of base of skull)
    4. Associations:
       a. Meningomyelocele
       b. Syringomyelia
    5. Treatment
       • Decompression surgery

C. Dandy-Walker malformation
    1. Partial or complete absence of the cerebellar vermis
    2. Cystic dilation of fourth ventricle
    3. Noncommunicating hydrocephalus
    4. Treatment
       • Shunt to treat hydrocephalus

D. Syringomyelia
    1. Degenerative disease of spinal cord
       a. Symptoms appear in the third and fourth decades.
       b. Fluid-filled cavity (syrinx) within the cervical spinal cord (Fig. 25-8)
       c. Produces cervical cord enlargement
       d. Cavity expands and causes degeneration of spinal tracts.
    2. Associated with Arnold-Chiari malformation
    3. Pathogenesis
       a. Obstruction of outflow from fourth ventricle
       b. Birth injury
    4. Clinical findings
       a. Disruption of the crossed lateral spinothalamic tracts
          (1) Loss of pain and temperature sensation in the hands
            • Tactile sense preserved

Margin notes:

Spina bifida occulta: dimple/tuft of hair overlying L5–S1

Meningocele: cystic mass with meninges

Meningomyelocele: cystic mass with meninges and spinal cord

Arnold-Chiari: caudal extension medulla/ cerebellar vermis through foramen; hydrocephalus; meningomyelocele; syringomyelia

Dandy-Walker: partial/ complete absence of cerebellar vermis; cystic dilation of 4th ventricle; hydrocephalus

Syringomyelia: degenerative disease of spinal cord; usually cervical cord

Syringomyelia: cervical cord enlargment; fluid-filled cavity

Syringomyelia: ↓ pain/ temperature sensation in hands; loss intrinsic muscles of hand

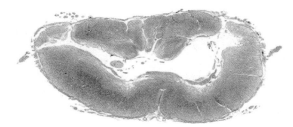

25-8: Syringomyelia. Note the collapsed cystic cavity (syrinx) in the center of the cervical spinal cord. *(From Burger PC, Scheithauer BW, Vogel KS: Surgical Pathology of the Nervous System, 4th ed. London, Churchill Livingstone, 2002, p 554, Fig. 11-70.)*

(2) Patient can burn hands *without* being aware of the burn.

b. Destruction of anterior horn cells

  (1) Atrophy of intrinsic muscles of the hands

  (2) Often confused with amyotrophic lateral sclerosis (ALS)

   • *No* sensory changes in ALS

c. Charcot joint shoulder, elbow, wrist

5. Diagnosis

 • MRI shows enlarged cervical cord and cystic cavity.

6. Treatment

 • Drainage of syrinx slows progression.

E. Phakomatoses (neurocutaneous syndromes)

1. Epidemiology

  a. Neurocutaneous syndromes

  b. Disordered growth of ectodermal tissue

  c. Malformations or tumors of the CNS

  d. Includes the following in descending order of incidence:

   • Neurofibromatosis, tuberous sclerosis, Sturge-Weber syndrome

2. Neurofibromatosis (NF)

  a. Autosomal dominant (AD) disorder with incomplete penetrance

  b. No gender predominance

  c. Type 1 (NF1; most common) and type 2 (NF2) variants

   (1) NF1—mutation on chromosome 17 coding for neurofibromin

   (2) NF2—mutation on chromosome 22 coding for merlin

   (3) Both proteins act as tumor suppressors.

  d. NF1 (peripheral type) associated with:

   (1) Café au lait coffee-colored macules (Fig. 25-9)

    (a) Occur in both types

    (b) Occur in 100% of children *before* 2 years of age

   (2) Optic gliomas (2–5%); astrocytomas

   (3) Lisch nodules (>90%)

    • Hamartoma of the iris

   (4) Axillary and inguinal freckling (70%)

   (5) Mild scoliosis

   (6) Pigmented plexiform neurofibromas (*not* in NF2)

    • May progress into neurofibrosarcoma involving large nerves

   (7) Pigmented cutaneous/subcutaneous neurofibromas

    (a) Occur in both types

    (b) Occur anywhere on the body except palms, soles

    (c) Appear in late adolescence and increase in size with age

    (d) Focal or diffuse

   (8) Tumor associations

    (a) Pheochromocytoma; Wilms' tumor

     • Both produce hypertension.

    (b) Juvenile chronic myelogenous leukemia (CML)

   (9) Neurodevelopment problems (30–40%)

  e. NF2 (central type); associated with:

   (1) Bilateral acoustic neuromas (schwannoma; >90%)

Syringomyelia: MRI shows cervical enlargement and cavity

Phakomatosis: neurocutaneous syndromes

NF: AD; incomplete penetrance

Both types: café au lait macules; neurofibromas

NF1: optic gliomas; Lisch nodules; axillary/inguinal freckling

NF1 tumor associations: pheochromocytoma; Wilms' tumor; CML (juvenile)

NF2: bilateral acoustic neuromas; juvenile cataracts; meningiomas

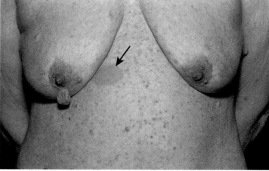

25-9: Neurofibromatosis showing café-au-lait macule (*arrow*) and numerous pigmented, pedunculated neurofibromas. (*From Forbes C, Jackson W: Color Atlas and Text of Clinical Medicine, 2nd ed. St. Louis, Mosby, 2003, p 104, Fig. 2-86.*)

    (a) Cranial nerve (CN) VIII tumor
    (b) Benign tumor
    (c) Sensorineural hearing loss; tinnitus
   (2) Meningiomas
   (3) Spinal schwannomas
   (4) Juvenile cataracts (~80%)
  f. Genetic testing available for both types
  g. Treatment is mainly surgical.
 3. Tuberous sclerosis
  a. AD disorder
  b. Second most common phakomatosis after neurofibromatosis
  c. Mental retardation and seizures (infantile spasms) beginning in infancy
  d. Angiofibromas (adenoma sebaceum) on the face (Fig. 25-10)
  e. Hypopigmented skin lesions ("ash leaf" lesions; Fig. 25-11)
   (1) Best identified with Wood's lamp
   (2) Occur in >80% of cases
  f. Hamartomatous lesions
   (1) Astrocyte proliferations in subependyma
    • Look like "candlestick drippings" in the ventricles
   (2) Angiomyolipomas in the kidneys (80%)
  g. Rhabdomyoma in the heart (50–60%)
   • Almost 100% predictive of tuberous sclerosis
 4. Sturge-Weber syndrome (SWS; refer to Chapter 9; see Fig. 9-9D)
  a. Somatic mosaicism or sporadic
  b. Vascular malformation on the face
   • In a trigeminal nerve distribution
  c. Some patients have ipsilateral arteriovenous malformation in the meninges.

III. Head Trauma
 A. Cerebral contusion
  1. Permanent damage to small blood vessels and the surface of the brain

Margin notes:

Tuberous sclerosis: AD; mental retardation; hamartomas in brain, kidneys

Triad: seizures, mental retardation, angiofibromas, ash leaf lesions

Rhabdomyoma of heart: highly predictive of tuberous sclerosis

SWS: vascular malformation of face; ipsilateral arteriovenous malformation in meninges in some patients

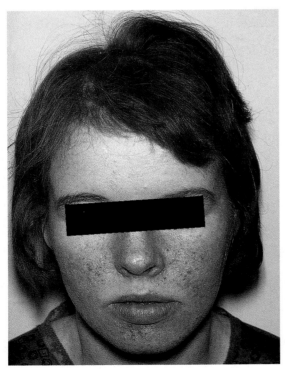

25-10: Adenoma sebaceum (angiofibromas) in tuberous sclerosis. Note the reddish brown papules on the nose, cheeks, and chin. *(Courtesy of R.A. Marsden, MD, St. George's Hospital, London.)*

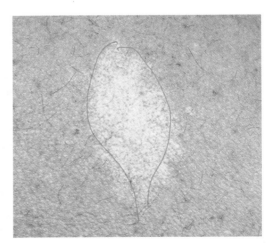

25-11: Shagreen patch in tuberous sclerosis. Note the irregular area of white skin (leukoderma) with the typical ash-leaf pattern of a shagreen patch. *(From Lookingbill DP, Marks JG: Principles of Dermatology, 3rd ed. Philadelphia, Saunders, 2000, p 234, Fig. 14-7.)*

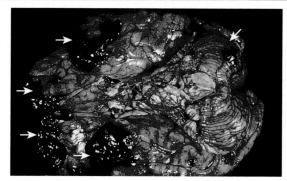

25-12: Brain contusion. The contrecoup injury involves the frontal and temporal lobes (*left arrows*), while the coup lesion (site of impact) involves the cerebellum (*right arrow*). *(From Damjanov I, Linder J: Pathology: A Color Atlas. St. Louis, Mosby, 2000, p 403, Fig. 9-6.)*

Coup injuries: site of impact

Contrecoup injuries: opposite site of impact

2. Most often secondary to an acceleration-deceleration injury
3. Coup injuries occur at the *site* of impact (Fig. 25-12).
4. Contrecoup injuries occur *opposite* the site of impact.
   • Common sites are at the tips of the frontal and temporal lobes.
   B. **Acute epidural hematoma**
      1. Epidemiology
         a. Occurs in 1% to 2% of head injuries
         b. Arterial bleed creates a blood-filled space between the bone and dura (Fig. 25-13A and B).

Epidural hematoma: temporoparietal skull fracture; tear of middle meningeal artery

         c. Caused by a fracture of the temporoparietal bone
            (1) Causes—hammer; baseball bat; any focused blow to head
            (2) Severance of the middle meningeal artery
            (3) Vessel lies between the dura and inner table of bone.
      2. Some patients have lucid interval after trauma followed later by neurologic deterioration.
      3. Intracranial pressure increases, leading to herniation and death.
      4. Diagnosis

CT scan: imaging test of choice

         a. Head CT scan is the imaging test of choice.
         b. Hematoma rarely crosses the suture line due to firm attachment of dura at these sites.
      5. Treatment consists of creating burr holes to relieve pressure.
   C. **Subdural hematoma**
      1. Epidemiology

Subdural hematoma: venous bleed between dura and arachnoid membranes

         a. Venous bleeding between the dura and arachnoid membranes
         b. Causes
            (1) Most often the result of blunt trauma
               • Examples—car accident, baseball bat

Subdural hematoma: most often caused by trauma; increased risk with cerebral atrophy

            (2) Other causes
               (a) Medical anticoagulation
               (b) Hemophilia
               (c) Child abuse; shaken baby syndrome
               (d) Spontaneous
            (3) Risk factors
               (a) Elderly patients and alcoholic with atrophy of brain
               (b) Loss of brain mass leads to excess traction on the inflexible bridging veins
      2. Pathogenesis
         a. Tearing of bridging veins between brain and dural sinuses (Fig. 25-13C and D)

Subdural hematoma: tear of bridging veins producing venous blood clot

         b. Slowly enlarging blood clot covers the convexity of the brain.
      3. Clinical findings
         a. Fluctuating levels of consciousness
         b. Herniation and death may occur.
         c. Chronic subdural hematomas may produce dementia.

CT scan: imaging test of choice

      4. CT scan is best imaging study
      5. Treatment consists of creating burr holes to relieve pressure.

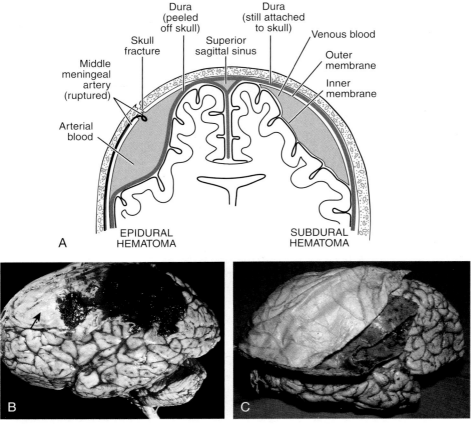

25-13: A, Schematic of epidural hematoma and subdural hematoma. **B,** Epidural hematoma. Note the blood is located on top of the dura *(arrow)*. **C,** Subdural hematoma. The reflected dura shows the outer membrane of an organized venous clot covering the convexity of the brain. *(A from Kumar V, Abbas AK, Fausto N, Mitchell RN: Robbins Basic Pathology, 8th ed. Philadelphia, Saunders Elsevier, 2007, p 871, Fig. 23-13A; B courtesy of Dr. Raymond D. Adams, Massachusetts General Hospital, Boston; C from Damjanov I, Linder J: Pathology: A Color Atlas. St. Louis, Mosby, 2000, p 405, Fig. 19-20.)*

IV. **CNS Vascular Disorders**
   A. **Global hypoxic injury**
      1. Causes of global hypoxic injury (refer to Chapter 1)
         a. Cardiac arrest
         b. Hypovolemic shock; septic shock
         c. Chronic carbon monoxide (CO) poisoning

> Repeated episodes of **hypoglycemia** have the same effects on the brain as does global hypoxic injury. Hypoglycemia most commonly occurs in type 1 diabetes mellitus.

      2. Complications
         a. Cerebral atrophy (see Fig. 1-10A)
            (1) Due to apoptosis of neurons in layers 3, 5, and 6 of the cerebral cortex
               • Produces laminar necrosis
            (2) Neurons are the most susceptible cell to hypoxic injury.
            (3) Neurons undergo apoptosis ("red" neurons; Fig. 25-14).
         b. Watershed infarcts (refer to Chapter 1; see Fig. 1-4)
            (1) Occur at the junctions of arterial territories
            (2) Example—junction between the anterior and middle cerebral arteries
         c. Cerebrovascular accident (e.g., stroke)
   B. **Strokes**
      1. Epidemiology
         a. Increased incidence with age
         b. Peak incidence is between 80 and 84 years of age.
         c. More common in men than women

Global hypoxic injury: hypotensive episodes; chronic CO poisoning

Complications: cerebral atrophy; watershed infarcts; stroke

Red neurons: apoptotic neuron

Hypoglycemia: ~effect on brain as global hypoxia

Strokes: ↑ incidence with age

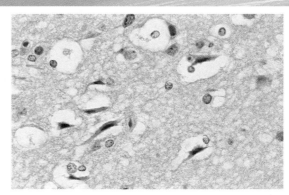

25-14: Red neurons. Note the brightly eosinophilic staining cells with the pyknotic nuclei within spaces representing apoptotic neurons. *(From Burger PC, Scheithauer BW, Vogel KS: Surgical Pathology of the Nervous System, 4th ed. London, Churchill Livingstone, 2002, p 415, Fig. 7-34.)*

d. Types of strokes
 (1) Ischemic (70–80%)
  (a) Atherosclerotic
   • Most common type
  (b) Embolic
 (2) Intracerebral hemorrhage
 (3) Subarachnoid hemorrhage
 (4) Lacunar stroke
2. Atherosclerotic (thrombotic) stroke
 a. Most common overall type of stroke
  • Ischemic type of stroke due to thrombosis
 b. Usually pale infarcts (liquefactive necrosis)
  (1) Platelet thrombus develops over a disrupted plaque. Sites:
   (a) Middle cerebral artery (MCA)
   (b) Internal carotid artery near the bifurcation
  (2) Reperfusion does *not* usually occur.
   • Hemorrhagic infarction develops if reperfusion occurs.
 c. Most occur in the distribution of the MCA.
 d. Gross and microscopic findings
  (1) Wedge-shaped area of pale infarction
   • Develops at the *periphery* of the cerebral cortex (Fig. 25-15)
  (2) Swelling of the brain occurs.
   (a) Loss of demarcation between gray and white mater
   (b) Myelin begins to break down.
  (3) Gliosis is the reaction to injury.
   (a) Astrocytes proliferate at the margins of the infarct.
   (b) Microglial cells (macrophages) remove lipid debris.
  (4) Cystic area develops after 10 days to 3 weeks.
   • Example of liquefactive necrosis
 e. Clinical findings
  (1) Most atherosclerotic strokes are preceded by transient ischemic attacks (TIAs).
   (a) Transient neurologic deficits last <24 hours.
    • Visual loss, paresthesias, hemiparesis, loss of speech
   (b) Usually caused by microembolization of plaque material
  (2) Deficits that do *not* resolve within 24 hours are called strokes.
  (3) Amaurosis fugax
   • Temporary loss of vision due to embolization of atherosclerotic material to bifurcation of retinal arteries; called Hollenhorst plaque (Fig. 25-16)
  (4) Treatment of TIA
   • Aspirin; clopidogrel; ticlopidine
  (5) Strokes involving the MCA
   (a) Contralateral hemiparesis and sensory loss in the face and upper extremity
   (b) Expressive aphasia
    • If Broca's area is involved in the dominant (left) hemisphere

Atherosclerotic stroke: most common overall stroke; ischemic type of stroke

Atherosclerotic stroke: pale infarction extending to periphery of cerebral cortex

Atherosclerotic stroke: most occur in MCA distribution

Atherosclerotic stroke: infarction with liquefactive (not coagulative) necrosis

TIA: transient neurologic deficit lasting <24 hours; microembolization of plaque material

Amaurosis fugax: temporary loss of vision; embolic material trapped at bifurcation of retinal vessels

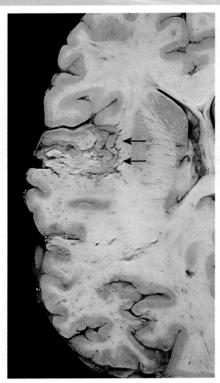

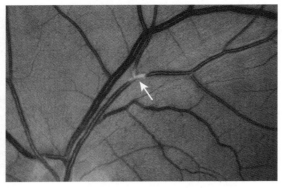

25-16: Cholesterol embolus to retinal artery. Note the yellow embolus trapped at the bifurcation of the retinal artery (*arrow*). This produces a sudden, painless loss of vision ("curtain coming down") followed in a variable period of time by restoration of vision ("curtain coming up") as the embolus dislodges. This is called amaurosis fugax. *(From Swartz MH: Textbook of Physical Diagnosis, 5th ed. Philadelphia, Saunders Elsevier, 2006, p 271, Fig. 10-113.)*

25-15: Atherosclerotic stroke showing necrotic areas at the periphery of the cerebral cortex in the distribution of the middle cerebral artery. *Arrows* are located at the line of demarcation between normal and infarcted tissue. *(From Damjanov I, Linder J: Pathology: A Color Atlas. St. Louis, Mosby, 2000, p 408, Fig. 19-25A.)*

            (c) Visual field defects
            (d) Head and eyes deviate *toward* the side of the lesion.
        (6) Strokes involving anterior cerebral artery (ACA)
            • Contralateral hemiparesis and sensory loss in the lower extremity
            • ACA stroke: contralateral paresis/sensory loss in lower extremity
        (7) Strokes involving vertebrobasilar arterial system
            (a) Vertigo, ataxia
            (b) Ipsilateral sensory loss in face
            (c) Contralateral hemiparesis and sensory loss in the trunk and limbs
    f. Prevention of atherosclerotic strokes
        • Aspirin; clopidogrel if allergic to aspirin
3. Embolic (hemorrhagic) stroke
    a. Ischemic type of stroke due to embolization
    b. Source of emboli
        • Most often originate from the left side of the heart (refer to Chapter 4)
    c. Produces a hemorrhagic infarction
        (1) Most occur in the distribution of the MCA (Fig. 25-17).
        (2) Vessel reperfusion after lysis of embolic material produces hemorrhage.
4. Intracerebral hemorrhage
    a. Most often due to stress imposed on vessels by hypertension
        (1) Branches of lenticulostriate vessels develop Charcot-Bouchard macroaneurysms.
        (2) Rupture of aneurysms produces intracerebral hemorrhage (hematoma).
            • Intracerebral hematoma pushes the brain parenchyma aside (Fig. 25-18).
    b. Common sites of hemorrhage
        (1) Basal ganglia (35–50% occur in the putamen)
        (2) Thalamus (10%)
        (3) Pons and cerebellar hemispheres (10%)

MCA stroke: contralateral paresis/sensory loss in face/upper extremity; head/eyes deviate to side of lesion

ACA stroke: contralateral paresis/sensory loss in lower extremity

Embolic stroke: ischemic type of stroke due to embolization

Embolic stroke: hemorrhagic infarction extending to periphery of cerebral cortex

Intracerebral hemorrhage: complication of hypertension; rupture of aneurysm

Rx hypertension reduces the incidence of stroke by more than 40%.

Intracerebral hemorrhage: basal ganglia most common location

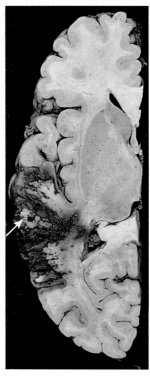

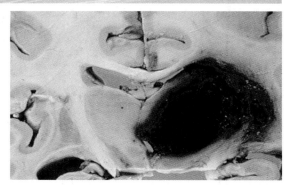

25-18: Intracerebral hemorrhage, showing a large blood clot within the basal ganglia area of the brain. *(From Damjanov I: Pathology for the Health-Related Professions, 2nd ed. Philadelphia, WB Saunders, 2000, p 506, Fig. 21-7.)*

25-17: Embolic stroke showing a wedge-shaped hemorrhagic infarction *(arrow)* along the periphery of the cerebral cortex in the distribution of the middle cerebral artery. It is hemorrhagic because blood flow was reestablished when the embolus dislodged and converted a pale infarct to a hemorrhagic infarct. *(From Damjanov I, Linder J: Pathology: A Color Atlas. St. Louis, Mosby, 2000, p 408, Fig. 19-25B.)*

5. Subarachnoid hemorrhage

   a. Causes

      (1) Majority are secondary to rupture of a congenital berry aneurysm.

      (2) Bleeding from an arteriovenous malformation is a less common cause.

   b. Congenital berry aneurysm

      (1) May develop from normal hemodynamic stress or hypertension

      (2) Most develop at junctions of communicating branches with main cerebral artery (Fig. 25-19).

         (a) Junction lacks internal elastic lamina and smooth muscle.

         (b) Most common site for berry aneurysm is junction with ACA.

      (3) Rupture releases blood into the subarachnoid space.

         • Blood covers the surface of the brain (Fig. 25-20).

      (4) Blood in the CSF is broken down into bilirubin pigment.

         • Imparts a yellow color to CSF called xanthochromia (see Box 25-1)

   c. Clinical findings

      (1) Sudden onset of severe occipital headache

         (a) Described as "worst headache ever"

         (b) Nuchal rigidity is present.

      (2) About 50% of patients die soon after the hemorrhage.

      (3) Complications

         (a) Further hemorrhage

         (b) Hydrocephalus

            • Blockage of arachnoid granulations; block foramina

         (c) Permanent neurologic deficits

6. Lacunar infarcts

   a. Cystic areas of microinfarction < 1 cm in diameter (Fig. 25-21)

   b. Caused by hyaline arteriolosclerosis

      • Secondary to either hypertension (most common) or diabetes mellitus

---

Subarachnoid hemorrhage: rupture of congenital berry aneurysm

Berry aneurysms: junction of communicating branch with main cerebral artery

Subarachnoid hemorrhage: severe occipital headache; described as "worst headache ever"

Lacunar strokes: microinfarction < 1 cm

Lacunar strokes: hyaline arteriolosclerosis due to hypertension/diabetes

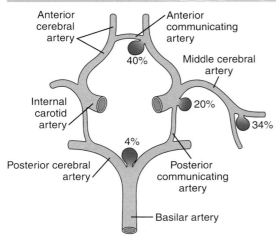

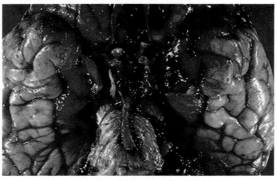

25-20: Subarachnoid hemorrhage. Note the presence of blood covering the surface of the brain. *(From Klatt E: Robbins and Cotran's Atlas of Pathology. Philadelphia, WB Saunders, 2006, p 470, Fig. 19-77.)*

25-19: Schematic of locations of berry aneurysms in the circle of Willis. See text for discussion. *(From Kumar V, Abbas AK, Fausto N, Mitchell RN: Robbins Basic Pathology, 8th ed. Philadelphia, Saunders Elsevier, 2007, p 867, Fig. 23-9.)*

    c. Stroke syndromes
        (1) Pure motor strokes with or without dysarthria
           • Occur if the posterior limb of the internal capsule is involved
        (2) Pure sensory strokes
           • Occur if the thalamus is involved
   7. Diagnosis
    a. CT scan without contrast
        (1) Overall best imaging technique
        (2) Distinguishes hemorrhage from nonhemorrhagic strokes
    b. MRI is most useful for identification of posterior fossa infarcts.
   8. Treatment
    a. Acute treatment
        (1) Depends on the type of stroke and elapsed time to arrival at a hospital
        (2) Thrombolytic therapy in thromboembolic strokes
           (a) Depends on the time interval of symptoms (<3 hours is ideal)
           (b) Usually *not* implemented if stroke is hemorrhagic
        (3) In some cases, intracerebral hemorrhages can be evacuated.
    b. Chronic treatment
        (1) Antiplatelet treatment (e.g., aspirin, clopidogrel)
        (2) Warfarin for embolic types of strokes
        (3) Treat risk factors for strokes (e.g., hypertension, diabetes)

V. CNS Infections
  A. Pathogenesis
    1. Hematogenous spread (most common)

> Diagnosis of strokes: CT without contrast best test

> CNS infections: most are due to sepsis

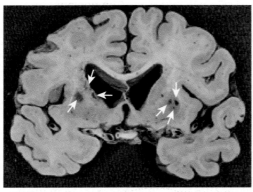

25-21: Lacunar infarcts. The *arrows* show multiple small cystic spaces (liquefactive necrosis) that are most prominent in the basal ganglia. Sections under these lesions showed hyaline arteriolosclerosis. *(From Damjanov I, Linder J: Pathology: A Color Atlas. St. Louis, Mosby, 2000, p 408, Fig. 19-28.)*

2. Traumatic implantation
3. Local extension from nearby infection
4. Ascent of peripheral nerve

B. Meningitis

1. Inflammation of pia mater covering the brain (Fig. 25-22)
2. Usually due to hematogenous spread; mechanism for bacterial meningitis:
   a. Adherence of bacteria to mucosa of nasopharynx
   b. Bacteremia
   c. Translocation through blood-brain barrier (BBB)
      • Involves bacterial lysins
   d. Bacteria in subarachnoid space attract neutrophils.
   e. Acute meningitis
3. Risk factors in children
   a. Undernutrition; otitis media
   b. Pneumonia; immunodeficiency
   c. Viral infection; sickle cell disease
   d. Craniofacial abnormality
4. Viral meningitis
   a. Most transmitted by fecal-oral route
   b. Respiratory route less common
5. Clinical findings in meningitis
   • Fever, nuchal rigidity, headache
6. Complications of meningitis
   a. Seizures; focal neurologic deficits
   b. Cranial nerve palsies
   c. Sensorineural hearing loss
   d. Communicating and noncommunicating hydrocephalus
7. Laboratory findings in viral meningitis (Table 25-1; see also Box 25-1)
   a. Increased CSF protein
      • Due to increased vessel permeability
   b. Increased total CSF leukocyte count
      • Initially neutrophils but converts to lymphocytes in 24 hours
   c. Normal CSF glucose
8. Laboratory findings in bacterial meningitis (see Table 25-1 and Box 25-1)
   a. Increased CSF protein
   b. Increased total CSF leukocyte count
   c. Decreased CSF glucose

Meningitis: inflammation of pia mater

Bacterial meningitis: majority of organisms originate in nasopharynx

Viral meningitis: most often transmitted by fecal-oral route

Meningitis: nuchal rigidity

Meningitis: ↑ CSF protein (viral, bacterial, fungal); ↓ CSF glucose (bacterial, fungal)

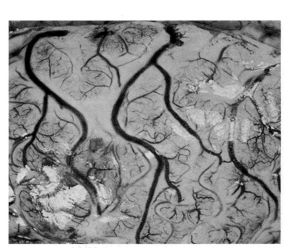

25-22: Bacterial meningitis showing engorged blood vessels and a creamy exudate covering the surface of the pia mater. *(From Perkin GD: Mosby's Color Atlas and Text of Neurology. St. Louis, Mosby, 2002, p 196, Fig. 11-1.)*

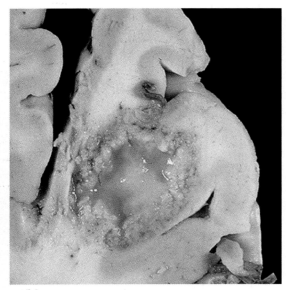

25-23: Cerebral abscess showing a cystic mass lined by necrotic, purulent material. *(From Burger PC, Scheithauer BW, Vogel KS: Surgical Pathology of the Nervous System, 4th ed. London, Churchill Livingstone, 2002, p 121, Fig. 3-17.)*

TABLE 25-1. CEREBROSPINAL FLUID (CSF) FINDINGS IN VIRAL, BACTERIAL, AND FUNGAL MENINGITIS

CSF FEATURE	BACTERIAL/FUNGAL	VIRAL
Total cell count	1000–20,000 cells/mm³	<1000 cells/mm³
Differential count	>90% neutrophils (>80%)	First 24–48 hours, neutrophils, then switches to lymphocytes/monocytes after 48 hours
CSF glucose	Decreased (<40 mg/dL)	Normal: exceptions—mumps, herpes
CSF protein	Increased (>50 mg/dL)	Increased
Gram stain	Frequently positive (60–90%) Culture positive (65–90%)	Negative

C. **Encephalitis**
   1. Inflammation of the brain
   2. Clinical findings
     a. Fever, headache
     b. Impaired mental status, drowsiness

    Encephalitis: inflammation of brain; headache; drowsiness; coma

D. **Cerebral abscess**
   1. Pathogenesis
     a. Spread from an adjacent focus of infection (e.g., sinuses)
     b. Hematogenous spread (e.g., infective endocarditis)
   2. Single or multiple lesions (Fig. 25-23)

    Cerebral abscess: hematogenous; contiguous spread

E. **Viral CNS infections** (Tables 25-2 and 25-3 and Figs. 25-24 and 25-25)
F. **Bacterial CNS infections** (Table 25-4)
G. **Fungal and parasitic CNS infections** (Table 25-5 and Fig. 25-26)

VI. **Demyelinating Disorders**
  A. **Pathogenesis**
   1. Destruction of normal myelin
     • Example—multiple sclerosis
   2. Production of abnormal myelin
     • Example—leukodystrophy
   3. Destruction of oligodendrocytes
     • Examples—multiple sclerosis, slow virus infections

    Demyelination: destruction normal myelin/oligodendrocyte; abnormal myelin

  B. **Acquired disorders**
   1. Multiple sclerosis (MS)
     a. Epidemiology
       (1) Most common demyelinating disease
       (2) Most common debilitating disease among young adults
       (3) Female predominance
         • Occurs most often in women 20 to 40 years of age
     b. Many subtypes
     c. Pathogenesis
       (1) Autoimmune disease initiated by:
         (a) Genetic factors (e.g., HLA-DR2)
         (b) Environmental triggers
           • Microbial pathogens (e.g., Epstein-Barr virus, human herpes virus 6, *Chlamydophilia pneumoniae*), vitamin D, sun exposure
       (2) Environmental trigger activates helper T cells whose antigen-specific receptors recognize CNS myelin basic protein (other antigens as well) as an antigen.
       (3) T cells release cytokines that activate macrophages, which also release cytokines (e.g., tumor necrosis factor-α) that destroy the myelin sheath as well as oligodendrocytes that synthesize myelin (type IV hypersensitivity).
       (4) Antibodies directed against the myelin sheath and oligodendrocytes may also be involved (type II hypersensitivity).
     d. Gross and microscopic findings
       (1) Demyelinating plaques occur in white mater of brain/spinal cord (Fig. 25-27A and B).
         • White mater looks like gray mater in areas of demyelination.
       (2) Inflammatory infiltrate in plaques is composed predominantly of CD4 T cells and microglial cells with phagocytosed lipid.
     e. Clinical findings
       (1) Episodic course punctuated by acute relapses and remissions (80–90%)

    MS: most common demyelinating disease

    MS: CD4 T cells react against self antigens in myelin sheath; cytokines activate macrophages that destroy myelin

    MS: genetic factors and environmental triggers

    Demyelinating plaques: white mater looks like gray mater

TABLE 25-2. **VIRAL INFECTIONS OF THE CENTRAL NERVOUS SYSTEM**

VIRUS	DISEASE	COMMENTS
Arboviruses	Encephalitis	Mosquitoes are the vector Wild birds are the reservoir for the virus West Nile virus: crows and other birds have spread the disease from New York to the West Coast Encephalitis can be fatal
Coxsackievirus	Meningitis	Enterovirus: most common cause of viral meningitis Viral meningitis peaks in late summer and early autumn
Cytomegalovirus (see Fig. 25-24A)	Encephalitis	Most common viral CNS infection in AIDS Primarily intranuclear basophilic inclusions Periventricular calcification in newborns Treatment: ganciclovir + foscarnet; or valganciclovir
Herpes simplex virus type 1 (see Fig. 25-24B)	Meningitis and encephalitis	Causes hemorrhagic necrosis of temporal lobes Treatment: IV acyclovir
HIV (see Fig. 25-24C)	Encephalitis	Most common cause of AIDS dementia Microglial cells fuse to form multinucleated cells
Lymphocytic choriomeningitis Meningitis and encephalitis		Endemic in the mouse population Transmission: food or water contaminated with mouse urine/feces Meningoencephalitis: combination of nuchal rigidity and mental status abnormalities (encephalitis) CSF findings: increased protein, lymphocyte infiltrate, normal to decreased glucose
Poliovirus	Encephalitis and myelitis—spinal cord	Destroys upper and lower motor neurons Causes muscle paralysis Post-polio syndrome: occurs in ~50% of people with previous poliomyelitis; usually occurs 15–30 years after original infection; increased muscular weakness/pain in muscle groups already affected; excessive fatigue
Rabies virus (see Fig. 25-24D)	Encephalitis	Most often transmitted by raccoon bite (40% of cases) Other vectors are dog, skunk, bat, and coyote Viral receptor is acetylcholine receptor Initially replicates at site of the bite; moves by axonal transport to the CNS; after CNS replication, it migrates to the saliva Animal transmits virus when in the agitated state (encephalitis stage) Incubation period 10–90 days Prodrome: fever, paresthesias in and around the wound site Hydrophobia: due to spasms of throat muscles when swallowing Followed by flaccid paralysis Encephalitis: death of neurons; eosinophilic intracytoplasmic inclusions called Negri bodies; seizures, coma, death Treatment: wash wound site (quaternary ammonium compound); give passive immunization (immune globulin) mostly into wound site (where virus initially replicates); give active immunization (human diploid vaccine) Universally fatal if not treated

TABLE 25-3. **SLOW VIRUS DISEASES OF THE CENTRAL NERVOUS SYSTEM**

DISEASE	COMMENTS
Creutzfeldt-Jakob disease (see Fig. 25-25)	Unconventional slow virus encephalitis due to prions (proteinaceous material devoid of RNA or DNA); noninfectious prion protein normally found on surface of neurons (function unknown) Transmitted by corneal transplantation, contact with human brain, use of improperly sterilized cortical electrodes, or ingestion of tissues from cattle with bovine spongiform encephalopathy ("mad cow" disease) Brain has "bubble and holes" spongiform change in cerebral cortex Death usually occurs within 1 year
Progressive multifocal leukoencephalopathy	Conventional slow virus encephalitis due to papovavirus Intranuclear inclusion in oligodendrocytes Occurs in AIDS when CD4 T$_H$ count < 50 cells/mm^3
Subacute sclerosing panencephalitis	Conventional slow virus encephalitis associated with rubeola (measles) virus Intranuclear inclusions in neurons and oligodendrocytes Death usually occurs within 1–2 years

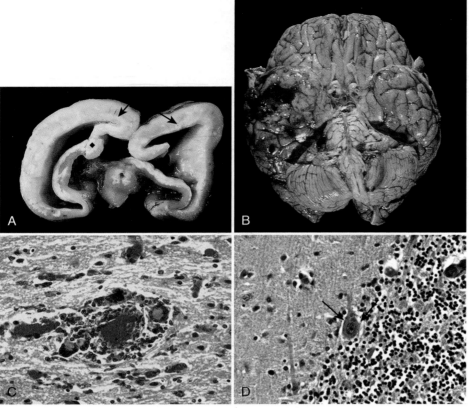

25-24: **A,** Congenital cytomegalovirus encephalitis. The *arrows* show many chalky periventricular calcifications (dystrophic calcification). **B,** Herpes simplex encephalitis. The basal view shows hemorrhagic necrosis of the right temporal lobe. Cerebral edema is also present. **C,** HIV encephalitis. Note the numerous multinucleated microglial cells, which is a characteristic finding in HIV encephalitis, the cause of AIDS dementia. **D,** Rabies. The Purkinje cells have intracytoplasmic, eosinophilic inclusions (*arrows*) called Negri bodies. *(**A** and **C** from Klatt E: Robbins and Cotran's Atlas of Pathology. Philadelphia, WB Saunders, 2006, pp 476, 477, Figs. 19-94, 19-97, respectively; **B** from Perkin GD: Mosby's Color Atlas and Text of Neurology. St. Louis, Mosby, 2002, p 208, Fig. 11-15; **D** from Kumar V, Fausto N, Abbas A: Robbins and Cotran's Pathologic Basis of Disease, 7th ed. Philadelphia, WB Saunders, 2004, p 1375, Fig. 28-25.)*

(2) Sensory dysfunction
    (a) Paresthesias
    (b) Loss of pain/temperature sensation
    (c) Loss of vibratory sensation
(3) Upper motor neuron (UMN) dysfunction
    (a) Spasticity
    (b) Increased deep tendon reflexes (DTRs)
    (c) Muscle spasms
    (d) Extensor plantar response (Babinski)

Sensory dysfunction: paresthesias; loss pain/temperature/vibratory sensation

UMN dysfunction: spasticity; ↑ DTRs; muscle spasm; Babinski; weakness

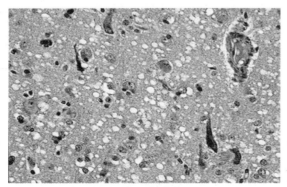

25-25: Spongiform encephalopathy in Creutzfeldt-Jakob disease showing classic "bubbles and holes" of the neuropil cell bodies. *(From Damjanov I, Linder J: Pathology: A Color Atlas. St. Louis, Mosby, 2000, p 412, Fig. 19-41.)*

TABLE 25-4. BACTERIAL INFECTIONS OF THE CENTRAL NERVOUS SYSTEM

BACTERIUM	DISEASE	COMMENTS
Group B streptococcus (*Streptococcus agalactiae*)	Neonatal meningitis	Gram-positive coccus Most common cause of neonatal meningitis (49%) Spreads from a focus of infection in maternal vagina *Empiric treatment* (culture negative): ampicillin + cefotaxime *Specific treatment:* penicillin G or ampicillin
Escherichia coli	Neonatal meningitis	Gram-negative rod Second most common cause of neonatal meningitis (18%) *Empiric treatment* (culture negative): ampicillin + cefotaxime *Specific treatment:* ceftazidime + gentamicin
Listeria monocytogenes	Neonatal meningitis	Gram-positive rod with tumbling motility; actin rockets help organism to move from cell to cell Pathogen found in soft cheese, hot dogs *Empiric treatment* (culture negative): ampicillin + cefotaxime *Specific treatment:* ampicillin ± gentamicin
Neisseria meningitidis	Meningitis	Gram-negative diplococcus; locates in posterior nasopharynx Most common cause of meningitis in those between 1 month and 18 years of age *Treatment:* ceftriaxone Prophylaxis for people in close contact: ciprofloxacin or rifampin or ceftriaxone
Streptococcus pneumoniae	Meningitis	Gram-positive diplococcus Most common cause of meningitis in patients > 18 years of age (some authors say *N. meningitidis* is the most common and *S. pneumoniae* the 2nd most common) *Treatment:* penicillin G or ampicillin
Mycobacterium tuberculosis	Meningitis	Complication of primary tuberculosis Involves base of brain Vasculitis (infarction) and scarring (hydrocephalus) *Treatment:* isoniazid, rifampin, ethambutol, pyrazinamide, dexamethasone (prevent scarring)

Treponema pallidum	Meningitis, encephalitis, myelitis	Spirochete
		Types of neurosyphilis:
		  Meningovascular: vasculitis causing strokes
		  General paresis: dementia
		  Tabes dorsalis: involves posterior root ganglia and posterior column; causes ataxia, loss of vibration sensation, absent deep tendon reflexes, Argyll-Robertson pupil (pupils accommodate but do *not* react)
		Treatment: penicillin G (difficult to treat)

TABLE 25-5. FUNGAL AND PARASITIC INFECTIONS OF THE CENTRAL NERVOUS SYSTEM

FUNGUS/PARASITE	DISEASE	COMMENTS
Cryptococcus neoformans (see Fig. 25-25A)	Meningitis and encephalitis	Occurs in immunocompromised host Most common fungal CNS infection in AIDS Budding yeasts visible with India ink *Treatment:* fluconazole non-AIDS, amphotericin + flucytosine
Mucor species (see Fig. 25-25B)	Frontal lobe abscess	Occurs in diabetic ketoacidosis; spreads from frontal sinuses *Treatment:* amphotericin B
Naegleria fowleri	Meningoencephalitis	Protozoa (amoeba) Involves frontal lobes Contracted by swimming in freshwater lakes *Treatment:* amphotericin B
Trypanosoma gambiense/ rhodesiense	Encephalitis	Protozoa (hemoflagellate) Transmission: bite of an infected tsetse fly (*Glossina*) Trypanosomes invade the blood and lymphatics early in the disease; initial drainage into the posterior cervical nodes produces lymphadenopathy (Winterbottom's sign); encephalitis occurs in later stages Diffuse encephalitis: somnolence ("sleeping sickness") due to the release of sleep mediators by the organisms Trypanosomes are capable of antigen variation (cyclical fever spike) Starvation is the most common cause of death Diagnosis: trypanosomes in blood, CSF; serologic tests; characteristic increase in IgM early in the disease *Treatment:* pentamidine early in the disease; melarsoprol in encephalitis stage

TABLE 25-5. FUNGAL AND PARASITIC INFECTIONS OF THE CENTRAL NERVOUS SYSTEM—cont'd

FUNGUS/PARASITE	DISEASE	COMMENTS
Taenia solium (see Fig. 25-25C)	Cysticercosis	Helminth (tapeworm; cestode); pig transmitted disease Patient (intermediate host) ingests food or water containing eggs; eggs develop into larval forms (cysticerci) that invade brain, producing calcified cysts causing seizures; hydrocephalus *Treatment*: albendazole + dexamethasone
Toxoplasma gondii (see Fig. 25-25D and E)	Encephalitis	Protozoa (sporozoan) Most common CNS space-occupying lesion in AIDS; ring-enhancing lesions on CT Congenital toxoplasmosis produces basal ganglia calcification *Treatment*: pyrimethamine + sulfadiazine + folinic acid (leucovorin)

AIDS, acquired immunodeficiency syndrome; CNS, central nervous system; CT, computed tomography.

(e) Weakness
  • Shoulder abduction; finger extension; foot dorsiflexion; hip/knee flexion
(4) Autonomic dysfunction
  (a) Urge incontinence
    • Hyperactive detrusor muscle (refer to Chapter 20)
  (b) Sexual dysfunction
  (c) Bowel motility problems
(5) Optic neuritis
  (a) Inflammation of the optic nerve
    • MS is the most common cause of optic neuritis.
  (b) Blurry vision or sudden loss of vision
(6) Cerebellar ataxia
(7) Scanning speech (sound drunk)
(8) Intention tremor, nystagmus
(9) Bilateral internuclear ophthalmoplegia (INO; Fig. 25-27C)
  • Demyelination of medial longitudinal fasciculus (MLF)
(10) Flexion of the neck produces an electrical sensation down the spine.
f. Laboratory findings (see Box 25-1)
  (1) Increased CSF leukocyte count
    • Primarily CD4 T lymphocytes
  (2) Increased CSF protein
    • Primarily an increase in γ-globulins
  (3) Increased CSF myelin basic protein
    • Indicates active disease
  (4) Normal CSF glucose
  (5) High-resolution electrophoresis shows oligoclonal bands.
    (a) Discrete bands of protein in the γ-globulin region (Fig. 25-27D)
    (b) Sign of demyelination
  (6) MRI is extremely sensitive in detecting demyelinating plaques (Fig. 25-27E).
g. Diagnosis
  (1) Spinal tap (see earlier text and Box 25-1)
  (2) MRI with gadolinium (most sensitive test)
h. Treatment
  (1) Acute relapse
    • High dose methylprednisolone
  (2) Chronic
    (a) Disease modifying drugs—e.g., interferon-beta
    (b) Monoclonal antibody—natalizumab
    (c) Cytotoxic—cyclophosphamide; methotrexate; azathioprine
i. Prognosis
  (1) Varies with the type of disease
  (2) On average, ~70% of patients with MS are alive 25 years after their diagnosis.
2. Central pontine myelinolysis (CPM; Fig. 25-28)
  a. Most often occurs in alcoholics who have hyponatremia
  b. Rapid intravenous correction causes demyelination in the basis pontis.
  c. Treatment is supportive.
3. Viral infections with direct infection of oligodendrocytes
  • Examples—subacute sclerosing panencephalitis, progressive multifocal leukoencephalopathy

Autonomic dysfunction: urge incontinence; sexual dysfunction; bowel motility dysfunction

MS: blurry vision due to optic neuritis; MS most common cause

SIN: scanning speech, intention tremor, nystagmus

Bilateral INO: pathognomonic for MS; demyelination of MLF

Lab: ↑ CSF lymphs, CSF protein, CSF MBP; normal CSF glucose

Oligoclonal bands in high-resolution electrophoresis: sign of demyelination

CPM: due to rapid IV correction of hyponatremia

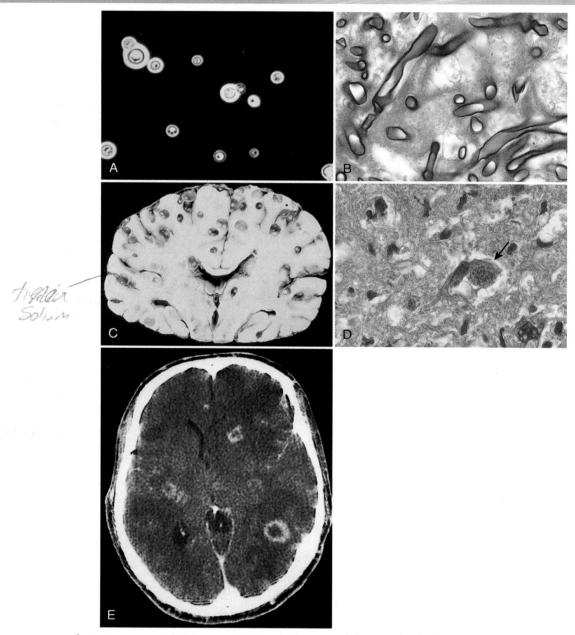

tylair Solium

25-26: A, *Cryptococcus.* India ink preparation showing large capsules surrounding budding yeast cells. **B,** *Mucor* species (zygomycosis). Note the broad, aseptate hyphae that have wide-angled branching. **C,** Neurocysticercosis. Note the multiple cysts located between the gray and white mater. **D,** Toxoplasmosis. Note the cyst (*arrow*) filled with bradyzoites. **E,** Toxoplasmosis. The computed tomographic scan shows multiple enhancing lesions. Toxoplasmosis is the most common space-occupying lesion in the brain in AIDS. It can be confused with primary central nervous system lymphoma. (*A and B from Murray PR, Shea YR: Medical Microbiology, 2nd ed. St. Louis, Mosby, 2002, pp 787, 794, Figs. 75-8, 75-18, respectively; C from Damjanov I, Linder J: Pathology: A Color Atlas. St. Louis, Mosby, 2000, p 411, Fig. 19-38; D from Burger PC, Scheithauer BW, Vogel KS: Surgical Pathology of the Nervous System, 4th ed. London, Churchill Livingstone, 2002, p 143, Fig. 3-78; E from Perkin GD: Mosby's Color Atlas and Text of Neurology. St. Louis, Mosby, 2002, p 216, Fig. 11-23.*)

C. Hereditary disorders

- Leukodystrophies are inborn errors of metabolism.

1. Adrenoleukodystrophy

   a. X-linked recessive (XR) disorder

   b. Enzyme deficiency in β-oxidation of fatty acids (FAs) in peroxisomes
      - Results in accumulation of long-chain fatty acids

   c. Causes generalized loss of myelin in the brain and adrenal insufficiency

2. Metachromatic leukodystrophy

   a. Autosomal recessive disorder
      - Lysosomal storage disease (LSD)

Adrenoleukodystrophy: XR; peroxisomal enzyme deficiency in β-oxidation of FAs

Metachromatic leukodystrophy: LSD; deficiency arylsulfatase A

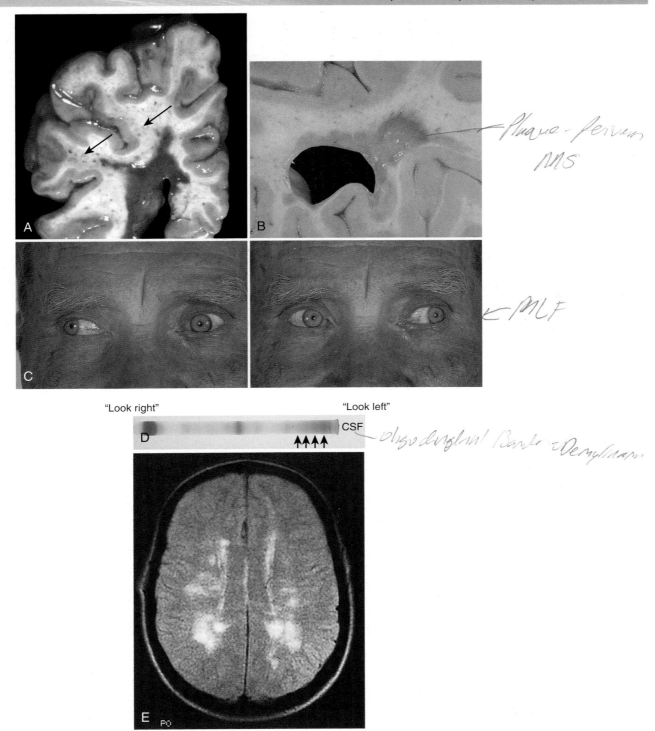

Plaque-periven MMS

← MLF

"Look right"   "Look left"

oligodendrial Bands = Demyelination

25-27: A, Multiple sclerosis, gross appearance. The brain shows multiple areas of demyelinated white mater (*arrows* pointing to gray-brown plaques). **B,** Multiple sclerosis, gross appearance. Note the periventricular location for the demyelinating plaques. **C,** Bilateral internuclear ophthalmoplegia in multiple sclerosis. When the patient is asked to look right, the right eye moves to the right and exhibits jerk nystagmus, while the left eye remains stationary. When the patient is asked to look left, the left eye moves to the left and shows jerk nystagmus, while the right eye remains stationary. These findings are due to bilateral demyelination of the medial longitudinal fasciculus. **D,** High-resolution electrophoresis of spinal fluid showing oligoclonal bands (*arrows*). Oligoclonal bands indicate the presence of demyelination. **E,** Magnetic resonance image showing extensive demyelination (white areas). (*A from Kumar V, Fausto N, Abbas A: Robbins and Cotran's Pathologic Basis of Disease, 7th ed. Philadelphia, WB Saunders, 2004, p 1383, Fig. 28-32; B from Klatt E: Robbins and Cotran's Atlas of Pathology. Philadelphia, WB Saunders, 2006, p 480, Fig. 19-105; C, D, and E from Perkin GD: Mosby's Color Atlas and Text of Neurology. St. Louis, Mosby, 2002, pp 183, 187, 188, Figs. 10-8, 10-14, 10-17, respectively.*)

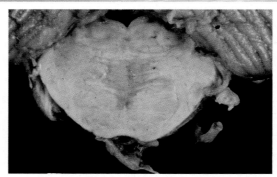

25-28: Central pontine myelinolysis. Note the central area of demyelination in the pons. *(From Damjanov I, Linder J: Pathology: A Color Atlas. St. Louis, Mosby, 2000, p 413, Fig. 19-45.)*

b. Deficiency of arylsulfatase A
• Results in accumulation of sulfatides
3. Krabbe's disease
a. Autosomal recessive disorder
• LSD
b. Galactocerebroside β-galactocerebrosidase deficiency
• Leads to accumulation of galactocerebroside
c. Brain shows large, multinucleated, histiocytic cells (globoid cells).

VII. Degenerative Disorders
• Degenerative diseases involve neurons in the brain or spinal cord.
A. Alzheimer's disease (AD)
1. Epidemiology
a. Most common cause of dementia (50–75% of all cases)
(1) Sporadic late onset type of AD (most common)
(2) Sporadic early onset type of AD (before age 65)
• Related to apolipoprotein gene E, allele ε4
(3) Familial early onset type of AD (<1% of cases)
(a) Mutations of amyloid precursor protein (APP) on chromosome 21
(b) Mutations in presenilin 1 on chromosome 14
(c) Mutations in presenilin 2 on chromosome 1
b. Prevalence increases with age.
(1) It is <1% in the 60- to 64-year-old age group.
(2) It is 40% to 50% by the age of 95.
c. Trisomy 21 (Down syndrome) has a strong association with AD.
• By 40 years of age, most Down syndrome patients have AD.
2. Role of β-amyloid (Aβ) protein in causing AD
a. Aβ is neurotoxic and damages neurons in the following sites:
(1) Medial temporal lobe structures
(2) Frontal cortex, especially the entorhinal cortex and hippocampus
b. Pivotal role of activated glycogen synthase kinase-3β (GSK) in neurotoxicity of Aβ
(1) Activation of GSK causes phosphorylation of Aβ, which in turn, produces:
(a) Neuronal and synaptic dysfunction
(b) Signaling for neuronal apoptosis
(2) Phosphorylated Aβ also has a positive feedback on GSK; hence, keeping the cycle of neurotoxicity in motion
(3) Initial activation of GSK has been traced to dysfunction within the Wnt (Wingless integration pathway), which is a family of genes normally involved in:
(a) Neuronal development during embryogenesis
(b) Normal neuronal function
(4) Normally, the Wnt signaling pathway inactivates GSK, hence preventing phosphorylation of Aβ and its harmful effect on neurons.
(5) However, if the Wnt signaling pathway is dysfunctional, GSK remains activated leading to phosphorylation of Aβ and its neurotoxic effects (e.g., apoptosis of neurons).
c. Aβ also deposits in the wall of cerebral vessels.
• Important in producing amyloid angiopathy (see later text)
d. Aβ stains positive with Congo red and has apple-green birefringence with polarization (refer to Chapter 3).

Krabbe's disease: LSD; deficiency galactocerebroside β-galactocerebrosidase

AD: most common overall cause of dementia

AD: sporadic late onset type most common type

AD: prevalence increases with age

AD: ↑ Aβ → neurotoxic

Activated GSK-3β: phosphorylates Aβ → neurotoxic

Aβ: can be converted into amyloid; deposits in cerebral vessels

e. Aβ is a metabolic product of APP.
   (1) APP is normally coded for on chromosome 21.
   (2) Defects in metabolism of APP by secretases cause an increase in Aβ.
   (3) α-Secretases cleave APP into fragments that *cannot* produce Aβ.
   (4) β-Secretases followed by γ-secretases cleave APP into fragments that are converted to Aβ.
   (5) In the sporadic early onset type of AD, apolipoprotein gene E, allele ε4 codes for a product that cannot eliminate Aβ from the brain leading to early onset of neurotoxicity.
f. Insulin degrading enzyme
   (1) Involved in the clearance of Aβ
   (2) Insulin resistance syndromes (type 2 diabetes; metabolic syndrome) have increased risk for AD, because increased insulin lowers insulin degrading enzyme, which increases Aβ.
3. Role of tau protein in AD
   a. Normal function is to maintain microtubules in neurons.
      • Assembles and supports scaffolding important in neuron structure and function
   b. Activated GSK enhances hyperphosphorylation of tau protein.
      (1) This process causes the protein to change shape and cluster into fibers.
      (2) Fibers appear as neurofibrillary (NF) tangles (twisted fibers) in the cytoplasm.
         • Best visualized with silver stains (Fig. 25-29)
      (3) NF tangles produce neuronal dysfunction including death of the neuron.
      (4) Pin 1 enzyme (prolyl isomerase) normally strips excess phosphate molecules from NF, restoring it to its original shape; however, in some cases of AD, this enzyme is absent or dysfunctional.
4. Gross and microscopic findings
   a. Cerebral atrophy with dilation of ventricles (hydrocephalus ex vacuo)
      (1) Due to loss of neurons in the temporal, frontal, and parietal lobes
      (2) Occipital lobe is usually spared.
   b. Presence of NF tangles in the cytoplasm of neurons
      (1) Best visualized with silver stains (see Fig. 25-29)
      (2) They may occur in other disorders.
         • Elderly patients *without* dementia, Huntington's disease, Niemann-Pick disease
   c. Senile (neuritic) plaques
      (1) Core of Aβ surrounded by neuronal cell processes containing tau protein, microglial cells, and astrocytes (Fig. 25-30)
         • Located in the gray mater.
      (2) Aβ stains with Congo red (refer to Chapter 3).
      (3) Best visualized with silver stains
      (4) Are also normally present in the brains of elderly people

Margin notes:

Aβ: metabolic product of APP; coded for on chromosome 21

Secretases: β-secretases followed by γ-secretases cleave APP to produce Aβ

Insulin degrading enzyme: involved in clearance of Aβ

Apo gene E, allele ε4: sporadic early onset AD

Activated GSK-3β: hyperphosphorylates tau protein

NF tangle: hyperphosphorylated tau protein in neuron

PIN 1 enzyme: dephosphorylates hyperphosphorylated tau protein; deficient in some cases of AD

AD: ↑ density of NF tangles and senile (neuritic) plaques in the brain

Senile (neuritic) plaques: core of Aβ surrounded by neuronal cell processes with tau protein

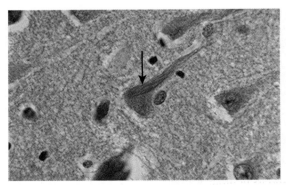

25-29: Neurofibrillary tangle. The stain shows a neuron with neurofilaments *(arrow)* composed of hyperphosphorylated tau protein. These are present in Alzheimer's disease. *(From Klatt E: Robbins and Cotran's Atlas of Pathology. Philadelphia, WB Saunders, 2006, p 481, Fig. 19-110.)*

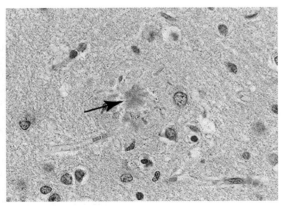

25-30: Senile plaque *(arrow)* shows an eosinophilic center with peripherally located distended neuronal processes (neurites). Like neurofibrillary tangles, these are present in Alzheimer's disease. *(From Burger PC, Scheithauer BW, Vogel KS: Surgical Pathology of the Nervous System, 4th ed. London, Churchill Livingstone, 2002, p 428, Fig. 8-9.)*

d. Amyloid angiopathy
   (1) Aβ is present in cerebral vessels.
   (2) Causes weakening of vessels with increased risk for hemorrhage
e. Confirmation of Alzheimer's disease
   (1) Requires postmortem examination of the brain
   (2) Must be widespread presence of NF tangles and senile plaques

5. Clinical findings
   a. Prominent early sign is the decline in short-term memory.
   b. Another early sign is loss of smell.
      • Dysfunction in entorhinal cortex
   c. Patients with mild to moderate disease have only cognitive defects.
   d. Additional deficits accumulate, including changes in behavior, judgment, language, and abstract thought.
   e. Even later in the course, functional deficits manifest in the patient not being able to care for themselves.
   f. *No* focal neurologic deficits are present early in the disease.
   g. Patients usually die of an infection.
      • Example—intercurrent bronchopneumonia

6. Presumptive diagnosis is made with mental status testing; tests for:
   a. Orientation
   b. Attention
   c. Verbal recall
   d. Language
   e. Visual-spatial skills

7. Positron emission tomography (PET) is useful the differential diagnosis of dementia.

8. Treatment
   a. Cholinesterase inhibitors
      • Increase synaptic transmission
   b. Memantine (blocks glutamate receptors)

B. Parkinsonism

1. Epidemiology
   a. Group of disorders that alter dopaminergic pathways involved in voluntary muscle movement
      (1) Striatal system is involved in voluntary muscle movement.
         • Substantia nigra, caudate, putamen, globus pallidus, subthalamus, thalamus
      (2) Dopamine is the principal neurotransmitter in the nigrostriatal tract.
         • Connects the substantia nigra with the caudate and putamen
   b. Incidence increases with age.
   c. Idiopathic Parkinson's disease is the most common type (see below).
   d. Other causes of parkinsonism
      (1) Encephalitis, ischemia
      (2) Chronic carbon monoxide poisoning
         • Causes necrosis of globus pallidus
      (3) Wilson's disease
      (4) Addiction to MPTP, a derivative of meperidine
         • 1-Methyl-4-phenyl-1,2,3,6-tetrahydropyridine
      (5) Antipsychotic drugs (e.g., phenothiazines)

2. Idiopathic Parkinson's disease
   a. Epidemiology
      (1) Occurs between 45 and 65 years of age
      (2) Distribution is equal in men and women.
      (3) Most cases are sporadic.
   b. Pathophysiology
      (1) Degeneration/depigmentation of neurons in substantia nigra (Fig. 25-31)
      (2) Causes deficiency of dopamine
      (3) Neurons contain intracytoplasmic, eosinophilic bodies called Lewy bodies.
         • Ubiquinated damaged neurofilaments (refer to Chapter 1)
   c. Clinical findings
      (1) Muscle rigidity
         (a) Slowness of voluntary muscle movement (bradykinesia)
         (b) Cogwheel rigidity on physical examination

Margin notes:

Amyloid angiopathy: risk for cerebral hemorrhage

Confirmation of AD: must be made at autopsy

AD: prominent early sign is decline in short-term memory

AD: presumptive diagnosis with mental status testing; rule out all other causes of dementia

Parkinsonism: alteration in dopaminergic pathways involved in voluntary muscle movement

Dopamine: principal neurotransmitter in nigrostriatal tract

Idiopathic Parkinson's disease: most common cause of parkinsonism

Idiopathic Parkinson's disease: depigmentation substantia nigra neurons; ↓ dopamine

Clinical: rigidity, resting tremor, bradykinesia

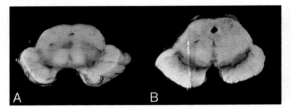

25-31: Substantia nigra in Parkinson disease. **A,** The pigmentation in the substantia nigra of the midbrain is markedly diminished, when compared to the normal amount of pigmentation (**B**). *(From Damjanov I, Linder J: Pathology: A Color Atlas. St. Louis, Mosby, 2000, p 419, Fig. 19-67.)*

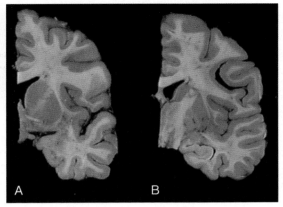

25-32: Huntington's disease. The coronal section (**B**) shows atrophy of the caudate, putamen, and globus pallidus when compared with a normal coronal section (**A**). *(From Perkin GD: Mosby's Color Atlas and Text of Neurology. St. Louis, Mosby, 2002, p 156, Fig. 8-19A and B.)*

(2) Resting tremor
    (a) "Pill rolling" between thumb and index fingers
    (b) Illegible handwriting
(3) Expressionless face ("poker face"), stooped posture
(4) Difficulty in initiating first step; shuffling gait
(5) Blepharospasm; postural instability
(6) Commonly have severe seborrheic dermatitis (refer to Chapter 24)
(7) Dementia in some cases

> Idiopathic Parkinsonism: expressionless face; blepharospasm; seborrheic dermatitis

3. Treatment
  a. Avoid drugs that worsen parkinsonism—neuroleptics, antiemetics, monoamine oxidase (MAO) inhibitors
  b. Levodopa—transformed into dopamine
  c. Carbidopa, benserazide—dopa decarboxylase inhibitors
  d. Bromocriptine, pergolide—dopamine agonists
  e. Selegiline, rasagiline—inhibit monoamine oxidase-B, which inhibits breakdown of dopamine
  f. Specialized surgical procedures

C. Huntington's disease (HD)
1. Epidemiology
  a. Autosomal dominant disease
  b. Trinucleotide repeat disorder (CAG) involving chromosome 4 (refer to Chapter 5)
  c. Delayed appearance of symptoms until 30 to 40 years of age
  d. No gender dominance

> HD: AD; trinucleotide repeat disorder

2. Atrophy/loss of striatal neurons
  • Caudate, putamen, globus pallidus (Fig. 25-32)

> HD: atrophy of caudate nucleus, putamen, globus pallidus

3. Clinical findings
  a. Chorea
    (1) Irregular, rapid, nonstereotyped involuntary movements
    (2) Called choreoathetosis if it has a writhing quality
  b. Oculomotor abnormalities
  c. Parkinsonism in later stages
  d. Depression

> HD: chorea; oculomotor abnormalities

4. Diagnosis
  a. Genetic testing is available
  b. Imaging studies (CT, MRI)
    • Atrophy of caudate and putamen
5. Treatment is supportive.

D. Friedreich's ataxia
1. Epidemiology
  a. Autosomal recessive (AR) disease
    (1) Trinucleotide repeat disorder (GAA)

(2) Frataxin deficiency
    (a) Leads to impaired mitochondrial iron homeostasis
    (b) Cells are more prone to apoptosis.
  b. Most common neurodegenerative hereditary ataxic disorder
  c. Sites of degeneration
    (1) Dorsal root ganglia
    (2) Posterior columns
    (3) Spinocerebellar tract
    (4) Lateral corticospinal tracts
    (5) Large sensory peripheral neurons
  d. Hypertrophic cardiomyopathy
  e. Type 1 diabetes mellitus (10%)
 2. Clinical findings
  a. Progressive gait ataxia
  b. Loss of deep tendon reflexes
    • Initially at the ankles
  c. Loss of vibratory sensation and proprioception
  d. Muscle weakness in the legs
 3. Diagnosis
  a. Gene testing is available.
  b. Imaging (MRI) shows spinal cord atrophy.
 4. Treatment is supportive.

E. Lou Gehrig's disease (amyotrophic lateral sclerosis [ALS])
 1. Epidemiology
  a. Degenerative disease involving upper and lower motor neurons
  b. Symptoms usually appear between 40 and 60 years of age.
  c. Most cases are sporadic (90–95%).
  d. Familial cases involve mutations on chromosome 21.
    (1) Defective superoxide dismutase 1
    (2) Produces superoxide free radical injury of neurons

 2. Clinical findings
  a. Upper motor neuron (UMN) signs
    • Spasticity, Babinski's sign
  b. Lower motor neuron (LMN) signs
    (1) Muscle weakness
      • Begins with atrophy of intrinsic muscles of the hands
    (2) Eventual paralysis of respiratory muscles

  c. No sensory changes
  d. Preservation of bowel and bladder function
 3. Diagnosis
  • Electromyography and nerve conduction studies
 4. Treatment
  • Riluzole (glutamate antagonist)
 5. Average survival time is 3 to 5 years.

F. Werdnig-Hoffmann disease
  • Lower motor neuron disease that occurs in children

VIII. Toxic and Metabolic Disorders
 A. Wilson's disease (refer to Chapter 18)
  1. Autosomal recessive disease
    a. Defect in copper excretion in bile
    b. Defect incorporation of copper into ceruloplasmin
    c. Leads to liver cirrhosis and excess free copper in blood

  2. CNS findings
    a. Atrophy and cavitation of basal ganglia, particularly globus pallidus and putamen (Fig. 25-33)
    b. Signs of parkinsonism, chorea, and dementia
 B. Acute intermittent porphyria (AIP)
  1. Epidemiology
    a. Autosomal dominant disorder
    b. Defect in porphyrin metabolism
      (1) Deficiency of uroporphyrinogen synthase (porphobilinogen deaminase)
      (2) Proximal increase in porphobilinogen (PBG) and δ-aminolevulinic acid (ALA)

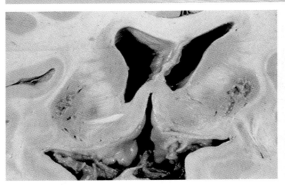

25-33: Wilson's disease. Note cavitary necrosis of the putamen on both sides of the brain. *(From Damjanov I, Linder J: Pathology: A Color Atlas. St. Louis, Mosby, 2000, p 413, Fig. 19-43.)*

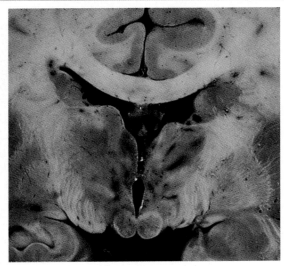

25-34: Wernicke's encephalopathy showing hemorrhage and discoloration of mamillary bodies and the wall of the third ventricle. *(From Damjanov I, Linder J: Pathology: A Color Atlas. St. Louis, Mosby, 2000, p 413, Fig. 19-43.)*

    (3) Urine is *colorless* when first voided.

        (a) Exposure to light causes oxidation of PBG to porphobilin producing port-wine color.

        (b) Classic "window-sill test"

    (4) Heme has a negative feedback relationship with ALA synthase.

      • ALA synthase is the rate-limiting enzyme of porphyrin metabolism.

    (5) Decreasing heme precipitates porphyric attacks by increasing porphyrin synthesis.

      • Example—drugs enhancing liver cytochrome P-450 system (e.g., alcohol)

  2. Clinical findings

    a. Neurologic dysfunction

      (1) Recurrent bouts of severe abdominal pain simulating acute abdomen

      (2) Often mistaken for a surgical abdomen

        • Patient has "bellyful of scars."

    b. Psychosis

    c. Peripheral neuropathy

    d. Dementia

  3. Diagnosis

    • Enzyme assay in RBCs

  4. Treatment

    a. Avoid drugs that precipitate attacks

    b. Carbohydrate loading with glucose

      • Inhibits ALA synthase

C. Vitamin B$_{12}$ deficiency (refer to Chapter 11)

  1. Subacute combined degeneration of the spinal cord

    • Posterior column and lateral corticospinal tract demyelination

  2. Dementia, peripheral neuropathy

D. CNS findings associated with alcohol abuse

  1. Cortical and cerebellar atrophy

  2. Central pontine myelinolysis (see Fig. 25-28)

  3. Wernicke-Korsakoff syndrome

    a. Most often due to thiamine deficiency (refer to Chapter 7)

    b. Gross and microscopic findings

      (1) Hemorrhages with hemosiderin deposits

        • Mamillary bodies, wall of the third and fourth ventricles (Fig. 25-34)

      (2) Neuronal loss, gliosis, vessel hemorrhage

    c. Wernicke's encephalopathy; reversible findings:

      • Confusion, ataxia, nystagmus, ophthalmoplegia (eye muscle weakness)

Margin notes:

AIP: urine colorless when first voided; exposure to light produces color

AIP: deficiency uroporphyrinogen synthase; "bellyful of scars"; peripheral neuropathy; dementia

Rx AIP: carbohydrate loading inhibits ALA synthase

Vitamin B$_{12}$ deficiency: subacute combined degeneration; dementia

Wernicke-Korsakoff syndrome: hemorrhage in mamillary bodies

Wernicke's encephalopathy: confusion, ataxia, nystagmus, ophthalmoplegia

d. Korsakoff's psychosis
   (1) Advanced irreversible stage of Wernicke's encephalopathy
      • Targets the limbic system
   (2) Anterograde amnesia (inability to form new memories)
   (3) Retrograde amnesia (inability to recall old memories)
   (4) Confabulation
   (5) Hallucinations
4. Treatment
   • Thiamine supplementation

Alcoholics receiving IV infusion with glucose: supplement IV with thiamine to prevent acute Wernicke's encephalopathy

Most common primary CNS tumor in adults: glioblastoma multiforme

Childhood tumors: cystic astrocytoma and medulloblastoma, both in cerebellum

Clinical: headache, seizures, intracranial hypertension

Astrocytoma: most common neuroglial tumor

GBM: grade IV astrocytoma; often crosses corpus callosum; hemorrhagic/cystic

Meningioma: most common benign brain tumor in adults

Meningioma: female predominance; psammoma bodies

IX. **CNS Tumors**
   A. **Epidemiology**
      1. Primary brain tumors in adults
         a. Approximately 70% occur above the tentorium cerebelli.
         b. In order of decreasing frequency:
            • Glioblastoma multiforme, meningioma, ependymoma
      2. Primary brain tumors in children
         a. Second most common cancer in children
         b. Approximately 70% occur *below* the tentorium cerebelli.
         c. In order of decreasing frequency:
            • Cystic cerebellar astrocytoma, medulloblastoma, brainstem glioma
      3. Risk factors
         • Turcot's syndrome, neurofibromatosis, cigarette smoking
      4. General clinical findings
         a. Headache (20% initially, 60% later)
            (1) Tend to be worse during the night; wakes person up
            (2) Accompanied by nausea and vomiting
         b. Seizures (>30%)
         c. Symptoms/signs of intracranial hypertension (see section I)
      5. Imaging studies
         a. MRI with gadolinium enhancement
         b. CT scan useful if calcium or hemorrhage is present
         c. Functional MRI for lesions in vital areas
         d. PET
      6. Treatment modalities
         • Surgery, irradiation, chemotherapy
   B. **Astrocytoma**
      1. Accounts for about 70% of all neuroglial tumors
         a. Usually involves frontal lobe in adults
         b. Usually involves the cerebellum in children
         c. Grades I and II are low-grade cancers.
         d. Grades III and IV are high-grade cancers.
      2. Glioblastoma multiforme (GBM)
         a. High-grade astrocytoma
            (1) May arise de novo
            (2) May arise from dedifferentiation of a low-grade astrocytoma
         b. Hemorrhagic tumor (Fig. 25-35A)
            (1) Multifocal areas of necrosis and cystic degeneration
            (2) Commonly cross the corpus callosum
         c. May seed the neuraxis via the CSF
            • Rarely metastasize outside the CNS
         d. Generally poor prognosis
   C. **Meningioma**
      1. Most common benign brain tumor in adults
         • Female predominance (tumors have estrogen receptors)
      2. Derived from arachnoidal cells
         • Locations—parasagittal location, olfactory groove, lesser wing of sphenoid
      3. Associated with neurofibromatosis, history of radiation
      4. Gross and microscopic findings (Fig. 25-35B and C)
         a. Firm tumors
            (1) May indent *(not invade)* the surface of brain

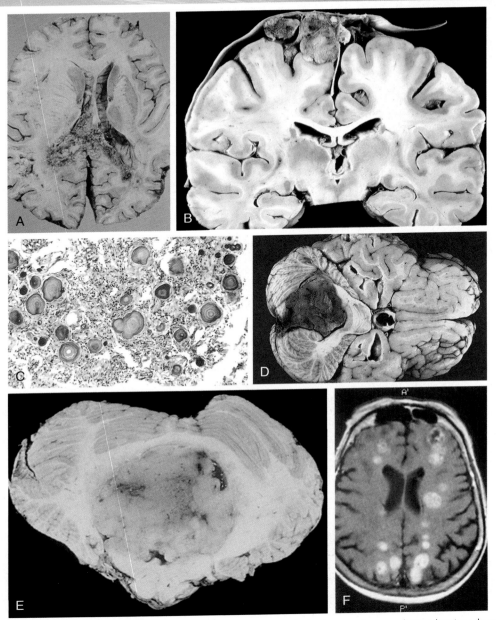

25-35: **A,** Glioblastoma multiforme showing hemorrhage and necrosis in the brain parenchyma and spreading into the adjacent hemisphere via the corpus callosum. **B,** Meningioma. Note the parasagittal multilobular tumor that is attached to the overlying dura. The tumor compresses the underlying surface of the brain. **C,** Meningioma. Note the swirling meningothelial cells and numerous basophilic staining psammoma bodies. **D,** Ependymoma of fourth ventricle. Note the hemorrhagic mass filling and expanding the fourth ventricle. **E,** Medulloblastoma. In the cerebellum there is a centrally located hemorrhagic tumor with necrosis that has almost compressed shut the fourth ventricle. **F,** Brain metastasis. The magnetic resonance image shows multiple nodular enhancing masses of varying sizes representing metastases from a breast cancer. *(A from Damjanov I, Linder J: Anderson's Pathology, 10th ed. St. Louis, Mosby, 1996, p 2750, Fig. 77-120; **B** and **C** from Kumar V, Fausto N, Abbas A: Robbins and Cotran's Pathologic Basis of Disease, 7th ed. Philadelphia, WB Saunders, 2004, p 1409, Fig. 28-48A and 28-48B, respectively; **D** from Klatt E: Robbins and Cotran's Atlas of Pathology. Philadelphia, WB Saunders, 2006, p 487, Fig. 19-127; **E** from Damjanov I, Linder J: Pathology: A Color Atlas. St. Louis, Mosby, 2000, p 424, Fig. 19-82; **F** from Katz D, Math K, Groskin S: Radiology Secrets. Philadelphia, Hanley & Belfus, 1998, p 349, Fig. 1.)*

(2) Often infiltrate overlying bone
- Causes increased bone density

    b. Swirling masses of meningothelial cells encompass psammoma bodies (calcified bodies).

5. Common cause of new-onset focal seizures

D. Ependymoma

    1. Benign tumor derived from ependymal cells (Fig. 25-35D)

Ependymoma: fourth ventricle in children; cauda equina in adults

2. Arises in cauda equina in adults
3. Arises in fourth ventricle in children

E. Medulloblastoma

Medulloblastoma: small cell tumor of cerebellum

1. Malignant small cell tumor
   - Primarily occurs in children
2. Arises from the external granular cell layer of the cerebellum (Fig. 25-35E)
3. Often seeds the neuraxis and invades the fourth ventricle

F. Oligodendroglioma

Oligodendroglioma: frontal lobe calcifications in an adult

1. Benign tumor derived from oligodendrocytes
   - Primarily occurs in adults
2. Frontal lobe tumor that frequently calcifies

G. CNS lymphoma

Primary CNS lymphoma: occurs in AIDS; EBV-mediated cancer

1. Majority are metastatic high-grade B-cell non-Hodgkin's lymphomas.
2. Primary CNS lymphomas
   a. Most often associated with AIDS
   b. Epstein-Barr virus (EBV)–mediated B-cell lymphomas
   c. Rapidly increasing due to the increase in AIDS

H. Metastasis

Most common brain malignancy

1. Most common brain malignancy: metastasis (Fig. 25-35F)
2. In order of decreasing frequency:
   - Lung, breast, skin (melanoma), kidney, gastrointestinal tract

X. Peripheral Nervous System Disorders

A. Peripheral neuropathies

Sensory changes: demyelination—paresthesias; "glove and stocking" distribution

Motor changes: axon degeneration—muscle fasciculations, atrophy

1. Associated with demyelination and axonal degeneration
   a. Demyelination is often segmental.
      - Sensory changes (e.g., paresthesias), often in a "glove and stocking" distribution
   b. Axonal degeneration
      - Muscle fasciculations leading to muscle atrophy

CMT: most common hereditary neuropathy

CMT: lower legs have "inverted bottle" appearance

2. Charcot-Marie-Tooth (CMT) disease
   a. Most common hereditary neuropathy
      - Autosomal dominant disease
   b. Peroneal nerve neuropathy
      (1) Causes atrophy of muscles of lower legs
      (2) Legs have an "inverted bottle" appearance.
   c. Treatment is supportive.

GBS: most common acute peripheral neuropathy

3. Guillain-Barré syndrome (GBS)
   a. Epidemiology
      (1) Most common acute peripheral neuropathy
      (2) Most common cause of acute flaccid paralysis
      (3) Predominantly motor involvement
      (4) Variants can be motor and sensory
      (5) Autoimmune demyelination syndrome
         (a) Involves nerve roots and peripheral nerves
         (b) Common preceding infections

Preceding infections: *M. pneumoniae, C. jejuni*, viruses

            - *Mycoplasma pneumoniae* pneumonia, *Campylobacter jejuni* enteritis, viral infection (HIV, EBV, cytomegalovirus, influenza)
   b. Rapidly progressive ascending motor weakness
      (1) Less commonly descending motor weakness
      (2) Usually starts in proximal muscles and eventually includes distal muscles
      (3) Danger of respiratory muscle paralysis and death

GBS causes ascending paralysis.

   c. Depressed or absent deep tendon reflexes in arms and legs
   d. "Glove and stocking" paresthesias/anesthesia
   e. Laboratory findings (see Box 25-1)
      (1) Increased CSF protein
         - Oligoclonal bands present on high-resolution electrophoresis
      (2) CSF glucose, cell count normal
   f. Diagnosis
      (1) Spinal tap with increased CSF protein
      (2) Electromyography and nerve conduction studies

Rx GBS: IV immunoglobulin or plasma exchange

   g. Treatment
      (1) Infusion IV immunoglobulin or plasma exchange
      (2) Mechanical ventilation if required

h. Prognosis
   (1) Mortality 5% to 10%
   (2) Full motor recovery 60%
   (3) Residual weakness 15%
4. Diabetes mellitus (DM)
   a. Most common cause of peripheral neuropathy
   b. Due to osmotic damage of Schwann cells (refer to Chapter 22)
5. Toxin-associated neuropathies
   • Alcohol, heavy metals, diphtheria
6. Idiopathic Bell's palsy
   a. Lower motor neuron palsy causing unilateral facial paralysis
   b. Inflammatory reaction of facial nerve (CN VII)
      • Near the stylomastoid foramen or in the bony facial canal
   c. May be associated with herpes simplex virus (HSV, most common), HIV, sarcoidosis, Lyme disease, pregnancy
      • Often bilateral in Lyme disease
   d. Clinical findings in LMN disease (Figs. 25-36 and 25-37)
      (1) Ipsilateral upper and lower face involvement
      (2) Drooping of the corner of the mouth
      (3) Difficulty speaking
      (4) Inability to close the eye
      (5) Hyperacusis in some cases
   e. Clinical findings in UMN disease (see Fig. 25-37)
      (1) Contralateral lower face involvement
      (2) Contralateral sparing of the upper face
7. Drugs producing peripheral neuropathy
   • Examples—vincristine, hydralazine, phenytoin
8. Vitamin deficiencies producing peripheral neuropathy
   • Examples—deficiency of thiamine, vitamin B$_{12}$, pyridoxine
9. Treatment of peripheral neuropathies; reduce nerve pain:
   a. Antiseizure medications—gabapentin, carbamazepine, phenytoin
   b. Lidocaine patch
   c. Tricyclic antidepressants—amitriptyline, nortriptyline

Margin notes:

DM: most common cause of peripheral neuropathy

Idiopathic Bell's palsy: facial muscle paralysis due to inflammation of CN VII

Idiopathic Bell's palsy: HSV most common association

LMN Bell's palsy: ipsilateral weakness upper/lower face

UMN Bell's palsy: contralateral weakness lower face; sparing of upper face

Drugs: vincristine, hydralazine, phenytoin

Vitamin deficiencies: thiamine, pyridoxine, vitamin B$_{12}$

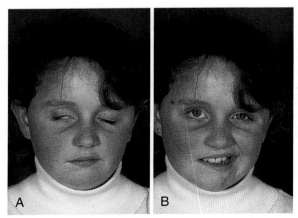

"Close your eyes."   "Open your eyes and smile."

25-36: Right-sided Bell's palsy showing inability to fully close the eye (**A**) and drooping of the corner of the mouth (**B**). *(From Perkin GD: Mosby's Color Atlas and Text of Neurology. St. Louis, Mosby, 2002, p 77, Fig. 4-24A and B.)*

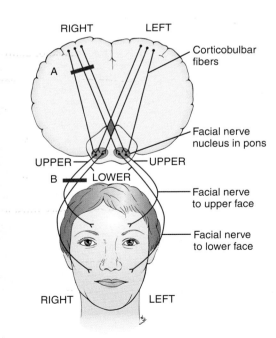

RIGHT   LEFT
Corticobulbar fibers
Facial nerve nucleus in pons
UPPER   UPPER
LOWER
Facial nerve to upper face
Facial nerve to lower face
RIGHT   LEFT

25-37: Schematic of lower and upper motor neuron Bell's palsy. See text for discussion. *(From Swartz MH: Textbook of Physical Diagnosis, 5th ed. Philadelphia, Saunders Elsevier, 2006, p 677, Fig. 21-16.)*

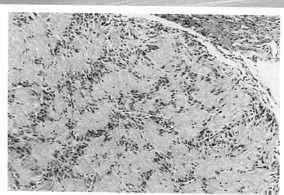

25-38: Acoustic neuroma showing spindle-shaped cells with alternating dark and light areas. *(From Damjanov I, Linder J: Pathology: A Color Atlas. St. Louis, Mosby, 2000, p 432, Fig. 19-107.)*

Schwannoma: benign tumor of Schwann cells

Acoustic neuroma: schwannoma of CN VIII

B. Schwannoma (neurilemoma)
1. Benign tumor derived from Schwann cells
   a. CN V (trigeminal) and VIII (acoustic) may be involved.
   b. Spinal nerve roots, peripheral nerves may be involved.
2. Acoustic neuroma
   a. Schwannoma of CN VIII
   b. Majority are located in the cerebellopontine angle.
      (1) Encapsulated tumors
      (2) Usually unilateral
      (3) Microscopic view shows alternating dark and light areas (Fig. 25-38).
   c. Clinical findings
      (1) Associated with neurofibromatosis (NF2)
         • Usually bilateral tumors

TABLE 25-6. SELECTED NERVE INJURIES

INJURY	COMMENTS
Ulnar nerve (C8–T1) (see Fig. 25-39A)	Fracture of medial epicondyle of the humerus Injury produces a "claw hand" (loss of interosseous muscles)
Radial nerve (C5–T1) (see Fig. 25-39B)	Midshaft fractures of humerus Draping the arm over a park bench (called "Saturday night palsy") Injury produces wrist drop
Axillary nerve (C5-6)	Fracture of surgical neck of humerus; anterior dislocation of the shoulder joint (may also injure the axillary artery) Cannot abduct the arm to horizontal position or hold the horizontal position when a downward force is applied to the arm (paralysis of deltoid muscle)
Median nerve (C6–T1) (see Fig. 25-39C and D)	Most commonly due to entrapment in the transverse carpal ligament of the wrist or between the bellies of the pronator teres muscle Rheumatoid arthritis and pregnancy two most common causes; also overuse of hands and wrist (e.g., in barbers), amyloidosis, hypothyroidism, supracondylar fracture of humerus Clinical: nocturnal pain; pain, numbness, or paresthesias in the thumb, index finger, third finger, and radial side of fourth finger; thenar atrophy produces an "ape" hand appearance and difficulty in opposing the thumb with the 5th finger Tinel's sign: pain reproduced by tapping over the median nerve Phalen's sign: pain reproduced with forced flexion of the wrist for 1 minute Diagnosis: nerve conduction studies; electromyography to rule out muscle degeneration related to nerve compression

Common peroneal nerve (L4–S2) (see Fig. 25-39E) *PRO*	Common peripheral neuropathy; lead poisoning; fractured neck of the fibula; cast tightness
	Motor deficits:
	   Loss of foot eversion due to weakening of the peroneus longus and brevis muscles
	   Loss of foot dorsiflexion due to weakening of the tibialis anterior muscle produces "slapping gait" or "high-stepping gait" like a horse
	   Loss of toe extension due to weakening of the extensor digitorum longus and hallucis longus muscles
	   Combined effect of all the above produces an equinovarus deformity, where there is plantar flexion with foot drop and inversion of the foot
	Sensory deficits involve the anterolateral aspect of the leg and dorsum of the foot
	Loss of the ankle jerk reflex

Erb-Duchenne palsy (see Fig. 25-39F)	Brachial plexus lesion involving C5 and C6 "Waiter's tip deformity"

(2) Tinnitus (ringing in the ears)
(3) Sensorineural deafness
(4) Sensory changes in CN V distribution
  • Due to tumor impingement on CN V
  d. Treatment is surgery.
C. Selected peripheral nerve injuries (Table 25-6 and Fig. 25-39)

XI. Selected Eye Disorders (Table 25-7 and Fig. 25-40)
XII. Selected Ear Disorders (Table 25-8 and Figs. 25-41 and 25-42)

Acoustic neuroma: tinnitus and sensorineural hearing loss

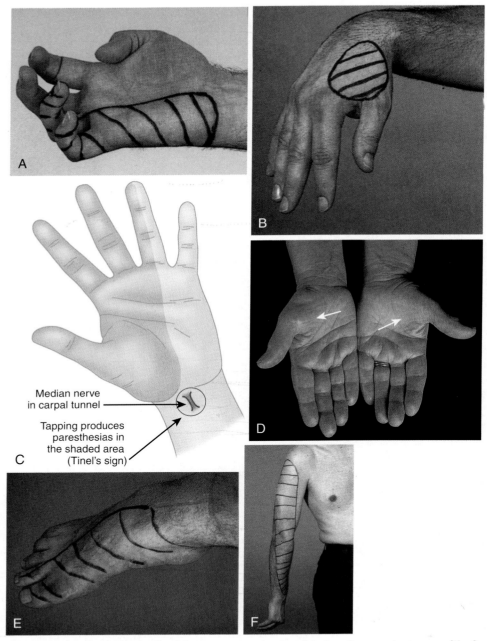

Median nerve in carpal tunnel

Tapping produces paresthesias in the shaded area (Tinel's sign)

25-39: A, Ulnar nerve injury. Note the claw hand due to an opposed action of the long flexors and extensors of the fingers. The ink markings show the distribution of impaired sensation. **B,** Radial nerve injury. Note the wrist drop. The ink markings show the distribution of impaired sensation. **C,** Effect of carpal tunnel syndrome on the median nerve. See text for discussion. **D,** *Arrows* show atrophy of thenar eminence. **E,** Common peroneal nerve injury. Note the foot drop. The ink markings show the distribution of impaired sensation. **F,** Erb-Duchenne palsy. Note how the arm is internally rotated and the forearm pronated producing a "waiter's tip" deformity. The ink markings show the distribution of impaired sensation of the outer side of the upper arm. *(A, B, E, and F from Grieg JD: Color Atlas of Surgical Diagnosis. London, Mosby-Wolfe, 1996, pp 337, 334, 338, 332, Figs. 42.8, 42.4, 42.9, 42.2, respectively; C from Goldman L, Ausiello D: Cecil's Textbook of Medicine, 23rd ed. Philadelphia, Saunders Elsevier, 2008, p 2008, Fig. 285-5; D from Perkin GD: Mosby's Color Atlas and Text of Neurology. St. Louis, Mosby, 2002, p 224, Fig. 12.10A.)*

TABLE 25-7. **SELECTED EYE DISORDERS**

EYE DISORDER	DISCUSSION
Arcus senilis (see Fig. 25-40A)	Most often occurs in elderly Gray-opaque ring at the corneal margin (periphery of cornea) Cholesterol deposits in corneal stroma; may indicate hypercholesterolemia if patient is <50 years old and a smoker

Ophthalmia neonatorum	Conjunctivitis in newborn
	Pathogens: *Neisseria gonorrhoeae* (first week; 2–4 days), *Chlamydia trachomatis* (second week; 3–10 days)
	Treatment:
	    N. gonorrhoeae: ceftriaxone
	    C. trachomatis: erythromycin
	    Erythromycin eye drops (chemical irritation)

Bacterial conjunctivitis (see Fig. 25-40B)	Purulent conjunctivitis; pain but *no blurry vision* Pathogens: *Staphylococcus aureus* (most common), *Streptococcus pneumoniae, Haemophilus influenzae* (*H. aegyptius*, pink eye) *Treatment:* gatifloxacin ophthalmic solution
Viral conjunctivitis (see Fig. 25-40C)	Watery exudates Adenovirus: viral cause of pink eye, preauricular lymphadenopathy No treatment HSV-1: keratoconjunctivitis with dendritic ulcers noted with fluorescein staining *Treatment:* trifluridine ophthalmic
Allergic conjunctivitis	Seasonal itching of eyes *Treatment:* antihistamine ophthalmic solutions; olopatadine (mast cell stabilizer)
Acanthamoeba infection	Severe keratoconjunctivitis in patients who do not clean their contact lenses properly *Treatment:* propamidine + polymyxin/neomycin/gramicidin ophthalmic
Stye (see Fig. 25-40D)	Infection of eyelid most commonly due to *S. aureus* *Treatment:* hot packs + dicloxacillin
Chalazion (see Fig. 25-40E)	Granulomatous inflammation involving the meibomian gland in the eyelid; usually disappear on their own within 2 months *Treatment:* if do not disappear; intralesional corticosteroid injection or surgical removal
Orbital cellulitis	Periorbital redness and swelling that is often secondary to sinusitis (e.g., ethmoiditis in children) Pathogens: *S. pneumoniae, H. influenzae* Fever, proptosis (eye bulges out), periorbital swelling, ophthalmoplegia (eye movement impaired), normal retinal examination *Treatment:* nafcillin + ceftriaxone + metronidazole
Orbital fracture (see Fig. 25-40F)	Most often associated with blunt trauma to the eye that produces an orbital floor fracture Often associated with edema and ecchymoses of the eyelids and periorbital region ("raccoon" eyes) Vertical diplopia, prolapse of orbital contents into the maxillary sinus (sunken eye), damage to infraorbital nerve may occur in severe fractures *Treatment:* varies according to degree of severity
Pterygium	Raised, triangular encroachment of thickened conjunctiva on the nasal side of the conjunctiva; may grow onto cornea Due to excessive exposure to wind, sun, and sand *Treatment:* surgical removal
Pinguecula (see Fig. 25-40G)	Yellow-white conjunctival degeneration at the junction of cornea and sclera on the temporal side of the conjunctiva Does not grow onto the cornea like a pterygium does Usually requires no treatment
Optic neuritis	Inflammation of optic nerve Causes: multiple sclerosis (most common), methanol poisoning Blurry vision or loss of vision, may cause optic atrophy *Treatment:* corticosteroids

TABLE 25-7. **SELECTED EYE DISORDERS—cont'd**

EYE DISORDER	DISCUSSION
Central retinal artery occlusion (see Fig. 25-40H)	Causes: embolization of plaque material from ipsilateral carotid or ophthalmic artery; giant cell temporal arteritis involving the ophthalmic artery Sudden, painless, complete loss of vision in one eye, pallor of optic disk due to narrowed arteries, "boxcar" segmentation of blood in retinal veins, cherry red macula *Treatment*: acetazolamide to lower intraocular pressure; carbogen (CO_2 dilates + O_2); hyperbaric O_2 therapy
Central retinal vein occlusion (see Fig. 25-40I)	Causes: hypercoagulable state (e.g., polycythemia vera) Sudden, painless, unilateral loss of vision, swelling of optic disk, engorged retinal veins with hemorrhage ("blood and thunder" appearance) *Treatment*: intravitreal injections; laser photocoagulation
Glaucoma (see Fig. 25-40J)	Increased intraocular pressure *Chronic open angle type:* Decreased rate of aqueous outflow into the canal of Schlemm; bilateral aching eyes; pathologic cupping of optic disks; night blindness and gradual loss of peripheral vision leading to tunnel vision and blindness *Treatment*: 1st: β-blockers (e.g., timolol; decrease rate of flow into eye); 2nd: prostaglandins, α-adrenergic agonists, pilocarpine, carbonic anhydrase inhibitors; if drugs fail, laser trabeculoplasty *Acute angle-closure type:* Due to narrowing of anterior chamber angle, precipitated by mydriatic agent, uveitis, lens dislocation; severe pain associated with photophobia and blurry vision; red eye with a steamy cornea; pupil fixed and nonreactive to light *Treatment*: pilocarpine + systemic carbonic anhydrase inhibitor to lower pressure to allow for laser surgery
Optic nerve atrophy (see Fig. 25-40K)	Pale optic disk Most commonly due to optic neuritis or glaucoma No effective treatment
Uveitis	Inflammation of uveal tract (iris, ciliary body, choroid) Causes: sarcoidosis, ulcerative colitis, ankylosing spondylitis Pain with blurry vision, miotic pupil, circumcorneal ciliary body vascular congestion, normal intraocular pressure, adhesions between iris and anterior lens capsule *Treatment*: corticosteroids (oral or topical), atropine
Macular degeneration (see Fig. 25-40L)	Most common cause of permanent visual loss in the elderly. Disruption of Bruch's membrane in the retina *Dry type*: thinning of retina and formation of yellowish white deposits called drusen *Wet type*: extension of dry type; vessels under retina hemorrhage causing retinal cells to die, creating blind spots or distorted central vision Antioxidants may decrease risk *Treatment*: antiangiogenics (drugs that block vascular growth factors); insertion of special intraocular lens
CMV retinitis (see Fig. 25-40M)	Most common cause of blindness in AIDS; usually occurs when CD4 T helper cell count < 50 cells/μL Cotton-wool exudates and retinal hemorrhages *Treatment*: oral, IV, intraocular ganciclovir or foscarnet
Cataracts (see Fig. 25-40N)	Opacity in the lens Causes: advanced age (most common), diabetes mellitus (osmotic damage), infection (e.g., rubella), corticosteroids Common in congenital infections (e.g., CMV, rubella) *Treatment*: cataract extraction
Malignant tumors (see Fig. 25-40O)	Retinoblastoma in children ("white eye reflex") Malignant melanoma in adults *Treatment*: enucleation

CMV, cytomegalovirus; HSV, herpes simplex virus.

CMV→ CW = Cotton wool

25-40: A, Arcus senilis. Note the gray-white ring around the perimeter of the cornea. **B,** Bacterial conjunctivitis. Note the conjunctival hemorrhage and pus. **C,** Herpes simplex virus keratoconjunctivitis. The special stain highlights the dendritic ulcers associated with this infection. **D,** Stye. Note the swelling, erythema, and pus from this infection of the lower eyelid. **E,** Chalazion. Note the swelling of the eyelid and absence of pus and conjunctival irritation, which distinguishes a chalazion from a stye. **F,** Orbital fracture. Note the periorbital swelling and ecchymoses giving the appearance of "raccoon" eyes. **G,** Pinguecula. Note the yellow-white conjunctival tissue on the temporal side of the conjunctiva. It extends to the junction of the cornea and sclera but it does *not* extend onto the cornea, unlike a pterygium. **H,** Central retinal artery occlusion. Note the generalized pallor of the optic disk and narrowed arteries. There is a cherry red spot on the macula, which is to the right of the optic disk. There is no boxcar segmentation in the retinal veins. **I,** Central retinal vein occlusion. Note the numerous flame hemorrhages in the retina as well as swelling of the optic disk. **J,** Schematic of the eye. Aqueous humor is produced by the ciliary body from which it flows into the anterior chamber and then out through a spongy tissue at the front of the eye called the trabecular meshwork into a drainage canal (*circle*). Glaucoma is an increase in aqueous pressure. In open-angle glaucoma, fluid cannot flow effectively through the trabecular meshwork. In acute angle-closure glaucoma there is narrowing of the anterior chamber caused by forward displacement of the ciliary body (*arrow*). **K,** Optic nerve atrophy showing a pale optic disk. **L,** Macular degeneration. Note the yellow-white deposits (drusen) in the macula. **M,** Cytomegalovirus retinitis in AIDS. Note the numerous cotton-wool exudates in the retina. **N,** Cataract. Note the opacity in the left eye. **O,** Retinoblastoma in the right eye of a child showing a white eye reflex. (*A, D, E,* and *G* from Kanski JJ, Nischal KK: *Ophthalmology: Clinical Signs and Differential Diagnosis.* St. Louis, Mosby, 2000; *C, H, I, J,* and *N* from Swartz MH: *Textbook of Physical Diagnosis,* 5th ed. Philadelphia, Saunders Elsevier, 2006, Figs. 10-57, 10-110, 10-116, 10-2, 10-67A, respectively; *B* from Newell F: *Ophthalmology: Principles and Concepts,* 8th ed. St. Louis, Mosby, 1996; *F* from Mir MA: *Atlas of Clinical Diagnosis.* London, WB Saunders, 1995; *K* from Perkin GD: *Mosby's Color Atlas and Text of Neurology.* St. Louis, Mosby, 2002, p 64, Fig. 4-3; *L* from Goldman L, Ausiello D: *Cecil's Medicine,* 23rd ed. Philadelphia, Saunders Elsevier, 2008, p 2855, Fig. 449-12; *M* courtesy of Douglas A. Jobs, MD, The Wilmer Opthalmological Institute, The Johns Hopkins University and Hospital, Baltimore; *O* from Damjanov I, Linder J: *Pathology: A Color Atlas.* St. Louis, Mosby, 2000, p 445, Fig. 20-39.)

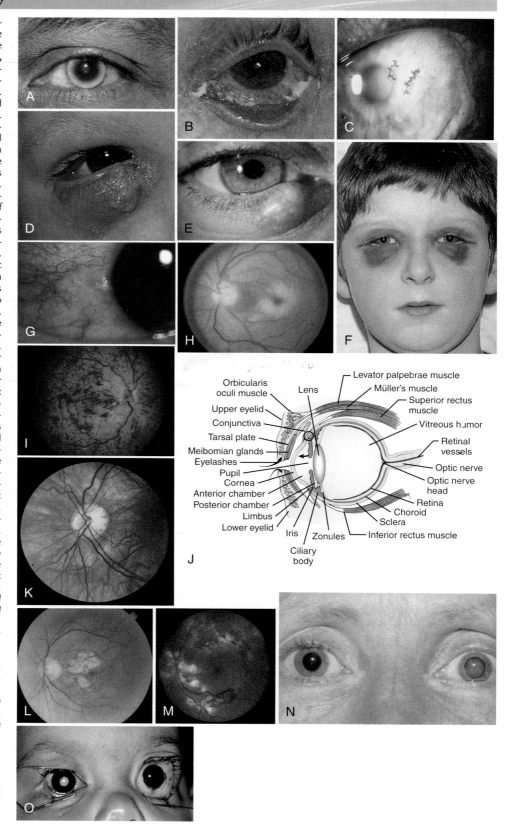

Nervous System and Special Sensory Disorders

TABLE 25-8. **SELECTED EAR DISORDERS**

EAR DISORDER	DESCRIPTION AND COMMENTS
Meniere's disease	Increased endolymph in inner ear and loss of cochlear hairs Dizziness, vertigo, tinnitus, sensorineural hearing loss *Treatment:* hydrochlorothiazide + triamterene; surgery in resistant cases
Sensorineural defect	Weber test: lateralizes to normal ear (contralateral ear is affected) Rinne test: air conduction > bone conduction in both normal and affected ear
Presbycusis	Most common cause of sensorineural hearing loss in elderly Due to degeneration of cochlear hairs *Treatment:* amplification devices; cochlear implants
Otosclerosis	Most common cause of conduction deafness in elderly Due to fusion of middle ear ossicles Other causes of conduction defects: impacted cerumen in outer ear canal; otitis media *Treatment:* amplification devices; surgery
Conduction defect	Weber test: lateralizes to affected ear Rinne test: bone conduction > air conduction
Otitis media (see Fig. 25-41)	Most common cause of conduction deafness in children Most commonly due to *Streptococcus pneumoniae* Other causes: *Haemophilus influenzae, Moraxella catarrhalis* *Treatment:* antipyrine and benzocaine ear drops for pain; controversy regarding antibiotics—those that use antibiotics usually use amoxicillin-clavulanate
External otitis (see Fig. 25-42)	Inflammation of outer ear canal "Swimmer's ear": due to *Pseudomonas aeruginosa, Staphylococcus aureus, Aspergillus* species *Treatment:* ear drops—polymyxin B + neomycin + hydrocortisone + selenium sulfide shampoo Malignant external otitis: severe infection of outer ear canal in patients with diabetes mellitus; *Pseudomonas aeruginosa* most common cause *Treatment:* imipenem-cilastatin

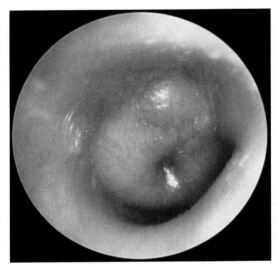

25-41: Otitis media. Note the bulging, erythematous tympanic membrane. *(From Swartz MH: Textbook of Physical Diagnosis, 5th ed. Philadelphia, Saunders Elsevier, 2006, p 314, Fig. 11-29.)*

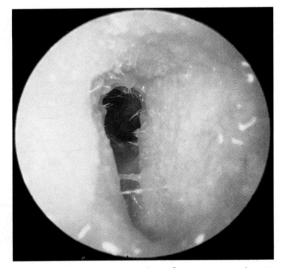

25-42: Otitis externa. Note the inflammatory exudate in the external canal. *(From Swartz MH: Textbook of Physical Diagnosis, 5th ed. Philadelphia, Saunders Elsevier, 2006, p 314, Fig. 11-26.)*

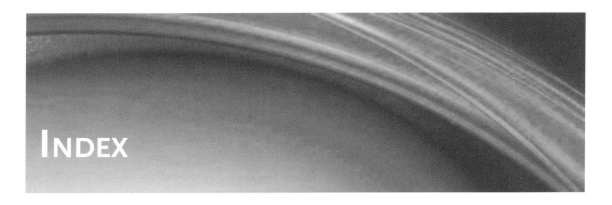

INDEX

Note: Page numbers followed by *f* indicate figures; those followed by *t* indicate tables; those followed by *b* indicate boxes.

A

A blood group, characteristics of, 265
a wave, in jugular venous pulse, 160
AA amyloid, 53
AB blood group, characteristics of, 265
ABCD criteria, for malignant melanoma, 552*f*, 553
Abciximab, 252
Abdominal aortic aneurysm, 143, 144*f*
Abdominal colic, lead poisoning causing, 204, 204*f*
Abdominal radiography, of lead chips, 204, 204*f*
Abdominal striae, in Cushing's syndrome, 502
Abetalipoproteinemia (apolipoprotein B deficiency), 142
ABL gene, 131*t*
ABO blood group, determination of, 265, 266*f*
ABO blood group antigens, definition of, 265
ABO hemolytic disease of newborn, 269, 270*f*
Abortion, spontaneous, 97
Abrasions, 105
Abruptio placentae, 462, 462*f*
Abscess
  Bartholin gland, 436
  cerebral, 580*f*, 581
  frontal lobe, *Mucor* in, 584*t*, 586*f*
  liver, 365*t*
  lung, 291, 292*b*, 292*f*
  pancreatic, 387
  periappendiceal, 355
  peritonsillar, 316*t*
  pilonidal sinus and, 356
  skin, 544
  subphrenic, 355
Acanthamoeba infection, of eye, 600*t*
Acantholysis, definition of, 541*t*
Acanthosis nigricans, 135*t*, 554, 555*f*
Accidental needle stick transmission, of AIDS, 49
Acetaminophen, adverse effects of, 104, 105*t*
Acetaminophen free radicals, 8
Acetyl coenzyme A, as product of alcohol metabolism, 102, 102*f*
Achalasia, 324, 325*f*
Achilles tendon xanthoma, 140, 140*f*
Achlorhydria
  in pernicious anemia, 208
  in Plummer-Vinson syndrome, 199
Achondroplasia, 86, 515
Acid-base disorders, 68
  aspirin-induced, 104
  mixed, 73
    formulas identifying, 73
  primary alterations in HCO₃- in, 70, 71*t*, 72*t*
  primary alterations in PCO₂ in, 68, 68*t*, 69*t*
Acid-base homeostasis, renal maintenance of, 390
Acidosis
  metabolic. *See* Metabolic acidosis.
  potassium shifts related to, 67, 67*f*
  renal tubular, 72*t*
  respiratory. *See* Respiratory acidosis.
Acne rosacea, 558*f*, 562
Acne vulgaris, 544*f*, 546
Acoustic neuroma, 598, 598*f*
Acquired immunity, 37

Acquired immunodeficiency syndrome (AIDS), 49. *See also* Human immunodeficiency virus (HIV).
  clinical findings in, 49
  laboratory tests for, 49*t*
  organ systems affected by, 50, 50*f*, 50*t*
  transmission of, 49
Acquired polycystic kidney disease, 398*t*
Acral lentiginous melanoma, 552*f*, 553
Acromegaly, 479, 480*f*
Actinic (solar) keratosis, 556, 556*f*
Actinomyces israeli, 285*t*
Actinomycosis, cervicofacial, 316*t*, 317*f*
Acute blood loss, in normocytic anemia, 210, 222*t*
Acute chest syndrome, in sickle cell anemia, 215
Acute hemorrhagic (erosive) gastritis, 327
Acute intermittent porphyria, 592
Acute lung injury, 282
Acute lymphoblastic leukemia (ALL), 234, 235*f*, 237*t*
Acute mountain sickness, 110
Acute myeloblastic leukemia (AML), 233, 234*f*
  French-American-British (FAB) classification of, 234*t*
Acute myocardial infarction (AMI), 17*f*, 167
  clinical findings in, 168
  complications of, 168, 169*f*
  crushing retrosternal pain in, 168
  ECG patterns in
    classic, 170
    correlation of microscopic changes and, 170, 170*f*
  gross and microscopic findings in, 167, 168*f*
  laboratory diagnosis of, 169*f*, 170
  less common causes of, 167
  nonpharmacologic and pharmacologic therapy for, 171
  non–Q wave, 168
  Q wave, 168
  reperfusion injury in, 167
  right ventricular, 170
  silent, 168
Acute rejection, in transplantation, 42
Acute respiratory distress syndrome (ARDS), 282
Acute tubular necrosis (ATN), 405
  ischemic, 405, 405*f*
  nephrotoxic type of, 406
Addison's disease, 43, 499, 500*f*
  electrolyte changes in, 64
  electrolyte profile in, 74*t*
  oral manifestations of, 318
Adenoacanthoma, endometrial, 455
Adenocarcinoma
  bladder, 421
  endometrial, 455, 455*f*
  esophageal, 326, 326*f*
  gallbladder, 385
  gastric, 331, 331*f*
  papillary, of thyroid, 490, 490*f*
  pulmonary, 308, 309*f*, 310*t*
  sigmoid colon, 353*f*
  sites of, 123, 124*f*
Adenoma
  follicular thyroid, 490
  growth hormone, 479, 480*f*
  liver cell, 380
    drug/chemical–induced, 370*t*

D